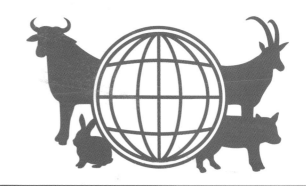

TRANSBOUNDARY
AND EMERGING
DISEASES OF ANIMALS

ISBN # 978-0-9846270-5-9

This material is based on work supported by the Cooperative State Research Education and Extension Service (Now National Institute of Food and Agriculture), U.S. Department of Agriculture, under Agreement No. 00384119278 and Agreement No. 2005-38411-15859 and by the U.S. Department of Agriculture, Animal and Plant Health Inspection Service, Veterinary Services under Agreement No. 14-9100-1472 CA and 15-9100-1504 CA. This material was made possible, in part, by a Cooperative Agreement from the United States Department of Agriculture's Animal and Plant Health Inspection Service (APHIS). It may not necessarily express APHIS' views.

Published by the Center for Food Security and Public Health and the Institute for International Cooperation in Animal Biologics, Iowa State University, College of Veterinary Medicine, Ames Iowa 50011

Printed by Walsworth, Marceline, MO USA

To purchase copies of this book, go to *www.cfsph.iastate.edu* and select Products. For questions, call 515 294 7189 or fax 515 294 8259. Email: cfsph@iastate.edu

Mailing address:

Center for Food Security and Public Health
Iowa State University, College of Veterinary Medicine,
1800 Christensen Drive, Ames, IA 50011-1134.

TRANSBOUNDARY AND EMERGING DISEASES OF ANIMALS

Edited by:

Anna Rovid Spickler, DVM, PhD
James A. Roth, DVM, PhD, DACVM
Gayle Brown, DVM, PhD
Jane Galyon, MS

Project Management:

Glenda Dvorak, DVM, MS, MPH, DACVPM
Dani Ausen, BFA
Andrew Kingsbury, BFA
Maria Victoria Lenardón, DVM, MPH

Disease Images:

Claire B. Andreasen, DVM, PhD, DACVP
Steven D. Sorden, DVM, PhD, DACVP

Graphic Design:

Dara Neubauer, BLS

Center for Food Security and Public Health

Institute for International Cooperation in Animal Biologics
An OIE Collaborating Center for the Diagnosis of Animal Diseases and
Vaccine Evaluation in the Americas

College of Veterinary Medicine, Iowa State University, Ames, Iowa USA

DEAR VETERINARY COLLEAGUE,

I am pleased to introduce the first edition of the Transboundary and Emerging Diseases of Animals textbook. Whether you are just starting your career in veterinary medicine or have been in the profession for years, you will find this important reference textbook to be a valuable resource.

The U.S. Department of Agriculture, Animal and Plant Health Inspection Service (APHIS) conducts about 500 foreign animal disease (FAD) investigations per year. Our success depends on more than the vigilance of our Federal workforce: veterinarians in private practice serve as our first line of defense against disease introduction. Recent worldwide events, such as the global dispersion of the Asian strain of highly pathogenic avian influenza (HPAI), have demonstrated the importance of awareness and education. The recent emergence of zoonotic animal diseases has changed veterinary medicine from an individual endeavor to a team effort with our public health colleagues and homeland security officials.

Whether intentional or unintentional, introduction of a FAD will require an efficient response to eradicate it before it affects our agricultural viability. In addition to updated clinical information in this textbook, the first chapter provides information on some of the important issues facing the profession and the role veterinarians play in human health, animal health, and environmental health. Chapters 2-4 contain information on the U.S. systems for disease diagnosis and response. Chapter 5 contains information about actual disease outbreaks and how they were managed, and the fact sheets contain extensive information on selected diseases.

In anticipation of the need to staff future incidents with animal health professionals, APHIS created the National Animal Health Emergency Response Corps (NAHERC). NAHERC provided critical personnel resources during the 2001 United Kingdom foot-and-mouth disease incident and the 2015 HPAI outbreak. When mobilized, NAHERC volunteers become temporary Federal employees and receive full salary and benefits. However, event participation is voluntary. I encourage you to visit the NAHERC Web site at *www.aphis.usda.gov/naherc* to learn more about this important initiative.

In addition to learning more about NAHERC, I invite you to consider a career in the exciting world of public practice veterinary medicine, which often involves cutting-edge work with many of the diseases described in this textbook. Veterinarians in private practice should also consider completing the voluntary Federal accreditation process: visit *www.aphis.usda.gov/nvap*. Federal accreditation is approval of private veterinarians to perform official regulatory functions on behalf of the U.S. government. We have 66,000 accredited veterinarians in the United States.

For information on accreditation in the United States or a career with APHIS, please visit *www.aphis.usda.gov/wps/portal/aphis/home*.

Finally, I encourage you to keep this reference textbook in a central spot on your bookshelf. APHIS counts on its network of veterinary professionals to succeed in its mission of protecting the health and value of animal agriculture.

Sincerely,

John R. Clifford, D.V.M.
Deputy Administrator, Veterinary Services
Animal and Plant Health Inspection Service
United States Department of Agriculture

PREFACE

This is the first edition of *Transboundary and Emerging Diseases of Animals,* published by the Center for Food Security and Public Health (CFSPH) and the Institute for International Cooperation in Animal Biologics (IICAB). The CFSPH and IICAB are located at the Iowa State University College of Veterinary Medicine in Ames, Iowa, USA. This book is based on four previous editions of *Emerging and Exotic Diseases of Animals,* also published by the CFSPH and IICAB.

The purpose of this book is to provide veterinary students and veterinarians in the United States with an overview of transboundary and emerging animal diseases, their routes of introduction and spread, and the role of local, state, national and international agencies in controlling these diseases (Section 1). It is also meant to serve as a ready resource for information on important diseases that do not exist in North America or that are rare. The 34 disease fact sheets in Section 2 and the annotated images of diseases in Section 3 provide important information to enable veterinarians to become familiar with these diseases.

This book is a companion textbook to the Emerging and Exotic Diseases of Animals (EEDA) web-based course that is used by all U.S. Colleges of Veterinary Medicine. The content of Chapters 1 through 4 is similar to EEDA lessons 1 through 4. Chapter 5 contains nine examples of disease incursions; there are additional incursions in the EEDA course. The web-based course also contains four veterinary accreditation lessons and 20 interactive scenarios. To learn more about the EEDA course that is used by veterinary colleges, contact the CFSPH at cfsph@iastate.edu.

The EEDA course was initially created with funding from the USDA Cooperative State Research, Education, and Extension Service (CSREES) by faculty and staff from three colleges of veterinary medicine: Iowa State University (James Roth), the University of California, Davis (David Hird), and the University of Georgia (Corrie Brown, Susan Little). USDA Animal and Plant Health Inspection Service (APHIS) personnel (Aida Boghossian, Paula Cowen) assisted with course development. Beginning in 2004, the USDA APHIS funded a grants program to encourage colleges of veterinary medicine to adopt the course. APHIS has continued to provide funding for colleges to use the course and for ISU to update and enhance the course annually. Another CSREES grant in 2005 to Iowa State University (Claire Andreasen, Steve Sorden, James Roth) provided funding for the acquisition of most of the images and annotations featured in Section 3. The Veterinary Information Network (vin.com) partnered with ISU to offer the course to veterinary students and for continuing education from 2003 – 2009 and continues to offer the course to veterinarians. Beginning in July 2011, the USDA required all veterinarians seeking initial accreditation to complete components of the EEDA web-based course as one step in the process to be eligible for accreditation. For more information visit: *www.aphis.usda.gov/nvap*.

The CFSPH/IICAB website *(www.cfsph.iastate.edu)* contains a library of resources related to infectious diseases of animals, disease prevention, animal emergency response, disinfection, and zoonotic diseases. Visit the website for the most up to date versions of the disease fact sheets in this book, plus fact sheets on more than 125 additional diseases, additional annotated disease images, and additional in depth information on diseases, emergency response and infection control.

For more information, contact James A. Roth, DVM, PhD, Director, Center for Food Security and Public Health, College of Veterinary Medicine, Iowa State University, Ames, Iowa 50011; Phone 515 294 7189; Fax 515 294 8259; email: cfsph@iastate.edu.

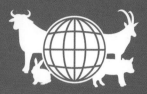

CONTENTS

SECTION 1
CHAPTER RESOURCES

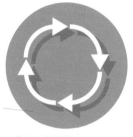

CHAPTER 1

14

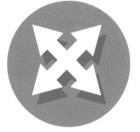

CHAPTER 2

28

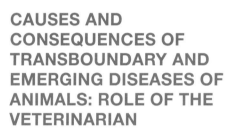

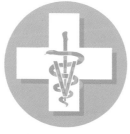
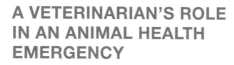

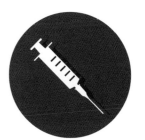

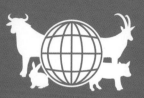

CONTENTS

SECTION 2
FACT SHEETS

Diseases listed in gray can be found online at
http://www.cfsph.iastate.edu/DiseaseInfo/

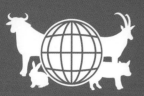

CONTENTS

SECTION 2
FACT SHEETS (CONT'D)

Diseases listed in gray can be found online at
http://www.cfsph.iastate.edu/DiseaseInfo/

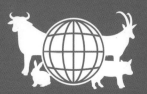

CONTENTS

SECTION 3
ANNOTATED IMAGES

SECTION 4
REFERENCE CHARTS

CHAPTER 1

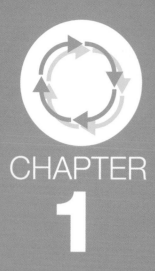

Authors:
James A. Roth, DVM, PhD, DACVM
Jane Galyon, MS
Gayle B. Brown, DVM, PhD
Center for Food Security and Public Health
Iowa State University,
College of Veterinary Medicine
Ames, IA 50011 USA

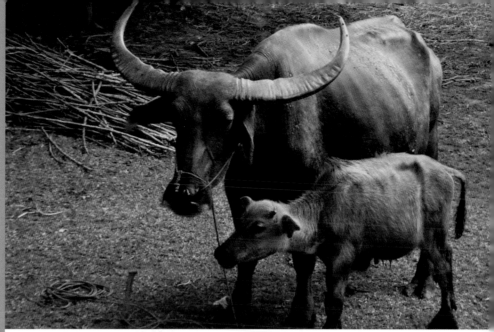

Many rural societies are highly dependent on livestock as sources of milk, meat, transportation, fiber and more
Source: Kristen Obbink, Iowa State University

Causes and Consequences of Transboundary and Emerging Diseases of Animals:
Role of the Veterinarian

EXAMPLES OF DISEASES AND THEIR IMPACT

Transboundary and **emerging diseases** of animals (TEDA) are a threat to human and animal health and jeopardize food security. Increases in human and animal populations, and international trade and travel enhance opportunities for pathogens to move within and between species. In most of the world, increased demand for animal protein has resulted in intensified commercial food animal production and/or expanded "backyard" production. Both present unique opportunities for disease emergence and difficulties in disease control.

Infectious diseases of animals jeopardize food security, and zoonotic diseases (those that may be passed from animals to humans) are also a major threat to public health. It is inevitable that the world will continue to experience disease outbreaks in the coming decades. Veterinarians play a key role in preventing, detecting, and controlling transboundary and emerging diseases. The veterinarian's oath embodies these responsibilities. No matter what career path a veterinarian chooses, it will involve some responsibility for the protection of animal health and welfare, the relief of animal suffering, the conservation of livestock resources and the environment, the protection of public health, and the advancement of medical knowledge.

This chapter will briefly explore the impact of transboundary and emerging diseases on animal health, public health, and food security. The causes of disease emergence and the role of the veterinary profession in preventing, detecting, and controlling these diseases will also be discussed.

Perhaps the best way to understand the causes and consequences of these types of diseases is to consider examples from the distant and recent past.

PLAGUE

In the 14th century, plague (*Yersinia pestis*) was carried from outbreaks in India and China to Italy by merchants returning home. It quickly spread to the rest of Europe. Over one third of the European human population died during the ensuing "Black Death" epidemic. The decline in the population was a factor in the fall of the feudal system and the emergence of the Industrial Revolution. At the time, no one understood where the Black Death came from or how it could be acquired. There was

mass panic as some people fled from the cities to the country; others shut themselves into closed communities, and still others thought the cure lay in drinking and merriment and went from tavern to tavern. The scientific understanding of this disease's mechanisms, its routes of transmission, and its animal reservoirs has evolved. Scientists now know that more than 200 species of mammals can be infected with *Y. pestis*. Rodents are the reservoir hosts, and fleas can transmit the plague bacillus from rodents to humans. Scientists have also discovered that humans or other mammals can sometimes spread this organism directly to others without the intervention of fleas. This knowledge allows public health professionals to monitor and prevent the transmission of this disease, thus avoiding further devastating, large-scale outbreaks. For example, in 2014, a pit bull in eastern rural Colorado developed a fever, ataxia, and hemoptysis that resulted in humane euthanasia. Four days later, the owner was hospitalized with pneumonia and, shortly after, two veterinary employees who were in close contact with the dog developed similar signs. A fourth person, who was in close contact with the dog's owner, also fell ill. After an epidemiological study and laboratory tests were conducted by the state health department, the causative

EMERGING DISEASES AFFECTING VARIOUS ANIMAL SPECIES

AQUACULTURE
Viral hemorrhagic septicemia
Infectious salmon anemia
White spot disease

DOGS
Canine influenza
Nipah virus infection
Rift Valley fever
Leishmaniasis

HORSES
West Nile encephalitis
Hendra virus infection
Equine herpesvirus
  myeloencephalopathy

POULTRY
High pathogenicity avian influenza
Newcastle disease
West Nile encephalitis (geese)

SWINE
Porcine reproductive and
  respiratory syndrome virus
Porcine circovirus associated disease
Foot and mouth disease
African swine fever
Classical swine fever
Swine influenza
Nipah virus infection
Menangle virus infection
Reston Ebolavirus infection
Porcine enteric corona viruses

CATS
High pathogenicity
  avian influenza (H5N1)
Plague *(Y. pestis)*
Rift Valley fever

RUMINANTS
Foot and mouth disease
Rift Valley fever
Brucellosis
Prion diseases
  BSE, CWD, Scrapie
Bluetongue
Tuberculosis, bovine
Schmallenberg

Transboundary animal disease Highly contagious or transmissible and has the potential for very rapid spread irrespective of national borders, causing serious socio-economic and/or public health consequences. This term is used in the global setting, as nothing is technically exotic or foreign. (UN Food and Agriculture Organization)

Emerging disease A new occurrence in a species of a disease, infection or infestation, causing a significant impact on animal or public health. Emerging diseases occur when there is a change in a known pathogenic agent or it spreads to a new geographic area or species, or a previously unrecognized pathogenic agent or disease is diagnosed for the first time. (World Organization for Animal Health)

agent was identified as *Y. pestis.* The four people with confirmed cases were hospitalized and treated with a course of antibiotics. Overall, 114 people were exposed to *Y. pestis,* and 88 were put on prophylactic antibiotics. Though the outbreak was not correctly diagnosed until 13 days after the dog was euthanized, there were no human deaths because of advances in science. It also serves as a reminder that plague remains a public health threat in endemic areas.

RINDERPEST

Rinderpest is an acute, highly contagious, viral disease of cattle, domesticated buffalo, and some species of wildlife. It is not a zoonotic disease, yet its introduction into Africa in the 19th century caused starvation and resulted in massive human fatalities. In 1889, cattle shipped from India carried the rinderpest virus to Africa, causing an epidemic that established the virus on the continent. Initially, approximately 90 percent of the cattle in sub-Saharan Africa died as well as many sheep and goats. Wild buffalo, giraffe, and wildebeest populations were decimated. The loss of draft animals, domestic livestock, and wildlife resulted in mass starvation, killing a third of the human population in Ethiopia and two-thirds of the Maasai people of Tanzania. The reduced number of grazing animals allowed thickets to form in grasslands. These thickets served as breeding grounds for tsetse flies, the vectors for most trypanosomes, resulting in an outbreak of trypanosomiasis (African sleeping

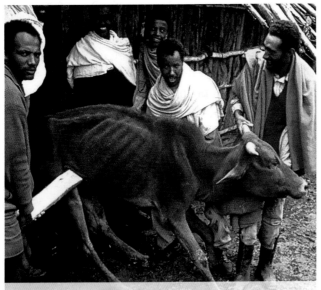

Rinderpest clinical signs included dehydration, emaciation and collapse.
Source: FAO EMPRES

sickness) in humans. The rinderpest epidemic and the subsequent outbreak of trypanosomiasis is considered by some to have been the most catastrophic natural disaster ever to affect Africa. The Global Rinderpest Eradication Program, started in 1992, was a large-scale international collaboration, involving vaccination, local and international trade restrictions, and surveillance. Rinderpest was declared eradicated from the world in May 2011; it is only the second disease (after smallpox) to be globally eradicated. This effort is one of veterinary medicine's greatest achievements. However, virus stocks, vaccines and biologic samples, which may contain the virus, are still stored in many laboratories worldwide, and there is a risk of a reoccurrence through an accidental release or a deliberate terrorist attack. Although rinderpest has been eradicated from the animal population, it must not be forgotten.

FOOT AND MOUTH DISEASE

Foot and mouth disease (FMD) is perhaps the most important disease of livestock worldwide. It is a highly contagious viral disease that primarily affects cloven-hooved livestock and wildlife. FMD was once found worldwide, but has been eradicated from approximately 70 countries. However, approximately 100 countries are still considered either endemically or sporadically infected with the disease. Where FMD is endemic, it affects animal production and performance, including the capacity of draft animals to help farmers produce their crops. Countries where the infection occurs are unable to access international markets. Outbreaks of FMD in countries that were previously free of the disease can be devastating to the economy, due to loss of trade and the cost of eradication. An outbreak in the Republic of Korea in 2010-2011 is estimated to have cost $2.8 billion. Approximately 3.5 million cattle, pigs, goats, and deer were culled, and a nationwide vaccination campaign was initiated to assist with FMD control. As of 2015, the Republic of Korea is considered to be FMD-free where vaccination is practiced. In 2012, the Food and Agriculture Organization (FAO) and the World Organization for Animal Health (OIE) launched a global campaign to improve the control of FMD and eradicate this disease, using tools developed by these two organizations. A key component of the Global FMD Control Strategy is strengthening veterinary services worldwide and providing opportunities to better control and prevent other major diseases of livestock as well as FMD. In the Americas, the Hemispheric Program for the Eradication of FMD (PHEFA) has a goal of eradicating this disease from the hemisphere by 2020.

WEST NILE VIRUS

In 1999, the New York City area of the United States experienced an outbreak of encephalitis of unknown etiology in people. At the same time, increased deaths were observed in a variety of bird species. Dr. Tracy McNamara, a veterinarian at the Bronx Zoo, hypothesized a link between the disease in birds and humans and submitted samples from dead zoo birds to the USDA National Veterinary Services Laboratories (NVSL). NVSL, the U.S. Centers for Disease Control and Prevention (CDC), and the University of California, Irvine all identified the agent as West Nile virus (WNV), which was, at that time, endemic in parts of the Eastern Hemisphere, but had never before occurred in the Western Hemisphere. This virus primarily replicates in birds, including many wild species, but it can also affect reptiles and mammals, particularly horses and humans. Most infected people either have no symptoms or develop a flu-like illness (West Nile fever); however, serious complications including encephalitis, meningitis, or a paralytic syndrome occur in less than one percent. WNV is mainly transmitted by mosquitoes although it can spread by direct contact in some species of birds and

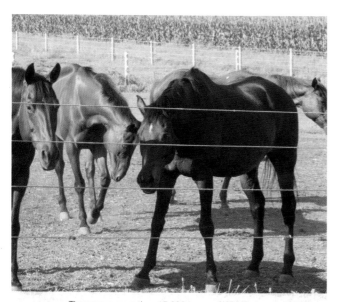

There were more than 15,000 cases of WNV in horses in 2002.
Source: Patricia Futoma, Iowa State University

reptiles. During the several years after it was introduced, West Nile virus progressed across the U.S. and into Canada and Mexico, and later into Central America; it is now considered endemic in the Americas, and there is no feasible way to eradicate it. Between 1999 and 2014, there were almost 42,000 diagnosed human cases of West Nile fever or neurological disease in North America, and 1,765 deaths. Additional cases are likely to have remained undiagnosed because the signs were mild and resembled other common illnesses. In 2000, there were 60 reported cases of equine disease caused by WNV; the number jumped to more than 15,000 cases in 2002. There have also been reports of WNV in Central and South America.

Shortly after the outbreak began, the veterinary vaccine industry, working in cooperation with the USDA Center for Veterinary Biologics, developed effective vaccines to prevent the disease in horses. WNV vaccine is now considered one of the core equine vaccines in the U.S. Use of the vaccine helped to reduce the number of reported equine cases to 141 in 2014. The vaccine has also been used off label to protect some endangered birds, such as California condors. There is currently no vaccine for humans, and recent experiences suggest that human outbreaks may continue to occur in North America at unpredictable intervals.

RIFT VALLEY FEVER

Rift Valley fever (RVF) is a zoonotic, mosquito-borne, viral disease that mainly affects ruminants. Rift Valley fever virus (RVFV) is primarily endemic in sub-Saharan Africa, but it has also been seen in North Africa and may have become established in Egypt. There are concerns that this virus might be spreading to new regions, after outbreaks were reported in Saudi Arabia and Yemen in 2000. The epidemiology of Rift Valley fever is thought to differ between ecosystems; in savannah regions, it tends to occur as periodic, explosive outbreaks, typically precipitated by heavy rainfalls. The rain floods shallow depressions in the soil that contain dormant, RVFV-infected mosquito eggs, which subsequently hatch. If the area also contains large numbers of susceptible mammalian amplifying hosts, an epidemic can result. Sheep, cattle, and goats are thought to be the primary hosts and amplifiers of RVFV, although other ruminants, and some nonruminant species, can also become ill. Clinical cases are generally most severe in young animals, with case fatality rates that may approach 100% in very young lambs and kids, while abortions, with or without clinical signs, predominate in adults. Both can result in severe economic impacts. In addition, an outbreak may cause losses from trade restrictions, or from movement bans implemented to help control the epidemic. Humans can become infected with RVFV after exposure to raw tissues from infected animals or a bite from an infected mosquito. Most people either show no clinical signs or have a febrile, flu-like illness with liver abnormalities, but a small number develop complications such as ocular lesions, renal dysfunction, hemorrhagic fever, or encephalitis. Because the number of human infections in some epidemics can be very large (e.g., possibly more than 180,000 in Kenya in 2006-2007), this can result in hundreds of serious cases and significant numbers of deaths. Vaccination protects ruminants from clinical signs and can reduce virus amplification if begun before an outbreak; however, controlling RVF is otherwise difficult. The breeding grounds for infected mosquitoes are usually extensive, making vector control impractical in many cases. RVF could spread to other countries outside of Africa via an infected mosquito, animal, or human and could become established in a new region, following a pattern similar to that of the spread of WNV throughout the Americas.

INFLUENZA

Influenza viruses are highly contagious, extremely diverse, and prone to mutation. In their numerous hosts, they cause respiratory or systemic signs of varying severity. Wild birds in aquatic habitats are thought to be the natural hosts for influenza viruses (avian influenza viruses), but a few viruses have adapted to circulate in domestic poultry, pigs (swine influenza viruses), horses (equine influenza viruses), people (human influenza viruses), and recently, dogs (canine influenza viruses). Such species "jumps" still happen occasionally, although they are rare. Influenza viruses can also reassort with each other, resulting in novel viruses that contain gene segments from multiple viruses. Expanding human and animal populations and movements of people and animals provide increased opportunities for these viruses to mutate and emerge in new species and/or new locations.

In 1997, a highly pathogenic H5N1 avian influenza virus emerged in Asia and became established in poultry. Despite control efforts, these viruses and their descendants have continued to circulate and evolve in some regions. They have

INFLUENZA A VIRUSES

→ Adapted to new species

----→ Rare infections

Wild aquatic birds are considered the reservoir species for influenza A viruses. Some subtypes have infected another species and become adapted to the new species. Occasionally, an influenza A virus will infect another species and cause a rare infection. This graphic does not represent the full spectrum of species influenza A can infect, but illustrates some of the different species and the interspecies transmissions that have occurred.

killed millions of birds, and sporadically infected various mammals including dogs, cats, pigs, zoo animals, and people. While human infections are uncommon, the case fatality rate is high, and the circulation of H5N1 viruses in poultry for nearly two decades has resulted in more than 600 human fatalities. A highly pathogenic H5N8 avian influenza virus, which spread widely in Asia and Europe reached the U.S. and Canada in 2014, apparently via wild bird migratory pathways on the West Coast. This H5N8 virus reassorted with North American avian influenza viruses, and some of the resulting viruses have infected wild birds and poultry. One, a highly pathogenic H5N2 virus, caused extensive and devastating outbreaks among turkeys and laying hens in the Midwest in 2015. There are currently no reports of human illnesses linked to this H5N2 virus; however, other avian influenza viruses throughout the world, most notably an H7N9 virus in China and the H5N1 previously mentioned, have caused symptoms ranging from conjunctivitis or mild upper respiratory signs to life-threatening systemic disease.

Swine influenza viruses have also caused occasional human illnesses, most mild and resembling human flu. Only one of these viruses has become established in human populations. This H1N1 virus, apparently the progeny of at least two swine influenza viruses circulating in different geographic areas (with gene segments that originated in swine, avian, and human viruses), caused a worldwide pandemic in 2009. It has since become a seasonal human influenza virus, joining others that previously entered human populations, such as H3N2 viruses.

Additional influenza viruses have affected animals, but not humans. Around the start of the 21st century, an H3N8 equine influenza virus jumped from horses to dogs in the U.S. This virus became adapted to dogs and continues to circulate, although its distribution seems to be patchy. It has not been found outside North America as of 2015. In approximately 2006, an H3N2 virus, apparently originating as one or more avian influenza viruses, became established among dogs in Asia. This virus spread regionally in parts of Asia and has caused a number of clinical cases in dogs, some severe and fatal. It has also been found in cats, and appears to be capable of causing illness in this species. The H3N2 canine influenza virus entered the U.S. in 2015 and has affected dogs in a number of states. While a vaccine is available for H3N8 canine influenza, there is currently no vaccine for the H3N2 virus.

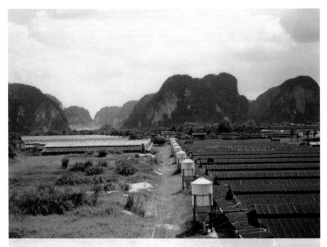

Emerging diseases are often seen in areas where human or agriculture activity expands into previously undeveloped areas, such as this farm in Malaysia where the Nipah virus emerged. Source: James Roth, Iowa State University

NIPAH VIRUS

In 1998, a never-before-observed virus emerged in the Malaysian pig population, causing severe respiratory and neurologic signs. The virus spread to swine farmers and caretakers, resulting in more than 265 cases and over 105 human deaths in Malaysia and Singapore. There were also reports of infections and illnesses in some other mammals in contact with pigs. A novel paramyxovirus, which was named Nipah virus, was isolated from a human patient. Both the CDC and the Australian Animal Health Laboratory sent teams of veterinarians and other specialists to Malaysia within days of isolation of the virus. Working closely with the Malaysian government and scientists, these teams developed diagnostic tests and control strategies (including the culling of more than one million pigs) that resulted in eradication of the virus from the swine population. Scientists also discovered that the virus is carried by healthy fruit bats; pig farming was banned in certain high-risk areas where the concentrations of bats are high. There were no new cases of Nipah virus infection in Malaysia between 2001 and 2015. However, the virus is still present in fruit bats in Southeast Asia, and in 2015 was detected on the Pacific island of New Caledonia. Human cases of Nipah virus encephalitis have been reported repeatedly since 2000 in Bangladesh, in some cases due to eating fruit or drinking unpasteurized fruit juices contaminated by fruit bat urine or saliva. Subsequent human-to-human transmission has also occurred.

INFECTIOUS SALMON ANEMIA

Infectious salmon anemia (ISA) is another example of an economically devastating emerging disease. First described in Norway in 1984, the causative orthomyxovirus has caused outbreaks in Atlantic salmon in Canada, Scotland, Denmark, the U.S., Ireland, and Chile. The outbreak in Chile was one of the largest and had a major impact in the country. Atlantic salmon were introduced in Chile in the early 1980s, and by the late 1990s, salmon farming was growing into a major industry in Chile. Farming of Atlantic salmon increased due to market demand, and by October 2006, Atlantic salmon comprised 63 percent of salmon production in Chile. In June 2007, ISA was identified for the first time in the country and rapidly expanded throughout the Atlantic salmon farming industry. The number of farms affected peaked at the end of 2008, but the economic impact of the crisis was not completely felt until 2009-2010 when harvest and production of Atlantic salmon were at their lowest, dropping nearly two-thirds due to ISA mortality and culling. In addition, the loss of export markets resulted in the laying off of nearly 25,000 workers, causing a significant social impact. Coordinated efforts and collaboration between industry and the government resulted in the establishment of best management practices (e.g., improved environmental, biosecurity and sanitary conditions), voluntary control measures, and regulations to control the disease. By 2011, the industry began to see reduced mortalities and improved growth rates, good indicators of recovery of the industry.

TRADE: ROLE OF THE OIE

The international organization responsible for tracking diseases in animals worldwide is the World Organization for Animal Health (OIE). It was formed in 1924 as the Office International des Epizooties, in response to an outbreak of rinderpest in Europe. Although the name of this organization has changed, it kept its previous acronym. The OIE is comprised of 180 member countries and territories. Its most important function is to inform governments of the occurrence and course of epizootics (outbreaks of animal disease) that could endanger animal

or human health. The OIE maintains a list of the most important animal diseases for international trade and distributes information about the presence or absence of these diseases in each country. The OIE also publishes the *Terrestrial Animal Health Code* and the *Aquatic Animal Health Code*. These "Codes" describe the health measures to be used by the veterinary services or other authorities of importing and exporting countries to ensure the safe trade of animals and animal products. The Codes are the primary references for international trade. Member Countries of the World Trade Organization (WTO) use these documents to meet their obligations under the WTO Agreement on the Application of Sanitary and Phytosanitary (SPS) Measures. This Agreement, known as the SPS Agreement, sets out the basic rules for food safety and animal and plant health standards. More information, as well as the list of diseases reportable to the OIE, can be found at www.oie.int.

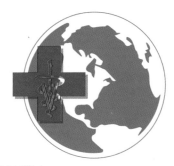

ONE HEALTH

Today, there is a growing understanding that human health, animal health, and the environment are inextricably linked. In addition to causing illness and death among animals, all of the diseases described in the previous section of this chapter threatened human health because they were zoonotic, threatened the food supply, or resulted in social and economic disruption. Since 1980, more than 75 percent of new emerging human infectious diseases have been vector-borne or zoonotic. In addition, over 60 percent of the approximately 1,460 infectious diseases found in humans are caused by multi-host pathogens that are recognized for their ability to move across species lines.

A recent example is Middle East Respiratory Syndrome (MERS), caused by a strain of coronavirus (MERS-CoV) that was first identified in Saudi Arabia in 2012. MERS-CoV antibodies have been found in camels in the

Middle East and Africa. Scientists believe that the virus was initially transferred from bats to camels in Africa, and that it may have been circulating in camels in East Africa since 1983. Genetic sequences from humans and camels in the same geographic areas show a close link, and people who work closely with camels are at higher risk of infection. In 2014, the virus was mainly confined to the Middle East with 679 cases in Saudi Arabia, 57 cases in United Arab Emirates and a few cases in Jordan, Iran, Kuwait, Lebanon, Oman, and Qatar. There were a handful of exported cases in Europe, Asia and North America. In May 2015, the first case of MERS was reported in the Republic of Korea. The case occurred in an individual who had recently traveled to four countries in the Middle East. The patient sought care at two out-patient clinics and two hospitals before being diagnosed with MERS. More than 185 MERS cases, including 36 deaths, were subsequently reported in South Korea, as the result of transmission in healthcare facilities where MERS patients were treated. As of July 2015, there were 1368 laboratory confirmed cases of MERS reported to the World Health Organization (WHO).

Organizations such as the WHO, the FAO and the OIE are working to improve human and animal health by collaborating to address critical global needs, including enhancing public health and veterinary infrastructures in developing countries. Other initiatives involve enhancing cooperation and collaboration among physicians, veterinarians, and other health professionals.

FACTORS LEADING TO DISEASE EMERGENCE AND REEMERGENCE

Diseases may emerge and re-emerge around the world for a number of interconnected reasons, which can vary in importance depending on the specific region, the disease, and other factors. Factors that may be involved in disease emergence include:

- Growing human population;
- Increasing numbers of food producing animals;
- Encroachment of people and domestic animals into wildlife habitats, resulting in increased exposure to wild animals;
- Changing climate;
- Environmental degradation;
- Transfer of pathogens between species;
- Global travel and trade; and
- Accidental or deliberate introduction of disease agents into new areas.

HUMAN POPULATION

In the 1940s, Norman Borlaug, who is considered the father of the Green Revolution, conducted research in Mexico to develop new disease-resistant, high-yield varieties of wheat. At that time, the world population was under 2.5 billion people. The development of new crop varieties, mechanized agriculture, and the increased use of fertilizers and irrigation, dramatically increased crop yields and the areas where crops could be successfully grown. These changes were major factors in the success

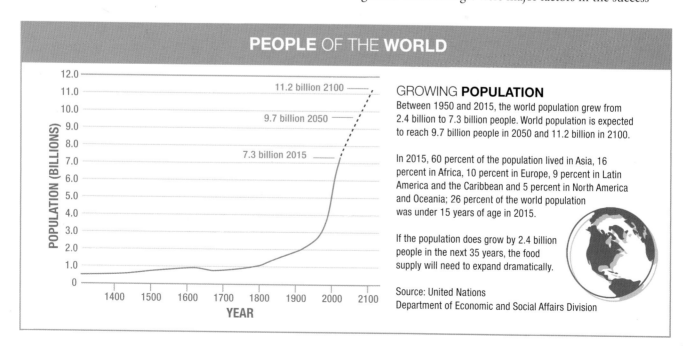

PEOPLE OF THE WORLD

11.2 billion 2100

9.7 billion 2050

7.3 billion 2015

POPULATION (BILLIONS)

YEAR

GROWING **POPULATION**

Between 1950 and 2015, the world population grew from 2.4 billion to 7.3 billion people. World population is expected to reach 9.7 billion people in 2050 and 11.2 billion in 2100.

In 2015, 60 percent of the population lived in Asia, 16 percent in Africa, 10 percent in Europe, 9 percent in Latin America and the Caribbean and 5 percent in North America and Oceania; 26 percent of the world population was under 15 years of age in 2015.

If the population does grow by 2.4 billion people in the next 35 years, the food supply will need to expand dramatically.

Source: United Nations
Department of Economic and Social Affairs Division

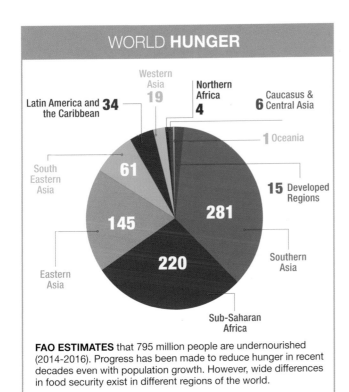

WORLD HUNGER

Western Asia **19**

Northern Africa **4**

Caucasus & Central Asia **6**

Latin America and the Caribbean **34**

1 Oceania

South Eastern Asia **61**

15 Developed Regions

281

145

Eastern Asia

220

Southern Asia

Sub-Saharan Africa

FAO ESTIMATES that 795 million people are undernourished (2014-2016). Progress has been made to reduce hunger in recent decades even with population growth. However, wide differences in food security exist in different regions of the world.

of the Green Revolution. Dr. Borlaug received the Nobel Peace Prize in 1970 for his work in reducing world hunger. Later, he established the World Food Prize to recognize those who have made the most significant contributions to improving the quality, quantity, and availability of food.

The Green Revolution prevented famine in countries like India and China and changed the face of agriculture forever. However, in the 1970s, Dr. Borlaug warned that if the human population continued to expand, the relief from hunger and the prevention of famine afforded by the Green Revolution would only be temporary. According to the United Nations Department of Economic and Social Affairs Population Division, in 2015 the world population was 7.3 billion. It is expected to reach 8.5 billion by 2030, 9.7 billion in 2050, and 11.2 billion in 2100. The median age of the world population in 2015 was 29.6 years with 26 percent of the world's people under 15 years of age. Africa has the highest rate of population growth and is expected to account for more than half of the world's population growth between 2015 and 2050.

If the population does grow by 2.4 billion people in the next 35 years, the food supply will need to expand dramatically. In 2014, an estimated 794.6 million people were undernourished (approximately one in nine) according to the FAO. However, progress to reduce

hunger has been made, even with significant population growth. Since 1990-92, the number of undernourished people has declined by 216 million at the same time that population as a whole increased by 1.9 billion.

Hunger is not limited to the developing world. In 2013, an estimated 14.3 percent of American households (17.5 million households) were food insecure at least some time during the year, meaning they lacked access to enough food for an active, healthy life for all household members. Of those, an estimated 6.8 million households had very low food security, meaning that the food intake of some household members was reduced, and normal eating patterns were disrupted at times, due to limited resources.

INTENSIVE ANIMAL PRODUCTION

The animal production industry has responded to the increased need and demand for protein by amplifying animal production. According to the FAO, in 1963 there were more than four billion chickens in the world (live animal production). In 2013, the number jumped to almost 21 billion. The global cattle population increased from more than 970 million in 1963 to almost 1.5 billion in 2013, and the global pig population grew from almost 450 million pigs in 1963 to 977 million in 2013.

In industrialized countries, it is not unusual to see a poultry laying facility with 150,000 or more birds per house and a dozen houses at one site, or 50,000 cattle in a feedlot. Large swine and poultry production facilities typically have good biosecurity and practice all-in, all-out management with cleaning, disinfection and down time between groups of animals, resulting in better infectious disease control. However, if a disease agent enters one of these facilities, it can spread rapidly within the unit with devastating consequences. This occurred during the highly pathogenic avian influenza outbreak in the upper Midwest in 2015. One infected egg layer site in Iowa had approximately 5.5 million hens, all of which had to be depopulated and disposed. A large number of animals on one site can also provide extensive opportunities for the infectious agent to replicate and perhaps mutate into a more virulent form.

At the same time, large modern food animal operations produce high-quality meat, milk, and eggs efficiently and at reduced cost. These operations help to meet the increasing world demand for inexpensive, high-quality

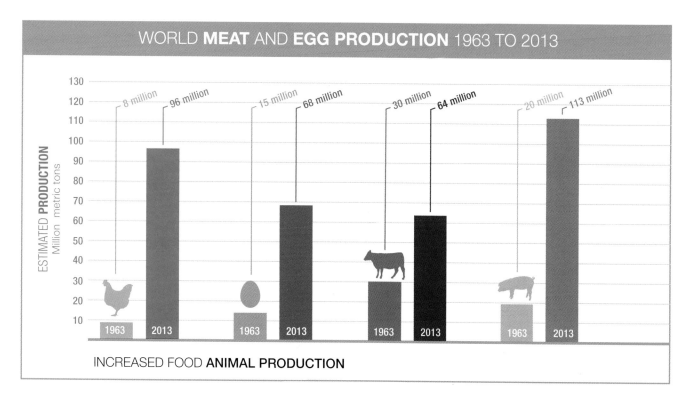

WORLD **MEAT** AND **EGG** PRODUCTION 1963 TO 2013

ESTIMATED PRODUCTION Million metric tons

8 million · 96 million · 15 million · 68 million · 30 million · 64 million · 20 million · 113 million

1963 · 2013 · 1963 · 2013 · 1963 · 2013 · 1963 · 2013

INCREASED FOOD **ANIMAL PRODUCTION**

protein. Also, increasing pressure is being placed on animal production to ensure it is carried out in an environmentally acceptable way that is mindful of animal welfare. Veterinarians and organized veterinary medicine must play a major role in finding a balance among the need for efficient food production, conservation of the environment, and animal welfare.

BACKYARD ANIMAL PRODUCTION

People in developing countries have also responded to the growing need and desire for animal protein. Both rural and urban dwellers are raising poultry, pigs, or small ruminants in their backyards or even inside their homes, in order to increase animal protein consumption. According to the FAO, family farms and small-scale farmers are crucial in the fight against world hunger because they increase food availability and create job opportunities in developing rural areas. More than 90 percent of the 570 million farms worldwide are managed by an individual or a family and depend on members of the family to work on the farm. These farms account for 80 percent of the value of all food produced globally.

This type of production allows the reuse of household waste and crop by-products as feed and has minimal need for transportation. While backyard animal production provides much-needed protein and income for many of

the world's poor, the close interaction between animals and people can facilitate the spread of zoonotic diseases. These small scale producers often lack knowledge of biosecurity and access to veterinary care, including diagnostic testing and vaccines. In particular, diseases such as H5N1 influenza in poultry and brucellosis in small ruminants present significant zoonotic disease challenges for backyard production in many regions of the world.

CAPTURE FISHERIES AND AQUACULTURE

Global aquatic animal food production has grown steadily since the 1960s and at a faster rate than world population growth. Globally, aquatic animals provide more than 1.5 billion people with almost 20 percent of their average per capita intake of animal protein, and three billion people with at least 15 percent of such protein. Protein from aquatic animals is an essential nutritional component in some densely populated areas where overall protein intake levels may be low.

In 2011, capture fisheries accounted for 93.7 million tonnes (a tonne is a metric ton/1t = 1,000 kg) of fish and in 2012, global aquaculture production accounted for 66.6 million tonnes of food. Aquaculture production in China alone accounted for 43.5 million tonnes of food in 2013. Approximately 58.3 million people worked in capture fisheries and aquaculture in 2012. FAO estimates that fisheries and aquaculture assure the livelihoods of 10-12 percent of the world's population.

Aquaculture is the fastest-growing sector of animal protein production and accounted for 42 percent of the world's aquatic animal food supply in 2012. Approximately 540 species are being produced around the world in intensive production systems, including multiple species of finfish, crustaceans, and mollusks. In China, 90 percent of food from aquatic animals comes from aquaculture farming. Similarly to terrestrial farming, aquaculture is susceptible to changes in the ecosystem, including natural disasters (floods, droughts, hurricanes, etc.), pollution and diseases. The El Niño phenomenon can frequently cause dramatic drops in fish production such as anchoveta (a species of anchovy) production. Diseases have emerged as significant problems as a result of the high fish-stocking densities common in intensive aquaculture. These diseases may devastate the farmed aquatic animals and spread to wild populations. Examples include sea lice, which have emerged as a problem in multiple locations, infectious salmon anemia in Chile, and white spot disease among shrimp in Asia.

Both capture fisheries and aquaculture face challenges for long-term sustainability. Challenges include illegal, unreported and unregulated fishing, harmful fishing practices, destruction of coastal habitats and unpredictable environmental fluctuations. The devastating effect pollution can have on fisheries and aquaculture was demonstrated following the 2010 oil spill in the Gulf of Mexico, where fisheries reported an estimated 100,000 tonnes loss of production.

CLIMATE CHANGE

Humans and animals are directly affected by climate change through altered weather patterns. They are indirectly impacted through changes in ecosystems, agriculture, industry, and the economy. A 2015 report in The Lancet stated that the indirect effects of climate change on water, food security and extreme climatic events are likely to have the biggest impact on global health. In addition, the expansion of vector-borne diseases and heat waves will also affect health. The report states that the impact of climate change is greatest on those who have the least access to the world's resources and less infrastructure to cope with current and future problems.

THE **EL NIÑO PHENOMENON** IS CHARACTERIZED BY UNUSUALLY WARM WATER TEMPERATURES IN THE PACIFIC OCEAN.

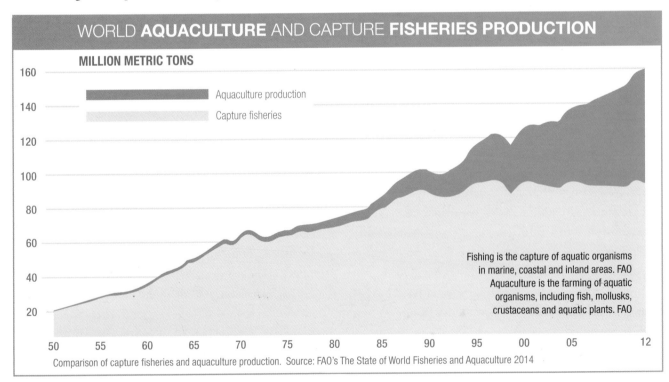

WORLD **AQUACULTURE** AND CAPTURE **FISHERIES PRODUCTION**

MILLION METRIC TONS

Aquaculture production
Capture fisheries

Fishing is the capture of aquatic organisms in marine, coastal and inland areas. FAO Aquaculture is the farming of aquatic organisms, including fish, mollusks, crustaceans and aquatic plants. FAO

Comparison of capture fisheries and aquaculture production. Source: FAO's The State of World Fisheries and Aquaculture 2014

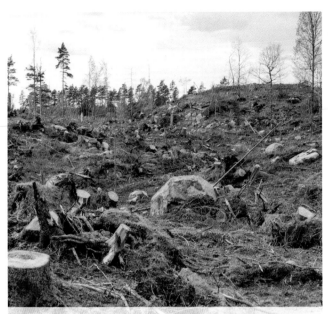
Environmental degradation and climate change impact disease emergence.
Source: iStock.com, kn1

ENVIRONMENTAL DEGRADATION

Environmental degradation includes deforestation, desertification, pollution, and climate change. The challenge of feeding the expanding human population puts pressure on natural resources and the environment. The conversion of marginal lands for food production often requires irrigation and can strain water supplies. Pressure for farmland expansion causes deforestation. The loss of trees leads to soil erosion, water runoff, flooding, and decreased biodiversity, all of which can result in unintended consequences, such as disease emergence or re-emergence. For example, loss of biodiversity following deforestation has caused insect vectors to adapt to human blood as an alternative food source. This adaptation has been linked with changes in the distribution of leishmaniasis in South America. Human activity generates waste and pollution, which affect the air, water, and soil, and damage the health of people, animals, and plants. The natural habitat, including tropical rainforests, old growth forests, coral reefs, and wetlands, is also threatened by environmental degradation.

INTERSPECIES TRANSFER OF PATHOGENS

Increased production of food animals, habitat encroachment, environmental degradation, and climate change are all leading to increased transfer of infectious agents between species. When domestic animals are raised in novel environments, such as land made farmable through destruction of portions of rain forests, both domestic and wild animals are exposed to species of animals and pathogens that they may have not encountered before. This can result in infectious agents being transferred to a new species. Sometimes, these agents may be carried subclinically or produce only mild disease in their original hosts, but result in severe illnesses when they enter new hosts. One example, discussed at the beginning of this chapter, described the interspecies transfer of Nipah virus from bats to pigs when a large pig farm was established in an area of Malaysia that has a large population of fruit bats. The Nipah virus was transmitted from the fruit bats to pigs, spread rapidly through the pig population, and was subsequently transmitted to people in close contact with the pigs.

GLOBAL TRADE AND TRAVEL

Global trade of products facilitates the transfer of infectious agents. The expansion of agricultural trade has helped provide a wider variety of food to increasing numbers of people at lower prices. World trade in agriculture is well over one trillion U.S. dollars annually. Approximately 23 percent of the world's food produced for human consumption is traded internationally. Both developed and developing countries have processes in place to control the import and export of food and agriculture products to meet sanitary and phytosanitary trade standards as mandated by the WTO. While these standards are important safeguards, not all animals or products carrying disease can be stopped at the borders between countries. Animals and animal products illegally transported between countries can cause disease outbreaks. For example, it is speculated that fighting cocks infected with Newcastle virus, a transboundary disease of birds, were smuggled from Mexico to Southern California in 2002. The outbreak resulted in the death of four million birds, and cost $160 million to eradicate and $395 million in trade losses. Poultry smuggling may also contribute to the ongoing spread of the Asian strain H5N1 influenza viruses.

Wildlife trade, both legal and illegal, is another important and often overlooked factor in potential disease transmission. Some estimates indicate that approximately 40,000 live primates, four million

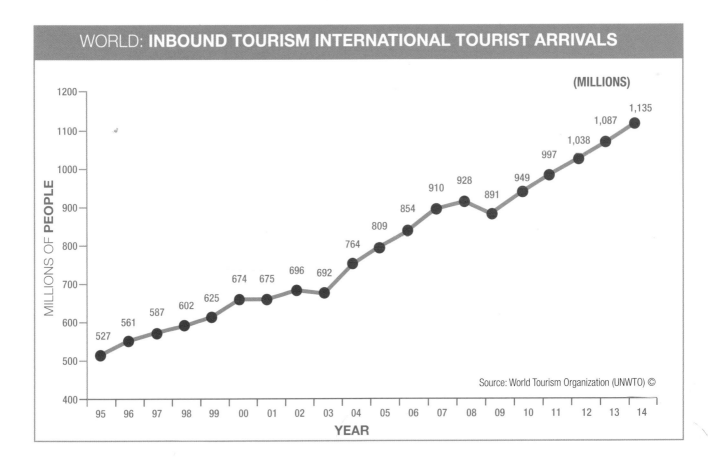

WORLD: **INBOUND TOURISM INTERNATIONAL TOURIST ARRIVALS**

(MILLIONS)

MILLIONS OF **PEOPLE**

527, 561, 587, 602, 625, 674, 675, 696, 692, 764, 809, 854, 910, 928, 891, 949, 997, 1,038, 1,087, 1,135

Source: World Tourism Organization (UNWTO) ©

YEAR

live birds, 640,000 live reptiles and 350 million live tropical fish are traded globally each year. When wild mammals, birds and reptiles flow through trading centers, they are in contact with people and dozens of other species before being shipped to other markets, sold locally, or sent back to the wild. Wildlife trade also introduces species of animals to new regions where they may compete with native species for resources or alter ecosystems.

The U.S. Fish and Wildlife Services estimates that the illegal trade of wildlife, live animals, and harvested by-products is a multibillion dollar business.

People also are constantly moving around the globe for business, tourism, or to immigrate to new areas. In 2013, there were 1.1 billion international tourist arrivals around the world. These travellers may inadvertently carry and spread both human and animal diseases. Worldwide travel can dramatically increase the speed with which a disease is spread across international borders.

In addition, migratory birds, wild animals, and insects cross international borders irrespective of import and export controls.

DELIBERATE ACTS OF DISEASE INTRODUCTION

Finally, pathogens could be deliberately introduced to create an impact on human health, animal health, food safety, food security, the economy, or to cause social disruption. Pathogens have been deliberately used against humans and animals for centuries. Criminals or terrorist groups can gain access to pathogens in nature or laboratories. Biological material can be disguised and transported undetected through security checks. The pathogens themselves can sometimes be propagated and dispersed with only a moderate level of technical expertise and equipment.

The mechanisms to detect an animal disease outbreak are the same whether an agent has been released deliberately, accidentally or as the result of a natural occurrence. Strong national veterinary services are essential to effectively respond to the introduction of a pathogen, including one that is deliberately released. It is also critical that laboratories holding high consequence and dangerous pathogens (including those that have been eradicated, e.g., smallpox and rinderpest) have a very high level of biosecurity to prevent these agents from falling into the wrong hands or being accidentally released.

PROSPECTS FOR THE EMERGENCE OF NEW DISEASES

All of the factors discussed above contribute to disease emergence/re-emergence and are reflective of ongoing trends. They are also difficult to reverse. Addressing the economic, social, health, and environmental issues related to animal production will be one of the greatest political challenges in the 21st century. The fact that so many people depend on livestock and poultry for their livelihoods and as a source of food limits policy options, complicates local and global trade decisions, and raises political sensitivities. It is inevitable that the world will continue to experience the emergence of new human and animal diseases in the coming decades. This challenge mandates the need for the medical, veterinary, public health, and environmental communities to work together locally and internationally to protect human health, animal health, food safety, food security, and the environment.

Information Sources for this chapter can be found at *http://www.cfsph.iastate.edu/TEDATextbookReferences/*.

ROLE OF THE **VETERINARIAN**

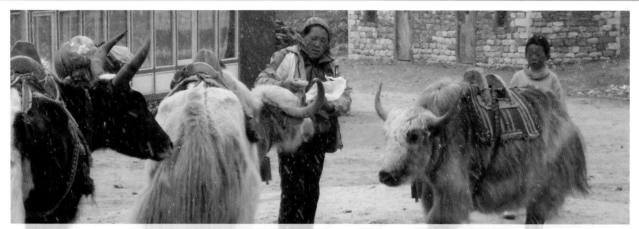

In many societies, livestock live in close proximity to humans and other animals, which may contribute to the emergency and spread of disease. A child observes a Sherpa woman feeding her family's yaks in the village center. Source: Kristen Obbink, Iowa State University

The multidisciplinary training that veterinarians receive provides the tools to help address the challenges described in this chapter. Clients and the public expect veterinarians, no matter what their job responsibilities, to be knowledgeable about transboundary and emerging diseases that affect both animals and humans.

VETERINARIANS CAN CONTRIBUTE TO MEETING THE CHALLENGES OF EMERGING DISEASES BY:

- Maintaining and improving the health and welfare of food-producing animals in the developed and developing world;
- Controlling food-borne and zoonotic diseases in food-producing animals;
- Providing health care to prevent and control zoonotic diseases in companion animals;
- Conducting research leading to improved vaccines, diagnostics, and pharmaceuticals;
- Working to reduce the impact of livestock, poultry, and aquatic animal production on the environment;
- Improving the health of aquatic animals, exotic animals, and zoo animals;
- Working to ensure the health of wildlife and to maintain biodiversity;
- Educating animal owners and the public on these critically important issues; and
- Engaging in the political and social discussions related to the factors leading to disease emergence.

CHAPTER 2

Authors:

Gayle Brown, DVM, PhD
Center for Food Security and Public Health
Iowa State University,
College of Veterinary Medicine
Ames, IA 50011 USA

Corrie Brown, DVM, PhD
The University of Georgia,
College of Veterinary Medicine
Athens, GA 30602 USA

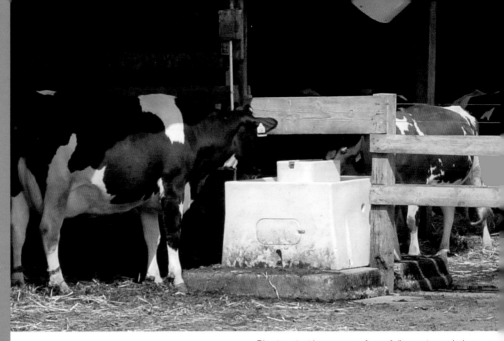

Direct contact is a common form of disease transmission.
Source: Danelle Bickett-Weddle, Iowa State University

Routes of Transmission and the Introduction of Transboundary Animal Diseases

PORTALS OF ENTRY

A number of transboundary and emerging infectious diseases constantly threaten to expand their geographic range and become established in new regions. Porcine epidemic diarrhea virus, a disease that had been circulating in Asia and Europe, was introduced into the United States for the first time in 2013. An H3N2 canine influenza virus, which was known to circulate in parts of Asia, entered the U.S. and spread in 2015. Heartwater, which is mainly confined to Africa, could become endemic in any country where suitable host populations and tick vectors exist. Where diseases have been eradicated, countries also face the ongoing threat of re-introduction. Foot and mouth disease (FMD), for example, has been re-introduced into several FMD-free countries, including the United Kingdom, Argentina and Uruguay. To prevent animal diseases from entering the U.S., authorities monitor all of the routes by which pathogens could cross their borders. This job is made more difficult by the existence of many diverse portals of entry, including livestock and pets, wildlife, animal products, arthropod vectors, inanimate objects, and humans. Veterinarians play an important role in supporting authorities that monitor the routes of transmission of diseases.

ANIMALS

Each year, the U.S. imports livestock and poultry from many countries. In 2014, for example, approximately 2.4 million cattle and five million pigs were imported into the U.S. People also return from many countries with pets, either following a vacation or after living abroad. Animals entering the U.S. must be screened to ensure that diseases are not entering the country with them, perhaps as hitchhikers on a flock of sheep or on the family dog. Although the system works well, occasionally a potential disease problem is missed. In one incident, screwworms were found in a group of horses imported from Argentina after they had left a U.S. quarantine facility. The risk is greater with animals that do not pass through inspection stations, such as smuggled animals or migratory wild animals. There is particular concern that wild birds, which can migrate great distances, might carry transboundary diseases across international borders. The introduction of H5 highly pathogenic avian influenza viruses from Eurasia into Canada and the U.S. in late 2014 was attributed to migratory wild waterfowl.

ANIMAL PRODUCTS

Animal products, in which disease agents can sometimes survive for long periods, are also a concern. Each year the U.S. imports millions of tons of edible and non-edible animal products. While it is not feasible to screen each and every individual product, a representative subset of these shipments are examined for infectious agents. Imported biologics, such as vaccines, embryos and ova for embryo transfer, and semen for artificial insemination, must also be screened to ensure freedom from pathogens.

VECTORS AND FOMITES

Pathogens can also enter the country on **fomites** (contaminated inanimate objects) and in **vectors** (living organisms that transmit diseases from one animal to another). Vectors capable of carrying some very serious diseases of livestock have been imported on reptiles. For example, *Amblyomma spp.* ticks, which can carry the transboundary livestock disease heartwater, have been discovered on tortoises imported into Florida. Fomites can also carry pathogens into the country. For instance, a livestock virus could be carried across international borders on the shoe of a traveler who had walked through an infected farm.

PEOPLE

Humans can act as fomites or incubators to bring animal diseases into disease-free countries or areas. For example, a fisherman or boater might inadvertently transfer viral hemorrhagic septicemia, a serious disease of fish, in mud or water taken from one lake to another. People could also introduce a foreign disease by importing an unscreened food product or a product they have mislabeled. This introduction could be devastating if the product contained a contagious disease. For example, classical swine fever could be re-introduced into the U.S. by a traveler carrying pork products from a Caribbean island or country in Central or South America, where this disease is still endemic. Feeding swine contaminated products, or discarding contaminated products in an area accessible to swine, has the potential to start an epidemic. In some cases, humans can be infected by the same pathogen that affects animals and could act as incubators to bring the disease into the country. This is a particular concern for arthropod-borne diseases such as Rift Valley fever, which can be transmitted from an infected person to mosquitoes, and subsequently to livestock or birds, without the person ever coming in contact with an animal.

Besides all of these unintentional means of introduction, consider the possibilities of a nefarious introduction; for instance, an agroterrorist using a foreign animal disease agent to decimate susceptible livestock species. Any of the routes mentioned above could be used by an agroterrorist. The economic consequences would be the same as those of an unintentional introduction and the only defense is to respond rapidly and effectively.

DEFINITIONS FOR UNDERSTANDING THE TRANSMISSION OF TRANSBOUNDARY DISEASES

While many portals of entry exist for transboundary diseases, each pathogen can use only some of these routes. This section of the chapter reviews some general concepts

---

Fomites inanimate objects that can carry infectious agents between animals

Vectors living organisms that transmit diseases from one animal to another

in animal disease transmission important for understanding how an agent's characteristics contribute to the likelihood that it will be introduced into a new location.

A **disease** is defined as any deviation from normal structure or function in a human, animal, or plant. Diseases may be described according to their transmission characteristics. An **infectious disease** is a disease caused by the invasion and multiplication of a living agent in a host. Infectious diseases can be described as viral, bacterial, mycotic, or parasitic, according to the type of etiologic agent responsible. When a parasite lives inside a host (endoparasites), it is an infection; however, when a parasite lives on the hair, fur, feathers, or skin (ectoparasite) of the host, it is an **infestation.** For example, a cat can be infected with roundworms and infested with fleas. As another example, the tick vector that transmits Lyme disease, *Ixodess capularis,* infests the host but the agent it transmits, *Borrelia burgdorferi,* infects the host.

A **contagious disease** is a disease that is transmissible from one human or animal to another via direct or airborne means. Agents that cause contagious diseases can be spread from animal to animal in excretions and secretions, including respiratory aerosols, scabs, and other body fluids or tissues. One example of a contagious disease is peste des petits ruminants (PPR), a serious viral disease of small ruminants found in parts of Africa, the Middle East, and Asia. Sheep and goats with peste des petits ruminants excrete infectious virus in their ocular, nasal, and oral secretions. Coughing and sneezing animals readily spread this virus in aerosols to nearby animals.

Infectious diseases can be communicable without being contagious. A **communicable disease** is caused by an agent capable of transmission from an infected person, animal, or plant to another by direct or indirect routes. Indirect routes include transmission via insects or fomites, such as food, water, clothing, vehicles, and equipment. Many important communicable diseases are not directly contagious but are transmitted between animals by arthropod vectors. African horse sickness is one example. This disease, a severe cardiac and pulmonary disease of horses and other Equidae, is caused by an orbivirus, transmitted by biting midges in the genus *Culicoides.* Infected horses can transmit the African horse sickness virus to new *Culicoides* vectors but do not spread it directly to other horses.

Understanding these terms is crucial to understanding how transboundary diseases are introduced into and spread in a country. For example, if a disease is highly contagious, contact between infected and susceptible

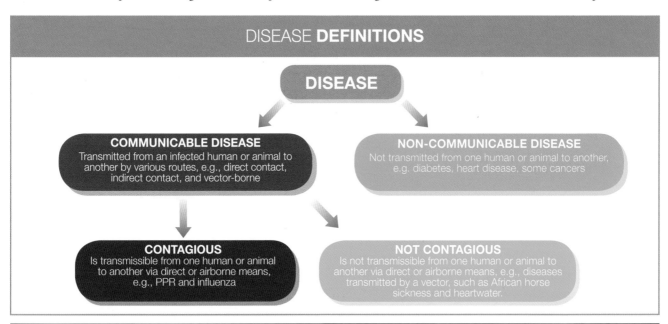

DISEASE **DEFINITIONS**

DISEASE

COMMUNICABLE DISEASE
Transmitted from an infected human or animal to another by various routes, e.g., direct contact, indirect contact, and vector-borne

NON-COMMUNICABLE DISEASE
Not transmitted from one human or animal to another, e.g. diabetes, heart disease, some cancers

CONTAGIOUS
Is transmissible from one human or animal to another via direct or airborne means, e.g., PPR and influenza

NOT CONTAGIOUS
Is not transmissible from one human or animal to another via direct or airborne means, e.g., diseases transmitted by a vector, such as African horse sickness and heartwater.

Disease any deviation from normal structure or function

Infectious disease a disease caused by a pathogen living and multiplying in a host

Infestation a parasite living on the hair, fur, feathers, or skin of a host

Contagious disease a disease that is transmissible from one human or animal to another via direct or airborne means.

Communicable disease A disease transmitted from an infected human or animal to another by various routes, e.g. direct and indirect contact, and vectors

Direct contact pathogens transmitted directly from animal to animal

Indirect contact pathogens transmitted through an intermediary such as a physical object or insect

animals must be prevented. Such prevention may take the form of quarantining animals, possibly slaughtering infected or exposed animals, and disinfecting equipment and vehicles that could transmit the organism from one farm to another. However, if the disease is communicable but not contagious, like many arthropod-borne diseases, transmission to the arthropod must be prevented, but animals that have been in direct contact with an infected animal may not have been infected.

ROUTES OF TRANSMISSION OF INFECTIOUS DISEASE AGENTS

The most likely route of introduction for a transboundary disease depends on its mode of transmission. A pathogen transmitted by mosquitoes can be spread between regions in an infected insect, while a virus that persists on fomites might enter a country on a contaminated shoe. Other more fragile pathogens may be able to enter new areas only in the infected host animal. A number of factors can influence the mode of introduction of a given pathogen. For example,

- Is it transmitted between unrelated animals or from parent to offspring?
- Is an intermediate host or vector required for transmission?
- Does it persist in the environment?
- Is it immediately infectious or does it require time in the environment to develop to the infectious stage?

VERTICAL TRANSMISSION

Vertical transmission is the transfer of a pathogen from the mother to offspring; the infectious disease may be transferred to the embryo, fetus, or newborn prior to, during, or shortly after parturition. Types of vertical transmission in animals include transplacental passage, infection within the birth canal, and the transmission of infectious agents through the colostrum or milk. Classical swine fever virus (CSFV) is an example of a disease agent that can be transferred vertically. If a sow becomes infected with CSFV while she is pregnant, the virus can cross the placenta, resulting in infection of the fetus and potentially the newborn; outcomes include abortion, stillbirths, and malformed piglets. And depending on the virus strain and timing, the infection could result in the birth of asymptomatic, persistently infected piglets. *Toxoplasma gondii,* the causative agent

of toxoplasmosis, can likewise be transmitted vertically through the placenta. Transplacental transmission of this agent can cause abortion in sheep and severe congenital abnormalities in humans. The transmission of hookworms in milk, from the bitch to the nursing pups, is an example of lactogenic vertical transmission.

HORIZONTAL TRANSMISSION

Horizontal transmission is the transfer of a pathogen from an infected animal to a susceptible animal, independent of the parental relationship of those individuals. Horizontal transmission can occur by either direct or indirect contact. Pathogens spread by **direct contact** are transmitted directly from animal to animal; pathogens spread by **indirect contact** are transmitted through an intermediary, such as a physical object or insect.

Disease agents transferred by direct contact may be spread by licking, rubbing, biting, and coitus. Ovine pulmonary adenocarcinoma, a lung tumor of sheep caused by a retrovirus, is an example of an agent that can be transmitted horizontally by direct contact via droplets or aerosols. **Airborne transmission** is often considered to be a form of direct horizontal transmission because animals must usually be in close contact since disease agents do not generally survive for extended periods within aerosolized particles. However, foot and mouth disease can be transmitted by aerosols and, under

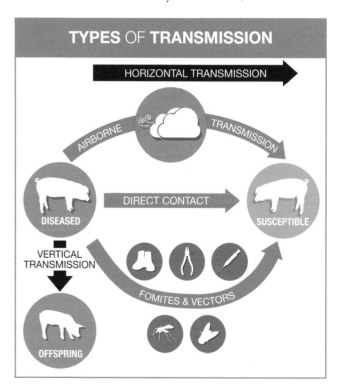

favorable conditions, this virus may travel up to 10 km. The direct and indirect routes are not mutually exclusive; some agents, such as foot and mouth disease virus, can be transmitted by direct and indirect routes.

FOMITES AND VECTORS

Pathogens transmitted by indirect contact are spread by fomites or vectors. A fomite is any inanimate object that carries an infectious agent from one animal to another. Examples of fomites include used needles, dirty clippers, contaminated clothing or vehicles, and contaminated food and water supplies. **Iatrogenic transmission** is a specific form of fomite-mediated transfer in which a medical professional accidentally spreads a disease agent via objects such as contaminated instruments or vaccines. Routine procedures, such as bleeding, tagging, dehorning, and vaccinating, can create an opportunity for iatrogenic transmission by contaminating medical equipment.

The term **vector** is sometimes used in a broad sense to signify anything that allows the transport and/or transmission of a pathogen. Some sources consider fomites to be vectors. However, according to a strict ecological definition, vector-borne transmission occurs when a living creature, because of its ecological relationship to others, acquires a pathogen from one living host and transmits it to another. Thus vector-borne transmission is a form of indirect horizontal transmission in which a biological intermediary, often an arthropod, carries a disease agent between animals. Vectors may be either mechanical or biological.

A **mechanical vector** carries the pathogen, but the pathogen is not altered while on the vector. Contamination of mechanical vectors tends to be short-lived, and they are considered to be little more than flying fomites.

A **biological vector** supports replication of the pathogen. The disease agent and its biological vector typically have a long-standing ecological relationship. Nevertheless, agents can sometimes enter new vectors that are similar. Biological vectors are usually persistently infected with the disease agent and may even be a required part of that organism's life cycle. *Anaplasma*

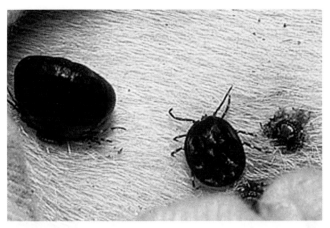

Amyblyomma variegatum. *Ticks feeding on goat skin can transmit the agent of heartwater (Ehrlichia ruminantium).*

marginale, the parasite that causes bovine anaplasmosis, is an example of an agent that can be transmitted by both vectors and fomites. In the southeastern and midwestern U.S., mechanical transmission by biting flies (mechanical vectors) and iatrogenic transmission by contaminated equipment and needles appear to be important in maintaining this disease. In the western U.S., A. *marginale* is transmitted via ticks that act as biological vectors. These ticks pick up the organism from an infected animal while feeding. A *marginale* then replicates in the tick's tissues, including the salivary glands. When the infected tick bites a new host, the organism is transferred to the animal during the blood meal.

TRANSSTADIAL AND TRANSOVARIAL IN VECTORS

The two major forms of transmission within vector populations, transstadial and transovarial, can be very important in maintaining a source of infection for animals. In **transstadial transmission,** the pathogen is maintained in the vector as it develops between life stages. A tick vector infected as a larva with *Borrelia burgdorferi,* the causative agent of Lyme disease, continues to harbor infectious *B. burgdorferi* when it molts to the nymph and then the adult stage. **Transovarial transmission** is a form of vertical

---

Fomites inanimate objects that can carry infectious agents between animals

Iatrogenic transmission a specific form of horizontal transmission by fomites in which the veterinarian or physician accidentally furthers the spread of a disease agent via routes such as contaminated instruments or vaccines

Mechanical vector a vector that carries a pathogen but does not alter the pathogen

Biological vector a vector that supports replication of the pathogen

transmission in which the female vector passes the infectious agent through her eggs to the next generation. Eggs laid by a *Rhipicephalus spp.* tick infected with *Babesia bigemina* will hatch infected larvae.

Transovarial transmission allows pathogens to resist conditions that kill the adult vectors but allow the eggs to survive. Transovarial transmission is a very important mechanism in Rift Valley fever, a mosquito-transmitted viral disease of ruminants. Mosquitoes infected by Rift Valley fever virus lay eggs that may lie dormant in dried-out depressions for long periods. After heavy rainfalls fill these depressions with water, the mosquitoes hatch and bite and infect susceptible hosts and the cycle continues. This can result in periodic, explosive outbreaks of Rift Valley fever in some regions.

CHARACTERISTICS OF PATHOGENS

The innate characteristics of pathogenic organisms play a huge role in determining their potential for introduction into a new area or species. Important characteristics influencing the risk for spread include the pathogen's persistence in the environment or in a host, the time required for it to become infective after it has been shed from a host, and other aspects of its life cycle. The diseases cited below serve as useful examples.

PERSISTENCE IN THE ENVIRONMENT

Disease agents vary in their ability to survive outside a living host. Some agents are quickly inactivated by sunlight, high temperatures, pH changes, or other environmental factors while others can withstand harsh conditions for months or even years. The persistence of the organism influences how long an environment will remain infectious for animals. Anthrax bacteria *(Bacillus anthracis),* for example, produce spores that persist in soil for many years. Cases of anthrax can occur for decades in a contaminated pasture, affecting animals that have had no direct contact with an infected host. Agents that remain viable in the environment for long periods, such as anthrax, can be particularly hard to eradicate.

PERSISTENCE IN THE HOST

Some pathogens enter the host temporarily; if they do not kill the host, they are eliminated by the immune response. Others can become permanent residents, persisting with or without clinical signs for the lifetime of the animal. The maedi-visna lentivirus (MVV), for example, can be transmitted to lambs or kids when they drink contaminated milk or colostrum. Once the animal is infected, the virus is incorporated into its DNA and becomes resident in that animal for life. Some animals infected with MVV develop dyspnea, neurologic signs, mastitis, or arthritis; however, many remain asymptomatic. These asymptomatic animals can, nevertheless, infect their offspring or other animals in close contact. Agents that persist in the host, such as MVV, can "hide" in asymptomatic hosts between clinical infections or epidemics. Asymptomatic carriers thus spread disease but are not readily detected as sources of the disease.

Some infections are maintained in a **reservoir** population between disease outbreaks. A reservoir is an

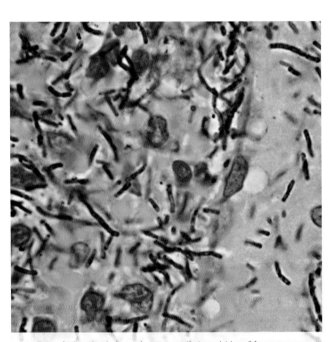

Anthrax bacteria produce spores that persist in soil for many years.
Source: ISU College of Veterinary Medicine

Transstadial transmission infection with a pathogen is maintained in the vector as it develops between life stages

Transovarial transmission a form of vertical transmission in which the female vector passes the infectious agent through her eggs to the next generation

animal or group of animals that continuously contains the disease agent and can spread it to other groups. In some cases, a single animal is persistently infected throughout its lifetime. In others, the agent is maintained in a population where it is spread from animal to animal. Reservoir hosts serve as a habitat for the pathogen to survive and may or may not become ill from the infection. Migratory waterfowl, for example, act as reservoir hosts for avian influenza viruses and can spread these viruses to poultry flocks.

MATURATION REQUIREMENT FOR INFECTIVITY

Some pathogenic agents are infectious when they are shed. *Giardia,* a protozoan that can cause diarrhea in numerous species, is an example of such an agent. Other organisms require time either within the environment or within another host or vector to develop into the infectious stage. *Toxocara canis,* an ascarid (roundworm) of wild canids and domestic dogs, is a good example. The eggs of this parasite are unembryonated when shed in the feces and must develop for two to four weeks in the environment before they become infectious.

THE LIFE CYCLE OF THE PATHOGEN

Many aspects of a pathogen's life cycle influence how easily it can be controlled and the points at which it can be destroyed. For example, some disease agents are found only in infected animals, passing directly from animal to animal. These pathogens can be controlled by destroying them within the host, or by preventing them from entering new hosts. The host range of an agent is also important. Pathogens that infect a single host species are usually easier to control than agents that infect many different species. The smallpox virus, which infects only humans, was eradicated by isolating infected humans and vaccinating their contacts. This approach is only successful if the pathogen does not

persist for long periods in the environment or in a host that must be kept alive (e.g., a person), and if it does not enter vectors. Rinderpest is another example of a virus with a very limited host range and poor survivability in the environment; these characteristics allowed it to be only the second disease to be eradicated from the world. In contrast, pathogens that infect and persist in wildlife can be particularly difficult to identify and control; once a pathogen enters native wildlife, eradication may become impossible.

Parasitic diseases present additional complications. The control of a parasitic infection is influenced by whether the parasite's life cycle is direct or indirect. Parasites with a **direct life cycle** can complete their entire developmental cycle in a single host. Parasites with an **indirect life cycle** require at least two hosts: one or more intermediate hosts and a definitive host. Most parasitic trematodes (flukes) and cestodes (tapeworms) and some nematodes have indirect life cycles. Intermediate hosts of some parasites may suffer greater consequences than the definitive host. *Echinococcus granulosus* infections are a good example. Canids, the definitive hosts for this tapeworm, usually carry *E. granulosus* asymptomatically in their intestines even when the parasite's numbers are large. However, its growth in various tissues of intermediate hosts, which can include humans, may eventually compress or damage tissues and organs. Furthermore, both definitive and intermediate hosts may introduce parasites into a new area. In the case of *E. granulosus,* the definitive host introduces the parasite by excreting tapeworm eggs in its feces. These eggs can subsequently infect any intermediate hosts that accidentally ingests them. Intermediate hosts can also introduce *E. granulosus;* however, this requires that their tissues be eaten by a definitive host.

Because of their complex life cycles and the large number of hosts they can infect or infest, some parasites can be difficult to control once introduced to an area.

Reservoir an animal or group of animals that continuously contains the disease agent and can spread it to other groups

Direct life cycle indicates a parasite that can complete their entire development within a single host

Indirect life cycle indicates a parasite that requires an intermediary host in which to develop but does not reach sexual maturity

Amblyomma variegatum, the tropical bont tick, is not found in the U.S., but poses a threat and is on the USDA's High-Consequence Foreign Animal Diseases and Pests list. This tick can be infected with pathogens such as the agent that causes heartwater disease.

A. variegatum, like many hard ticks, is a three-host tick: its larvae, nymphs, and adults feed on three different animals. Immature *A. variegatum* ticks feed on small mammals, ground–feeding birds, reptiles, cattle, sheep and goats. Adult ticks prefer cattle, but can also be found on sheep, goats, horses, camels, dogs and some large wildlife including antelope. Three-host ticks drop off the animal after each feeding and spend at least 90 percent of their life cycle in the environment. This also complicates control. Acaricides can eliminate the ticks from the animal, but do not prevent reinfestation and must be repeated periodically. To prevent entry of this tick, and diseases it may carry, animals imported from countries where this tick is endemic must be treated before entering the U.S.

Information Sources for this chapter can be found at: *http://www.cfsph.iastate.edu/TEDATextbookReferences/*

EXAMPLES OF **DISEASE TRANSMISSION**

The rest of this chapter presents examples of several introductions of diseases by different routes. Transboundary diseases can be introduced into a country by the movement of fomites, vectors, infected animals, animal products, or by the emergence of new diseases or new variants. The likelihood of these introduction events can be decreased through strict surveillance, precautionary practices, and good biosecurity. As you work through the examples, you may wish to review the definitions and examples presented in the first half of this chapter or explore the expanded information on the disease outbreaks in Chapter 5 or in the fact sheets in Section 2 of this book.

FOMITE AND DIRECT CONTACT: FOOT AND MOUTH DISEASE

A fomite is an inanimate object on which a pathogen can be conveyed. Disease transmission usually occurs via physical contact between the object and the animal. Classic examples of fomites are contaminated footwear, veterinary equipment, needles, clothing, eating or drinking containers, cages, bedding, dander, restraint devices, and transportation vehicles. The control of fomites can be vital in preventing the spread of some diseases, such as foot and mouth disease (FMD).

An outbreak of FMD in the U.K. in 2001 illustrates how rapidly and widely some diseases can spread from a single infected herd when the pathogen can be transmitted by both fomites and direct contact. In February 2001, a veterinary inspector found lesions suggestive of FMD on several pigs in an abattoir. The movement of animals in the U.K. was halted to prevent direct transmission by infected animals to uninfected animals. The infected pigs were traced back to an infected farm. But by this time the FMD virus had spread to sheep and other animals. Even though animal movement had stopped, the disease continued to spread. It is estimated that 80 percent of infected premises in some areas were infected because of indirect transmission via fomites and movement of people. This epidemic devastated the livestock industry and economy of the U.K. Before the outbreak was finally brought under control, more than 2,000 cases of FMD had been diagnosed, more than four million animals had been slaughtered, and foci of infection had spread to France, Ireland, and the Netherlands. For more information about the 2001 UK FMD outbreak, see Chapter 5.

For some diseases, such as FMD, transmission via fomites can be the major route of spread. Under the right conditions, the FMD virus can persist for days to weeks in the environment. Virus particles that contaminate footwear, clothing, transportation equipment, and other objects can be transported long distances. People may transport the virus on their hands, clothing, footwear or other items. Because the risk of transmission by humans and fomites is so high, border control officials work to prevent the virus from being introduced. Travelers who have visited farms or contacted farm animals in FMD-positive countries are required to declare this information at customs. Officials inspect their baggage and disinfect soiled footwear. In addition, travelers are instructed to wash their clothing before returning home to an FMD-free area and to stay off all farms for at least five days after their return. Infectious virus can also be found in animal products such as bone-in-meat, milk, bones, glands, and cheese. Ruminant and swine products found on travelers or in luggage are confiscated.

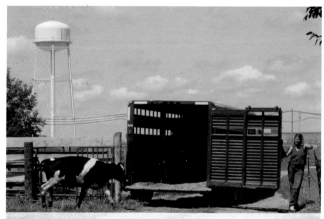

Livestock trailers can serve as fomites to transmit diseases.
Source: Danelle Bickett-Weddle, Iowa State University

TRANSMISSION VIA FOMITE AND DIRECT CONTACT

A pathogen is picked up on one of many fomites.

Examples of Fomites: Footwear, Cages, Needles, Bedding, Clothing, Vehicles, Food Containers, Restraint Devices.

The fomite carries the pathogen to other animals.

Animals transfer the pathogen through direct contact.

VECTORS: WEST NILE VIRUS

Biological vectors are living organisms, usually an arthropod, infected with an agent and transmit the agent from one animal to another. Biological vectors are capable of introducing transboundary disease agents to new areas and/or spreading a disease once it is introduced. Mosquitoes are biological vectors for West Nile virus (WNV) and played a major role in the spread of West Nile virus after it was introduced into the U.S.

WNV is a zoonotic pathogen that can cause encephalitis in humans, horses, some other species of mammals, and some birds and reptiles. Mosquito vectors mainly transmit this virus between birds, which are the primary reservoir hosts; however, mosquitos can also spread the virus from birds to other animals. People and horses are the species most commonly diagnosed with disease caused by the virus. Until 1999, West Nile encephalitis was found only in the Eastern Hemisphere. In the summer and fall of 1999, WNV was identified in dead birds in and around the Bronx Zoo and, concurrently, in several cases of human and equine encephalitis in New York. It is still unclear how it was introduced but it was possibly by an infected person, an infected bird or infected mosquito. Although it was detected soon after its introduction, control efforts could not stop its spread across the U.S. The mosquitoes in the U.S. were competent vectors and the bird – mosquito cycle kept the virus alive. With each passing year, the virus spread westward across the entire U.S. Stopping the spread of a disease with mosquitos as the vector and wild birds as the reservoir is virtually impossible. West Nile virus is now endemic in the U.S. and horses in the U.S. are routinely vaccinated for it.

More details about the incursion of West Nile virus into the U.S. can be found in Chapter 5.

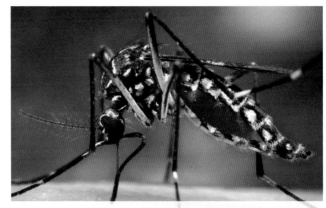

Mosquitoes can serve as vectors for pathogens such as West Nile virus.
Source: Centers for Disease Control and Prevention

TRANSMISSION VIA BIOLOGICAL VECTORS

Vector transmission

Vector

Vector transmission

PATHOGEN CYCLES BEWEEN THE RESERVOIR AND VECTOR

Dead end hosts do not pass the pathogen back to the vector

Dead end host

Reservoir

Dead end host

CONTAMINATED ENVIRONMENT:
ELAPHOSTRONGYLUS RANGIFERI

When a healthy-looking animal enters a country, it may be incubating a foreign disease or serving as an asymptomatic reservoir for a pathogen. Susceptible animals may then become infected by direct or indirect contact with the animal. The introduction of infected animals is thought to have been responsible for bringing cerebrospinal elaphostrongylosis to native Canadian caribou in Newfoundland.

Cerebrospinal elaphostrongylosis is a severe neurological disease of cervids, sheep, and goats, caused by the nematode *Elaphostrongylus rangiferi. E. rangiferi* has an indirect life cycle. Caribou or reindeer are the definitive hosts and shed larvae in their feces. The larvae penetrate the footpad of a snail or slug (intermediate hosts) to develop into the infective stage. Caribou or reindeer then ingest infected snails or slugs while feeding. Once in the host, the parasites migrate through the spinal cord and brain before reaching the muscles of the shoulder and hindlimbs where they mature and lay eggs. The eggs are carried via the bloodstream to the lungs where they hatch into larvae, cross the alveoli, travel up the respiratory tree, are swallowed, and are then excreted in the feces.

Cerebral elaphostrongylosis was first recognized in Newfoundland in the 1970s. It had been introduced to Newfoundland in the early 1900s when infected reindeer were imported from Norway to establish herds for food and draft animals. Once in Newfoundland, the reindeer traveled across native caribou range, most likely leaving feces in areas where snails were present and caribou grazed.

At present, most of the caribou herds in Newfoundland are infected with *E. rangiferi* although Canada's mainland herds appear to remain free of infection. To prevent introductions such as this, animals entering a country are quarantined and tested for transboundary diseases before they are allowed to mingle with native populations.

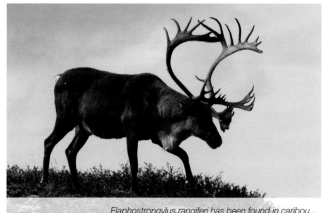

Elaphostrongylus rangiferi has been found in caribou in Newfoundland, Canada. Source: Dmitry Chulov, istock.com

---

TRANSFER THROUGH INGESTION OF AN **INTERMEDIATE HOST**

The pathogen is shed in feces and contaminates the environment.

The pathogen is picked up by an intermediate host and develops to the infectious stage.

Susceptible animals ingest the intermediate host and become infected and shed the pathogen in their feces. The cycle continues.

ANIMAL PRODUCTS: AFRICAN SWINE FEVER AND CSF

Animal products can transmit disease agents when they are discarded near farms or are deliberately fed to susceptible animals. The practice of feeding uncooked or improperly cooked scraps (swill) to pigs is a risk for introduction for several high consequence swine diseases, including African swine fever (ASF) and classical swine fever (CSF). ASF and CSF are both highly contagious diseases of swine that cause hemorrhagic systemic disease.

Transmission of these two viruses occurs via oral/nasal route by direct or indirect contact with infected animals, animal products, and fomites. ASF virus can also be transmitted by the soft ticks of the *Ornithodoros* spp. ASF and CSF viruses can be hardy in some environments and can survive for months or longer within some pork products.

Countries who are free of these diseases have strict regulations on the importation of pigs and pork products from countries known to harbor these diseases and regulations on feeding swill to pigs. In addition, constant vigilance to prevent disease introduction by other means is also important; for example, animal products are confiscated from travelers returning to the U.S. from countries where these diseases exist.

To read more about the introduction of CSF in the UK and ASF in the Caucasus and Eastern Europe, see Chapter 5.

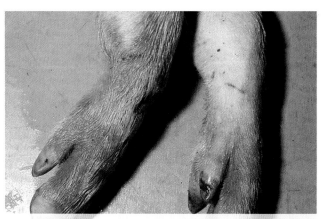

Pigs with African swine fever may have hyperemia of the distal limbs.
Source: Plum Island Animal Disease Center

SURVIVABILITY OF AFRICAN SWINE FEVER AND CLASSICAL SWINE FEVER IN DIFFERENT PRODUCTS

ASF virus has been reported to survive:

- 150 days in refrigerated boned meat;
- Several years in frozen carcasses;
- 40 days in salted dried hams.

CSF virus has been reported to survive:

- 90 days in refrigerated meat;
- More than four years in frozen meat;
- 17 days to more than 180 days in cured and smoked meats depending on the technique.

An outbreak of CSF in the U.K. in 2000 was most likely started when contaminated pig meat in food was discarded by people on a walking path near a pig holding. ASF was most likely introduced into the Caucasus region in 2007 in discarded food waste (swill) from an international ship docked at a Caucasus port; the ship had come from a country where ASF is present.

TRANSMISSION VIA ANIMAL PRODUCTS

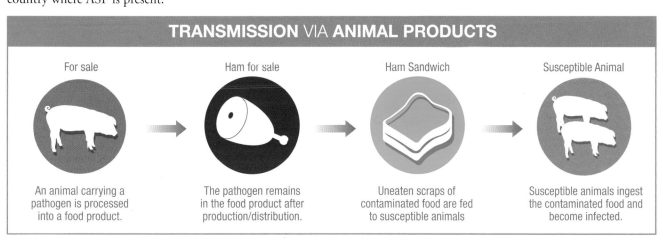

For sale	Ham for sale	Ham Sandwich	Susceptible Animal
An animal carrying a pathogen is processed into a food product.	The pathogen remains in the food product after production/distribution.	Uneaten scraps of contaminated food are fed to susceptible animals	Susceptible animals ingest the contaminated food and become infected.

NEW DISEASE EMERGENCE:
BOVINE SPONGIFORM ENCEPHALOPATHY

The transmissible spongiform encephalopathies (TSEs) are examples of a novel pathogen type that has emerged in several forms over the last few decades. TSEs are fatal neurologic diseases that have been detected in a number of species, including sheep, goats, cattle, elk, deer, cats, mink, and humans. Infected animals develop progressive, irreversible neurologic signs. The causative agents are infectious proteins called prions, which are usually acquired by ingestion.

Bovine spongiform encephalopathy (BSE), commonly referred to as mad cow disease, was first diagnosed in the United Kingdom in 1986. Epidemiological evidence suggests that this outbreak occurred when the BSE agent was amplified by feeding cattle supplements that used contaminated meat-and-bone meal as a protein source. By the time the disease was recognized, a full-blown epidemic had begun. In spite of control measures, the number of cases escalated each year, peaking in 1992, before the disease was finally brought under control. The BSE agent also infected some housecats and zoo cats fed bovine tissues, resulting in approximately a hundred cases of feline spongiform encephalopathy. In people, it caused at least 160 cases of a new disease called variant Creutzfeldt Jakob disease (vCJD).

In the U.K. and many other countries, including the U.S., the use of mammalian meat-and-bone meal in feed for all food-producing animals is now prohibited. Testing requirements and/or prohibitions have also been placed on the use of certain bovine tissues for human food.

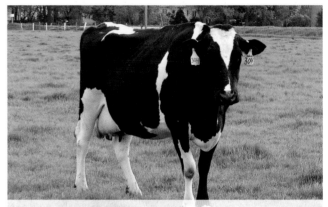

BSE was first diagnosed in the U.K. in 1986.
Source: Danelle Bickett-Weddle, Iowa State University

VARIOUS WAYS DISEASES EMERGE

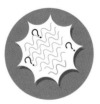

New agent can emerge, e.g. BSE

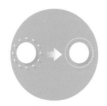

Infectious agents can mutate into a new, more pathogenic form, e.g. influenza

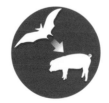

A pathogen can jump from one species to another, e.g. Nipah virus

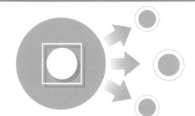

A disease that was previously under control re-emerges as a significant problem, e.g. bovine tuberculosis

CHAPTER 3

Prepare
International Agencies
National Agencies
- **Veterinary Services –**
  SPRS, NIES, STAS
Prevent
Import, Quarantine and
- **Border Protection**
Respond
National Response Framework
FAD Investigations
NVSL
Response Activities
- Quarantine, Movement
  Control, Epidemiological
  Investigations, Surveillance,
  Treatment, Stamping out,
  Disposal, Disinfection
Secure Food Supply
Recover

Authors:
Anna Rovid Spickler, DVM, PhD
Jane Galyon, MS
Center for Food Security and Public Health
Iowa State University
College of Veterinary Medicine
Ames, IA 50011 USA

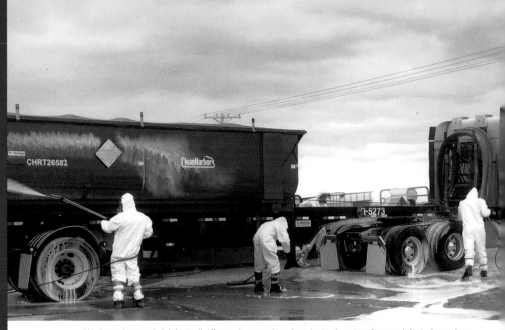

*Workers clean and disinfect roll-off containers and trucks prior to departure from an infected premises.
Source: USDA*

Response to a Foreign Animal Disease Outbreak in the United States

PREPARE, PREVENT, RESPOND, AND RECOVER

Animal agriculture is a major part of the U.S. economy. Protecting animal agriculture from the introduction of devastating diseases is an important function of the government. Maintaining the health and marketability of animals requires diligence and a strong integrated system. Many diseases considered to be foreign such as foot and mouth disease, were once present in the U.S. and could easily be re-established if surveillance, border controls, and eradication activities were relaxed. Some foreign animal diseases (FADs) are zoonotic and present a significant public health threat. Despite all efforts to exclude FADs, they occasionally enter the country.

Some FADs detected and reported in the U.S. since 2005 include highly pathogenic avian influenza in poultry and wild birds, vesicular stomatitis and contagious equine metritis in horses, white spot syndrome virus in shrimp, Old World screwworms and New World screwworms in dogs, and rabbit hemorrhagic disease. In the majority of cases, FADs are successfully eliminated. The strong U.S. veterinary infrastructure works both within the country and abroad to monitor animal diseases and protect animal health. This chapter describes how international agencies, the federal government and state governments work to prevent FAD agents from entering the country, investigate and diagnose suspicious cases, respond to confirmed findings, and assist with recovery from an outbreak.

INTERNATIONAL AGENCIES
INVOLVED IN DISEASE CONTROL

The World Organization for Animal Health (OIE) is the intergovernmental organization responsible for improving animal health worldwide; it includes approximately 180 member countries and maintains permanent relations with 45 other international and regional organizations. The OIE headquarters is in Paris, France, and supporting offices are maintained in each region of the world. Regional commissions work to strengthen surveillance, control animal diseases, and address problems specific to each region.

The OIE maintains a list of important diseases in livestock (including horses and camels), rabbits, birds, fish, mollusks, crustaceans, amphibians, and bees; these diseases are "notifiable" by its member nations. Each country is obligated to report which diseases are present or absent in its country. To collect and share information on animal disease outbreaks, the OIE uses a global health information system called the World Animal Health Information System or WAHIS.

Information on animal disease outbreaks collected by veterinarians, producers, hunters, and others, is submitted to state and/or national veterinary authorities on a regular basis. This information is then analyzed by the national authorities and reported to the OIE. This notification is mandatory, and all member countries are linked

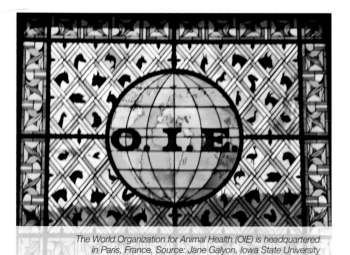

The World Organization for Animal Health (OIE) is headquartered in Paris, France. Source: Jane Galyon, Iowa State University

electronically to WAHIS. OIE specialists then analyze and organize the data. At the same time, the OIE tracks rumors and verifies other unofficial information to supplement the officially submitted data.

Events that must be reported immediately to the OIE include an outbreak of a disease normally absent from the country, or a change in an OIE-listed pathogen such as a new strain, an unexpected increase in morbidity or mortality, or a change in the epidemiology of the disease. Countries must also notify the OIE if they detect an emerging disease with significant morbidity, mortality or zoonotic potential, even if that disease is not listed by the OIE. In addition, every six months each country provides routine information on the presence or absence of listed diseases within its borders. An annual report submitted to the OIE compiles the information about the diseases listed in the six-month reports, other diseases that are not obligatory to report, and additional details, such as the diagnostic capabilities of the country's laboratories.

Next, the information is disseminated on an open access web interface. There are three parts to this system: 1) a monitoring system, which displays the global situation for about 120 diseases of terrestrial and aquatic animals (domesticated and wild); 2) an early warning system, which displays real time notification of potential animal health risks including emerging diseases; and 3) a summary of information specific to each country (e.g., animal population, human capacity in veterinary services and laboratories, vaccination, etc.).

For example, if an FAD occurs in the U.S., the country must immediately notify the OIE, which promptly reports the outbreak to all member nations. Likewise, the U.S. government receives reports concerning the disease status of other countries. This allows it to increase surveillance for a disease, undertake tracing activities or stop imports during an outbreak, and to make informed decisions on routine import restrictions and testing requirements.

THE OIE ALSO:

- Encourages international cooperation in the control of animal diseases;
- Develops and maintains health standards related to trade in animals and animal products, diagnostic tests, and vaccines. The World Trade Organization uses these standards as it oversees the rules of trade between nations;

- Provides technical support for disease control and eradication to member countries requesting assistance;
- Works to improve the national veterinary services, especially for developing and in-transition countries;
- Works to assure the safety of food of animal origin and to promote animal welfare through a science-based approach.

NATIONAL AGENCIES
INVOLVED IN DISEASE CONTROL

Keeping a country free of exotic diseases requires pre-border, at-border, and post-border controls, a process to screen imported animals and animal products, and mechanisms to identify, control, and eradicate introduced diseases. Multiple agencies may be involved in these processes.

In the U.S., the federal government has a critical role in controlling animal diseases. The Animal and Plant Health Inspection Service (APHIS), which is part of the U.S. Department of Agriculture (USDA), is the lead agency in an animal disease outbreak. APHIS has six

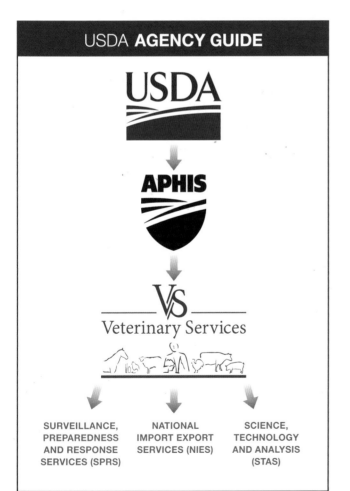

USDA **AGENCY GUIDE**

USDA → APHIS → VS Veterinary Services

| SURVEILLANCE, PREPAREDNESS AND RESPONSE SERVICES (SPRS) | NATIONAL IMPORT EXPORT SERVICES (NIES) | SCIENCE, TECHNOLOGY AND ANALYSIS (STAS) |

operational program units, including **Veterinary Services** (VS). VS protects and improves the health, quality, and marketability of the nation's animals, animal products, and veterinary biologics by preventing, controlling, and/or eliminating animal diseases, and monitoring and promoting animal health and productivity. VS has primary responsibility in a disease outbreak involving domestic livestock and/or poultry.

VS is divided into three operational units: Surveillance, Preparedness and Response Services (SPRS), National Import Export Services (NIES), and Science, Technology and Analysis Services (STAS).

Surveillance, Preparedness and Response Services (SPRS) activities include animal health incident management (disease outbreaks), commodity business planning, and the management of disease programs, surveillance programs, animal disease traceability programs, emergency preparedness programs, epidemiological investigations, One Health programs, and management of a Logistics Center which includes the National Veterinary Stockpile.

The National Preparedness and Incident Coordination Center (NPIC) is part of SPRS. NPIC has responsibility for animal disease traceability, the National Animal Health Emergency Response Corps (see Chapter 4), the National Veterinary Accreditation Program, and Preparedness and Incident Coordination. NPIC works closely with the APHIS animal health commodity centers and the six districts that are responsible for field operations across the U.S.

National Preparedness and Incident Coordination Center activities include:
- Developing and distributing emergency response guidelines based on the National Incident Management System and National Response Framework (see below and chapter 4);
- Developing the foreign animal disease preparedness and response plans (FAD PReP);
- Coordinating investigations and disseminating information about foreign animal disease investigations and events;
- Supporting the Secure Food Supply Plans (collaborating with public-private academic partnerships to facilitate business continuity in the event of an FAD incident); and

- Managing the Emergency Management Response System, a web-based information management system that stores data on FAD investigations, animal health incidents, epidemiological tracing, disease surveillance, and intrastate and interstate animal movements.

National Import Export Services (NIES) manages import and export activities from setting policy to inspection at ports of entry. This group develops policies related to permitting and regulatory services and manages Animal Import Centers and Port Services, the Agricultural Select Agent Program, and the International Animal Health Standards Services. NIES operates six service centers, several animal quarantine facilities, and multiple ports of entry.

Science, Technology and Analysis Services (STAS) includes the Center for Veterinary Biologics, the National Veterinary Services Laboratories, and the Center for Epidemiology and Animal Health. STAS provides analysis, expertise, and information to policy and decision makers.

While the USDA-APHIS VS is the main federal government agency responsible for protecting animal health, it does not work alone. Protecting animal health and responding to a foreign animal disease outbreak takes an integrated approach and may involve other USDA groups and other federal agencies such as the Department of Homeland Security (DHS), the Centers for Disease Control and Prevention (CDC), the Federal Bureau of Investigation (FBI), various state and local government agencies (agriculture, wildlife, natural resources, etc.), local emergency management, and private organizations like animal industry groups and veterinary response teams. The groups involved depend on many factors, including the specific situation, the animal species affected, and the disease agent. Additional federal agencies may be involved in regulating imports, and individual states may have special entry requirements for animals and animal products.

PREVENTING DISEASE INTRODUCTION

The first defense against a foreign animal disease is to prevent its entry into the country.

IMPORT RESTRICTIONS

Federal agencies establish the rules for the importation of many animals and animal products and issue import permits. Several agencies may be involved and import rules vary with the species, the disease, the animal product, the diseases present in the country of origin, and whether the product being imported has been treated or not. For example, fresh meats cannot be imported from countries that have foot and mouth disease but meats that have been cured or heat-processed may be allowed. Import policies take into account factors such as the epidemiology of the disease, the surveillance methods and veterinary infrastructure in the exporting country, and the end use of the commodity to be imported, as well as OIE guidelines and recommendations. For instance, more stringent requirements may be placed on poultry imports from a country that does not report Newcastle disease but has poor veterinary infrastructure, compared to similar imports from a country with good surveillance for Newcastle disease and excellent diagnostic laboratories. In addition to setting overall import guidelines, the U.S. federal agencies monitor OIE bulletins and stop imports from countries where outbreaks of certain diseases of concern have been reported.

QUARANTINE

The quarantine process is an important step in ensuring that animals, particularly inapparent carriers, do not carry exotic diseases into the U.S. Livestock and poultry deemed to be a significant risk must be imported through a USDA Import Center. This includes animals that could be carrying serious diseases or arthropod

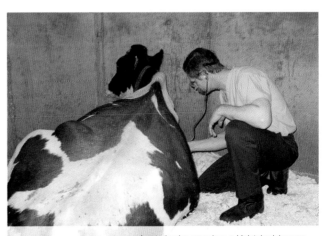

A veterinarian examines a Holstein dairy cow.
Source: Danelle Bickett-Weddle, Iowa State University

pests. The USDA operates quarantine facilities in Miami and New York and oversees private quarantine facilities at several other ports including Los Angeles, Chicago, and San Juan. USDA quarantine facilities handle a variety of species; private quarantine facilities are generally approved for specific species. Livestock imported from Canada and Mexico can usually enter the U.S. without quarantine.

An APHIS port veterinarian gives imported animals a preliminary examination and checks their identification, health certificates, and permits. If any information or documentation is missing, the animal is refused entry. Animals refused entry are held at the import center until the problem is corrected or the animal is removed from the U.S. Animals with appropriate documentation receive a thorough physical examination and may be sprayed for external parasites. They are then taken to isolation facilities for a set number of days, which can vary depending on the species of animal and its country of origin. Cattle, horses, birds, waterfowl, and zoo animals are housed separately in species-specific holding areas. Within each area, each animal or group of animals is segregated into units that are sufficiently separated to reduce the likelihood of disease transmission. Imported animals are tested for applicable diseases, depending on its species and the country of origin. When all required tests are negative and the quarantine period has passed with no signs of disease, the animal is released to its owner. The receiving state is notified when animals are being released from quarantine.

CDC regulations govern the importation of some animals; currently, the list includes pet dogs and cats, African rodents, turtles, monkeys, and civets. Pets are inspected at ports of entry, using a risk-based approach, but they are not usually quarantined except in Hawaii, which is free of rabies. Individual states also have entry requirements that must be satisfied for livestock, birds, dogs, cats, and other animals. For example, all states and the CDC require that dogs be vaccinated against rabies. Some states also mandate that cats have proof of rabies vaccination, although this is not a CDC requirement. Information on entry requirements for each state can be obtained from the State Animal Health Official (SAHO) in each state.

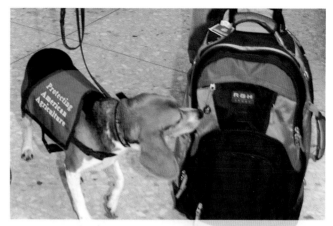

A beagle in the Beagle Brigade sniffs luggage for agricultural contraband.
Source: James Tourtellotte, U.S. Customs and Border Protection

BORDER PROTECTION

Border patrols and inspections ensure that animal products do not bypass the import and quarantine process. The U.S. Department of Homeland Security's (DHS) Customs and Border Protection (CBP) unit is responsible for carrying out inspections. CBP Agriculture Specialists screen passengers, all types of cargo, and international mail at ports of entry. At some ports, detector dogs (e.g. the Beagle Brigade), are used to screen passengers and cargo for hidden items that may contain harmful plant pests and FADs. At other ports, officials use low-energy x-rays to detect the presence of organic materials such as fruit and meats.

RESPONDING TO ANIMAL DISEASE OUTBREAKS

Despite the import and quarantine process and border controls, FADs occasionally enter the U.S. If an outbreak occurs, the most important goal is to return the country to a disease-free state as soon as possible. The disease must be identified, contained, and, if possible, eradicated. The animal industry must also recover and be able to resume trade. The most critical step in this process is the rapid <u>recognition</u> and <u>reporting</u> of suspicious cases. Prompt reporting can prevent a FAD from spreading, reduce the economic costs of an outbreak, reduce the risk that the disease will become established in wildlife or arthropod reservoirs, and, in some cases, prevent human disease. Conversely, delayed reporting can increase the cost and complexity of an outbreak and increase the risk that the disease may never be eradicated.

Private practitioners are usually the first to suspect an exotic disease. In some cases, the disease raises suspicions immediately because the morbidity or mortality rate is unexpectedly high or because the clinical signs are unusual. However, FADs can also resemble common diseases already present in the U.S. A horse with neurological signs from Japanese encephalitis, for example, does not look different clinically from a horse with equine herpes myeloencephalitis or Western equine encephalitis, both endemic to the U.S. Exotic pathogens can also have multiple strains, some of which are more virulent than others and thus, easier to recognize. For example, a highly virulent strain of classical swine fever virus (CSFV) can cause a hemorrhagic syndrome with morbidity and mortality rates approaching 100% in a naïve herd of pigs; however, moderately virulent strains of CSFV tend to cause a much less dramatic illness that may be indistinguishable from endemic diseases such as salmonellosis or erysipelas. All of these factors present a challenge for the practitioner in terms of when to report a suspected FAD. A history of possible recent contact with people or livestock returning from abroad should increase the suspicion of an exotic disease, as should a syndrome that does not follow the expected clinical or treatment response patterns. If there is any doubt about whether a disease is exotic or not, it is better to report it rather than delay and let it spread.

Once a disease has been reported as suspicious, trained FAD specialists are sent by the U.S. government to investigate. Many reported diseases turn out to be indigenous diseases masquerading as something more exotic. Between 1997 and 2014, FAD specialists investigated more than 9,500 potential FAD or emerging disease incidents. All but a small percentage were found to be caused by agents endemic to the U.S. If an incursion is found to be caused an FAD, the consequences can vary widely. In many cases, the disease is identified early and the response is rapid, simplifying eradication. Occasionally, however, a pathogen has disseminated more widely before its discovery, or it has entered wildlife or invertebrate populations, making eradication much more difficult.

The process of investigating an FAD is complex, and can involve different agencies, and, in some cases, different procedures. Veterinarians should be knowledgeable about what to do when an FAD is suspected and understand how a response effort will unfold.

NATIONAL RESPONSE FRAMEWORK

The National Response Framework is a guide to how the nation responds to all types of disasters and emergencies. Preparedness for these events is a shared responsibility across the whole community. Under the NRF, the USDA coordinates the protection of agriculture and natural resources in all types of emergencies. APHIS VS is responsible for leading responses to animal disease outbreaks. APHIS may receive help in carrying out the response from other federal agencies, state governments, industry, and private groups.

When the disease is zoonotic or a food safety concern, agencies such as the Office of Public Health and Science (OPHS), the CDC, the Food and Drug Administration (FDA), and the USDA's Food Safety and Inspection Service (FSIS) may be involved. Assistance may also be requested from Department of Defense (DOD) and the Federal Emergency Management Agency (FEMA). If the outbreak involves agro- or bioterrorism, the FBI and the DHS will become major participants. State departments of agriculture, boards of animal health, industry groups, and other agencies have also developed emergency plans that complement the federal response, and universities often provide additional assistance.

The National Incident Management System (NIMS) standardizes procedures and ensures that responders from a variety of agencies will be able to work together quickly and efficiently. All of these responders use a common framework, the Incident Command System (ICS), which establishes job responsibilities and the organizational structure of the response. The ICS is described in Chapter 4.

FAD INVESTIGATIONS IN THE U.S.

Federally accredited veterinary practitioners are obligated to report a variety of diseases to state and federal authorities. OIE-listed diseases not present in the U.S. are always reported immediately. Each state maintains a list of diseases that are reportable within a specific timeframe. e.g., 72 hours, a week, or a month. Such diseases might include, for example, an illness that is being monitored

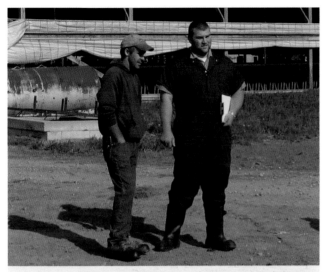
Private veterinary practitioners and producers are usually the first to recognize a FAD. Source: Tara Wellman, Iowa State University

but is not unusual. In addition, zoonotic diseases may be reportable to the health department.

Sometimes diseases are not initially regulated or reportable, but later change their status. Porcine epidemic diarrhea virus (PEDV), a coronavirus that primarily affects piglets, was first diagnosed in the U.S. in 2013. The disease was considered production-related and not a restriction on trade. However, PEDV persisted and spread through many states, despite federal, state, and industry actions. In 2014, the USDA issued a Federal Order requiring that this disease be reported to USDA or state animal health officials and requiring affected premises to work with officials to develop and implement management plans for the virus.

Most suspected FADs are first recognized by private veterinary practitioners and livestock producers. Practitioners who suspect an FAD should immediately contact both the State Animal Health Official's (SAHOs) office and the APHIS Assistant Director (AD) in the District Office for their state. Practitioners should not submit laboratory samples or attempt to diagnose a suspected FAD themselves. APHIS and the state office also receive reports of possible FADs from other sources, such as producers or county extension specialists. Veterinary diagnostic laboratories play an important role in early detection; laboratory workers may find exotic disease agents in samples submitted by practitioners who believe they are investigating an endemic condition. In addition, trained diagnosticians at APHIS-approved laboratories conduct routine surveillance for certain

FADs, such as classical swine fever, that are at a high risk of entering the country.

Once the suspicion of a foreign animal disease has been raised, the case is entered into the computerized national Emergency Management Response System (EMRS), which is used to report and track possible foreign and/or emerging animal disease investigations. APHIS also sends a Foreign Animal Disease Diagnostician (FADD) to investigate. FADDs are USDA, state, or university-affiliated veterinarians who have been trained to recognize and diagnose exotic diseases. FADDs respond as quickly as possible, normally within just a few hours. The assigned investigator contacts the affected facility and visits the premises to perform a herd/flock exam, conduct necropsies if necessary, and collect laboratory samples. The FADD also ships necessary diagnostic samples to a federal laboratory and informs the laboratory that the samples are on the way. Some high priority samples may be personally delivered by courier and rapid transport.

In addition, the FADD helps the producer establish biosecurity measures that will prevent the disease from spreading; in most cases, all clothing, equipment, and vehicles must be thoroughly cleaned and disinfected before leaving the premises. Information from the investigation is entered into EMRS where it can be viewed by appropriate state and federal animal health authorities.

THE NATIONAL VETERINARY SERVICES LABORATORIES AND THE NATIONAL ANIMAL HEALTH LABORATORY NETWORK

USDA APHIS National Veterinary Services Laboratories (NVSL) has primary responsibility for FAD testing. The NVSL consists of three laboratories in Ames, Iowa, and the Foreign Animal Disease Diagnostic Laboratory (FADDL) at Plum Island, New York. Only the NVSL can confirm an outbreak of an FAD.

Each NVSL laboratory specializes in specific diseases. The three NVSL-Ames laboratories diagnose foreign animal diseases affecting poultry, swine, and equids, as well as transmissible spongiform encephalopathies (TSEs). The fourth NVSL laboratory, FADDL-Plum Island, has particularly secure containment facilities. FADDL diagnoses vesicular infections and other highly contagious exotic diseases. It is operated by DHS. Plum

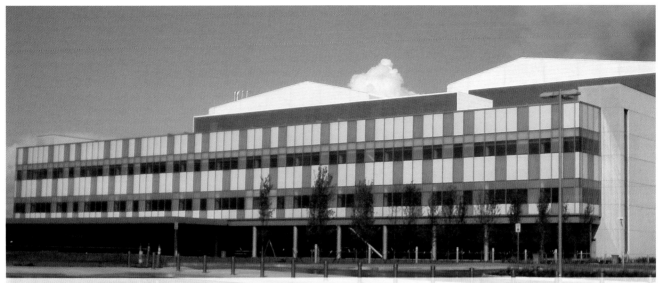

The National Centers for Animal Health in Ames, Iowa, houses the USDA ARS National Animal Diseases Center, three of the APHIS National Veterinary Services Laboratories, and the Center for Veterinary Biologics. Source: Larry Elsken, USDA

Island is also where FADDs are trained and where the USDA's Agricultural Research Service (ARS) conducts research on highly contagious FADs. DHS is in the process of building a new state-of-the-art biocontainment facility, which will assume much of the work currently conducted at Plum Island. This facility is called the National Bio and Agro-Defense Facility (NBAF) and is located in Manhattan, Kansas.

After an FAD has been confirmed, state and university laboratories that are part of the National Animal Health Laboratory Network (NAHLN) may assist the NVSL.

NATIONAL VETERINARY SERVICES LABORATORIES

Conducts almost 500 specific diagnostic tests and is the federal reference laboratory for "program diseases" (i.e., those that are designated for control or eradication, such as brucellosis)

Serves as an OIE reference laboratory for 15 diseases and a Food and Agriculture Organization reference laboratory for a number of diseases

Supports testing for export certification, as well as surveillance, eradication, and control programs for domestic diseases

Certifies State and university National Animal Health Laboratory Network laboratories to conduct diagnostic tests for regulated diseases, such as equine infectious anemia, equine viral arteritis, brucellosis, and bluetongue.

During an outbreak, these laboratories test suspect herds, help determine the extent of the outbreak, and conduct follow–up surveillance to verify that a state or area is disease-free. They also perform routine targeted surveillance testing. U.S. laboratories that have been classified as OIE international reference laboratories are sometimes asked to help diagnose exotic disease outbreaks in other countries. The U.S. can, likewise, request assistance from another country's OIE reference laboratory that has expertise in a particular disease.

RESPONSE TO A CONFIRMED OUTBREAK

The USDA-APHIS NPIC has developed a set of guidelines, called the Foreign Animal Disease Preparedness and Response Plan (FAD PReP), to manage outbreak responses for FADs. These materials are flexible and can be adapted to meet each unique situation. The goals of FAD PReP are to 1) control and contain the FAD as quickly as possible; 2) eradicate the FAD using strategies that are designed to stabilize animal agriculture, the food supply, the economy and to protect public health and the environment; and 3) provide science- and risk-based approaches and systems to facilitate continuity of business for non-infected animals and non-contaminated animal products.

FAD PReP materials include Strategic Plans, National Animal Health Emergency Management System Guidelines, Industry Manuals, Disease Response Plans,

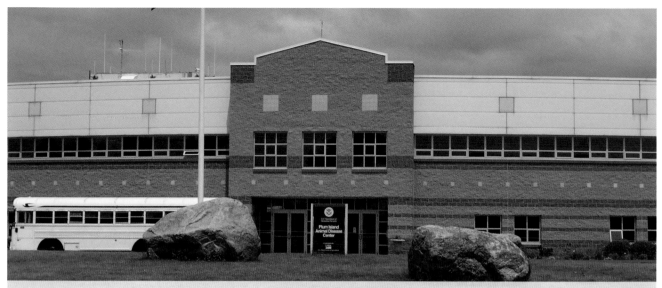

The Plum Island Animal Disease Center on Plum Island, New York, is operated by the U.S. Department of Homeland Security. The USDA Agriculture Research Service and APHIS conduct research and diagnostic activities in this facility. Source: USDA

Standard Operating Procedures, Secure Food Supply Plans, and Ready Reference Guides. These materials are available at *www.aphis.usda.gov/fadprep.*

In situations where the case history, clinical signs, and epidemiological evidence suggest the case is likely to be an FAD, state and federal authorities begin planning for a possible response, even while testing is still ongoing at NVSL. Final laboratory confirmation of some diseases may take more than 48 hours; planning can minimize delays once this confirmation is available. In some high-risk situations, responses may even be initiated and/or animal movement restrictions placed while authorities are waiting for the test results. If the test results then reveal that the infection is not an FAD, the case is closed and any restrictions that would not have ordinarily been placed on the premises, based on the diagnosis, are lifted. If, however, NVSL confirms the presence of an FAD, federal and state officials implement full-scale response plans.

Federal authorities notify the OIE immediately of the findings. In addition, they inform neighboring countries and major trading partners. To protect their own animal industries and human populations, other countries may place bans on the importation of certain animals or animal products from the infected country, or the affected regions of the country. Throughout the eradication process, OIE, state, and federal officials receive continual updates on the progress of the eradication effort and the disease status of affected regions. APHIS provides information to agricultural officials in other countries about the status of the outbreak, biosecurity measures, and surveillance activities. These updates and consultations help to ensure that trading partners will not place unnecessary restrictions on the exportation of animals and animal products from disease-free areas.

An operations center is established in the area of the outbreak, and incident management teams are dispatched to perform specified activities needed to bring it under control. The response to a foreign animal disease outbreak may involve any or all of the following restrictions and surveillance.

QUARANTINES AND MOVEMENT RESTRICTIONS

The foreign animal disease must be contained, if possible, within a defined area. Movement restrictions are placed on animals within the area, and quarantines are placed on infected and exposed herds. Quarantines are generally imposed by the states. The federal government ordinarily has authority to intervene only in matters of foreign or interstate commerce. However, if the U.S. Secretary of Agriculture has declared an animal health emergency, the federal government can also apply quarantines. As the disease comes under control and is eradicated from some locations, the remaining affected areas are regionalized if possible. This allows trade and animal transport to resume from locations that have regained FAD-free status – an important consideration for animal welfare and

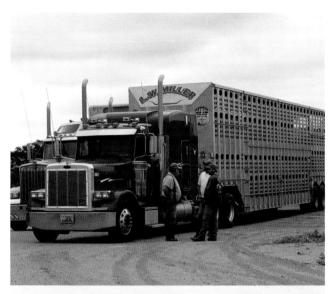
During an FAD investigation, animal movement may be restricted or stopped, depending on the disease. Source: Renee Dewell, Iowa State University

economic reasons. Animal movement restrictions and eradication activities continue inside the affected areas until the disease is eradicated.

EPIDEMIOLOGICAL INVESTIGATIONS

During a disease investigation, federal and state officials trace the movements of infected animals to determine whether the disease has spread and, if so, where. The case, herd or flock discovered first, called the index case or index herd/flock, is used to identify other animals and herds that may be infected. The movements of animals into and out of affected herds are traced, and contacts with other animals are investigated. This can be a daunting task because livestock production in the U.S. depends on extensive movement of animals. For example, an estimated 40 million swine are shipped into a new state each year, with one million swine on the road in trucks each day, about half of them being sent to packing plants. Many of the animals being moved cross multiple state lines. Other factors leading to disease spread are the extensive movements of people, feed, manure, and equipment onto and off livestock premises each day. Biological insect vectors are also a concern with some FADs.

SURVEILLANCE

All susceptible animals/herds that may have been exposed must be tested for the FAD. These assays may be conducted by either NVSL or NAHLN laboratories.

Depending on the disease and its transmission methods, samples may be collected from animals in contact with infected herds, all susceptible animals within a defined area, or some other subset of animals. In any outbreak, constant reassessment is a necessity. Determining that an agent has been completely eradicated may be difficult, particularly if it is vector-borne, can be carried in asymptomatic animals, or can enter wildlife reservoirs. For this reason, extensive surveillance usually continues after an outbreak. Such surveillance is also necessary to substantiate the country's post-outbreak disease-free status to international trading partners.

WILDLIFE AND INVERTEBRATE RESERVOIRS

Wildlife can serve as hosts for a number of FADs, such as highly pathogenic avian influenza (HPAI), classical swine fever, or foot and mouth disease. Wild populations may propagate some agents only temporarily, with spontaneous clearance of the infection once it has been eradicated from domesticated animals. In other cases, wild species can act as true maintenance hosts, and their populations remain infected indefinitely. In the latter situation, eradication may become very difficult or impossible. West Nile virus, which entered the U.S. in 1999 and has since become endemic in wild birds, is a good example of such a disease. Likewise, agents may persist long-term if they propagate in cycles involving invertebrate vectors, such as ticks.

In December 2014, an H5N8 HPAI virus, which had caused outbreaks across Asia and Europe, was detected in the Pacific flyway in the U.S. This virus reassorted with low pathogenic avian influenza viruses normally carried among U.S. birds, and these viral variants were detected among wild birds in the Pacific, Central and Mississippi flyways, and in captive wild birds, backyard and/or commercial poultry flocks in these regions. The outbreaks caused by this virus are, to date, the largest and most costly animal disease outbreaks in the U.S. While eradication from poultry was accomplished by the summer of 2015, it is still uncertain whether these particular viruses will be maintained long-term in North American wild bird populations. If they are, this would pose a continuing threat of introduction to poultry.

Preventing an FAD from entering wildlife populations generally depends on preventing any contact with infected domesticated animals or their carcasses, infectious fomites, or in some cases, invertebrate vectors. Federal and state wildlife agencies may be consulted for help in monitoring wildlife species during an outbreak. Control of an FAD that has entered wildlife is difficult, although vaccines administered orally in bait have been helpful for some diseases such as classical swine fever.

TREATMENT

Treatment of FADs is uncommon. It tends to be limited to exotic arthropods such as screwworms or ticks, where there is a high degree of confidence that the treatment will eliminate the agent.

VACCINATION

Vaccines may be used as a tool to help control the spread of the disease in some outbreaks. Vaccination can decrease the severity of the clinical signs, reduce transmission, and/or help insulate disease-free areas from affected regions. Many factors can influence a decision to vaccinate, such as the availability of an effective vaccine in sufficient quantities to control the outbreak; the availability and reliability of tests to detect infections in vaccinated animals; and the risk that vaccination will mask clinical signs and allow the agent to replicate "silently" in the population. If the U.S. decides to immunize animals against an FAD, vaccines will be distributed and administered as directed by state and federal officials.

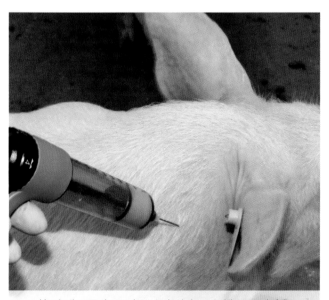

Vaccination may be used as a tool to help control the spread of disease in some outbreaks. Source: Alex Ramirez, Iowa State University

STAMPING OUT

Most FADs have traditionally been eradicated by depopulating exposed and affected animals. The government provides affected producers with indemnity, at the fair market value, for animals that must be culled. Most FADs are highly contagious, and entire affected and exposed herds must usually be euthanized. A few FADs are not contagious. BSE, for example, is acquired by eating contaminated feed. As BSE develops only after a very long incubation period, there is no reason to assume that other animals in the current herd are automatically infected and, typically, the rest of the herd is not euthanized. Similarly, horses infected with West Nile virus are dead end hosts and do not transmit the virus further.

CARCASS DISPOSAL

It is important to destroy any remaining infectious agent in the carcass or to keep the carcass from coming into contact with uninfected animals while the agent is naturally deactivated. Carcasses may be buried, incinerated, rendered, entered into landfills, or composted, depending on the agent and its susceptibility to inactivation. Burial, which is quick and requires fewer resources than most other techniques, may be chosen for carcasses, animal products, feed, and organic wastes. However, space considerations, soil type, a high water table, or other impediments may prevent burial from being an effective option, and other methods can be the best alternative in specific situations. Carcass disposal can be very challenging aspect to manage when the number of animals is large. During the HPAI outbreak in the Midwest in 2015, the enormous number of poultry carcasses made rapid, effective disposal difficult.

DISINFECTION

Infected premises and equipment are thoroughly cleaned and decontaminated as soon as possible after the disposal of infected animals, bedding, animal waste, and other materials. This reduces the chance that fomites and wild animals will spread the disease agent to new areas. The stringency and timing of the decontamination process varies with the agent and its resistance to inactivation. Delays in restocking animals may also be necessary when an agent is difficult to destroy and persists for longer periods in the environment.

VECTOR CONTROLS

Diseases spread by mosquitoes, ticks, or other vectors may require spraying programs or other vector control measures, as well as surveillance of susceptible vector populations. Effective control of arthropod vectors can be difficult, particularly long-term or in large areas. In addition, there may be concerns about the environmental effects of some chemicals, and the costs and sustainability of such programs. Arthropods can develop resistance to some agents used for their control.

SECURE FOOD SUPPLY PLANS

While stamping out continues to be used to manage many FAD outbreaks, it can be difficult to accomplish effectively and rapidly when herds are large. The U.S. contains some very large herds, including feedlots with more than 50,000 head of cattle, dairies with more than 5,000 lactating cows, dairy calf ranches with more than 70,000 head of calves, and swine farms with more than 20,000 sows. These premises are too large to rapidly depopulate. Even if this were possible, carcass disposal would present enormous logistical and environmental challenges. Alternative methods are being developed to control FADs when rapid depopulation is not feasible, as part of the Secure Food Supply business continuity plans. In a large outbreak where rapid depopulation is not possible, the response will focus on quarantines, managed movement by permit, biosecurity, surveillance, marketing of recovered animals that return to health, and vaccination (if available). The goal will still be to return the U.S. to disease-free status; however, it will be through a long-term disease control program.

The Secure Food Supply Plans are commodity-specific plans that use science-and risk-based information to facilitate market continuity for specific products in an FAD outbreak. Plans are developed or in process for eggs, turkeys, milk, pork, broilers, and beef. These plans are the result of discussions between federal, state, industry, and academia on best approaches to:

- Avoid interruptions in animal/animal product movement to commercial processing from farms with no evidence of infection during a foreign animal disease outbreak;
- Provide a continuous supply of safe and wholesome food to consumers; and
- Maintain business continuity for producers, transporters, and food processors through response planning.

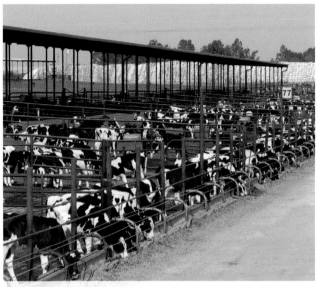
Large production operations should have plans in place to manage animals during a disease outbreak. Source: Mark Kirkpatrick

PUBLIC EDUCATION

During an outbreak, websites and hotlines are set up to inform the public. Information may also be disseminated directly to specific groups such as producers or veterinarians. In addition to keeping the public informed, these campaigns can help raise awareness and identify new cases of the disease. Federal and state protocols are in place to inform the media.

RECOVERY

The OIE's *Terrestrial Animal Health Code* and *Aquatic Animal Health Code* outline the recommendations for determining when a country (or compartment) will be classified as free of a specific FAD. The OIE standards, which should be satisfied before full international trade resumes, serve to reassure trading partners that a country's animal exports are likely to be safe.

The OIE is the only world organization to grant an official status on freedom from specified animal diseases. In 2015, the diseases on the OIE list include:
- Foot and mouth disease (FMD);
- Contagious bovine pleuropneumonia (CBPP);
- Bovine spongiform encephalopathy (BSE);
- African horse sickness (AHS);
- Peste des petits ruminants (PPR); and
- Classical swine fever (CSF).

For FMD only, countries or zones can be given a free status with or without vaccination.

APHIS VS works towards recovery from a disease outbreak through partnerships with local and state governments and other organizations, including livestock industries. Recovery activities include prompt payment for euthanized livestock and destroyed materials, the lifting of quarantines and movement controls, the renegotiation of international export protocols, and federal government and industry reassurances and reinforcement of consumer expectations.

The ultimate costs of an outbreak for a country, its producers, and affiliated industries can be high. In addition to the direct costs of eradication, there will be other losses. Trade restrictions may prevent producers from selling products from healthy animals and the value of these products may also fall in the domestic markets. Industries such as meat packers and shipping companies, as well as producers, may suffer losses. In extreme cases, even industries such as tourism may be affected.

Lastly, every eradication effort may not be successful. West Nile virus first appeared in the Western Hemisphere when it was found in New York City in 1999. Although the U.S. made a concerted effort to eradicate this virus, it overwintered in mosquito and bird populations, reappeared in 2000, and eventually became established throughout much of North America. It has also found its way into Central America and continues to spread. There is no guarantee that such an event will not happen again, particularly with an arthropod-borne and/or a wildlife disease; however, the chances of another FAD becoming established can be decreased by maintaining a strong emergency management system to exclude, detect, and respond to all outbreaks.

CONCLUSION

An effective response to an outbreak requires prompt recognition and reporting of the initial cases, and a fast, efficient, and flexible response that can evolve with the outbreak if it spreads. The current emergency management system in the U.S. requires cooperation among local, state, federal, and tribal agencies, as well as industry. Practicing veterinarians can contribute to FAD detection and response by becoming knowledgeable about the FADs most likely to enter the country, by being aware of clinical or necropsy findings that should raise the suspicion of a FAD, and by routinely including FADs in their list of differential diagnoses. Private veterinarians play an important role in FAD surveillance and control by immediately reporting suspicious cases, by remaining on site until a government veterinarian arrives, and by continuing to refer suspicious cases during an outbreak. Lastly, private veterinarians can assist in the local and federal response to a disease outbreak. The ways veterinarians can participate in these responses will be discussed in Chapter 4.

Information Sources for this chapter can be found at *http://www.cfsph.iastate.edu/TEDATextbookReferences/*.

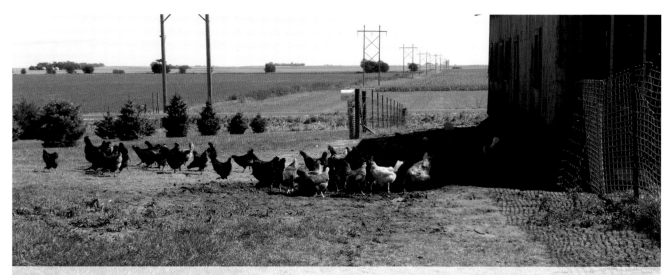

Poultry can be infected with avian influenza or Newcastle disease through contact with wild birds.
Source: Jane Galyon, Iowa State University

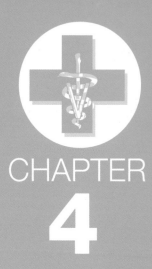

CHAPTER
4

Teams and Training
- National Animal Health Emergency Response Corps (NAHERC)
- National Veterinary Response Team (NVRT)
- Veterinary Medical Assistance Teams (VMAT)
- State Animal Response Teams
- Non Profit Organizations

The Incident Command System
- Incident Command
- Operations Section
- Planning Section
- Logistics Section
- Finance/Administration Section

Emergency Management Incident Typing System

Experiences
- Pamela Kramer
- Dr. Pam Hullinger
- Dr. Michelle Schroeder

Authors:
Anna Rovid Spickler, DVM, PhD
Jane Galyon, MS
Center for Food Security and Public Health
Iowa State University
College of Veterinary Medicine
Ames, IA 50011 USA

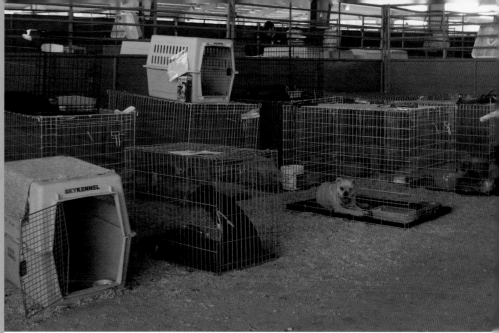

Veterinarians may set up temporary housing and care for displaced animals during hurricanes or floods. Source: Heather Case, American Veterinary Medical Association.

A Veterinarian's Role
in an Animal Health Emergency

TEAMS AND TRAINING

Veterinarians are important responders to animal disease outbreaks, natural disasters, and manmade disasters. They play a vital role in protecting animal health, the food supply, and public health. To best assist during an emergency, veterinarians should be part of a team with a clearly defined role.

The U.S. Animal and Plant Health Inspection Service (APHIS), a part of the Department of Agriculture (USDA), is the lead agency in an animal disease outbreak. APHIS Veterinary Services (VS) has primary responsibility in outbreaks involving domestic livestock and/or poultry, but coordinates its activities with other federal and state government organizations, as described in Chapter 3. Emergency responders from federal, state, and local organizations also assist at other types of incidents affecting animals, such as natural or man-made disasters. These incidents sometimes include pets as well as livestock. The Pets Evacuation and Transportation Standards Act (PETS Act) of 2006 was established in the aftermath of Hurricane Katrina, when the lack of provisions for pets or service animals in existing evacuation plans became apparent.

The PETS Act requires that plans for state and local emergency preparedness take into account the needs of individuals with household pets and service animals before, during and after a major disaster or emergency.

When a disease outbreak or other incident is small, it may be easily managed by a few state and/or federal government employees. However, a large, multi-location or extended incident can quickly overwhelm these responders, and additional help may be needed. Veterinarians in private practice can assist with response efforts, by participating in various federal, state, or non-governmental emergency response teams.

This chapter describes some organizations that may be open to veterinarians, and in some cases, also to animal health technicians and students. In addition, it provides an overview of the the Incident Command System (ICS), the organizational system that is used to manage emergency responses in the U.S., and gives a firsthand look at the experiences of some volunteers who participated in outbreak responses.

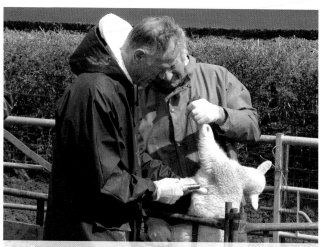
Veterinarians can have many duties in an animal health emergency Source: Pam Hullinger, University of California, Davis

THE NATIONAL ANIMAL HEALTH EMERGENCY RESPONSE CORPS

The National Animal Health Emergency Response Corps (NAHERC) is a pool of paid volunteers, including private veterinarians, veterinary technicians, and students who operate under APHIS and can be brought into federal government service quickly to supplement an emegency response. NAHERC was activated in 2015

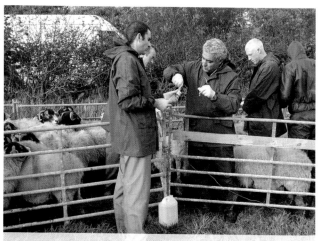
Veterinarians and animal health technicians work as a team in response situations. Source: Pam Hullinger, University of California, Davis

during the outbreak of highly pathogenic avian influenza in the Upper Midwest. NAHERC is managed by APHIS National Preparedness and Incident Coordination Center (NPIC), the federal organization that also coordinates, investigates, and disseminates information about suspected outbreaks.

When an outbreak requires more responders than state and APHIS employees can provide, NAHERC members who are able and willing to participate are activated by APHIS as temporary federal employees. Activated NAHERC members are assigned as either Veterinary Medical Officers (VMOs) or Animal Health Technicians (AHTs). AHT positions are for animal health technicians, students and others with animal-handling expertise, while VMO positions are restricted to veterinarians. VMOs may carry out a variety of duties, such as performing physical examinations or necropsies, collecting laboratory samples, vaccinating animals, performing euthanasia, supervising the disposal of carcasses, collecting epidemiological information, and inspecting livestock markets and vehicles used to transport animals. AHTs participate in similar activities within the scope of their knowledge and skills. The NAHERC members activated for each incident are chosen based on their specific skills and areas of expertise. Most tours of duty are expected to last 21-30 days. Members may accept more than one consecutive tour of duty but may not serve for more than a year. For the duration of their service, NAHERC members receive a government salary, overtime pay (when authorized), travel and per diem expenses, and worker's compensation. Although most assignments are within the U.S., members may occasionally be asked to assist in outbreaks in other countries.

During the emergency response, NAHERC members rely primarily on the experience and veterinary skills they have acquired at work and in school. Volunteers are not expected to be knowledgeable about exotic diseases before applying to the program; however, all NAHERC members must learn emergency response procedures and acquire other necessary knowledge through online training provided by APHIS. At the time of the outbreak, APHIS also provides additional instruction, such as information on the clinical signs and lesions for a specific disease. Veterinarians and others interested in participating in NAHERC can apply online through the APHIS website (search APHIS NAHERC).

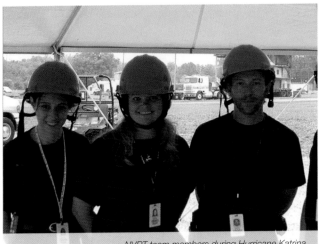

NVRT team members during Hurricane Katrina
Source: Gary Goemann, NVRT

OTHER VETERINARY RESPONSE TEAMS

Veterinarians and technicians can also use their skills and knowledge in an outbreak by working with the Department of Health and Human Services' National Veterinary Emergency Response Team, the American Veterinary Medical Association's Veterinary Medical Assistance Teams, state animal response teams, and non-profit groups such as the American Society for the Prevention of Cruelty to Animals.

THE NATIONAL VETERINARY RESPONSE TEAM

The National Veterinary Response Team (NVRT) is part of the National Disaster Medical System (NDMS). The NDMS is operated under the Department of Health and Human Services (HHS), Office of Preparedness and Response. The NVRT includes veterinarians, animal health technicians, epidemiologists, safety officers, logisticians, communication specialists, and other support personnel.

NVRT responsibilities in a disaster include assessing the veterinary medical needs of a community, providing veterinary medical support to working animals, treating injured or ill large and small animals, providing veterinary medical support for sheltered animals, and conducting veterinary health screenings. This organization also provides veterinary public health

support, including environmental and zoonotic disease assessment, and research animal support (lab animals), and supports USDA efforts in outbreaks involving livestock and poultry.

NVRT personnel are private citizens who are approved as intermittent federal employees and activated in a disaster. These individuals are assigned to specific teams that train together to prepare for emergencies. Deployed individuals are compensated for their time by the Federal government. The National Disaster Medical System will advertise and accept applications for available team positions on USAjobs.gov. Members are selected on criteria including the ability to be on call for deployment, work experience, skill level, team experience, etc. Individuals who have served in the military receive preference. Search National Veterinary Response Team for additional information.

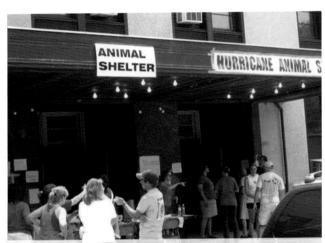

Animal shelters provide veterinary care for displaced animals and help to reunite pets and owners during a disaster. Source: Gary Goemann, NVRT

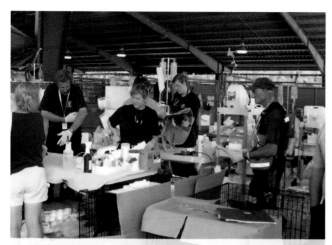
Veterinary hospitals may be established in warehouses and other available facilities during a disaster response. Source: Gary Goemann, NVRT

VETERINARY MEDICAL ASSISTANCE TEAMS

The American Veterinary Medical Association's (AVMA) Veterinary Medical Assistance Teams (VMAT) is a private non-governmental organization funded by the American Veterinary Medical Foundation (AVMF). VMAT teams serve as first responders during disasters and emergencies. The VMAT teams are a state-level resource and deploy to a state upon its request for assistance. In order to request VMAT assistance, a state must have a Memorandum of Understanding with the AVMA. The VMAT program has three primary functions:

- Early Assessment – Self-sufficient volunteer teams of 4-6 persons initially deploy for 72 hours, not including travel time, to assess veterinary conditions and infrastructure and gather data to help the state deploy appropriate resources;
- Basic Treatment – Self-sufficient volunteer teams of 4-6 persons initially deploy for five days, not including travel time, to provide primary field care to augment overwhelmed local capabilities; and
- Training – VMAT volunteers provide training on a wide range of emergency preparedness and response topics to veterinary response organizations, veterinary medical associations, veterinary students and other related organizations. In 2013, AVMA launched "VMAT U" which standardizes and formalizes the training VMAT has been offering for many years.

AVMA VMAT members are volunteers and do not receive a salary. AVMF provides funding for travel, housing and per diem expenses for the AVMA VMAT program. Additional information about the AVMA VMAT program can be found on the AVMA website *https://www.avma.org.*

STATE ANIMAL RESPONSE TEAMS

Veterinarians, students, and veterinary technicians can also participate in animal emergency response teams in their state. Because each region of the country has different animal populations and priorities, veterinary response teams may have different priorities and training requirements. State response organizations go by different names and may be supported through a state agency, the state veterinary medical association or a non-governmental organization. Veterinarians interested in participating in a response team should contact their state veterinary medical association or State Animal Health Official (SAHO) for more information.

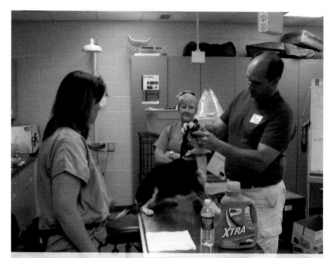
Veterinarians work to assess the health of displaced animals during natural disasters. Source: Kevan Flaming, Iowa State University

NON PROFIT ORGANIZATIONS

Private organizations also respond to disasters. Participating individuals may be involved in activities such as animal decontamination, animal evacuation and transportation, animal search and rescue, disaster veterinary care, and emergency animal sheltering. The National Animal Rescue and Sheltering Coalition (NARSC), established in 2006, is a coalition of agencies that cooperatively respond both nationally and internationally to wildfires, floods, ice storms, tornadoes, hurricanes, and other disasters, as well as to settings where groups of animals are being abused

ANIMAL RESPONSE ORGANIZATIONS

	Employer/Organization	Salaried	Basic Role
NAHERC	USDA-APHIS	YES	Responsibilities are primarily in the operation section of the ICS response. Some basic training in response is required.
NVRT	HHS/NDMS	YES	Roles include early assessments, treatment, and the provision of training on a variety of emergency response topics to others. Training in teams is required.
VMAT	AVMA/AVMF	NO	Roles include assessment of situations and needs, support and treatment, assistance to USDA as needed and requested. Training in teams is required.
State Animal Response Teams	State organized and run	NO	Roles may vary depending on the state, but responders are primarily activated to help with operations section. Training requirements vary by state.
Non Profits	Various organizations: for example, NARSC	NO	Roles include assisting with sheltering, evacuations, rescues, and supply needs.
Freelance Volunteer	None	NO	There is no defined role for freelance volunteers.

and/or lack basic care, such as in a hoarding situation. NARSC members include organizations such as the American Society for the Prevention of Cruelty to Animals (ASPCA) and the Best Friends Animal Society. Veterinarians, veterinary technicians, and veterinary students can play a role in these organizations. To learn more, visit the NARSC website at *narsc.net*.

THE INCIDENT COMMAND SYSTEM

To participate effectively in the emergency response, volunteers in the NAHERC, NVRT, VMAT, NARSC and other emergency response organizations must have a basic understanding of how these events are managed. The response system used in the U.S. is called the Incident Command System (ICS).

An emergency response system must be able to deal with a wide variety of incidents. Outbreaks may be small or large, simple or complex, localized or widespread. Small outbreaks limited to a single farm can be controlled by a few personnel, but many agencies need to work together in a major outbreak. The ICS is a framework that establishes job responsibilities and an organizational structure to facilitate this effort. Although originally developed for wildfire responses, this system has been adopted by emergency management organizations that respond to other types of disasters.

One of the strengths of the ICS is its adaptability; it is effective in both large and small incidents, planned events, and disasters such as fires, hazardous material

spills, earthquakes, hurricanes, and floods. It is also employed in search and rescue missions, biological pest eradication programs, disease outbreaks and containment, and responses to acts of terrorism. ICS uses the same general terminology for all incidents, which provides a common vocabulary for responders from different organizations and disciplines. One of the advantages of the ICS is that it is cost-effective and efficient. By establishing a unit that provides logistical and administrative support to all responders, this system reduces the duplication of effort that occurs if each agency must provide such services to its own personnel.

In the U.S., the Incident Command System is part of the National Incident Management System (NIMS), which is part of the National Response Framework (NRF). The ICS is modular; it is separated into sections,

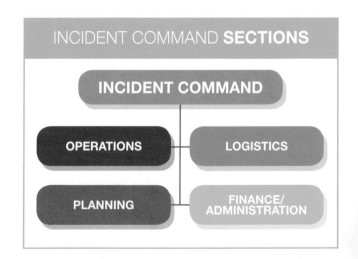

INCIDENT COMMAND SECTIONS

INCIDENT COMMAND

OPERATIONS — LOGISTICS

PLANNING — FINANCE/ADMINISTRATION

each of which performs specific duties. The five sections of the ICS, which are termed "major management functions," are called Incident Command, Operations, Planning, Logistics, and Finance/Administration.

INCIDENT COMMAND

The Incident Command section has the overall responsibility for managing the disease outbreak or other incident. The head of Incident Command is called the Incident Commander. In some incidents that involve multiple agencies, there may be a Unified Command with representatives from each agency. The Incident Commander or Unified Command sets the incident objectives, strategies, and priorities. The Incident Command section is also responsible for ensuring the safety of the responders, providing information to internal and external stakeholders, including the media, and establishing and maintaining liaisons with the other agencies involved. Small incidents may be run entirely by the Incident Commander. However, if an incident grows, the Incident Commander can assign some duties to other personnel. These individuals report to the Incident Commander and are called the Command Staff. The Command Staff includes a Public Information Officer, a Safety Officer, and a Liaison Officer. The Liason Officer serves as the primary contact for supporting agencies assisting at an incident.

The Incident Command section supervises the other sections: Operations, Planning, Logistics, and Finance/Administration. Each of these sections also has a command structure. The person in charge of each section is designated as a Chief. Under the ICS structure, each person is accountable to only one designated supervisor. In addition, there is an orderly chain of command within the ICS ranks. An important operating guideline, called the "span of control," specifies the number of individuals that one supervisor can effectively manage during an emergency response. One supervisor managing five individuals is the recommended ratio, but an effective span of control can vary from three to seven..

OPERATIONS SECTION

The Operations Section is where the tactical fieldwork is conducted. In an animal disease outbreak, the Operations Section would carry out vaccination, depopulation, carcass disposal, and other activities involved in

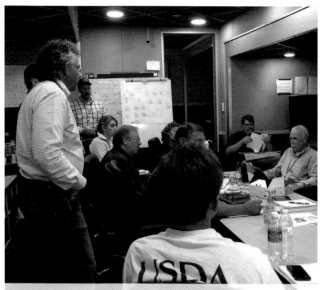
Members of a USDA APHIS Incident Response Team discuss plans for the next operational period. Source: USDA

eradicating the disease. Most VMOs, AHTs, and veterinary students are assigned to this section.

The Operations Section may be divided into groups, divisions, branches, strike teams, and task forces. Groups are used to describe functional areas of operation. For example, NAHERC members assigned to help with

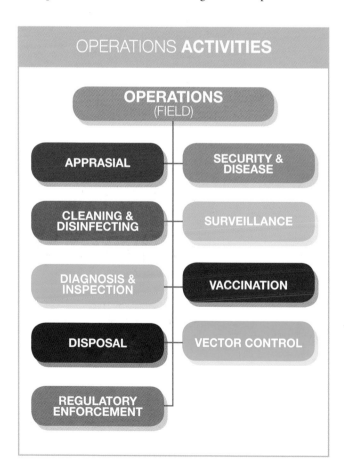

vaccination would belong to the Vaccination Group. Larger incidents may also be separated geographically by Divisions. Each Division responds to the incident in a specific location, such as a region of the country, the floor of a building, or a specific farm. Divisions are usually identified with alphabetic characters (e.g., Division A or Division B). Divisions and Groups may both be used in an incident and are at equal levels in the Incident Command organization. The person in charge of each Division or Group is called a Supervisor. Supervisors must work together and closely coordinate their activities. Branches are used when additional organization is needed. Branches can be either geographical or functional. For example, the Vaccination Group could have a "North Branch" and a "South Branch." Branches can also be used to create supervision levels within the Operations Section. The person in charge of each Branch is called a Director.

Strike Teams or Task Forces may also be established. Strike Teams consist of like resources. For example, a Strike Team might consist of several very similar trucks with drivers assigned to haul carcasses. Task Forces are teams that contain mixed resources. A team that consists of an epidemiologist, a microbiologist, and a wildlife biologist with a pickup truck is considered to be a Task Force. These teams operate under the direct supervision of the Strike Team Leader or Task Force Leader, respectively.

PLANNING SECTION

The Planning Section prepares and documents the Incident Action Plan. The Incident Action Plan gives all supervisors their instructions for each operational period, typically 12 or 24 hours. The Planning Section keeps track of the overall resources, including personnel and equipment needed and used in the incident. This section also collects and evaluates information and maintains documentation for the incident records.

LOGISTICS SECTION

The Logistics Section provides services and support to the incident response. This unit might, for example, set up computers or provide food, lodging, and basic first aid for the ICS participants. It also distributes supplies to responders.

FINANCE/ADMINISTRATION SECTION

The Finance and Administration Section monitors the costs related to the incident and provides accounting and procurement services. This section takes care of paychecks, overtime, reimbursement for meals and other expenses, forms for workman's compensation claims, and similar needs.

In a small incident, the Incident Commander may carry out the planning, logistics, and finance/administration sections' duties and supervise the operations section. In a larger incident, one or more of these sections may be established as separate units.

EMERGENCY MANAGEMENT INCIDENT TYPING SYSTEM

In a local or limited outbreak, the response is usually managed by regional state, federal, and industry officials, with consultation at the national level on issues such as trade and consequence management. In more extensive outbreaks, greater involvement by state and federal agencies becomes necessary, and the command structure becomes more complex. The Emergency Management and Incident Typing System is used to quantify incidents. This system has five categories, with Type 5 incidents being the simplest and most easily managed, and Type 1, the most complex, resource-intensive, and long lasting. In an animal disease outbreak, factors that are considered include the number and location of nearby livestock populations, the history of disease in the area, the current conditions, and management requirements. If a disease outbreak escalates, the incident type can be changed to a higher level, and additional resources can be brought in to manage it.

Free ICS training is available on the Federal Emergency Management Agency website, *www.fema.gov.*

EXPERIENCES IN ANIMAL HEALTH EMERGENCIES

The following stories illustrate how veterinarians and veterinary students can use their education and training to assist in animal emergencies. Pamela Kramer, a veterinary student who participated in the 2003 exotic Newcastle disease outbreak in California, Pam Hullinger, a veterinarian who helped eradicate foot and mouth disease from the United Kingdom in 2001, and Michelle Shroeder, a veterinarian who helped with tuberculosis testing, share their stories in this section.

PAMELA KRAMER

Pamela Kramer was a first-year veterinary student at Iowa State University when she learned about the opportunity to work with NAHERC on the exotic Newcastle disease (END) outbreak in southern California in 2003, **NOTE:** now refered to as Newcastle Disease (ND). The following is an account of her experience.

I am just a small town Iowa girl who didn't travel much at all, especially by myself. In spite of this, I found myself being taken to the Des Moines airport by a friend and flying to California to spend two months working with the USDA trying to eradicate END. Truthfully, I was scared but yet excited all at the same time. Scared partially because I was going somewhere that I had never been before, but for the most part, I was very excited to get this once-in-a-lifetime opportunity and get the chance to participate in a disease eradication program in California. I had the pleasure of working with veterinarians, technicians, interpreters, and clerical people in Southern California for two months -- from Memorial Day through the end of July 2003.

When I arrived in southern California, I spent the first day completing all the necessary paperwork, including getting my ID card and cell phone. I had to take a defensive driving class before I could get my rental car. The USDA arranged for my hotel and provided funds for food and related expenses.

During the first two weeks, I was assigned to the surveillance group and worked as the leader of four people. Every morning we met at Orange County headquarters at 7 a.m. to be briefed on what was going on. We were informed of new birds or premises that had tested positive or other relevant news. Following the morning briefings, each day my team received a map of a section of a community to cover. Our job was to go door to door and speak with someone at every house about pet birds and game birds. If the residents owned birds, we filled out a form indicating types and numbers of birds and whether or not they were sick. If no one was home, we left flyers about END and a number to call if they wanted more information or if they wanted their birds

tested. The USDA-APHIS would pay for all birds to be tested once. It was very interesting to go to the different neighborhoods, especially since this was my first time in California. Most of the people were very nice and didn't mind us inquiring about whether or not they had birds. However, in some areas where positive birds or flocks had been eradicated, people were hesitant to talk to us because they thought we were coming to take their birds. Surprisingly, not very many people knew much about END. The interpreters were quite helpful to have along because in some areas, many people spoke only Spanish. We were told that if we did not feel safe in an area to return to headquarters, and we would be reassigned to a different area.

For my next assignment, I worked at the Orange County APHIS headquarters for a week, entering all the surveillance results in the computer database. While it may not have been the most exciting work, it gave me an understanding of what it was like to work at headquarters and the important role of the support staff in supporting an animal health emergency.

The remainder of my time with the NAHERC was spent collecting cloacal and tracheal swabs from pet birds and chickens in San Diego, Lancaster, and Santa Clarita,

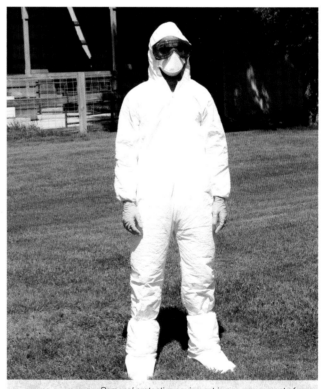

Personal protective equipment is one component of an overall safety, infection control and biosecurity program.
Source: Andrew Kingsbury, Iowa State University

California. I was with a group of 15-20 people, made up mainly of veterinary students, a couple interpreters and one to two veterinarians. We were trained in the field by a veterinarian on biosecurity and collecting samples. Then, we were split into smaller groups, consisting of two or more vet students and one to two interpreters. As with the surveillance unit, we were given maps of the area where we were to go to test birds. As a part of our daily duties, we routinely gowned up in biosecurity suits (Tyvek® suits), boots, gloves, and masks. After we were finished at each premise, each outfit was discarded into a garbage bag, sealed, and disinfected before placing it into another garbage bag. My team started on the outside of the infection zone and worked its way in to reduce the size of the quarantine zone.

I met and worked with veterinary students from Auburn University, Colorado State, Georgia, Iowa State, Kansas State, Minnesota, and Virginia/Maryland and have maintained contact with both veterinary students and veterinarians that I worked with in California.

The most important thing I learned from this experience is how things are done in the real world. Watching the federal and volunteer teams approach each situation was really interesting. Veterinary students received a lot of respect and people listened to them. I also liked the responsibilities I was given (like being in charge of a team). We routinely worked 12-14 hour days, so overtime pay became a big benefit for all the students.

The Newcastle disease outbreak primarily affected backyard birds and game birds. Source: Jane Galyon, Iowa State University

But we also got some time off to interact as a group and to do a little sightseeing on holidays.

This opportunity was a once-in-a-lifetime chance to be involved in a large-scale eradication program. This was an experience that I will never forget. It was so incredible getting to know and work with other veterinary students, veterinarians, and USDA APHIS staff from all over the country. If given the opportunity to do this again, I would jump at it.

PAM HULLINGER

Dr. Pam Hullinger, formerly a Veterinary Medical Officer and University Liaison with the California Department of Food and Agriculture (CDFA) and now the Large Animal Clinic Director with the UC Davis School of Veterinary Medicine, worked in the United Kingdom (U.K.) in 2001 assisting in the eradication of foot and mouth disease (FMD). She initially volunteered through the CDFA and then went back to the U.K. through the NAHERC. An account of Dr. Hullinger's experience follows.

This was an experience that I will never forget, and that has significantly shaped my veterinary career since that experience. There is no substitute for firsthand experience in gaining respect for the devastation that a foreign animal disease can inflict upon a naïve nation. An opportunity such as this was both personally and professionally rewarding. I would encourage anyone who has even a slight interest to make the time to participate if the opportunity arises.

At the time the FMD outbreak began in the U.K., I was both working for CDFA and finishing my winter quarter in the Masters in Preventive Veterinary Medicine Program (MPVM) at UC Davis. When I found out that CDFA veterinarians might be eligible to participate in the eradication efforts, I rapidly signed up. Little did I know that I would be on a plane three days later, about to begin an unforgettable, and life changing experience. It was probably the anticipation of seeing, first-hand, a legendary and much-feared disease, along with a sense of duty that inspired me to act so quickly. It wasn't until I was bound for London that I really started to think about what I might be getting myself into, and started having some apprehensive thoughts…How would U.K. farmers react to foreign veterinarians, etc.?…How would they react when their herds or flocks had to be destroyed?…

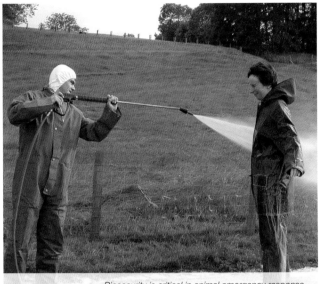
Biosecurity is critical in animal emergency response.
Source: Pam Hullinger, University of California, Davis

Would they let us on their farms?...Did they have guns?...Fortunately, all my apprehensions were largely unwarranted, although I did have to learn to "drive stick" on the "proper side" with my left hand and speak (or at least understand) proper British English.

My initial arrival in Carlisle, Cumbria (northwest England) occurred at a time when the regional Ministry of Agriculture, Fisheries and Food (now called DEFRA – Department for Environment, Food and Rural Affairs) office was expanding from a normal staff of 10-12 to well over 300 veterinarians, plus support staff. Things were very chaotic. The logistical support needed to effectively manage and support a field staff of that magnitude was mind-boggling. Acquisition of simple necessities like lodging, vehicles and cell phones was a challenge as local resources became rapidly depleted.

I had an uneasy feeling as I headed out on my first assignment, which was to inspect some potentially FMD infected cattle. While I was hoping to see "true" clinical FMD, I did not relish the thought of having to destroy the animals, nor the impact that it undoubtedly would have on the farmers. I also wondered how a "Yank" would be received by British farmers under the circumstances. I soon learned that the British farmers were an incredible group of warm, generous and gracious individuals, even in the face of personal and national tragedy. Some of these farmers and their families lost animals, herds and flocks that had been in their families for generations. Most situations were very emotional and stressful as individuals struggled with their

grief and sense of hopelessness at losing their stock and their livelihoods. They say that it is not just one's experiences in life, but how one reacts to them, that truly defines one's character. I will forever be impressed by both the grace and the fortitude of the farmers I worked with in the United Kingdom – they were truly inspirational in the face of chaos and national tragedy.

I also will never forget my initial image of Cumbria, one of the hardest hit areas of the United Kingdom. As I crested the "Pennines," a central mountain and hill range (driving for the first time on the "other" side of the road) and descended toward the town of Carlisle, I entered what resembled a "war zone." Smoke filled the air, burning my eyes and lungs as burning pyres of twisted cattle and sheep carcasses dotted the countryside. It was a haunting image, like nothing I could have imagined. I still remember the smell. The challenge of disposing of up to 80,000 carcasses a day was unimaginable and monumental.

Working in the field, veterinarians were usually asked to make a decision on whether or not a flock or herd was infected, based solely on clinical signs seen at the time of the initial visit (without the aid of any testing or laboratory support). The greatest challenge was in evaluating flocks of possibly infected sheep grazing coarse feed/pasture (that caused minor oral ulcerations or trauma) or flocks that may have been exposed more than three weeks prior to the initial visit (lesions would have healed on these animals). Destroying a person's farm and livelihood, based solely on a few oral ulcers in the mouths of a few sheep without laboratory confirmation was a very uncomfortable decision. While during an outbreak one must always err on the side of caution, we now know that many uninfected animals (>50%) were destroyed due to the lack of scalable, rapid diagnostics for FMD. I hope that many have learned from that unfortunate U.K. lesson, and I have worked hard and believe we are now much better prepared to face the diagnostic challenges of a large-scale FMD outbreak.

Most impressive was the overall magnitude and impact that FMD had on the U.K. and specifically the farming community, livestock populations, and tourism industry. While the direct impact of FMD was largely regionalized within the country, the indirect effects (primarily loss of tourism) were felt throughout the U.K. In the end, all the livestock on 9,677 farms were destroyed to control the spread of FMD. Of these, 2,030 were actually declared

FMD-infected premises and the remainder designated as dangerous contacts, either direct or indirect. Estimates are that 6-10 million animals were slaughtered, approximately 10 percent of the U.K. national herd. The widespread dissemination of FMD throughout the U.K. highlighted the need for continuous vigilance in both the public and private sector, and the importance of early detection of disease in minimizing the overall scale of an outbreak. Although U.K. farmers were eventually able to restock, they all suffered immeasurable personal losses that never will be quantified.

It is hard to describe the camaraderie, friendship, and understanding that develops among individuals who share such an experience. There are many individuals, U.K. veterinarians, U.K. farmers and the other veterinarians (from all over the world) who I will never forget. People of great character unselfishly gave up personal time to help those in need. Among those who were there to witness the situation and participate in the response, there is a unique bond and understanding that cannot be explained.

The time I spent working in the U.K was truly a memorable and rewarding experience. In my mind, the challenge that faces us is to take the experiences and lessons learned in the U.K. and use them to strengthen and enhance the detection, response, control and mitigation of foreign animal diseases in the U.S.

Addendum 2015: The U.K. 2001 FMD outbreak has immeasurably impacted my career. Following

that experience, I had the opportunity to passionately pursue FMD preparedness efforts on behalf of the U.S. through programs supported by the Department of Homeland Security Science and Technology Directorate (DHS, S and T) and the USDA, Veterinary Services. Approximately 300 U.S. veterinarians went to the U.K. to help with the response. In addition to helping with the outbreak, these veterinarians brought home valuable information and ideas to improve U.S. response plans. The U.S. owes great gratitude to the U.K. for the opportunity for so many U.S. veterinarians to have learned through working as part of that outbreak.

In 2011, I traveled back to Carsile, Cumbria to reunite with some of the individuals who I had worked with over the course of the outbreak. It also gave me a chance to seek out and speak with several of the farmers and farming families whose animals I had destroyed. While apprehensive, the experience was so rewarding, confirming my impression of the resiliency of the British livestock industry and farmers in general.

"The greatest tragedy is one that nobody learn from." In life, one gets few second chances. An ounce of prevention is worth a pound of cure!

DR. MICHELLE SCHROEDER

Dr. Michelle Schroeder is a small animal practitioner in Oregon and a NAHERC member. When Dr. Don Herriott, the APHIS Area Veterinarian in Charge in Oregon, needed a NAHERC member, Dr. Schroeder volunteered. She accepted an in-state NAHERC deployment. Dr. Schroeder was the only NAHERC member among the 20-person team tasked to conduct tuberculosis (TB) testing on about 24,000 dairy cows. The team was allotted two weeks to complete this daunting task but finished within a week. Dr. Schroeder credits the leadership of Dr. Don Hansen, Oregon State Veterinarian, Oregon Department of Agriculture, for the team's success.

Dr. Schroeder's role in the testing process was that of the "reader." She stood at the head of the cattle and scanned their tags as another member of the team injected the tuberculin into the caudal fold of the cow's tail. This role was good for Dr. Schroeder because, having had little previous experience with cattle, she had "some trepidation about doing cattle work." The team made sure Dr. Schroeder was

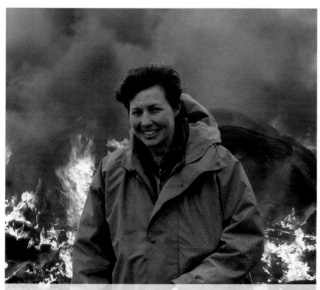

Dr. Pam Hullinger stands in front of a burning pyre of cattle and sheep carcasses. Source: Dr. Pam Hullinger, University of California, Davis

comfortable with what she was doing and taught her how to do the injections. The team also allowed her to palpate negative and suspect responders. According to Dr. Schroeder, this experience helped her brush up on her large animal skills. She now feels comfortable enough that, if called again, she would be able to work on tasks required for TB testing.

While this was Dr. Schroeder's first NAHERC deployment, she is no stranger to this concept. She has been a member of the Oregon Veterinary Emergency Response Team "pretty much since its inception." She is also part of several animal rescue groups in the countries of Namibia and Botswana. Dr. Herriott said, "I would gladly have Dr. Schroeder as part of an incident response team I was involved with putting together."

Dr. Schroeder is a graduate of a dual program between Oregon State University and Washington State University.

This story originally appeared in the NAHERC Quarterly Newsletter, Volume 1, Issue 2, February 2011, and was used with permission of NAHERC and Dr. Schroeder.

Information sources for this chapter can be found at *http://www.cfsph.iastate.edu/TEDATextbookReferences/*

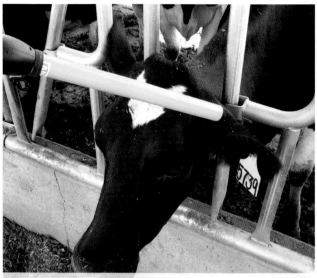

An individual radio frequency identification tag is read to identify this cow for reporting purposes. Source: Mark Kirkpatrick

CHAPTER
5

Highly Pathogenic Avian
  Influenza in the U.S.
Canine Influenza in the U.S.
Porcine Epidemic Diarrhea Virus
  in the U.S.
New World Screwworm
  in the U.S.
African Swine Fever
  in Eastern Europe
Monkeypox in the U.S.
Foot and Mouth Disease in the
  UK and Uruguay
Classical Swine Fever in the UK
West Nile Virus in the U.S.

Authors:

Gayle B. Brown, DVM, PhD
Anna Rovid Spickler, DVM, PhD
Jane Galyon, MS
James A. Roth, DVM, PhD
Center for Food Security and Public Health
Iowa State University,
College of Veterinary Medicine
Ames, IA 50011

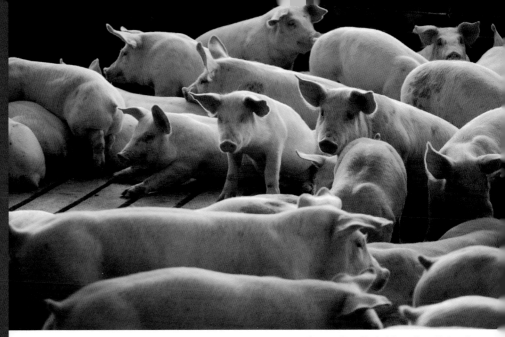

Source: Pam Zaabel, Iowa State University

Descriptions of Incursions
of Foreign, Transboundary and Emerging Animal Diseases

All countries experience outbreaks of foreign, transboundary, or emerging diseases. Some incidents are limited to one or a few cases and are quickly controlled. Others involve massive outbreaks that take months, or even years, to resolve. In the worst-case scenario, a foreign or transboundary disease becomes established, or re-established, in a country. The effects of epizootics on a nation's animal populations and economy may be devastating. This chapter describes a number of outbreaks of foreign and transboundary animal diseases that have occurred. These descriptions illustrate some of the many ways an agent may be introduced, the potential scope of disease outbreaks and their impact on the country, and how the response was handled in each situation.

HIGHLY PATHOGENIC
AVIAN INFLUENZA (HPAI)

In the spring of 2015, an outbreak of highly pathogenic avian influenza (HPAI) in the upper Midwest resulted in the largest U.S. animal disease outbreak to date. Approximately 50 million laying hens, turkeys and pullets were affected and depopulated. A total of 211 commercial and 21 backyard flocks were affected. The USDA spent over $900 million during the response for indemnity, disposal, cleaning and disinfection, and in preparation for a reemergence of the virus.

WHERE DID IT COME FROM?

Between January and April 2014, a highly pathogenic H5N8 virus emerged in Asia, most intensely in South Korea and Japan, resulting in the death of millions of chickens and ducks. The virus disappeared in April 2014, most likely because influenza virus does not survive in warm weather. After five months of no reported cases, highly pathogenic H5N8 was again detected in South Korea and later in Japan. In November, HPAI H5N8 was isolated in Germany in commercial poultry and a wild duck. By mid-December, HPAI H5N8 was isolated from commercial poultry in the Netherlands, the UK and Italy.

The virus made its way to North America and earned the designation of intercontinental influenza because of its ability to move around the world. Scientists believe that HPAI H5N8 was carried to Alaska by infected migratory waterfowl migrating on the East Asia/Australia flyway.

Things began to change in late 2014 and early 2015 when British Columbia, Washington, Oregon, Idaho, and California reported sporadic outbreaks of H5N8, H5N1 and H5N2 HPAI viruses in wild birds and backyard poultry. There were also a few cases in commercial poultry flocks. The H5N1 and H5N2 HPAI viruses were reassortant viruses. At some point birds were co-infected with H5N8 HPAI and a North American low pathogenicity (LP) AI virus, enabling the eight gene segments from both viruses to reassort and emerge as a new virus. The H5N1 and H5N2 HPAI viruses contained the H5 from the H5N8 HPAI virus and N1 and N2 genes from North American LPAI viruses. These new reassortant viruses have been named Eurasian American (EA/AM) H5N2 and EA/AM H5N1.

OUTBREAK IN THE U.S.

Within three months, HPAI H5 viruses from the Pacific Americas flyway were detected in the Mississippi/Central flyways.

In March 2015, the EA/AM H5N2 virus caused infection in a backyard flock in Kansas and two commercial turkey premises in Missouri and one in Arkansas. These flocks were depopulated, and there were no additional outbreaks in these states.

The initial detection of EA/AM H5N2 HPAI in the upper Midwest in a commercial turkey flock was in Minnesota in early March 2015. The virus became highly adapted to commercial poultry and spread rapidly from commercial premises to commercial premises. By April there were daily reports of commercial turkey premises being infected in Minnesota.

The first detection in a large commercial layer facility in northwest Iowa occurred in April, and the outbreak rapidly expanded. Between April and June in Iowa, 31.5 million poultry died or were depopulated, including almost 25 million laying hens, 5.6 million pullets, and 1.1 million turkeys. Seventy-one of the affected sites were commercial properties. Six "backyard" flocks became infected and lost a little more than 5,000 birds. The last detection in Iowa was on June 16, 2015.

Scientists and poultry producers did not expect the virus to primarily infect commercial flocks, which are indoors and protected from waterfowl exposure. They expected most outbreaks to be in backyard flocks that have little or no biosecurity and protection from exposure to waterfowl. However, the infections were largely in commercial poultry, apparently due to the movement of people and equipment without adequate biosecurity.

RESPONSE

There were a number of challenges in responding to this huge outbreak. The mean population among commercial farms with infections was more than 800,000 birds, with some farms having more than four million laying hens in cages. The logistics of depopulating the birds, disposing of the carcasses and cleaning and disinfecting the barns was initially

INFLUENZA VIRUSES belong to three genera in the Orthomyxoviridae family. Viruses in the genus Influenzavirus A, which are also known as influenza A viruses, infect birds and mammals. Waterfowl and shorebirds are considered the reservoir species for the influenza A viruses.

Influenza A viruses are classified into subtypes based on two proteins, the hemagglutinin (HA) and neuraminidase (NA). In birds, there are at least 16 different hemagglutinin proteins (H1 to H16) and nine neuraminidase proteins (N1 to N9); H17, H18, N10, and N11 have been isolated from bats. Influenza viruses are highly variable, and viruses that share a subtype are not necessarily closely related and may differ greatly in their virulence, host specificity, or other factors. For example, one virus with the subtype H1N1 is a human influenza virus, another is a swine influenza virus, and others are found only in birds. Waterfowl and shorebirds carry many different influenza A subtypes, potentially 144 different combinations. These reservoir species shed significant quantities of virus in their feces but rarely become ill from the virus.

The genome of influenza viruses consists of eight RNA segments and each segment codes for a different protein or proteins. The HA and NA proteins are coded for by different segments. Due to poor proofreading during gene replication, influenza viruses can quickly accumulate small mutations, a process called antigenic drift. In addition, they can exchange genes with other influenza viruses, and this is called genetic reassortment. Genetic reassortment is facilitated by the segmented genome. It is essentially a reshuffling of gene segments from two influenza viruses, resulting in genes from both viruses being packaged into a single, novel virion during virus assembly. An important aspect of reassortment is that it can generate viruses containing either a new H, a new N, or both. Such abrupt changes are called antigenic shifts. If two influenza viruses infect a cell simultaneously, the segments may mix when new virus particles are assembled. An influenza virus can reassort with any other influenza virus, regardless of its origin. For example, if a cell is infected by a H5N8 and an H3N2, the new viruses budding from that cell might contain some pieces from the H5N8, including the H5, and some genes from the H3N2, including the N2. The new reassortant virus is an H5N2.

Many wild birds carry influenza A viruses asymptomatically, however in turkeys and chickens, influenza viruses cause disease. The viruses that cause serious illness in poultry, or carry the genetic potential to do so, are known as highly pathogenic avian influenza (HPAI) viruses. Flocks infected with these viruses usually have severe clinical signs, and up to 90-100 percent of the birds may die. All other avian influenza viruses, which are associated with much milder clinical signs or asymptomatic infections in poultry, are known as low pathogenicity avian influenza (LPAI) viruses. HPAI viruses almost always have an H5 or H7 hemagglutinin. The hemagglutinin in HPAI viruses allow the virus to infect and spread systemically; the hemagglutinin of LPAI viruses are limited to infecting the gastrointestinal and respiratory tract. LPAI viruses can be of any subtype. For example, if an H3N2, H2N1 or H8N5 virus is found in a chicken, it is almost certain to be an LPAI virus; however, an H5N1 virus might be either LPAI or HPAI, and this can be determined only by testing it. H5 and H7 LPAI viruses can mutate into HPAI viruses when they are circulating among poultry, which makes them a concern.

ZOONOTIC ASIAN H5N1 HPAI

In 2004 to 2005, a highly pathogenic H5N1 virus emerged in Asia, killing millions of poultry. This Asian H5N1 HPAI virus is zoonotic and caused serious human illness in over 600 people. It has a fatality rate in humans of approximately 50 percent. There was great concern that the H5N1 would spread through migrating waterfowl from the flyways in Europe and Asia to the Western hemisphere. An extensive surveillance program was established in the U.S. For 10 years, this strain was undetected in the Western hemisphere. One explanation for this is that this zoonotic strain of H5N1 avian influenza made the migrating waterfowl sick enough that they could not make the long migration to the summer breeding grounds in the Arctic, where they could mingle with and transmit the virus to waterfowl from the Americas, thus transmitting the virus. This H5N1 is different than the EA/AM H5N1 in the U.S. No human infections with EA/AM H5N1 have been detected.

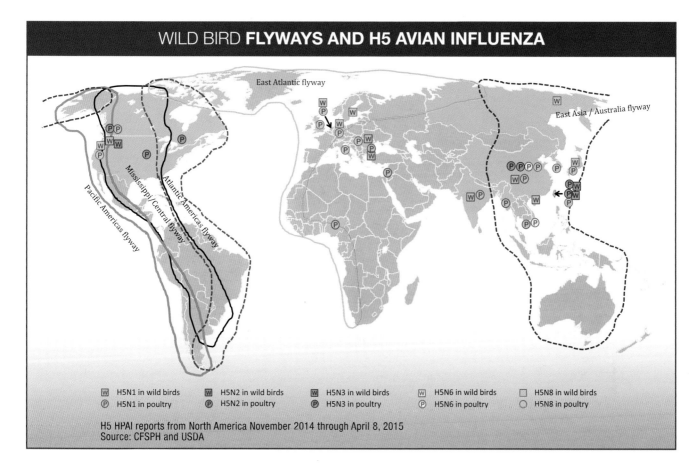

WILD BIRD **FLYWAYS AND H5 AVIAN INFLUENZA**

| W | H5N1 in wild birds | W | H5N2 in wild birds | W | H5N3 in wild birds | W | H5N6 in wild birds | ☐ | H5N8 in wild birds |
| P | H5N1 in poultry | P | H5N2 in poultry | P | H5N3 in poultry | P | H5N6 in poultry | ○ | H5N8 in poultry |

H5 HPAI reports from North America November 2014 through April 8, 2015
Source: CFSPH and USDA

beyond the capabilities of the industry, State, and Federal responders. It took time to gather the essential resources for such a huge outbreak.

More than 1,060 APHIS staff members were involved in the response, including 770 individuals working in the field for 21 straight days, sometimes 14-hours per day. Another 290 staff worked from headquarters. APHIS trained 100 members of the National Animal Health Emergency Response Corps (NAHERC); 65 individuals were deployed for 21-day assignments, some for more than one assignment. In addition, 3,000 individuals worked as contractors on various aspects of the outbreak. State government officials in each affected state also were involved in the response.

IMPACT
Prior to the outbreak, Iowa had 59.5 million layers in 3,821 laying facilities, produced 16.5 billion eggs annually, and also had 11 million turkeys.

The economic impact of the HPAI outbreak in Iowa was estimated at $1.2 billion. Thousands of poultry workers were laid off when production stopped for depopulation and cleaning and disinfection. Affiliated businesses such as processing plants, feed mills, trucking companies, food production companies that relied on eggs, and retail stores were affected.

NEXT STEPS
By the end of June, the virus had been eliminated, due to the response effort and assisted by the arrival of hot weather. The USDA enhanced its HPAI preparedness and response planning effort, based on lessons learned in anticipation of the virus returning in the fall with migrating waterfowl. USDA recommends that each farm have a biosecurity plan and that each state have an animal depopulation and disposal plan. The USDA also developed additional guidance documents to help producers and states be prepared.

CANINE INFLUENZA IN THE U.S.

Before 2004, no influenza viruses were known to circulate in dogs. Since then, two different influenza A viruses have emerged in dogs. One is an H3N8 virus, which jumped from horses to dogs in the U.S. and became adapted to circulate in canine populations. The second is an H3N2 virus, which originated from avian influenza viruses in Asia. Canine influenza is an example of the emergence and spread of a disease resulting from interspecies transmission and movements of companion animals.

EMERGENCE OF H3N8 CANINE INFLUENZA VIRUS IN 2004

As early as 1992, a respiratory disease described as "kennel cough" began circulating among racing greyhounds across the United States. While many affected dogs suffered only a mild cough and recovered, others quickly died from severe hemorrhagic pneumonia. In the late 1990s, additional sporadic outbreaks led to the quarantine of all racing greyhounds and the closure of U.S. racetracks for several weeks. When 22 racing greyhounds at a Florida racetrack became ill with a similar respiratory disease in January 2004, Dr. Cynda Crawford, an immunology and infectious disease specialist at the University of Florida, took action. An initial search for the common causes of kennel cough, *Bordetella bronchiseptica* and canine parainfluenza virus, had turned up empty. Using lung tissue samples from eight dogs that had died from the disease, Dr. Crawford and her collaborators discovered an H3N8 influenza A virus, very similar to an H3N8 influenza virus that circulates in horses. Serology, using paired acute and convalescent sera, demonstrated that the recovered dogs had also been infected by this virus. Looking at stored serum from U.S. greyhounds, it became apparent that the H3N8 virus had been circulating undetected in dogs for several years.

WHERE DID THE H3N8 CANINE INFLUENZA VIRUS COME FROM?

The evidence suggests that an H3N8 equine influenza virus was probably transmitted whole from horses to dogs as a one-time event. It is most closely related to the "Florida lineage" of H3N8 equine influenza viruses, which emerged in the early 1990s. Though the exact crossover event has not been identified, early speculation centered on the practice of feeding raw horse meat to greyhounds in the 1980s and early 1990s. Horses and dogs raced at different tracks, and the potential for spread by contact seemed less likely. When H3N8 canine influenza first emerged, the virus was thought to only affect greyhounds; however, all breeds of dogs are now known to be susceptible. This virus has been identified in most states in the U.S., but its distribution is patchy and it seems to be maintained mainly in environments such as animal shelters, kennels, and dog day care centers. Infections in household pets generally seem to be sporadic and infrequent. Most affected dogs develop a mild illness that resembles other upper respiratory diseases such as kennel cough, although bacterial or mycoplasmal coinfections can cause more serious cases with pneumonia. The hemorrhagic syndrome reported initially in racing greyhounds has not been reported from pets. The H3N8 canine influenza virus has also diverged considerably from equine influenza viruses, and no longer seems to be capable of replicating efficiently in horses.

WHAT IS CANINE INFLUENZA?

CANINE INFLUENZA is a highly contagious respiratory disease of dogs caused by influenza A viruses adapted to circulate in dogs. As of 2015, this includes two viruses, an H3N8 virus that has only been detected in North America and an H3N2 virus that originated in Asia, but is now also found in the U.S. Canine influenza viruses are spread in respiratory secretions by direct contact or fomites. The transmission of the virus is most efficient where groups of susceptible animals are in close contact (e.g., in a kennel). The clinical signs are similar to influenza in other species. Dogs typically present with respiratory signs, such as a coughing and nasal discharge, and may also have nonspecific signs of illness (e.g., fever, anorexia). Some dogs can develop severe pneumonia, especially when the infection is complicated by bacterial coinfections. Cats infected at animal shelters in South Korea and experimentally infected cats also developed respiratory signs, which were sometimes severe.

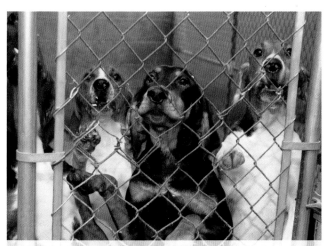

There is an increased risk of exposure to canine influenza in places where groups of dogs congregate, such as animal shelters.
Source: Dani Ausen, Iowa State University

EMERGENCE OF H3N2 CANINE INFLUENZA IN 2007 IN ASIA

In 2007, a cluster of clinical cases in dogs was reported in South Korea. Five dogs with similar cases of severe respiratory disease were seen at three veterinary clinics, and only one survived. An H3N2 influenza virus was isolated from these animals. Initially, it was unclear whether this was an isolated outbreak or a new virus had adapted to dogs. There have been instances where influenza viruses briefly affected small groups of dogs, but disappeared without spreading any further. Over the next decade, however, additional reports from clinics and animal shelters in South Korea, China and Thailand described clinical cases and outbreaks of respiratory disease affecting dogs, and sometimes cats. Some of these outbreaks were severe, with high mortality. Antibodies to H3N2 viruses were also found in healthy dogs and cats in some affected areas, suggesting that some animals had been mildly infected without clinical signs.

WHERE DID THE H3N2 CANINE INFLUENZA VIRUS COME FROM?

The H3N2 influenza virus isolated from the dogs contained gene segments from several different avian influenza viruses and may have crossed over into dogs as early as 2005. Further examination of several of the new canine influenza isolates from 2007 indicated that the event most likely occurred by a rare direct transfer of one or more complete avian influenza viruses. This jump from birds to dogs could have resulted from the feeding of raw, infected bird by-products to dogs in kennels or fattening farms or by aerosol transmission from infected birds to susceptible dogs in live-animal markets, where a number of different species are confined in close quarters.

THE SPREAD OF H3N2 CANINE INFLUENZA TO NORTH AMERICA

The H3N2 canine influenza virus made its first appearance in the United States in the spring of 2015, causing an outbreak affecting over 1,000 dogs in the Chicago area. The outbreak was originally thought to be caused by the endemic H3N8 canine influenza virus, but researchers at Cornell University and the University of Wisconsin confirmed on April 12 that the virus was an H3N2 strain and very closely related to the viruses circulating among dogs in South Korea and southern China. While the virus was rumored to have arrived in dogs rescued and imported from Asia, the exact mode of entry into the United States remains unknown.

Three months after the introduction of the virus into the Midwestern U.S., the H3N2 canine influenza virus caused an outbreak in dogs in Georgia, especially around the Atlanta area. By November 2015, the virus had spread to 25 states. The virus has continued to spread to new states; cases were reported in Washington and Montana at the end of 2015 and early 2016. By the end of 2015, more than 2,000 dogs across the United States had tested positive for the H3N2 influenza virus. Most cases in the U.S. have been characterized by relatively mild upper respiratory signs, and only a few deaths have been reported.

CONDITIONAL LICENSURE OF VACCINES

USDA APHIS conditionally licenses veterinary vaccines to meet an emergency condition, limited market, local situation, or other special circumstance, e.g. no vaccine available for an emerging disease. Conditionally licensed vaccines must meet the same safety and purity requirements as a fully licensed product, but they only need to demonstrate a reasonable expectation for efficacy. The conditional license is effective only for a limited time, usually one year. Additional data is then required for the vaccine to receive full licensure.

PREVENTION AND CONTROL OF CANINE INFLUENZA

Canine influenza is reportable in some states but not others. In states where it is reportable, veterinarians and/or laboratories who suspect or diagnose canine influenza must notify their State Animal Health Official.

The first vaccine for canine influenza was an H3N8 whole virus killed vaccine. USDA granted a conditional license to this vaccine in 2009, and it was fully licensed in 2010. As of January 2016, two licensed vaccines for canine H3N8 are available in the U.S. Both are whole virus killed vaccines.

In November 2015, the USDA provided conditional licensing to two companies to supply an H3N2 canine influenza vaccine for use in dogs at high risk of exposure to this virus.

Canine influenza vaccines are not part of the core vaccines for dogs but are considered "lifestyle" vaccines. They are intended to be used in dogs at increased risk of exposure to canine influenza. Places where dogs are more likely to encounter influenza viruses include dog kennels, animal shelters and other locations where large groups of dogs congregate.

Reports indicate that the virus may survive on hands and clothing for up to a few days, and possibly longer on some surfaces, depending on factors such as temperature, moisture, and the presence of organic material. Infection control measures are similar to those used for other contagious respiratory diseases and include isolation of infected animals; cleaning and disinfection of cages, bowls and other fomites; and hygiene measures, including hand washing. Clothing can be cleaned by washing it with detergent at normal laundry temperatures. When outbreaks occur at establishments, quarantines and the isolation of infected animals can reduce virus dissemination to the community and within the facility.

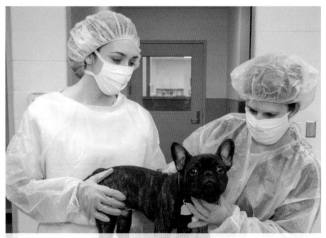

Canine influenza is not known to infect humans; however, using veterinary standard precautions reduces risks of spreading the virus.
Source: Dani Ausen, Iowa State University

The H3N2 canine influenza virus is a different virus than the seasonal human H3N2 influenza viruses circulating in human populations. To date, there is no evidence that humans have been infected by either this new canine influenza virus or the H3N8 canine influenza virus. However, some experts are concerned that, due to their close associations with humans, dogs might become a source of novel influenza virus transmission to humans. As a general practice, it is prudent for immunocompromised people, the elderly, young children and pregnant women to avoid contact with animals that are ill. Physicians, veterinarians, and others have been asked to report any cases of human influenza that seem to be linked to exposure to canine influenza.

This emergence of canine influenza highlights the changeability of influenza A viruses. It is certain that influenza viruses will continue to change and provide surprises. Prevention practices are very important, and equally important is a veterinary workforce ready to rapidly detect and report suspicious disease outbreaks in both companion animals and production animals.

PORCINE EPIDEMIC DIARRHEA VIRUS
INTRODUCTION INTO THE UNITED STATES

On April 28, 2013, a 2,400 sow breed-to-wean farm in Central Iowa reported an outbreak of explosive diarrhea affecting 90% of piglets in some of their farrowing rooms. By the next day, it had spread to all farrowing, breeding and gestation rooms with piglets experiencing watery diarrhea and vomiting. Animals became rapidly dehydrated and died 2–3 days after the onset of clinical signs; the piglet mortality rate was 95%. The referring veterinarian made a preliminary diagnosis of transmissible gastroenteritis (TGE) and sent tissue and fecal samples to the Iowa State University Veterinary Diagnostic Laboratory (ISU-VDL) in Ames, IA.

Eight days later, the ISU-VDL received samples from a 1,200 sow breed-to-wean farm in Northeastern Iowa and samples from a 400 sow breed-to-wean farm in Northwestern Iowa. Both of these submissions had nearly identical clinical signs and pathologic lesions as the first farm. The next day, the ISU-VDL received a similar submission from a farm in Indiana.

The four farms were more than 100 miles apart from each other and did not share personnel, equipment, or transportation companies, but each farm experienced severe outbreaks of diarrhea and high piglet mortality within a 10-day period. Samples submitted from the four farms tested negative for TGE. Negative electron microscopy stains indicated the presence of a coronavirus, so samples were tested for porcine respiratory coronavirus (PRCV); the results were also negative. A pan-coronavirus PCR was performed and the results suggested the causative agent was porcine epidemic diarrhea (PED) virus, a pathogen that had never been seen in the US. Because it was considered a novel enteric coronavirus in the US, the samples were sent to NSVL in Ames, IA for additional testing. On May 17, 2013, NVSL confirmed the diagnosis of PED.

WHERE DID PED COME FROM?

PED was first described in the United Kingdom in 1971 but it wasn't until 1978 that the etiologic agent

---

WHAT ARE **TGE AND PED?**

TRANSMISSIBLE GASTROENTERITIS (TGE) is an enteric coronavirus that causes severe, acute diarrhea and vomiting resulting in high mortality rates in piglets under 2 weeks of age. TGE was prevalent in the US after its discovery in 1946, however, became scarce when porcine respiratory coronavirus (PRCV) superseded its enteric counterpart in the late 80's. PRCV is enzoonotic worldwide, causing a mild respiratory disease that provides immunity from TGE with repeated exposure and is believed to have eliminated TGE from the majority of swine herds.

PORCINE EPIDEMIC DIARRHEA (PED) virus is an enveloped, single-stranded RNA virus in the Coronaviridae family, like TGE, that causes enteric disease in swine. Severity of clinical signs vary with the animal's age, virus strain, and herd susceptibility. PED is an acute disease with an incubation period of one to four days. Diarrhea and vomiting, resulting in severe dehydration, is most devastating in neonates and can cause mortality rates up to 100% with highly virulent strains. Milder clinical signs are seen with less virulent strains and in older animals; in these situations pigs generally recover within 7–10 days. PED is not zoonotic, not a food safety concern, and is not reportable to the OIE.

PED is transmitted by the fecal-oral route and the infectious dose is low. Pre-weaned piglets shed high amounts of virus in their feces resulting in rapid spread and high mortality rates. Older animals do not shed as much virus in their feces as piglets. Indirect contact from fomites also plays an important role in transmission of this disease; for example, the virus can be spread via contaminated livestock trailers, boots, other equipment, and personnel. In addition, a recent study has shown the virus can remain infectious when aerosolized and viral particles can disseminate up to 10 miles from the source of infection. However more research needs to be done to determine the extent of the role of aerosol transmission in the current outbreak. There are no vectors or reservoir species known for the virus, although some, such as starlings (Sturnus vulgaris), have been proposed.

Post-mortem findings in suckling animals include empty stomach contents with little milk curd. The intestines are thin-walled and distended, filled with a watery content. Diagnosis of PED is confirmed using PCR from feces or intestines of affected animals, or by immunohistochemistry on formalin-fixed tissue.

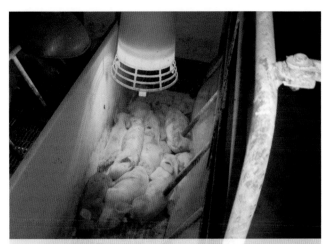
PED is most devastating in neonates and mortalities can reach 100%.
Source: Alex Ramirez, Iowa State University

was identified and confirmed as porcine epidemic diarrhea virus by researchers in Belgium. Since its discovery, PED has been documented in multiple countries in Europe and Asia including Hungary, Italy, Korea, Thailand, Czech Republic, the Philippines, Germany, Spain, Japan, and China.

China reported PED infections in swine beginning in the 1980's. The virus that was circulating had a relatively low impact on the Chinese swine industry. However, during 2010, a more virulent strain emerged causing higher morbidity and mortality that quickly spread throughout China. This resulted in serious economic loss in Asian countries where the pork industry is prominent, such as Thailand, the Philippines, and South Korea.

Analysis of the PED virus isolated from the initial

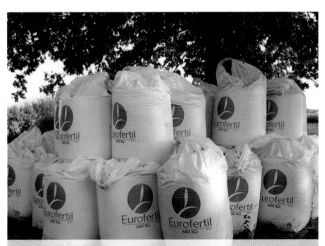
Flexible intermediate bulk containers (FIBCs) are used to transport a variety of products. Bags similar to this may be how porcine epidemic diarrhea virus entered the U.S., according to a USDA report.
Source: Wikimedia Commons

infections in the U.S. revealed a closely related genome to the virulent virus circulating in China. USDA-APHIS initiated a root-cause investigation and examined seventeen different potential ways the virus could have been introduced into the U.S. The exact route of entry was not proven, but the most likely scenario, after thorough investigation, was the introduction of PED through the use of Flexible Intermediate Bulk Containers (FIBCs). These containers are commonly used to transport a variety of products, including pig feed. The FIBCs may have been contaminated in the country of origin and then transported to the U.S., and the contaminated FIBC could have been used and reused for a variety of products, including pig feed or feed ingredients.

SPREAD AND RESPONSE TO THE OUTBREAK

PED is not reportable as an OIE-listed disease even though it can have a serious socio-economic impact. The U.S. did report the disease to the OIE as a new outbreak of an emerging disease. However, when it was confirmed in the U.S. there were no requirements for reporting cases to the state or federal animal health officials.

Shortly after its introduction, the virus rapidly spread to naïve herds throughout the U.S. The swine industry worked to disseminate information about the virus, its transmission, and important biosecurity practices to prevent introduction and spread. There were no PED vaccines approved for use in the U.S., but biologics companies began working to produce vaccines.

Despite all of the efforts by the producers, veterinarians, and the swine industry as a whole, the virus continued to spread. Approximately one year after its introduction to the U.S., the virus had spread to 31 states.

In February 2014, the first case of porcine delta coronavirus disease was confirmed in the U.S. causing a disease clinically indistinguishable from PED or TGE. Without mandatory reporting of these new coronaviruses, the USDA was unable to accurately track their incidence and geographic distribution. To address this, in June 2014, the USDA issued a Federal Order regarding cases of novel swine enteric coronaviruses. The Federal Order had two basic requirements:
- Producers, veterinarians, and diagnostic laboratories are required to report all cases of novel swine enteric

coronavirus diseases (SECD) to USDA or State animal health officials.

- Herds and premises confirmed to be affected with these viruses must work with a veterinarian—either their herd veterinarian, or USDA or State animal health officials—to develop and implement a reasonable herd/premises management plan to address the detected virus and prevent its spread.*

*On January 4, 2016, with concurrence from the swine industry, the Federal Order was amended. The requirements for the herd management plans were eliminated but the requirements for reporting remained in place.

In June 2014, the first U.S. PED vaccine was conditionally licensed, and in September 2014 a second conditionally licensed vaccine became available. These vaccines gave veterinarians and producers another tool to help control this disease.

Since it emergence in the U.S. in 2013, PED has crossed national borders into Canada, Mexico, and the Caribbean. Though the disease continues to spread, the increase in new cases has slowed, though the reason is unknown. Possible explanations include increased herd immunity, increased awareness, improved biosecurity, and/or mandatory reporting. During May 2015, the USDA reported 95 positive PED accessions in the U.S. compared to the near 300 reported during May 2014.

IMPACT

Fortunately, PED does not have any direct public health or food safety concerns; however, it has proven to be a serious threat to the U.S. swine industry. In the U.S., pork products constitute the second largest segment of meat and poultry production. During one year of the endemic period, nearly eight million piglets (approximately 10% of the swine population) were lost and pork prices increased to a record high.

The entrance of this disease took the industry by surprise and had a severe negative impact in a short period of time. PED demonstrated transboundary diseases can enter the U.S. and that biosecurity plans in place – while thought to be excellent – were not sufficient or not thoroughly implemented to stop the introduction of the virus. The outbreak also demonstrated that in the current world of global travel and commerce, identifying the point of disease introduction is complex and may be impossible. Since the PED outbreak, the U.S. National Pork Board has funded and launched the U.S. Swine Health Information Center. The mission of the Center is to protect and enhance health of U.S. swine herds through targeted research investments designed to minimize the impact of future disease threats, analyze swine health data, and monitor global swine diseases.

New World screwworms are larvae (maggots) of *Cochliomyia hominivorax* flies, and they feed on the flesh of living animals. New World screwworms were once found throughout the tropical and subtropical areas of North, Central, and South America, but they have been eradicated from many countries by a series of cooperative programs involving the release of sterile male flies. This approach, conducted and sustained by the USDA APHIS, has systematically eliminated screwworms from the U.S., Mexico, Puerto Rico, the Virgin Islands, Curacao, and all of Central America. Because screwworms are still widespread in South America, sterile fly releases across eastern Panama continue to be necessary even though screwworms were eradicated from there in 2006. The sterile flies create and maintain a biological barrier in Panama's Darien Gap, halting the pest's overall northward migration at the Panama-Colombia border. Small incursions are still detected occasionally in Panama.

In January of 2012, a New World screwworm *(Cochliomyia hominivorax)* infestation was discovered in a horse imported from Argentina to the United States while the horse was in quarantine. The following report describes the incursion and gives important information about screwworms.

This report appeared in the VMO Observer on February 16, 2012. The VMO Observer is a communication network for USDA Veterinary Services employees to share case reports, etc. We would like to thank these authors for permission to use the report: Percell M. Taylor, DVM (USDA APHIS Veterinary Services Miami Animal Import Center Assistant Director), James W. Mertins, PhD (USDA APHIS National Veterinary Services Laboratories Entomologist), Kendra Stauffer, DVM, DACVPM (USDA APHIS Veterinary Services Area Emergency Coordinator), and Elizabeth Enciso, DVM, MPH (USDA APHIS Veterinary Services Miami Animal Import Center Director).

HISTORY

In January 2012, a polo pony stallion was imported to the United States from Argentina with a load of approximately 30 other polo ponies. The horse arrived with a health certificate that stated that the required pre-import screwworm treatments had been applied. These treatments included oral administration of ivermectin three days prior to export, tranquilization to facilitate extension and inspection of the penis, and application of coumaphos solution to the penis and prepuce.

INVESTIGATION

While the horse was being held in quarantine at the animal import center, a caretaker noticed bloody discharge staining the dorsal aspect of the lower hind limbs (pastern area) of the horse. This sign is typically seen on recently castrated horses, due to drainage from the surgical wound in the inguinal area.

However, this male horse was intact and had no visible wounds. Through experience, animal import center personnel recognize this sign as a dead giveaway for another condition: screwworm infestation of the prepuce.

Import center personnel removed the horse from his stall to examine him on the clean floor of the barn aisle. They sprayed the prepuce of the horse with a pyrethrin solution, and, according to the Veterinary Medical Officer, the larvae fell onto the barn floor. The preputial area was examined, revealing a screwworm-infested wound in the fossa glandis.

LABORATORY FINDINGS

Maggots expelled and collected from the wound were overnighted to the USDA APHIS Veterinary Services, National Veterinary Services Laboratories (NVSL) in

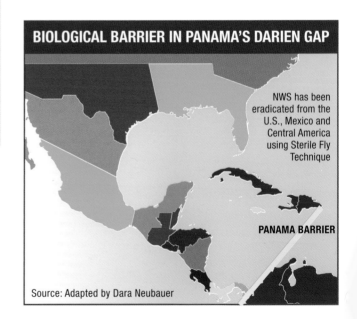

BIOLOGICAL BARRIER IN PANAMA'S DARIEN GAP

NWS has been eradicated from the U.S., Mexico and Central America using Sterile Fly Technique

PANAMA BARRIER

Source: Adapted by Dara Neubauer

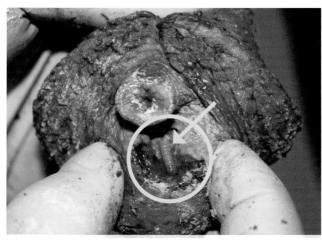

Cutaneous lesion with a screwworm in the fossa glandis.
Source: Cynthia Morales, USDA APHIS VS MAIC Animal Caretaker.

Ames, Iowa, for identification. Based upon standard morphological features (e.g., general somatic habitus, cuticular spinulation, spiracular conformation, darkened posterior tracheal trunks), origin, circumstances of collection, and expert opinion, the specimens were identified as eight second and 11 third instars of the New World screwworm *(C. hominivorax)*. Based upon their size, five of the maggots were deemed nearly mature and ready to leave the wound, but the range of maggot sizes present in the sample suggested that this infestation might have arisen from at least two separate fly strikes (bouts of oviposition) several days before host shipment.

REGULATIONS

APHIS regulations allow for the importation of horses to the United States from countries that APHIS recognizes as affected with screwworms, provided that the following conditions have been met (9 CFR 93.301).

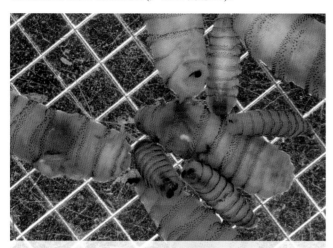

Part of the screwworm collection from the infested stallion from Argentina (grid pattern in 2-mm squares). Source: Dr. H. Joel Hutcheson

1. A veterinarian must treat the horse with ivermectin 3 to 5 days prior to the date of export to the United States, according to the recommended dose prescribed on the product's label.
2. The horse must be examined for screwworms by a full-time salaried veterinary official of the exporting country within 24 hours prior to shipment to the United States. The official must fully examine the horse, including its external genitalia. If the horse is found to be infested with screwworms, it must be treated until free from infestation.
3. At the time the horse is loaded onto a means of conveyance for export, a veterinarian must treat any visible wounds on the animal with a solution of coumaphos dust at a concentration of five percent active ingredient.

The veterinarian must state on the health certificate that he or she has thoroughly examined the horse, including its external genitalia, and found it to be free of screwworms and that the horse has been treated in accordance with numbers one and three above. The horse in this case did arrive with a health certificate stating that the required examination and treatments had been carried out in the country of origin.

A horse imported to the United States from a country that APHIS recognizes as affected with screwworms is required to be quarantined for a minimum of seven days at the port of entry.

According to standard operating procedures for the Miami Animal Import Center, a Veterinary Medical Officer inspects the horse upon arrival in the United States for wounds and ectoparasites, paying close attention to the false nostrils, ears, bulbs of the heels, and the navels of foals. After the examination, the horse is sprayed with a pyrethrin solution. All male horses (geldings and stallions) must be tranquilized by a private practitioner and checked for screwworms in the prepuce on the day before their release from quarantine.

The horse in this case remained in quarantine until he completed treatment to eliminate the infestation, which took about two weeks. Treatment consisted of a dose of invermectin, given orally, and topical application of coumaphos solution to the prepuce and penis. The lesion healed completely, and the horse was released from quarantine in time for the polo season.

SCREWWORM DETECTION & COLLECTION

Screwworms are either of two species of aggressive blow fly larvae (of the family Calliphoridae) that feed on the living flesh of any warm-blooded animal, commonly mammals and rarely birds. Screwworms infest wounds of any kind, from ones as small as tick bites to large cuts or surgical wounds. Common sites of infestation are the navels of newborns, perineal areas, or any orifice, including eyes, ears, and genitalia. In the first few days of the infestation, the larvae are hard to find. As they feed, the wound enlarges and deepens to create large pockets of larvae with only small openings in the skin. Infested livestock often isolate themselves from the rest of the herd and lie down. Untreated animals might die within a week or two from trauma or secondary infections.

New World screwworms *(C. hominivorax)* are found (endemic) only in the Western Hemisphere, where they were once widespread. Through eradication programs, screwworms have been eliminated from the United States, Mexico, and Central America. Warm-blooded animals in South America, however, continue to suffer from this aggressive, flesh-eating parasite. In Argentina, the annual economic loss attributed to screwworm myiasis (infestation of a living mammal with maggots) in livestock is estimated at $618 million U.S. dollars.

Old World screwworms *(Chrysomya bezziana)* occupy a similar ecological niche in certain warmer regions of the Eastern Hemisphere (e.g., the Middle East, Southeast Asia, and Africa). Old World screwworms have proven to be much less likely to be found in animals imported to the United States than New World screwworms (only one detection has ever been reported in the U.S., and that occurred in 2007), but any warm-blooded animal entering from affected Old World areas could be infested with them.

Screwworm myiasis should be suspected in a recently imported animal with draining and enlarging wounds. Female New World screwworm flies deposit their eggs in a distinctive shingle-like array on or near the edges of superficial wounds. The larvae, which resemble wood screws, emerge from the eggs 12 to 24 hours after oviposition (the act of laying or depositing eggs).

The best collections of suspected screwworms or other myiasis maggots for identification include a dozen or more specimens of various sizes (when present) taken from both superficial and deep areas of the wound. Always preserve the sample in alcohol (ethyl or isopropyl/rubbing); never use formalin. Submit samples in leakproof containers to the NVSL, accompanied by a completed VS Form 5-38 available on the NVSL website at *http://www.aphis.usda.gov/animal_health/lab_info_services/forms_publications.shtml.*

Our ability to detect and respond to screwworm infestations in animals imported to the United States relies upon collaboration of Federal, State, and accredited private veterinary practitioners.

The table below lists the detections of screwworm infestations in imported animals, along with the professions of the collectors from 2000 to 2012. Roughly half of the detections were made by Federal personnel and half by private practitioners.

SCREWWORMS INTERCEPTED FROM ANIMALS IMPORTED TO THE U.S.				
Year	Animal host	Origin	Screwworm species	Identified By
2000 (Feb)	Horse	Venezuela	New World	Federal veterinarian
2000 (Mar)	Horse	Argentina	New World	Private practitioner
2000 (Mar)	Horse	Argentina	New World	Federal veterinarian
2000 (Dec)	Domesticated dog	Cuba	New World	Private practitioner
2005 (Dec)	Horse	Argentina	New World	Federal animal health technician
2006 (Feb)	Horse	Argentina	New World	Federal veterinarian
2007 (Sep)	Domesticated dog	Trinidad	New World	Private practitioner
2007 (Oct)	Domesticated dog	Singapore	Old World[1]	Private practitioner
2008 (May)	Horse	Argentina	New World	Federal veterinarian
2010 (May)	Domesticated dog	Venezuela	New World	Private practitioner
2011 (Feb)	Horse	Argentina	New World	Federal veterinarian
2012 (Jan)	Horse	Argentina	New World	Federal animal caretaker

[1]This was the first (and is still the only) known incidence of Old World screwworm in the Western Hemisphere

Source: Re-created by Andrew Kingsbury, Iowa State University

Congratulations to the animal caretaker for sharp eyes and a good catch!

ONGOING RISK

Animals imported from countries affected by screwworms pose a risk for reintroduction of the parasite into the United States. If screwworm larvae are allowed to drop to the ground and pupate, the resulting adult flies could reestablish the species in North America; therefore, it is important to remain vigilant and quickly identify animals affected by this parasite.

AFRICAN SWINE FEVER

AFRICAN SWINE FEVER IN THE CAUCASUS, RUSSIAN FEDERATION AND EASTERN EUROPE

African swine fever (ASF) is a highly contagious viral hemorrhagic OIE-listed disease of pigs, with serious health, economic, and international trade consequences.

The European continent, except for the Mediterranean island of Sardinia, was free of ASF until 2007, when it was introduced to the Caucasus (a region bordering Europe and Asia). Since that time it has spread northward and westward. In an era where the global movements of people, products, and animals are common, the swine industry is on alert. The introduction and spread of ASF since 2007 illustrates the consequences and challenges of a virus that is fairly stable in both the environment and animal products and infects natural ranging wild boar who do not respect borders.

In Georgia, the first cases of ASF appeared on the west coast, suggesting a connection to the port city of Poti located on the Black Sea. Though details are lacking, it has been suggested that the ASF virus was introduced to Georgia via virus contaminated garbage (swill) from international ships. Virus-contaminated garbage from the ships may have been fed to pigs living near the port or ingested by free-roaming pigs.

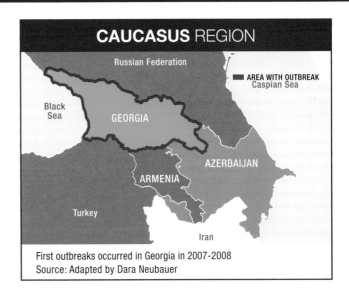

CAUCASUS REGION

First outbreaks occurred in Georgia in 2007-2008
Source: Adapted by Dara Neubauer

The feeding of garbage from international airplanes or ships has been implicated in other outbreaks of ASF, including those in Portugal (1957), Cuba (1971 and 1978), Malta, Sardinia, Brazil and the Dominican Republic (1978), and Belgium (1985.)

Georgia reported approximately 60 separate outbreaks with more than 64,000 cases. The case fatality rate was nearly 100 percent. Georgia implemented movement control, disinfection, quarantine, stamping-out and zoning, and they

WHAT IS AFRICAN SWINE FEVER?

AFRICAN SWINE FEVER is endemic in most of sub-Saharan Africa including the island of Madagascar and is caused by a large, enveloped, double-stranded DNA virus of the Asfarviridae family. The ASF virus is highly contagious, remains viable for weeks to months in pork products, and is highly resistant to environmental conditions. The virus infects domestic pigs, wild boar, and feral swine.

The clinical signs of ASF are variable. The clinical presentations have been classified into peracute, acute, subacute, and chronic. The clinical signs are relatively non-specific and include sudden death, fever, anorexia, lethargy and weakness. Erythema and cyanotic blotching on the ears, tail and legs may also occur. This disease is clinically indistinguishable from a number of other hemorrhagic diseases, including classical

swine fever, salmonellosis, erysipelas, and porcine multisystemic wasting syndrome.

African swine fever is not known to infect humans or other livestock.

African Swine Fever can be transmitted directly animal to animal, indirectly via fomites, or by vectors. In the Caucasus, Russia, and Baltic states, it appears the primary route of transmission is direct and indirect oronasal transmission. Infected animals shed the virus via all excretions, and the virus is relatively stable on fomites and in pork products.

In some areas where the disease is endemic (mostly southern and eastern Africa), transmission between soft ticks of the genus Ornithodoros and wild pig (mainly warthogs) is important. The role of ticks in the spread of the disease in Eastern Europe is not yet known.

declared the event resolved in January 2008.

However, the virus had already spread to the other Caucasus countries and Russia. The spread was most likely through the migration of infected wild boars. Russia was not able to eradicate the virus and it is now considered endemic in its southern region. The virus continued to spread and caused outbreaks in the Ukraine in 2012, Belarus in 2013, and the Baltic States and Poland in 2014. As of December 2015, reports of outbreaks continue (mainly in wild boar).

HOW IT BEGAN AND SPREAD

On May 17, 2007, Georgia notified the OIE of several disease outbreaks in domestic swine suspected to be postweaning multisystemic wasting syndrome (porcine circovirus type 2). However, on June 4 an OIE Reference Laboratory in the United Kingdom confirmed that ASF virus was present in submitted samples. The ASF virus isolate that was detected in the samples also underwent DNA sequencing to determine its genotype. Analysis showed that the Georgian isolate was closely related to strains circulating in Mozambique, Madagascar, and Zambia. Researchers concluded that a single introduction of the virus had likely occurred, and the source of the virus was eastern or southern Africa.

RISKS FOR TRANSBOUNDARY SPREAD

There are a number of factors that affect the likelihood of transboundary spread of ASF virus. The major risks for transmission of the virus include:

- Garbage feeding of food waste collected from international airplanes or ships from countries where the disease is found;
- Feral swine movements;
- Trucks moving between infected and free areas;
- Illegal movement of infected pigs or pork products which may be unintentional (e.g., tourists) or intentional (e.g., meat smuggling).

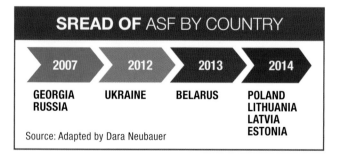

SREAD OF ASF BY COUNTRY

2007	2012	2013	2014
GEORGIA RUSSIA	UKRAINE	BELARUS	POLAND LITHUANIA LATVIA ESTONIA

Source: Adapted by Dara Neubauer

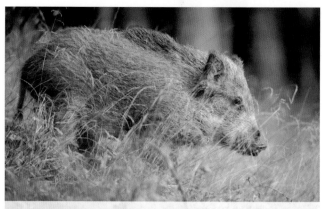

Feral swine or wild boars have played a major role in the spread of ASF.
Source: sduben, istock.com

SWINE INDUSTRY IMPACT

Overall, the ASF epidemic in the Caucasus region has led to a huge decrease in the swine population, both through infection and depopulation. From 2006–2010, the swine population in Georgia decreased 70% and in Armenia it decreased 56%. Pigs nearly disappeared from Azerbaijan, which only had a swine population of 22,000 before the epidemic. The swine population in Russia did not decrease initially, but has been shrinking since 2010 in areas affected by ASF.

It is difficult to estimate the economic impact of ASF in affected areas. Though data is generally lacking, it is estimated that in Russia alone, losses (direct and indirect) between 2007 and 2012 were $1 billion (in U.S. dollars).

PREVENTION AND CONTROL

Changes in production practices, increasing globalization, and increased outbreaks of this disease in Eastern Europe have increased the risk of introduction of ASF into North America.

If an incursion of ASF were to occur in the U.S., since there is no vaccine available, control measures must prevent disease spread and eliminate ASF from the U.S. as quickly as possible. This may include:

- Implementing aggressive stop movement, tracing, and stamping-out programs;
- Preventing ASF from becoming established in feral swine, including potentially eliminating feral swine in an area;
- Conducting surveillance to rapidly re-establish U.S. freedom from ASF, including tick surveillance to look for introduction of the pathogen into the potential vector populations.

The 2003 monkeypox outbreak in the U.S. demonstrates the importance of close cooperation between the medical, public health, and veterinary communities in addressing zoonotic diseases. In addition, this outbreak provides an opportunity to increase awareness about wildlife pet trade, the risk of introduction of disease from imported animals, and the importance of personal protection equipment (PPE) when working with an unknown disease.

HOW IT BEGAN

On May 11, 2003, a Wisconsin family purchased two prairie dogs from a pet swap meet. Two days after the purchase, the family's 3½-year-old child was bitten on the hand by one of the prairie dogs. At the time of the bite, the prairie dog was sick with lymphadenopathy, papular skin lesions and an ocular discharge. The prairie dog was examined at a veterinary clinic. It died, and its head was submitted for rabies testing, which was negative. A lymph node from the prairie dog was sent to the Marshfield Laboratory in Wisconsin for bacterial culture; but no pathogens were detected. The child who was bitten developed a fever. The bite wound became reddened and the child developed raised whitish lesions on her hand. She was taken to a physician who began treatment with antibiotics. Two days later, May 22, the child was hospitalized with fever, swelling around the eye, festering skin wounds, and new skin lesions on her scalp, extremities, and perineum.

On May 26, the child's mother became ill with fever, sweats, malaise, and a sore throat, as well as vesicles at the site of a skin wound. Marshfield Laboratory scientists performed electron microscopy on a skin biopsy from the mother, revealing the presence of a poxvirus, an unusual finding. The laboratory informed the Wisconsin Public Health Department (PHD) of its findings, and on the same day, the Wisconsin PHD received a report of an unusual illness from the Milwaukee Health Department. A Wisconsin man who distributed exotic animals had been bitten and scratched by a prairie dog on May 18. He later developed a skin nodule at the site of the scratch, fever, lymphadenopathy, chills, and sweats. His condition worsened to the point of hospitalization. An investigation revealed that the pet prairie dog that had bitten the child was purchased from this distributor.

On June 4, Marshfield Laboratory scientists informed the Wisconsin PHD that electron microscopy had detected an orthopoxvirus in tissues from the pet prairie dog. The following day, the Wisconsin PHD organized a teleconference between physicians and representatives from Federal, State, and local agencies. Plans were quickly made to ship specimens to the Centers for Disease Control and Prevention (CDC) Poxvirus Laboratory. The CDC analyzed samples from three patients and detected monkeypox virus. Monkeypox virus was also found in a virus culture of the prairie dog's lymph node. The epidemiological investigation that followed revealed that 11 people, including the exotic pet distributor, his wife, members of the public who bought prairie dogs, two veterinarians who had treated prairie dogs (and didn't use appropriate PPE), and employees of two different pet shops had symptoms consistent with monkeypox. On June 7, 2003, public health officials from the CDC and the states of Wisconsin, Illinois, and Indiana reported the first outbreak of human monkeypox outside of Africa.

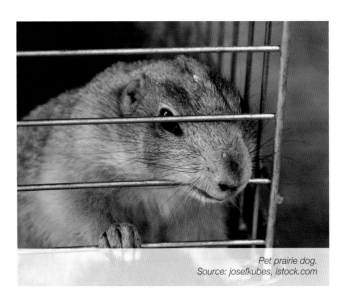

Pet prairie dog.
Source: josefkubes, istock.com

TRACING THE VIRUS IN THE U.S.

Traceback investigations found that the source of the infection in 2003 was a shipment of small mammals from Ghana, imported into Texas for pet trade on April 9 by an animal distributor. This shipment contained approximately 800 small mammals representing a variety of species, including six different genera of African rodents (rope squirrels, tree squirrels, Gambian giant rats,

MONKEYPOX U.S. DISTRIBUTION

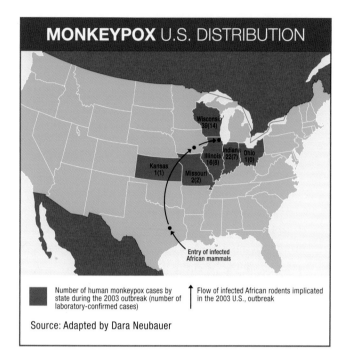

Number of human monkeypox cases by state during the 2003 outbreak (number of laboratory-confirmed cases)

Flow of infected African rodents implicated in the 2003 U.S., outbreak

Source: Adapted by Dara Neubauer

WHAT IS MONKEYPOX?

MONKEYPOX is a zoonotic disease that results from infection by the monkeypox virus, a member of the genus Orthopoxvirus in the family Poxviridae, and closely related to the smallpox virus.

Clinical signs in animals vary and can include skin lesions, lethargy and malaise, respiratory disease, diarrhea, and asymptomatic infections. Virus is found in skin lesions and most excretions and secretions of infected animals. Humans are usually exposed to the monkeypox virus via infected animals. This virus may be transmitted to people in animal bites, in aerosols during close contact, or by direct contact with lesions, blood, or body fluids

Monkeypox symptoms in humans usually resemble a milder form of smallpox. The initial symptoms of monkeypox are flu–like and are followed by a maculopapular rash. The skin lesions become vesicles and pustules ("pocks"), form scabs and are eventually shed.

Smallpox vaccine is effective at protecting people against monkeypox. According to the CDC, "because monkeypox virus is closely related to the virus that causes smallpox, the smallpox vaccine can protect people from getting monkeypox." It is recommended that the vaccine be given before exposure, but it can be given up to 14 days after exposure to help reduce symptoms of disease.

U.S. MONKEYPOX OUTBREAK

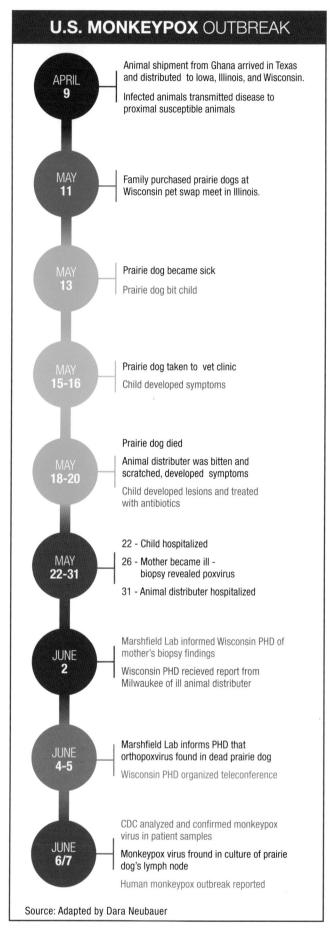

APRIL 9
Animal shipment from Ghana arrived in Texas and distributed to Iowa, Illinois, and Wisconsin.
Infected animals transmitted disease to proximal susceptible animals

MAY 11
Family purchased prairie dogs at Wisconsin pet swap meet in Illinois.

MAY 13
Prairie dog became sick
Prairie dog bit child

MAY 15-16
Prairie dog taken to vet clinic
Child developed symptoms

MAY 18-20
Prairie dog died
Animal distributer was bitten and scratched, developed symptoms
Child developed lesions and treated with antibiotics

MAY 22-31
22 - Child hospitalized
26 - Mother became ill - biopsy revealed poxvirus
31 - Animal distributer hospitalized

JUNE 2
Marshfield Lab informed Wisconsin PHD of mother's biopsy findings
Wisconsin PHD recieved report from Milwaukee of ill animal distributer

JUNE 4-5
Marshfield Lab informs PHD that orthopoxvirus found in dead prairie dog
Wisconsin PHD organized teleconference

JUNE 6/7
CDC analyzed and confirmed monkeypox virus in patient samples
Monkeypox virus fround in culture of prairie dog's lymph node
Human monkeypox outbreak reported

Source: Adapted by Dara Neubauer

brushtail porcupines, dormice and striped mice). Upon arrival into the U.S., the animals were not inspected for disease or quarantined.

Before the outbreak was detected, the animals infected with monkeypox were shipped to several states. Some of the imported animals were shipped from Texas to an Iowa distributor and then to a distributor in Illinois. In Illinois, the African Gambian rats and dormice were kept in close proximity to North American black-tailed prairie dogs, which were highly susceptible to this virus. It was estimated that more than 90 prairie dogs were infected or potentially infected while at the distributor in Illinois. The infected prairie dogs were then sold to other dealers and individuals in several states, including the Milwaukee animal distributor, who bought prairie dogs and a Gambian giant rat. Some prairie dogs were sold to pet shops, and others were sold or traded at the pet "swap meet" in northern Wisconsin. All of the humans infected in this outbreak had contact with infected prairie dogs, and most infections were associated with handling sick prairie dogs, getting bitten or scratched by prairie dogs, and/or cleaning the bedding/cage of the sick prairie dogs. There were no reports of infection in humans from exposure to only the infected African rodents, although some of these animals had high titers of virus. Why African rodents did not transmit the virus to humans is uncertain, but people might not have interacted closely with them as with prairie dogs. There were no reports of human-to-human transmission.

RESPONSE TO THE OUTBREAK

Several agencies worked together along with private practitioners, both medical and veterinary, to contain and eradicate this disease. The CDC was the lead agency in the response, and some of the major steps they took in the effort to contain and eradicate the disease are listed below *(from http://www.cdc.gov/poxvirus/monkeypox/outbreak.html)*.

- Activated the CDC Emergency Operations Center.
- Provided help for tracing and diagnosing the disease; it deployed teams to help investigate, conducted laboratory tests, distributed information about case definition in humans and animals, and assisted State, local, and Federal agencies.
  - Issued interim guidelines to prevent exposure and disease in humans. Recommendations included the following guidelines:

- Recomended all people who had close or intimate contact with a confirmed case of monkeypox should be vaccinated with the smallpox vaccine. (Seven people, including three veterinarians, two laboratory workers, and two health-care workers received pre-exposure prophylaxis. Another 23 people were vaccinated after exposure.)
- All animals with suspected monkeypox should be euthanized to prevent the further spread of the disease and the carcasses incinerated. All rodents from the April 9 shipment, and any prairie dogs on the premises at the same time as these African rodents, should be euthanized.
- Other mammals in contact with infected animals should be placed under quarantine for six weeks.

EXOTIC ANIMALS COMING TO THE U.S.

A positive outcome of the monkeypox outbreak was that a loophole in regulations was addressed; the loophole had allowed small mammals from Africa to be imported into the U.S. without quarantine and/or examination for disease. Once the source of the outbreak was identified, the CDC and the Food and Drug Administration (FDA) issued a joint order: the CDC prohibited the importation of all rodents from Africa, and the FDA prohibited the sale, distribution, transport, or release into the environment, of prairie dogs and six genera of African rodents. The CDC's import restrictions were effective, making the FDA rule unnecessary. The FDA section of the rule was rescinded in 2008. The result of these rulings is that African rodents may be imported only for

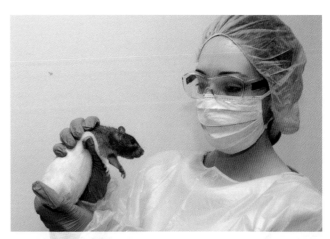

The most common route for transmission of monkeypox from animals to humans appears to be direct contact with infected animals.
Source: Dani Ausen, Iowa State University

scientific, exhibition, or educational purposes with a valid permit issued by CDC.

It is estimated that billions of wild animals and wild animal products are traded globally each year, both legally and illegally, amounting to tens of billions of dollars in trade yearly. These animals pose a risk of disease introduction; improvements in regulations, pathogen screening, and education help to minimize disease introductions. Fortunately, the prairie dogs and the humans were dead end hosts. The monkeypox virus infection was not maintained and did not continue to spread between animals or humans. Monkeypox does not circulate in the U.S. today, and regulations for importation of exotic animals have been strengthened. Fortunately, the human infections were all resolved; however, some of the infections that occurred could have been prevented if proper PPE had been used. The Compendium of Veterinary Standard Precautions for Zoonotic Disease Prevention in Veterinary Personnel, published by the National Association of State and Public Health Veterinarians, provides guidelines to help minimize risk of human infections from zoonotic diseases. *http://nasphv.org/Documents/VeterinaryStandardPrecautions.pdf*

FOOT AND MOUTH DISEASE

Of all the animal diseases foreign to the U.S., foot and mouth disease (FMD) presents the greatest threat to the livestock industry and economy; it is a priority for preparedness, response, and research. FMD is a viral disease that primarily affects cloven-hooved species, causing vesicles and erosions in the mouth, on the feet and at other sites. It is contagious and spreads rapidly to susceptible animals. Although FMD is not a life-threatening disease in most adult animals, the lesions are very painful and animals suffer. In addition, an outbreak of FMD results in loss of productivity and major economic and trading difficulties for the affected countries.

Every outbreak of FMD is different, and many factors, from practical considerations to socioeconomic conditions and public opinion, must be considered when designing a control plan. Stamping-out is often the quickest way for a country to return to FMD free status, but it may result in a very large number of animals being killed. Employing vaccination as a component of the control plan can result in fewer deaths; however, it can also have some detrimental effects on trade. The descriptions of two FMD outbreaks in 2001, one in the United Kingdom (U.K.) and the other in Uruguay, illustrate some of the factors involved in eradicating this virus and some of the control strategies and potential outcomes.

Although the U.K. and Uruguay are similar in size and were faced with a similar number of FMD-infected farms, they responded to FMD outbreaks in different ways. The U.K. used a stamping-out policy with no vaccination, while Uruguay culled few animals and concentrated its efforts on a massive vaccination campaign. More than six million animals were euthanized in the U.K. Uruguay, in contrast, euthanized approximately 6,900 animals, but used 24 million doses of vaccine. The two outbreaks lasted about the same amount of time, but the overall cost to control the epidemic was far less in Uruguay than in the U.K. In Uruguay the estimated direct and indirect costs were $730 million, and in the U.K. the estimates were around $9 billion. While the differences between these two outbreaks, and their respective costs, are intriguing, it should, nevertheless be kept in mind that factors other than vaccination differed between these two countries.

2001 FMD OUTBREAK IN THE UNITED KINGDOM

The 2001 outbreak of FMD in the U. K. was devastating, in part, because the initial infections were not detected and the virus had spread widely before control measures could be initiated. The U.K had not had a serious outbreak of FMD since 1968, and FMD was eradicated from the European Union in the late 1980s. This outbreak occurred with no forewarning.

On February 19, 2001, a veterinary inspector from the State Veterinary Service of the Ministry of Agriculture, Fisheries and Food (MAFF) was conducting routine inspections at an abattoir in Little Warley, Essex, and found vesicular lesions on 27 sows and one boar. While vesicles (blisters) are a characteristic sign of FMD, they can also occur in other diseases of livestock (e.g., vesicular stomatitis, swine vesicular disease, vesicular exanthema of swine, and Seneca Valley virus infections). In this case, however, laboratory tests confirmed the presence of a serotype O FMD virus belonging to the Pan-Asia lineage, a group of viruses that, since the 1990s, has caused a number of FMD outbreaks in Asia, which extended to parts of Africa and Europe.

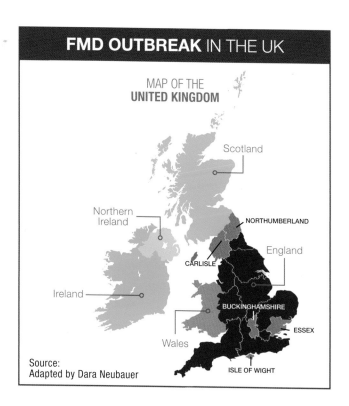

FMD OUTBREAK IN THE UK

MAP OF THE UNITED KINGDOM

Scotland

Northern Ireland

NORTHUMBERLAND

CARLISLE

England

Ireland

BUCKINGHAMSHIRE

ESSEX

Wales

ISLE OF WIGHT

Source: Adapted by Dara Neubauer

WHAT IS **FMD**?

FMD is a highly contagious viral disease that mainly affects cloven-hooved animals, such as cattle, swine, goats, sheep, deer and various other domesticated or wild hosts. Natural or experimental infections have also been reported in some other species, including hedgehogs, bears, armadillos, kangaroos, capybaras, and elephants. The FMD virus can be found in all secretions and excretions from acutely infected animals, which may begin shedding it before the onset of clinical signs. Many animals acquire the virus during close contact with infected animals, but it is also spread in aerosols and on fomites, such as manure-contaminated tires, boots, and clothing. The disease is characterized by fever and vesicles found mainly in the mouth, nares, muzzle, feet, or teats. The vesicles break quickly to become painful erosions. Affected animals can be lame or refuse to eat, can salivate profusely, and may lose weight. Adult sheep and goats tend to show very mild, if any, signs. Adult animals generally recover within a few weeks, but secondary infections may lead to a longer recovery time. High mortality rates are sometimes seen in young animals.

On February 20, MAFF announced an immediate "stop movement" of all susceptible livestock in the U.K., including the movement of animals to abattoirs, sale markets, and pastures. Efforts to trace the disease back to the infected farm and suppress the outbreak also began immediately. The infected pigs had arrived at the abattoir on February 16 from farms in Buckinghamshire and the Isle of Wight. They were traced back to a farm at Heddon-on-the-Wall, Northumberland. However, by the time the outbreak was discovered, FMD had spread to a cluster of holdings in the county of Essex, through the movement of pigs, people, fomites, and by localized airborne spread. Infected sheep from the farm at Heddon-on-the-Wall had also been moved to the Longtown market near Carlisle. Sheep often have minimal clinical signs when they are infected with FMD virus and can spread the virus unnoticed. Through various animal movements via markets and other channels, infected animals eventually spread the disease to thousands of additional sheep and cattle holdings in other parts of Great Britain.

SOURCE OF THE VIRUS

The source of the 2001 epizootic in the U.K. is thought to have been pig swill. The feeding of pig swill is a practice that has been going on for generations, as a way of producing protein (pork meat) from scraps that would otherwise be wasted. Pig swill can come from restaurants, schools, and anywhere humans eat and waste food on a large scale.

The feeding of pig swill has declined in industrialized nations because it is thought to be inefficient and outmoded and may be a risk for disease introduction, but for some areas, it is a reasonable method for farmers to produce protein for their families. In 1998, a government panel of agricultural experts in the U.K. advised that swill feeding be banned; however, the advice was rejected by ministers who did not want to impose new costs on hard-pressed farmers.

SPREAD OF FMD IN THE U.K. AND THE E.U.

By March 2, 2001, FMD had spread to 40 locations in the U.K. with many foci linked to infected markets. A total of 25,000 animals had been destroyed and incinerated on-farm. Cases were also confirmed in Northern Ireland. One week later, at least 127 locations were known to be affected, and this number continued to grow. The U.K. soon developed a shortage of qualified veterinarians to investigate suspect farms. Private practice veterinarians and government veterinarians from other nations were enlisted to help. The U.S. sent approximately 300 veterinarians to help over the course of the response. The MAFF provided educational materials to farmers and veterinarians on how to avoid spreading FMD and how to report suspected outbreaks. It also publicized the details of the clinical signs in sheep, as the illness in this species can be subtle.

The control measures established to stop FMD transmission resulted in a number of difficulties. Because animal movements were restricted, cows could not cross roads for milking or be moved to fresh grazing pastures. Pregnant ewes were, likewise, prevented from moving to shelter for lambing. This resulted in intense public criticism and an outcry to allow some animal movement for welfare reasons. Carcass disposal also became a problem. In spite of control measures, the epidemic continued to spread and cases began to appear outside the U.K. On March

13, FMD was confirmed at La Baroche-Gondouin in northwestern France, and a week later it was confirmed in four cows in the Netherlands. The virus is believed to have reached the Netherlands via a shipment of veal calves from the Republic of Ireland. Although the calves were thought to be uninfected when they left Ireland, they were rested for 12 hours near La Barouche Gondouin, where they were probably exposed to infected sheep coming from the U.K. All European Union (E.U.) countries were on high alert for FMD, so when the virus appeared in the Netherlands, the veterinary officials initiated stamping-out, and, in addition, E.U. officials in Brussels agreed to let the Netherlands conduct limited emergency vaccination around infected farms and animals awaiting slaughter. This overturned the 15-year E.U. policy of prohibiting vaccination for FMD.

Back in the U.K., the MAFF decided to initiate "ring depopulation." In ring depopulation, all susceptible livestock within a specified radius of infected premises are euthanized, whether they are diagnosed with the disease or not. Because approximately 850 infected premises had been identified by this time, ring depopulation resulted in the deaths of large numbers of animals. The farming and tourism industries were devastated, and even politics was affected. On April 2, Prime Minister Tony Blair announced that the general election scheduled for May 3 would be delayed until June 7 because of the FMD crisis.

Eventually, the control measures succeeded in controlling the epidemic. The last case of FMD was reported on September 30, 2001, bringing the total number of infected farms in the U.K. to 2,033. Approximately six million animals had been killed, either to prevent the spread of the disease or for welfare reasons (e.g. dwindling feed and space issues because animals couldn't be moved). On January 22, 2002, the OIE declared that the U.K. had regained its previously recognized FMD-free status without vaccination, clearing the way for international export trade in animals and animal products.

INTERNATIONAL REACTION

All FMD-free countries arc required to notify the World Organization for Animal Health (OIE) of FMD outbreaks within 24 hours of the first case. This notification helps other countries protect themselves from this disease, by stopping international trade from the affected area. On the day after the U.K. notified the OIE, the European Commission banned the export of live animals, germplasm, fresh meat, meat products, milk and milk products, hides, and skins of FMD susceptible species from all of the U.K. In the U.S., the United States Department of Agriculture (USDA) also stepped up its efforts to guard against this disease. The importation of swine, ruminants, any fresh swine or ruminant meat (chilled or frozen), and other products of swine and ruminant origin from the entire E.U. was temporarily prohibited. Travelers from the E.U. were stopped from carrying any agricultural products, particularly animal products, into the U.S. Also, security was tightened at ports of entry and airports to ensure that passengers, luggage, and cargo were checked as appropriate.

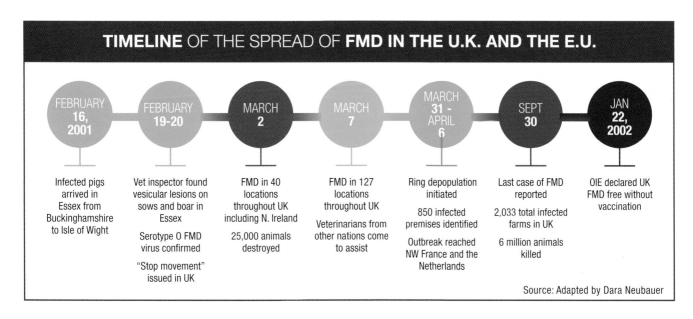

TIMELINE OF THE SPREAD OF **FMD IN THE U.K. AND THE E.U.**

FEBRUARY 16, 2001	FEBRUARY 19-20	MARCH 2	MARCH 7	MARCH 31 - APRIL 6	SEPT 30	JAN 22, 2002
Infected pigs arrived in Essex from Buckinghamshire to Isle of Wight	Vet inspector found vesicular lesions on sows and boar in Essex

Serotype O FMD virus confirmed

"Stop movement" issued in UK | FMD in 40 locations throughout UK including N. Ireland

25,000 animals destroyed | FMD in 127 locations throughout UK

Veterinarians from other nations come to assist | Ring depopulation initiated

850 infected premises identified

Outbreak reached NW France and the Netherlands | Last case of FMD reported

2,033 total infected farms in UK

6 million animals killed | OIE declared UK FMD free without vaccination |

Source: Adapted by Dara Neubauer

FOOT AND MOUTH DISEASE IN URUGUAY

BACKGROUND

The countries of South America established the Hemispheric Plan for the Eradication of Foot and Mouth Disease (PHEFA) in 1987. Under this plan, comprehensive vaccination was the backbone of eradication efforts, but stamping-out was also conducted if the disease threatened a disease-free region. The adoption of PHEFA led to a decrease in the number of FMD outbreaks reported in South America from 955 in 1990 to 130 in 1999. With the use of vaccine, Uruguay successfully eradicated FMD in the mid-1990s.

Use of vaccination placed restrictions on trade, and so, to acquire a more favorable trade status, Uruguay discontinued vaccine use and was recognized by the OIE as "FMD free without vaccination" in 1996. Argentina and Paraguay also stopped vaccinating in 1999, as did portions of Brazil in 2000. However, the change in policy, i.e., no vaccination, placed these countries at risk for FMD reintroduction. Some neighboring South American countries were not FMD free, and these countries continued to vaccinate. In this situation, viruses can sometimes still circulate while vaccination masks clinical signs. At the same time, animals in the FMD-free regions were losing their immunity from previous vaccinations and becoming more susceptible.

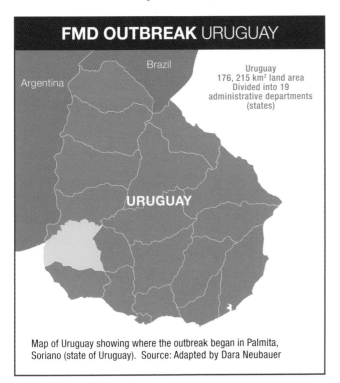

FMD OUTBREAK URUGUAY

Brazil

Argentina

Uruguay
176, 215 km² land area
Divided into 19
administrative departments
(states)

URUGUAY

Map of Uruguay showing where the outbreak began in Palmita, Soriano (state of Uruguay). Source: Adapted by Dara Neubauer

RE-INTRODUCTION OF FMD INTO URUGUAY

Livestock production is the major agricultural activity in Uruguay, representing more than 65 percent of all exports, and a significant contributor to its economy.

In February 2001, an FMD serotype A outbreak occurred in Argentina. It extended into Uruguay on April 23, 2001. The first infected farm was reported in Palmitas, Uruguay, which is located in the administrative department (state) of Soriano and is approximately 70 km from the Uruguay River, Uruguay's border with Argentina. Thirty-nine of the 430 cattle on the affected farm had signs of FMD, although lesions were not seen on the farm's 640 sheep. The affected and exposed animals were euthanized the following day. This area is economically integrated with the adjacent region of Argentina, which was experiencing FMD outbreaks. The virus is assumed to have spread from Argentina to Uruguay via fomites or people.

On April 26, FMD was found on a neighboring farm in Soriano, which had a mixed population of cattle, sheep, and pigs. At the same time, several infected premises were detected in the adjacent department of Colonia, 25 km from the Uruguay River and 40 km from the first cases. Quarantines were immediately placed on both affected departments, and the affected and exposed animals were destroyed and buried. In total, 5,093 cattle, 1,511 sheep, and 333 pigs were culled. On April 26, Uruguay began ring vaccination of cattle within a 10 km radius of the affected farms. The following day, all movement and trade of animals were prohibited throughout the country. Within a few days, the government was forced to suspend the stamping-out procedure because of strong resistance by local farmers and the discovery that the disease had spread to other areas of the country. Authorities learned that, a few days before the first cases were recognized, cattle had been sold at auction and delivered to other parts of Uruguay. The movement of people, agricultural equipment and machinery, and milk and beef trucks is also thought to have contributed to the spread of the virus. On April 30, vaccination was extended to form a protective barrier to prevent the virus from entering uninfected departments or neighboring countries.

VACCINATION PROGRAM

On May 5, Uruguayan authorities expanded the vaccinaton program to a massive, country-wide vaccination program for all cattle. It was completed by

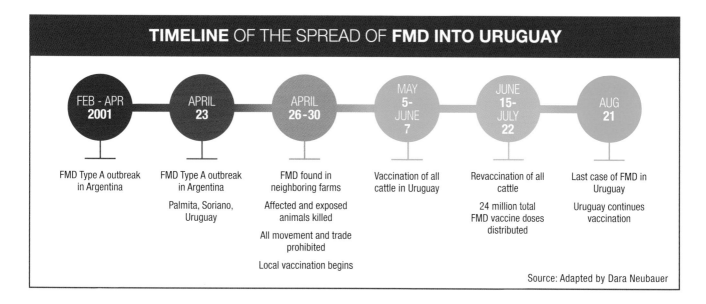

TIMELINE OF THE SPREAD OF **FMD INTO URUGUAY**

FEB – APR 2001
FMD Type A outbreak in Argentina

APRIL 23
FMD Type A outbreak in Argentina

Palmita, Soriano, Uruguay

APRIL 26–30
FMD found in neighboring farms

Affected and exposed animals killed

All movement and trade prohibited

Local vaccination begins

MAY 5– JUNE 7
Vaccination of all cattle in Uruguay

JUNE 15– JULY 22
Revaccination of all cattle

24 million total FMD vaccine doses distributed

AUG 21
Last case of FMD in Uruguay

Uruguay continues vaccination

Source: Adapted by Dara Neubauer

June 7, after which time animal movement restrictions were relaxed. The vaccine was provided to farmers free of charge, and they were responsible for vaccinating their animals within a given time period and identifying vaccinated cattle with ear-tags for tracking. Uruguay's 12 million sheep, which share pastures with the cattle, were not vaccinated; however, this did not seem to hamper the eradication of the virus. The country's approximately 270,000 pigs were also left unvaccinated, as the vaccine used was not thought to be effective in this species. At the height of the epidemic, 40-60 infected farms were being found each day; however, by the end of the first round of vaccination, there were fewer than 10 new foci per day.

From June 15 to July 22, Uruguay conducted a re-vaccination program. This revaccination effort boosted immunity in the cattle population to the optimum levels.

A total of 24 million doses of FMD oil-adjuvanted vaccines were distributed during these two vaccination rounds. The last case of FMD was found on a dairy farm on August 21, 2001. Uruguay submitted the required documentation and received OIE official recognition as "FMD free where vaccination is practiced."

COSTS OF THE OUTBREAKS
From April 23 to August 21, 2001, a total of 2,063 farms or facilities in Uruguay were affected by FMD, a number similar to the farms affected by the epidemic in the U.K. However, Uruguay was able to eradicate its extensive outbreak solely by restrictions on livestock movement and the vaccination of cattle, in spite of having a large and fully susceptible sheep population

in close contact with the cattle. The total direct cost of eradication was estimated at $240 million. Vaccine purchases accounted for $7.5 million, with the remainder used for compensation payments to farmers, cleaning and disinfection, and operating expenses. Indirect costs included the loss of export markets, which led to a pronounced decrease in livestock prices and movement restrictions on the entire livestock sector. This affected many workers and associated industries, such as packing plants that were forced to close. In total, the epidemic cost Uruguay approximately $730 million. This is, nevertheless, a much smaller figure than the approximately $9 billion in losses to agriculture, the food chain, and tourism during the outbreak in the U.K. Because there is still a threat that new FMD viruses could be introduced from neighboring countries, Uruguay has chosen to continue FMD vaccination for the present, despite eradicating the virus. However, this status of "FMD free where vaccination is practiced" puts some limitations on exports. In addition, maintaining this status requires that the country substantiate that FMD virus is not continuing to circulate "silently," with the vaccines masking its presence. This effort can require a substantial ongoing commitment to good surveillance and its associated costs.

RESPONSE PLANS IN THE EVENT OF AN FMD OUTBREAK
The type of response to any outbreak will depend on many factors, such as the structure of the livestock industry in the country, and the availability of personnel and resources for traditional stamping-out eradication efforts or vaccination

campaigns. Viruses that have spread over large regions may require different responses than ones in more localized areas. The goals of the outbreak response are also important. For instance, one country may prioritize rapid return to FMD-free status, while another desires to minimize the loss of animals. Even the region where the outbreak occurs can affect the approach. Pathogens are generally more difficult to eradicate from livestock-dense-areas, where they may spread more rapidly than infected and exposed animals can be euthanized and their carcasses buried or burned.

If a country chooses to vaccinate for FMD, selecting a vaccine is complicated by the existence of seven viral serotypes and at least 65 strains. There is no cross protection among the seven serotypes. There are over 60 strains within the serotypes. Protection between strains in a serotype varies.

A second issue is that most FMD-free countries do not routinely manufacture FMD vaccines, but large amounts of vaccine may be needed immediately in an outbreak. Some countries or organizations have established vaccine banks, which store a selection of FMD vaccine antigen concentrates at very low temperatures. The antigens stored are those expected to be protective against the currently circulating viruses considered to be of greatest threat. When they are needed, the concentrates can be formulated quickly into vaccines. However, the quantity of antigens held in vaccine banks is usually limited.

Historically, the U.S. plan for responding to FMD was exclusively based on stamping-out. The 2001 FMD outbreaks in the U.K. and Uruguay, and changes in the organization of the U.S. livestock industry prompted the U.S. to review and improve its preparedness and response plans for FMD. The U.S. response plans are contained in Foreign Animal Disease Preparedness and Response Plan (FAD PReP) materials. The FAD PReP materials were developed by USDA APHIS to raise awareness, develop capabilities, and enhance the coordinated response to an animal-disease outbreak. Guidelines for Classification of Phases and Types of an FMD Outbreak and Response are a part of the FMD Response Plan. This document provides guidance for making decisions about vaccination, stamping-out, or a combination. For example, if a focal FMD outbreak were to occur, it would likely be eliminated by stamping-out; whereas, if an outbreak were to spread nationally, stamping out would likely be discontinued and control measures would likely include vaccination to live (defined in text box).

DEFINITIONS FROM THE **FOOT AND MOUTH RESPONSE PLAN: RED BOOK**

Stamping-Out Depopulation of clinically affected and in-contact susceptible animals

Stamping-Out Modified with Emergency Vaccination to Live
Depopulation of clinically affected and in-contact susceptible animals and vaccination of at-risk animals, without subsequent depopulation of vaccinated animals. Vaccinated animals intended for breeding, slaughter, milking, or other purposes live out their useful lives

Stamping-Out Modified with Emergency Vaccination to Kill
Depopulation of clinically affected and in-contact susceptible animals and vaccination of at-risk animals, with subsequent depopulation and disposal of vaccinated animals. Depopulation and disposal of vaccinated animals may be delayed until logistically feasible, as determined by Incident Command (IC) and the VS Deputy Administrator (U.S. Chief Veterinary Officer [CVO])

Classical swine fever (CSF) is a systemic viral disease of swine that can result in mild to severe clinical signs, depending on the virulence of the outbreak strain. Like FMD, CSF is a disease of high consequence that spreads widely among naïve herds and has a devastating effect on international trade. An outbreak of CSF in the United Kingdom (U.K.) illustrates how a foreign animal disease can initially be mistaken for an endemic disease, and, once recognized, how it can be traced, controlled, and eradicated before it becomes widespread.

HOW IT BEGAN

On August 4, 2000, a suspected outbreak of CSF in a pig herd was reported to the Ministry of Agriculture, Fisheries, and Food (MAFF) Animal Health Divisional Office at Bury St Edmunds, Suffolk. The herd consisted of 3,500 weaned pigs in seven barns. The first signs of illness began on July 11 when a load of weaned pigs arrived from the breeding/multiplier unit. Initially, the pigs were thought to be affected by porcine dermatitis and nephropathy syndrome (PDNS), which had recently become a serious problem in Britain and has clinical signs similar to CSF. However, as the disease progressed and spread and mortalities increased, it became clear this was something else. By August 4, the disease had affected a total of 1,110 pigs, killing approximately 200. Given the concern that this could be CSF or another disease exotic to Britain, a MAFF veterinary officer visited the premises, examined the pigs, placed the holding under official movement restrictions, and took samples for testing. On August 7, the breeder unit that supplied weaned pigs to this farm, and another farm, which had received pigs from the breeder unit, reported pigs with similar clinical signs. These two herds were immediately placed under quarantine and samples submitted for laboratory testing, which confirmed the presence of CSF. An outbreak of classical swine fever was officially declared on August 8, 2000.

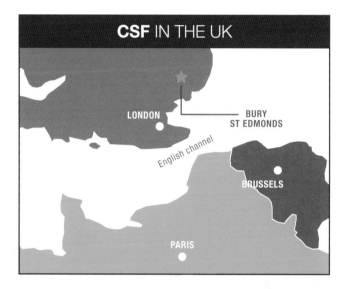

CSF IN THE UK

LONDON — BURY ST EDMONDS

English channel

BRUSSELS

PARIS

WHAT IS CLASSICAL SWINE FEVER?

CLASSICAL SWINE FEVER, also known as hog cholera, is a highly contagious disease of pigs caused by the CSF virus, a member of the genus Pestivirus. Wild suids are also susceptible to classical swine fever and can play a role in transmission. In an outbreak that began in 2012 in Latvia, the disease was first reported in wild boar and, subsequently, in domestic swine. Animals can become infected with CSF virus by ingestion, inhalation, genital (semen) infection, or wound contamination. CSF virus is often spread by contact with infected pigs or the feeding of contaminated, inadequately cooked garbage (swill), but the virus can also be transmitted on fomites. In addition, CSF virus can remain infectious for long periods in refrigerated, frozen, smoked or cured meat.

Virus shedding can begin before the onset of clinical signs, occurs throughout the course of acute or subclinical disease, and may go on continuously or intermittently for months in chronically infected pigs. The clinical signs vary with the strain of virus and the age and susceptibility of the animal. Acute cases, which are caused by highly virulent isolates and have a high mortality rate, are likely to be diagnosed rapidly. Infections with less virulent isolates can be more difficult to recognize, particularly in older pigs that have developed some immunity after exposure. These infections may be relatively mild and can resemble other diseases. In some herds infected with less virulent strains, the only sign of disease may be poor reproductive performance or the failure of some pigs to thrive. The wide range of clinical signs and similarity to other diseases, such as African swine fever, porcine dermatitis and neuropathy syndrome, or salmonellosis, can make CSF challenging to diagnose.

RESPONSE

National and local crisis centers were established to deal with the outbreak. Three-kilometer protection and 10-kilometer surveillance zones were established around the infected premises, and the movement of all pigs within the zones was prohibited. All pigs on the infected farms were killed, and the premises were cleaned and disinfected. The movements of pigs, feedstuffs, vehicles, and people onto and off each site were traced to identify possible sources of the virus and limit the spread of infection.

An epidemiological analysis found that CSF virus had probably entered the breeding unit first, likely in early May. However, the sows did not show significant clinical illness, which is not uncommon with some CSF strains in adult pigs. The sows were also housed outdoors, which may have slowed virus transmission, compared to pigs kept indoors. These factors probably helped mask the outbreak until the virus entered the all in/all out confinement facility, where its rapid spread and severe clinical signs in young animals raised the alarm.

All premises that had received pigs from the breeding unit, as of May 1, were traced, tested for CSF, and placed under official movement restrictions. All pigs on premises that had received pigs born after June 1 were treated as "dangerous contacts" and were destroyed. The production company that owned the breeding facility also owned or contracted with more than 45 other breeding herds; those facilities were traced, placed under quarantine, clinically inspected by a MAFF veterinary officer, and sampled for evidence of CSF. In addition, the government traced the movements of the transporter who took weaned pigs from the infected breeding premises. All premises that the transporter had visited were tested and placed under official movement restrictions, with 3 kilometer protection zones and 10 kilometer surveillance zones around each. Infected herds were depopulated, and, as the outbreak spread, dangerous contact herds and herds near infected herds were also depopulated.

Pigs kept outdoors on several farms near the grower became infected during this outbreak, although they had not received any infected pigs. It was suspected that, before CSF was diagnosed, some of the dead pigs from the grower barns had been placed outside, allowing wildlife to scavenge these animals and carry the disease to neighboring farms. Over the next few months, CSF was diagnosed on additional farms. A total of 16 infected sites were confirmed in Britain between August 4 and November 3, and around 75,000 animals were destroyed, 32,000 of which were in herds pre-emptively slaughtered because they were considered as dangerous contacts. By December the outbreak had been contained, and all control measures relating to the 16 infected premises were lifted.

SOURCE OF THE VIRUS

The origin of the virus in this outbreak and its route of introduction were not established with complete certainty. However, the evidence strongly suggested that CSF virus had not been introduced in infected pigs, contaminated vaccines or biological products or by contact with feral pigs, contaminated vehicles or personnel, or discharges of effluent. It is more likely that the infection was introduced in contaminated pig meat in food discarded by people; a public footpath ran adjacent to the outdoor paddocks containing dry sows on the breeding farm. Genetic typing showed that the outbreak strain was in the same genetic group that had been isolated during a CSF outbreak in Belgium, Italy, the Netherlands, and Spain in 1997-1998. Since this outbreak, many improvements have been made in diagnostics, preparedness and response plans. In 2014, U.K. veterinary authorities published a new "Disease Control Strategy for African and Classical Swine Fever in Great Britain."

U.S. PREPAREDNESS AND RESPONSE PLANS FOR CSF

The U.S. has a variety of ongoing preparedness and response activities with respect to CSF. Selected excerpts from the *Classical Swine Fever Response Plan, The Red Book, May 2013* about those activities are included in the text box (on the next page).

OUTBREAKS CONTINUE AROUND THE WORLD

CSF is still endemic in many regions, posing a threat to those that are disease-free. For example, in 2012, CSF was detected in two wild boars in Latvia, a country that had been free of CSF. An epidemiologic study suggested the origin of the virus likely came from Russia

CHAPTER 1

1.4.4.1 Economic Impact

"A U.S. outbreak would have a significant economic impact on the pork export market, with many exports of pork and pork products being halted for a significant period of time. In addition, a CSF response effort would involve direct costs for depopulation, indemnity payments, animal disposal, disinfection, and movement control measures. Additional indirect costs would be incurred by consumers and related sectors of the economy, such as feed producers and suppliers. Any CSF outbreak in the United States would have a sizeable and lingering economic impact.

CHAPTER 3

3.1.2 Domestic Activities

Domestically, the USDA works to prevent the introduction of CSF into the country, conducts proactive surveillance for CSF, and performs FAD investigations as needed for suspected cases. Some USDA activities include:

- Smuggling Interdiction and Trade Compliance (SITC) conducts risk management and anti-smuggling activities to prevent unlawful entry and distribution of prohibited agricultural commodities.
- National Center for Import and Export (NCIE) facilitates international trade, monitoring the health of animals presented at the border as well as regulating the import and export of animals and animal products.
- CSF surveillance, both active and passive, in cooperation with the National Animal Health Laboratory Network (NAHLN)
- USDA works to assist States in training and maintaining State Incident Management Teams and veterinary reserve corps, such as the National Animal Health Emergency Response Corps, (NAHERC). State groups will serve as early response teams for a CSF incident and can educate groups on the signs, symptoms, and reporting procedures."

CHAPTER 5

5.3 Surveillance.

CSF surveillance is proactively conducted in the United States through the Classical Swine Fever Surveillance Program. This program conducts surveillance in five swine populations through tissue and serology samples:

- Sick animals submitted to diagnostic laboratories,
- Swine condemned at slaughter by USDA FSIS,
- High-risk swine populations, including waste-feeding operations and high risk swine herds,
- Feral swine
- Swine FAD investigations submitted to FADDL as suspicious for CSF. In the event of a CSF outbreak, additional, targeted surveillance would occur with the objective of not only detecting CSF-infected swine, but to determine the extent of the outbreak.

The FAD PReP documents can be found at:

www.aphis.usda.gov/fadprep

or Belarus. These two countries were known to have infected wild boars, and the detection in Latvia was near the Russian and Belarus borders. The wild boar are largely asymptomatic when infected with the virus. In response to this finding, intensive hunting of wild boar was initiated, and veterinary teams began surveillance of domestic pigs, including backyard pigs. Weeks after the confirmation of CSF in the wild boars in Latvia, the disease was reported in backyard domestic pigs on three farms near where the wild boar were found. Epidemiologic investigation suggested the backyard pigs may have been infected by untreated food waste from hunter-killed wild boar.

Protection and surveillance zones were established, and all pigs in the infected premises were euthanized and destroyed. Despite control efforts, the virus continued to circulate in the wild boars. In May 2013, wild boar oral vaccination using bait was initiated. In June 2014, Latvia reported CSF in domestic swine in the infected zone, and these swine were killed. As of November 2015, the oral vaccination of wild boar in the infected zone continues, and the virus still circulates. This outbreak in Latvia illustrates the challenges associated with disease control when a disease enters the wildlife population. Wildlife were not a factor in the U.K. outbreak.

West Nile virus (WNV) is a mosquito-borne virus that, until 1999, was found only in the Eastern Hemisphere. In 1999, this virus was introduced in the New York City area. Despite eradication efforts, WNV became established in North America and eventually in Central and South America. This outbreak provides lessons about detecting and responding to a new disease, including the importance of local disease surveillance and response systems, and communication between public health agencies, animal health agencies and other groups. It also illustrates the particular difficulties posed by FADs that can become established in arthropod vectors and/or wildlife, especially the difficulty in preventing their establishment despite vigilance and a prompt response.

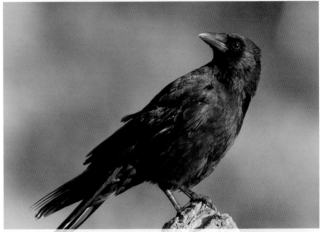

When WNV was introduced into the U.S. it killed large numbers of crows, along with several other types of birds.
Source: Art Wittingen, Shutterstock.com

HOW IT BEGAN

Tracy McNamara, DVM, head of the department of pathology at the Bronx Zoo, became concerned in early August 1999, when she heard that a large number of crows had been dying around the zoo. By late August, 40 crows had died. Then birds at the zoo began to die. Over the Labor Day weekend, the zoo lost a Guanay Cormorant, three Chilean flamingos, a pheasant, and a bald eagle. Because these deaths followed those of the crows, experts strongly doubted that the disease originated in the zoo. Necropsies of the birds revealed streaking in the heart and brain hemorrhages. Eastern equine encephalitis was suspected, but McNamara was skeptical because the emus in her care, which are very susceptible to eastern equine encephalitis virus, were thriving. "It was becoming more and more suggestive that this was not a regular bird disease," McNamara said. When two more flamingos died on September 9, she sent samples to the USDA's National Veterinary Services Laboratories (NVSL) in Ames, Iowa. The NVSL ruled out avian influenza and Newcastle disease viruses.

Meanwhile, on August 23, 1999, an infectious disease physician from a hospital in northern Queens contacted the New York City Department of Health (NYCDOH) to report two patients with encephalitis. On investigation, NYCDOH initially identified a cluster of six patients with encephalitis, five of whom had profound muscle weakness. Testing suggested that these patients had St. Louis encephalitis virus, an endemic mosquito-borne flavivirus. The earliest cases occurred among residents of a two-square-mile area in northern Queens. On the basis of these findings, aerial and ground applications of mosquito adulticides and larvacides were begun in northern Queens and South Bronx on September 3.

IDENTIFICATION OF WEST NILE VIRUS

In Ames, Iowa, the National Veterinary Services Laboratories isolated a virus from the birds' tissues and, after ruling out several viral agents that cause encephalitis in birds, performed electron microscopy to examine its structure. Forty nanometer virus particles with the morphology of togaviruses or flaviviruses were observed. On September 20, the NVSL forwarded the virus cultures to the U.S. Centers for Disease Control and Prevention (CDC) for identification and characterization. Testing at the CDC on September 23 indicated that the isolate was closely related to West Nile virus, which had never been isolated in the Western Hemisphere. CDC experts also detected flavivirus antigens in one of the human autopsy specimens by immunohistochemistry and found a West Nile-like virus genomic sequence in a human brain specimen from an encephalitis case. The genetic sequence was identical to that derived from the bird tissues. Concurrently, specimens of brain tissue from three human encephalitis cases, forwarded by the New York State Department of Health to the University of California, Irvine, were reported as positive for West Nile-like virus sequence by genomic analysis.

WHAT IS **WEST NILE VIRUS?**

WEST NILE VIRUS is a flavivirus that, like St. Louis encephalitis virus, belongs to the Japanese encephalitis subgroup of the Flaviviridae. WNV was first isolated in a febrile human in the West Nile province of Uganda in 1937 and in birds in the Nile delta region in 1953. It is a mosquito-transmitted virus that cycles between birds and mosquitoes in endemic regions. Many infected birds in the Eastern Hemisphere seem to carry this virus asymptomatically. In some birds, viremia can persist for more than three months, possibly contributing to the overwintering of the virus. When environmental conditions favor high viral amplification, mosquitoes can also spread the virus to mammals and reptiles. Horses, humans, and most other mammals are dead end hosts that cannot infect mosquitoes.

Among mammals, symptomatic infections mainly seem to occur in humans and horses. Approximately 80 percent of people who become infected with WNV remain asymptomatic, while 20 percent develop flu-like symptoms and less than one percent develops neurological signs. Like humans, most infected horses are asymptomatic, but some animals develop neurological signs and may die.

By September 28, 17 confirmed and 20 probable human cases with four deaths had been reported in New York City and the surrounding counties. Most cases, and all fatalities, occurred in older patients, although some cases occurred in patients as young as 15. In total, 62 human cases, with seven deaths, were recognized in 1999.

In October 1999, the NVSL first isolated WNV from the brain tissue of a Long Island horse with encephalitis. WNV was isolated at NVSL from two additional encephalitic horses, and WNV antibodies were identified in sick horses in Suffolk and Essex counties, New York. Retrospective classification of likely West Nile cases before October resulted in a total estimate of 25 equine cases.

In genetic sequencing studies, WNV isolates from the New York outbreak showed strong similarities to a pathogenic strain of the virus from Israel, suggesting that this region may have been the origin of the virus. How WNV was introduced into the United States is still unknown, but most speculation has centered on infected birds or mosquitoes.

RESPONSE TO THE OUTBREAK

Vector control measures had been initiated in northern Queens and the South Bronx on September 3. These measures were followed by a citywide pesticide application, after a laboratory confirmed West Nile encephalitis in a Brooklyn resident with no travel history to Queens. Surveillance of wild birds and sentinel chickens was used to assess WNV distribution in the region. Emergency telephone hotlines were established to address public inquiries about the encephalitis outbreak

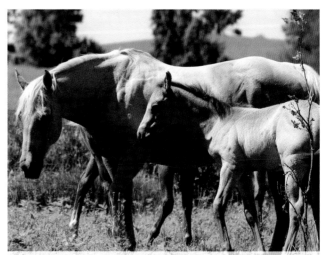

The West Nile Virus is a mosquito-transmitted virus that mostly cycles between birds and mosquitos. However, when environmental conditions are optimal the disease can be spread to mammals. Horses are susceptible.
Source: CFSPH

and pesticide application. Approximately 300,000 cans of DEET-based mosquito repellant were distributed citywide through local firehouses, and 750,000 public health leaflets were distributed with information about personal protection against mosquito bites. Recurring public messages were announced on radio, television, web sites, and in newspapers, urging personal protection against mosquito bites. Because horses do not play a role in the transmission of WNV, quarantines were never placed on any asymptomatic horses in the outbreak area. However, some horse movements were restricted, particularly the export of horses from affected areas to the European Union and the shipment of any horses to the E.U. via the Kennedy airport.

In 2000, the United States developed a national

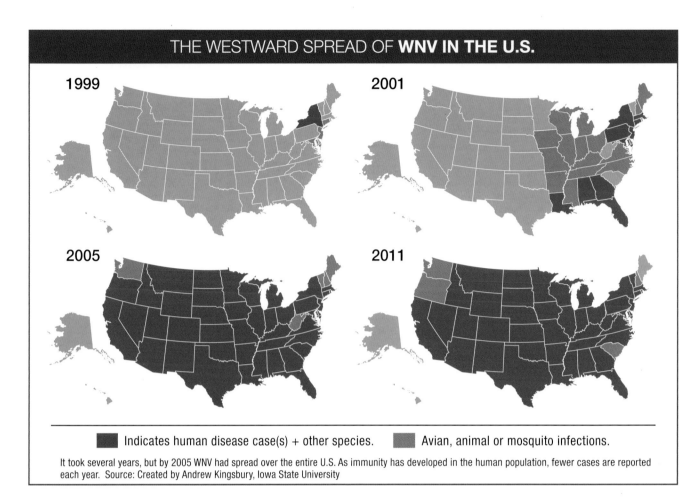

THE WESTWARD SPREAD OF **WNV IN THE U.S.**

1999

2001

2005

2011

■ Indicates human disease case(s) + other species.   ■ Avian, animal or mosquito infections.

It took several years, but by 2005 WNV had spread over the entire U.S. As immunity has developed in the human population, fewer cases are reported each year. Source: Created by Andrew Kingsbury, Iowa State University

electronic disease surveillance program called "ArboNET," managed collaboratively by the Centers for Disease Control and State health departments. It started as a surveillance system only for WNV. In 2003, this program expanded to include other human arboviral diseases, such as dengue virus and St. Louis encephalitis virus. Its goal is to monitor arboviruses throughout the United States and to provide timely information to government officials, health care providers, researchers, and the general public. ArboNET collects data from diagnostic laboratories that conduct surveillance testing on humans, mosquitoes, sentinel animals, dead birds, and veterinary species. This state and federal agency collaboration allows for weekly updates during the transmission season that can easily be disseminated to public health officials, government leaders, clinicians (medical and veterinary), and the public.

SPREAD OF WEST NILE VIRUS

By the end of 1999, WNV was identified in a limited area of the northeastern United States in wild birds, mosquitoes, humans, and horses. Illnesses in humans and horses occurred only from early August through

late October and were limited to the state of New York. WNV activity ended for the season because of various factors, including climate and vector control activities. Although authorities hoped that the outbreak had ended with the coming of winter and the resulting death of mosquito populations, WNV reemerged in the U.S. in 2000. Human and equine cases were reported in New York and other states, and birds were detected in 12 states and the District of Columbia. Evidence of WNV infection was also found in wild mammals. It was apparent that the virus was spreading westward and southward from New York. In 2001, WNV was transported through bird migration south to Florida and west to Iowa, and by 2005, it was found endemic in all continental U.S. states except Alaska. Through 2015, Alaska and Hawaii continued to remain free from locally-acquired WNV infection.

WNV also spread into Canada, where it was first detected in birds and mosquitoes in the provinces of Ontario and Quebec in 2001, with the first human and equine cases reported in 2002. In addition, these viruses reached Central and South America, and the Caribbean.

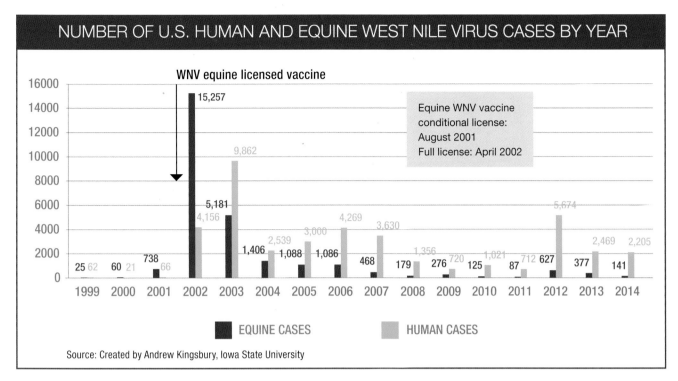

NUMBER OF U.S. HUMAN AND EQUINE WEST NILE VIRUS CASES BY YEAR

WNV equine licensed vaccine

Equine WNV vaccine
conditional license:
August 2001
Full license: April 2002

EQUINE CASES   HUMAN CASES

Source: Created by Andrew Kingsbury, Iowa State University

Recent genomic studies of avian isolates of WNV from 2001-2012 further demonstrate the explosive nature of its spread across North America. Limited clustering by geographic region and little evidence of adaptive evolution suggest this is a virus well-suited to existing mosquito vectors and avian hosts and has been able to spread rapidly and virtually unconstrained across the continent.

WILD BIRDS AND REPTILES

Most wild bird populations in the Eastern Hemisphere seem to be unaffected by endemic West Nile viruses circulating in the region. However, some North American birds, which were exposed for the first time, were severely affected by the introduction of WNV. The effects of this virus vary with the species, but by the end of 2012, WNV had been detected in over 300 species of dead birds in the United States. Initial outbreaks killed large numbers of crows, blue jays, and other corvids (birds in the crow family), as well as American robins, house wrens, eastern bluebirds, tufted titmice, chickadees, and sage grouse. With time, some species have apparently recovered or are recovering; other populations remain smaller than normal. Outbreaks have also been reported in domesticated geese, pheasants, and partridges, and occasional cases occur in captive psittacine (related to parrots) birds or zoo birds.

In North America, WNV has also revealed an unexpected ability to cause neurological disease in reptiles. At one U.S. alligator farm with more than 10,000 animals, 250 alligators died in an outbreak one year, and more than 1,000 died the following year. Young alligators were more severely affected than adults.

EPIDEMIOLOGY, CONTROL AND PREVENTION

West Nile virus continues to change and evolve as it becomes established in the Americas. The virus that was originally introduced to New York (NY99) evolved and has been replaced by variants. Infections caused by WNV in both animals and humans are notifiable disease in the U.S. In 2014, there were 2,205 reported human illnesses caused by WNV in the U.S., and many additional mild or asymptomatic infections go undetected. Without a vaccine, periodic outbreaks are expected to continue to occur. Far fewer clinical cases or deaths have been reported in Central and South America compared to the U.S. The reason for this difference is not known; however, it might involve protective immunity to cross-reactive flaviviruses, (e.g. dengue) circulating in those regions, the emergence of WNV isolates with decreased virulence, or lower levels of surveillance and specific diagnosis. In areas where dengue, another flaviviral disease, is present, some West Nile infections could be misdiagnosed as this disease.

Within two years of the WNV incursion, USDA Center for Veterinary Biologics conditionally licensed a killed virus vaccine for horses. Several fully licensed vaccines are now available, and are considered a core vaccination for horses in the U.S. As a result, the number of WNV cases in U.S. horses has decreased from more than 15,000 in 2002, to approximately 134 in 2014. Vaccines are sometimes used "off label" to protect sensitive birds or other species. For instance, in an effort to minimize the impact of West Nile virus on endangered California condors, captive condors have been vaccinated since 2003, and attempts have been made to vaccinate wild chicks in the nest.

At present, control measures for humans remain centered on continued surveillance and vector control, long-term trend analyses, continuing education, and careful monitoring of reservoir avian populations. Scientists are working on a vaccine for humans, and clinical trials are underway, as of 2015. Information Sources for this chapter can be found at: http://www.cfsph.iastate.edu/TEDATextbookReferences/.

CORE VACCINES

The AVMA defines core vaccinations as those "that protect from diseases that are endemic to a region, those with potential public health significance, required by law, virulent/highly infectious, and/or those posing a risk of severe disease. Core vaccines have clearly demonstrated efficacy and safety, and thus exhibit a high enough level of patient benefit and low enough level of risk to justify their use in the majority of patients."

SECTION

2

Transboundary and Emerging Diseases of Animals
FACT SHEETS

This section contains 34 fact sheets on animal diseases that are exotic or rare in the United States. Veterinarians are obligated to report the occurrence of most of these diseases to appropriate state, or federal authorities. Although these fact sheets contain information on diagnosis, veterinarians should not attempt to collect and submit samples from suspected foreign animal diseases directly to diagnostic laboratories. Instead, veterinarians who suspect an exotic disease should immediately contact the state, or federal authorities in their area for assistance. It is important to note that reportable diseases vary from state to state and province to province and the lists of these diseases may change. As a practicing veterinarian, you need to be familiar with the current list of reportable diseases for your area rather than rely on the general information in these fact sheets.

These fact sheets, plus approximately 115 additional fact sheets are available at www.cfsph.iastate.edu (click on animal disease information). The fact sheets are authored by Anna Rovid Spickler, DVM, PhD. Glenda Dvorak, MS, DVM, MPH, DACVPM, manages the fact sheets for the CFSPH website and coordinated conversion of the web-based fact sheets for this book. Since the fact sheets were originally developed beginning in 2000, many individuals have reviewed, contributed to, and enhanced the fact sheets. Comments and suggestions on the fact sheets are always welcome; send suggestions to cfsph@iastate.edu. The fact sheets are continually updated as new information becomes available. The most current versions can be found at *www.cfsph.iastate.edu*

To cite these fact sheets in publications, the following information can be used:

Spickler, Anna Rovid, "Title of fact sheet". In: Transboundary and Emerging Diseases of Animals, 1st Edition. 2016. Spickler, Anna Rovid; Roth, James A.; Brown, Gayle B., and Galyon, C. Jane (Eds). Center for Food Security and Public Health, Iowa State University, Ames, IA. USA. Pages: _____.

Author:
Anna Rovid Spickler, DVM, PhD
Center for Food Security and Public Health
Iowa State University
College of Veterinary Medicine
Ames, IA 50011

AFRICAN HORSE SICKNESS

Perdesiekte, Pestis Equorum, Peste Equina,
Peste Equina Africana

IMPORTANCE

African horse sickness (AHS) is a serious arthropod-borne viral disease of equids, with a mortality rate that can reach 95% in some species, such as horses. At present, AHS virus (AHSV) is only endemic in Africa; however, suitable vectors exist outside this area, and infected animals or vectors may carry the virus into AHS-free regions. The potential for dissemination is especially high in animals that tend to develop mild or subclinical infections, such as zebras (*Equus burchelli*) and donkeys, or horses with partial immunity. One extensive epidemic in 1959-1961 affected the Middle East and parts of Asia, as well as Africa, and is thought to have been responsible for the deaths of 300,000 equids. One outbreak in Spain lasted from 1987, when the virus was introduced in imported zebras, to 1990, and spread to Portugal and Morocco. Within Africa, additional AHSV serotypes have recently spread to some areas where only one serotype was previously found. Although vaccines are available, cross-protection between serotypes is limited, and the introduction of a new serotype into an area may result in outbreaks.

ETIOLOGY

African horse sickness results from infection with the African horse sickness virus (AHSV), a member of the genus *Orbivirus* in the family Reoviridae. There are nine serotypes of this virus, and while some serotypes are cross-protective (e.g., serotypes 6 and 9), others are not.

SPECIES AFFECTED

Equids including horses, donkeys, mules and zebras are the primary hosts for AHSV; however, this virus is also known to affect dogs. Among equids, the most serious infections occur in horses and mules, which are thought to be accidental hosts. Zebras, which are often asymptomatic, are thought to be the natural reservoir hosts in most regions of Africa.

Antibodies to AHSV have been reported in a number of other species, although there are sometimes inconsistencies between studies. Seropositive animals have included various wild carnivores, such as hyenas (*Crocuta crocuta*), jackals (various *Canis* spp.), African wild dogs (*Lycaon pictus*), cheetahs (*Acinonyx jubutus*), lions (*Panthera leo*) and large-spotted genets (*Genetta maculata*), which might be exposed by feeding on infected zebras. Some authors have reported that carnivores may have antibodies to AHSV serotypes (e.g., serotype 4) that are not necessarily common among equids

in the area. There are also reports of seropositive herbivores including dromedary camels (*Camelus dromedarius*), sheep, goats, African elephants (*Loxodonta africana*), black rhinocerus (*Diceros bicornis*) and white rhinocerus (*Ceratotherium simum*). Attempts to establish experimental infections resulted in seroconversion with no evidence of virus replication in African elephants, and seroconversion in hyenas, while mink (*Mustela vison*) did not seroconvert or replicate virus. The significance of seropositive animals is still unclear, and no animals other than equids are thought to be important in maintaining or amplifying AHSV.

Zoonotic potential

African horse sickness is not zoonotic.

GEOGRAPHIC DISTRIBUTION

African horse sickness is endemic in sub-Saharan Africa. Serotype 9 is widespread in the endemic region, while serotypes 1 to 8 occur in limited areas. The greatest virus diversity has been reported in southern and eastern Africa. Some serotypes have recently caused outbreaks in countries where they were not previously found. In particular, serotypes such as 2, 4, 6, 7 and 8 have been detected in regions where only serotype 9 was once common.

African horse sickness outbreaks have occurred outside Africa in the Middle East, the Mediterranean region of Europe and parts of Asia (e.g., the Indian subcontinent). Although all outbreaks, to date, were eventually eradicated, AHSV was able to persist for years in some areas.

TRANSMISSION

AHSV is transmitted by the midges *Culicoides imicola* and *C. bolitinos* in Africa. Additional species of *Culicoides* might also be able to act as vectors. They include species found outside the endemic region, such as *C. variipennis*, which occurs in North America and is an efficient AHSV vector in the laboratory, and *C. brevitarsis*, which is common in Australia. Wind has been implicated in the dispersal of infected vectors during some epidemics. AHSV is capable of overwintering, at least in milder climates where *Culicoides* adults can survive. Other arthropods might also be capable of transmitting AHSV, but are thought to be, at most, only minor sources of infection. Mosquitoes have been implicated as possible biological vectors, and biting flies in the genera *Stomoxys* and *Tabanus* may be able to transmit the virus mechanically. AHS virus was also isolated from the camel tick *Hyalomma dromedarii* in Egypt, and the dog tick, *Rhipicephalus sanguineus*, could transmit AHSV from dogs in the laboratory.

Zebras are thought to be the natural reservoir hosts for AHSV, but horses, mules and donkeys can also develop viremia sufficient to infect *Culicoides*. How long equids remain infectious for the vector is not certain; however, AHSV could be isolated from the blood of some experimentally infected zebras for up to 40 days, and from the spleen at 48 days. In experimentally infected horses, this virus has been recovered from blood for as long as 21 days, although viremia typically lasts only 4-8 days. Donkeys are reported to remain viremic for up to 28 days, and viral RNA has been detected longer in some studies (e.g., 47 days or more in some experimentally infected animals inoculated with serotype 4). African horse sickness is not transmitted between equids by casual contact.

Dogs can be infected if they eat contaminated horsemeat, and experimental infections have been established by the oral route as well as by subcutaneous or intravenous inoculation. AHSV is reported to persist for some time in frozen meat, and it is reported to survive for up to 6 months at 4ºC in medium containing serum, and for more than 2 years in putrid blood. Although arthropods including ticks can transmit AHSV from dogs to other dogs or horses in the laboratory, viremia is usually low and transient, and dogs are not thought to be significant in the epidemiology of African horse sickness. In addition, dogs are not usually hosts for *Culicoides* in the endemic region.

DISINFECTION

AHSV can be inactivated in the laboratory with formalin, β-propriolactone, acetylethyleneimine derivatives or radiation. It is resistant to liquid solvents such as ether. It is also destroyed at pH < 6 or pH ≥ 12. Acidic disinfectants such as 2% acetic or citric acid have been recommended for decontamination when it is warranted. AHSV is relatively heat stable, and it was not inactivated by heating in citrated plasma at 55-75°C for 10 minutes.

INCUBATION PERIOD

The incubation period for African horse sickness in equids is approximately 3 days to 2 weeks (usually < 9 days), with the cardiac form typically developing later than the pulmonary form. Experimental infections suggest that the incubation period might is potentially be as long as 21 days.

CLINICAL SIGNS

Four different forms of African horse sickness exist: the peracute (pulmonary) form, the subacute edematous (cardiac) form, the acute (mixed) form, and horsesickness fever. Sudden death can also occur without preceding signs. Symptomatic infections are seen most often in horses and mules, with the pulmonary and mixed forms usually predominating in susceptible populations of horses. Zebras and donkeys rarely develop serious clinical signs. The mildest form, horsesickness fever, tends to develop in resistant species such as donkeys, or in horses with partial immunity. This form can also occur in zebras, although most infections in this species are asymptomatic.

The peracute or pulmonary form

The pulmonary form of African horse sickness usually begins with an acute fever, followed within a day or two by the sudden onset of severe respiratory distress. Animals with this form often stand with forelegs spread, head extended, and nostrils fully dilated. Other clinical signs may include tachypnea, forced expiration, profuse sweating, spasmodic coughing, and a frothy serofibrinous nasal exudate. Dyspnea usually progresses rapidly, and the animal often dies within a few hours after the respiratory signs appear.

The subacute edematous or cardiac form

The cardiac form of African horse sickness usually begins with a fever that lasts less than a week. Shortly before the fever starts to subside, edematous swellings appear in the supraorbital fossae and eyelids. These swellings later spread to involve the face, tongue, intermandibular space, laryngeal region, and sometimes the neck, shoulders and chest. Edema of the lower legs is absent. Other clinical signs, usually seen in the terminal stages of the disease, can include severe depression, colic, petechiae or ecchymoses on the ventral surface of the tongue, and petechiae in the conjunctivae. Death often occurs from cardiac failure. If the animal recovers, the swellings gradually subside over a few days to a week.

The acute or mixed form

Clinical signs of both the pulmonary and cardiac forms are seen in the mixed form. In most cases, the cardiac form is subclinical and is followed by severe respiratory distress. Occasionally, mild respiratory signs may be followed by edema and death from cardiac failure. Although the mixed form is common, it may not be recognized except at necropsy.

Horsesickness fever

In horsesickness fever, the clinical signs are mild. This syndrome is characterized mainly by fever, often with morning remissions and afternoon exacerbations. Other signs are generally mild and may include mild anorexia or depression, edema of the supraorbital fossae, congested mucous membranes and an increased heart rate. Death would be unusual.

Infections in dogs

The pulmonary form is reported to be the most common form in dogs. Fatal cases have been described in dogs that ate infected meat during epidemics. In one outbreak, 13 of 17 dogs died with unspecified clinical signs, while two animals that survived longer had fever, depression, dyspnea, moist rales and white foam around the nostrils, and died within 24 hours despite intensive care. Some dogs living in endemic regions are seropositive, suggesting that milder cases or subclinical infections also occur, and AHSV has been isolated from feral dogs not reported to be ill. In early experiments, which used crude preparations of virus (e.g., filtered blood from infected horses), some dogs had no apparent signs of illness, while others developed febrile reactions and survived, or died with evidence of severe pulmonary disease.

POST MORTEM LESIONS

Horses

In the pulmonary form of African horse sickness, the characteristic lesions are interlobular edema of the lungs and hydrothorax. In the most acute cases, frothy fluid is present in the trachea and pulmonary airways, and may flow from the nostrils and the cut surface of the lungs. The lungs are typically mottled red (with distended interlobular septae) noncollapsed and heavy. In more prolonged cases, there may be extensive interstitial and subpleural edema, and hyperemia may be less apparent. Fluid may be found in the thoracic cavity (hydrothorax) and abdominal cavity. Occasionally, there can be extensive fluid accumulation in the thoracic cavity, with near normal appearance of the lungs. The lymph nodes, particularly the nodes in the thoracic and abdominal cavities, are usually enlarged and edematous. In some cases, there may also be subcapsular hemorrhages in the spleen, congestion in the renal cortex, edematous infiltration around the aorta and trachea, and petechial hemorrhages on various serosal and pleural surfaces. Gastrointestinal lesions can include hyperemia and petechiae in the small and large intestines, and hyperemia of the gastric fundus. Cardiac lesions are not prominent, although petechiae may be found on the pericardium, and there may be increased pericardial fluid.

In the cardiac form, a yellow gelatinous infiltrate can be seen in the subcutaneous and intermuscular fascia of the head, neck and shoulders, and occasionally the brisket, ventral abdomen and rump. Hydropericardium is common. The epicardium and endocardium often contain petechial and ecchymotic hemorrhages. Lesions may also be found in the gastrointestinal tract, resembling the pulmonary form. In addition, prominent submucosal edema may be noted in the cecum, large colon and rectum. Ascites can also be seen. The lungs are usually normal or slightly edematous/engorged in this form of AHS, and the thoracic cavity rarely contains excess fluid.

In the mixed form, the post mortem lesions are a mixture of typical findings from both the cardiac and pulmonary forms.

Dogs

The gross lesions reported in dogs have been consistent with pulmonary disease; the main lesions were hydrothorax and pulmonary congestion and edema. Red-tinged foam was noted in the airways of some animals. In some cases, the fluid in the lungs (clear and straw-colored) gelled on exposure to the air. Areas of emphysema and/or areas of hepatization were also reported in some lungs. Other lesions, such as hyperemia of the intestinal mucosa, petechiae and ecchymoses on the

endocardium, and congestion of the liver and other internal organs have been noted in experimentally infected or naturally infected dogs.

DIAGNOSTIC TESTS

African horse sickness is often diagnosed by virological methods. More than one test should be used to diagnose an outbreak (particularly the index case) whenever possible. AHSV can be isolated from the blood of live animals, or from tissue samples, especially spleen, lung and lymph nodes, collected at necropsy. Successful isolation from the blood is most likely if these samples are collected early during the febrile stage. AHSV can be recovered in various cell lines including baby hamster kidney (BHK-21), monkey stable (MS) or African green monkey kidney (Vero) cells, as well as *Culicoides* (e.g., KC cells) and mosquito insect cell lines, and in embryonated eggs, Intracerebral inoculation of newborn mice can also be performed. The isolate should be serotyped using virus neutralization or other methods, to allow the selection of an appropriate vaccine strain.

AHSV antigens can be detected in the blood and tissues (e.g., spleen) with enzyme-linked immunosorbent assays (ELISAs). Various reverse-transcription polymerase chain reaction (RT-PCR) assays are used to detect viral RNA. Some RT-PCR assays can also be used for rapid serotyping of field isolates.

Serology can also be used to diagnose African horse sickness, with antibodies usually detected within 8 to 14 days after infection. Paired serum samples are recommended, and are particularly important in areas where the disease is endemic. Available serologic tests include ELISAs, complement fixation, immunoblotting and virus neutralization. Complement fixation is now used infrequently in many areas, although is still employed in some endemic regions. The virus neutralization test is used for serotyping. Immunodiffusion and hemagglutination inhibition tests have also been described. Cross-reactivity between AHSV serotypes is variable, and AHSV does not cross-react with other known orbiviruses.

TREATMENT

There is no specific treatment for African horse sickness, other than supportive care. Treatment may also be needed for secondary infections.

CONTROL

Disease reporting

A quick response is vital for containing outbreaks in AHS-free regions. Veterinarians who encounter or suspect this disease should follow their national and/or local guidelines for disease reporting. In the U.S., state or federal veterinary authorities should be informed immediately.

Prevention

Live attenuated vaccines are routinely used to control African horse sickness in endemic regions. Monovalent or polyvalent vaccines may be employed, depending on the viruses circulating in the area. Reactivity to some vaccine strains is reported to be better than to others, and protection may be incomplete in some cases: clinical cases and mild or subclinical infections have been reported in some horses that had received as many as 5 vaccine doses in Africa. The currently available vaccines are teratogenic in pregnant mares, and vaccine strains may be transmitted by *Culicoides* vectors. No killed or subunit vaccines are currently manufactured commercially.

Stabling equids in insect-proof housing, especially from dusk to dawn (when *Culicoides* are most active), can also reduce the risk of infection. One study suggested that open stables might provide some degree of protection from *C. imicola*, but did not protect horses from *C. bolitinos*. Instead, concentrations of the latter vector seemed to increase inside open stables that contained horses. Vector control measures such as insect repellents and targeted applications of insecticides or larvicides might also be helpful.

When outbreaks occur in endemic areas, they have generally been controlled by vaccination and movement restrictions on equids. Some authors have recommended that surveillance systems be established to provide early warnings of outbreaks and detect the introduction of new serotypes in an area. Donkeys, which are not usually vaccinated for AHS, might be monitored by serology.

Most non-endemic countries test and quarantine imported equids to prevent them from introducing AHSV. The quarantine period may be extensive (e.g., 60 days in the U.S., if the horse is from an endemic country). If a virus is introduced into a non-endemic region, control measures may include the establishment of quarantine zones and movement controls, vaccination campaigns, and possibly the euthanasia of infected animals, depending on the situation. Stabling equids in insect-proof housing, at least overnight, can provide some protection to uninfected animals, as well as reduce the risk that infected animals will transmit the virus to vectors. Vector control measures may reduce the number of *Culicoides*, although they are unlikely to be completely eliminated. Monitoring for fever can be helpful in detecting cases early. Each susceptible animal should have its temperature taken regularly (optimally, twice daily). The onset of cold weather can end epidemics, but the virus has sometimes re-emerged in the spring, at least in climates with mild winters (e.g., in Spain).

MORBIDITY AND MORTALITY

Significant numbers of equids in Africa (e.g., 34% of equids and up to 50% of donkeys in Ethiopia) have been exposed to AHSV. Antibodies have also been documented in other animals, including 4-8% of dogs in some areas, although the significance of this finding is still unclear. Outbreaks of African horse sickness tend to occur in late summer and autumn, with cycles occurring at irregular intervals in some regions. Climatic conditions reported to favor epidemics are heavy rain alternating with hot, dry periods. Some countries have reported that there are fewer outbreaks since the number of free-ranging wild zebras decreased. In other regions, African horse sickness outbreaks seem to have increased recently, and have sometimes been caused by serotypes not usually found in that area.

Morbidity and mortality differ, depending on the viral strain, species of animal, previous immunity and form of the disease. In horses that develop clinical signs, the pulmonary form of African horse sickness is nearly always fatal, and the mortality rate in the cardiac form is usually 50% or higher. In the mixed form, mortality rate estimates vary from approximately 70% to greater than 80%, while horsesickness fever is not fatal. The mixed and pulmonary forms tend to predominate in naïve horse populations, and the mortality rate is usually 50-95%. African horse sickness is generally less severe in other equids. The mortality rate is approximately 50% in mules during epidemics, and 5-10% in European and Asian donkeys. Deaths are rare among donkeys and zebra in endemic areas of Africa. Little is known about morbidity and mortality rates in dogs, but both subclinical and fatal infections have been reported. Once pulmonary signs appear, the prognosis in this species also appears to be poor. In one outbreak, 15 of 17 dogs died after being fed horsemeat from a sick horse. Intensive treatment was attempted in 2 of these animals, but it was unsuccessful.

Equids that recover from African horse sickness develop good immunity to the infecting serotype and partial immunity to other serotypes.

PUBLIC HEALTH

Humans are not natural hosts for the African horse sickness virus, and no cases have been seen after contact with field strains. However, a neurotropic vaccine strain, adapted to mice, can cause encephalitis and retinitis in humans.

AFRICAN SWINE FEVER

Peste Porcine Africaine, Fiebre Porcina Africana, Pestis Africana Suum, Maladie de Montgomery, Warthog Disease, Afrikaanse Varkpes, Afrikanische Schweinepest

IMPORTANCE

African swine fever is a serious, highly contagious, viral disease of pigs. African swine fever virus (ASFV) can spread very rapidly in pig populations by direct or indirect contact.

It can persist for long periods in uncooked pig products, facilitating its introduction into new areas. This virus can also become endemic in feral or wild suids, and transmission cycles between these animals and *Ornithodoros* ticks can complicate or even prevent eradication. ASFV isolates vary in virulence from highly pathogenic strains that cause near 100% mortality to low-virulence isolates that can be difficult to diagnose. There is no vaccine or treatment.

African swine fever is a serious problem in many African countries. Changes in production practices and increasing globalization have also increased the risk of its introduction into other regions. Past outbreaks occurred in Europe, South America and the Caribbean, and the cost of eradication was significant. The swine herds of Malta and the Dominican Republic were completely depopulated during outbreaks in these countries. In Spain and Portugal, ASFV became endemic in the 1960s and complete eradication took more than 30 years. It still remains present on the island of Sardinia. In 2007, Africa swine fever was introduced into the Caucasus region of Eurasia, where it has spread widely among wild boar and domesticated pigs. This virus has caused outbreaks in pigs as far west as the easternmost countries of the E.U., and it has also been detected in wild boar in Iran.

ETIOLOGY

African swine fever results from infection by the African swine fever virus, which belongs to the genus *Asfivirus* in the family Asfarviridae. More than 20 genotypes of ASFV have been identified, most from wildlife cycles in Africa. The virus introduced into the Caucasus belongs to genotype II, while viruses endemic in Sardinia belong to genotype I. ASFV isolates differ greatly in virulence, from highly pathogenic viruses that kill most pigs to strains that result only in seroconversion.

SPECIES AFFECTED

African swine fever affects members of the pig family (Suidae). Species that can be infected include domesticated swine, Eurasian wild boars (*Sus scrofa scrofa*), warthogs (*Phacochoerus* spp.), bush pigs (*Potamochoerus larvatus* and *Potamochoerus porcus*) and giant forest hogs (*Hylochoerus* spp.). Warthogs and bush pigs, which are generally asymptomatic, are thought to be wildlife reservoirs for the virus in Africa. Some older reviews and textbooks suggest that peccaries (*Tayassu* spp.) may also become infected without clinical signs, although one attempt to infect collared peccaries (*Tayassu tajacu*) in 1969 was unsuccessful. Recent reviews state that that peccaries are not susceptible.

Zoonotic potential

There is no evidence that ASFV infects humans.

GEOGRAPHIC DISTRIBUTION

African swine fever is endemic in most of sub-Saharan Africa including the island of Madagascar. Outbreaks have been reported periodically outside Africa. The virus was eventually eradicated in most cases, although it remains endemic on the island of Sardinia (Italy) in the Mediterranean. In 2007, ASFV was introduced into the Caucasus region of Eurasia, via the Republic of Georgia, and it has spread to domesticated pigs and/or wild boars in a number of countries in this region. As of 2015, infections had been reported as far west as Lithuania, Latvia and Poland. Viruses that apparently originated from this outbreak have also been found in wild boar in the Middle East (Iran).

TRANSMISSION

African swine fever can be transmitted either with or without tick vectors as intermediaries. After direct (non-tickborne) contact with the virus, ASFV is mainly thought to enter the body via the upper respiratory tract. This virus has been found in all secretions and excretions of sick domesticated pigs, with particularly high concentrations in oronasal fluid. There may, however, be species differences among the Suidae. For instance, concentrations of ASFV appear to be much lower in adult warthogs, compared to pigs, and adult warthogs might not transmit the virus by direct contact. In pigs, aerosolized viruses may contribute to transmission within a building or farm, although current evidence suggests that this only occurs over relatively short distances. Because ASFV can persist in blood and tissues after death, it is readily spread by feeding uncooked swill that contains tissues from infected animals. Some reports suggest that the cannibalism of dead pigs may be important in transmission. In addition, massive environmental contamination may result if blood is shed during necropsies or pig fights, or if a pig develops bloody diarrhea. How long pigs can remain infected is still uncertain. Several studies have reported finding ASFV in the tissues of domesticated pigs for as long as 3 to 6 months, and virus shedding and transmission for at least 70 days after experimental inoculation. However, there are also studies where pigs could not transmit the virus for longer than a month. Currently, there is no evidence that the virus persists long-term in a latent state.

ASFV can spread on fomites, including vehicles, feed and equipment. In feces kept at room temperature, this virus was estimated to survive for several days in some reports, and for at least 11 days in one study where the sample was stored in the dark. One study reported that ASFV remained infectious longer in urine than feces, with estimated survival times of 3 days at 37°C and 15 days at 4°C. ASFV can also persist for a year and a half in blood stored at 4°C, 150 days in boned meat stored at 39°F, 140 days in salted dried hams, and several years in frozen carcasses.

Vector-mediated transmission is through the bites of *Ornithodoros* spp. soft ticks. In some regions of Africa, ASFV is thought to cycle between juvenile common warthogs (*Phacochoerus africanus*) and the soft ticks belonging to the *Ornithodoros moubata* complex, that live in their burrows. Transstadial, transovarial and sexual transmission have been demonstrated in these ticks. A similar cycle is thought to exist between domesticated pigs and the *Ornithodoros moubata* complex ticks that colonize their pig pens in Africa. *Ornithodoros erraticus* acted as a biological vector during an outbreak on the Iberian Peninsula in Europe, and additional species of *Ornithodoros* have been infected in the laboratory. *Ornithodoros* spp. ticks are long-lived, and colonies have been demonstrated to maintain ASFV for several years (e.g., 5 years in *O. erraticus*). However, the ticks can eventually clear the virus if they are not reinfected. There is no evidence that hard ticks act as biological vectors for ASFV.

Other bloodsucking insects such as mosquitoes and biting flies might be able to transmit ASFV mechanically. Stable flies (*Stomoxys calcitrans*) can carry high levels of the virus for 2 days. Under experimental conditions, these flies could transmit ASFV 24 hours after feeding on infected pigs.

DISINFECTION

Many common disinfectants are ineffective against ASFV; care should be taken to use a disinfectant specifically approved for this virus. Sodium hypochlorite, citric acid (1%) and some iodine and quaternary ammonium compounds are reported to destroy ASFV on some nonporous surfaces. In one recent experiment, either 2% citric acid or higher concentrations of sodium hypochlorite (e.g., 2000 ppm) could disinfect the virus on wood; however, citric acid was more effective.

Unprocessed meat must be heated to at least 70ºC for 30 minutes to inactivate ASFV; 30 minutes at 60ºC is sufficient for serum and body fluids. This virus can also be inactivated by pH < 3.9 or > 11.5 in serum-free medium.

INCUBATION PERIOD

The incubation period is 5 to 21 days after direct contact with infected pigs, but it can be less than 5 days after exposure to ticks. Acute disease typically appears in 3 to 7 days.

CLINICAL SIGNS

African swine fever can be a peracute, acute, subacute or chronic disease. Severe cases that affect large numbers of animals may be readily recognized; however, some herds develop milder symptoms that are easily confused with other diseases. Some animals can seroconvert without developing clinical signs.

Sudden deaths with few lesions (peracute cases) may be the first sign of an infection in a herd. Acute cases are characterized by a high fever, anorexia, lethargy, weakness and recumbency. Erythema can be seen, and is most apparent in white pigs.

Some pigs develop cyanotic skin blotching, especially on the ears, tail, lower legs or hams. Pigs may also have diarrhea, constipation and/or signs of abdominal pain; the diarrhea is initially mucoid and may later become bloody. There may also be visible signs of hemorrhagic tendencies, including epistaxis and hemorrhages in the skin. Respiratory signs including dyspnea, vomiting, nasal and conjunctival discharges, and neurological signs have also been reported. Pregnant animals frequently abort; in some cases, abortions may be the first signs of an outbreak. Leukopenia and thrombocytopenia of varying severity may be detected in laboratory tests. Death often occurs within 7 to 10 days.

Subacute African swine fever, caused by moderately virulent isolates, is similar to acute ASF but with less severe clinical signs. Abortions may be the first sign. Fever, thrombocytopenia and leukopenia may be transient; however, hemorrhages can occur during the period of thrombocytopenia. Affected pigs usually die or recover within 3 to 4 weeks.

Chronic disease was described in Europe when ASFV was endemic on the Iberian peninsula. Some authors speculate that the strains that cause this form might have originated from live attenuated vaccine strains investigated at that time. Pigs with the chronic form can have intermittent low fever, appetite loss and depression. The signs may be limited to emaciation and stunting in some animals. Other pigs develop respiratory problems and swollen joints. Coughing is common, and diarrhea and occasional vomiting have been reported. Ulcers and reddened or raised necrotic skin foci may appear over body protrusions and other areas subject to trauma. Chronic African swine fever can be fatal.

Signs in wild boar inoculated with a highly virulent isolate were similar to those in domesticated pigs; however, some runted animals infected with very low viral doses had few or no clinical signs, including fever, before death. Warthogs and bush pigs usually become infected asymptomatically or have mild disease.

POST MORTEM LESIONS

The gross lesions of African swine fever are highly variable, and are affected by the virulence of the isolate and the course of the disease.

Numerous organs may be affected, to varying extent, in animals with acute or subacute African swine fever. The carcass is often in good condition in animals that die acutely. There may be bluish-purple discoloration and/or hemorrhages in the skin, and signs of bloody diarrhea or other internal hemorrhages. The major internal lesions are hemorrhagic, and occur most consistently in the spleen, lymph nodes, kidneys and heart. In animals infected with highly virulent isolates, the spleen can be very large, friable, and dark red to black. In other cases, the spleen may be enlarged but not friable, and the color may be closer to normal. The lymph nodes are often swollen and hemorrhagic, and may look like blood clots; the nodes most often affected are the gastrohepatic and renal lymph nodes. Petechiae are common on the cortical and cut surfaces of the kidneys, and sometimes in the renal pelvis. Perirenal edema may be present. Hemorrhages, petechiae and/or ecchymoses are sometimes detected in other organs including the urinary bladder, lungs, stomach and intestines. Pulmonary edema and congestion can be prominent in some pigs. There may also be congestion of the liver and edema in the wall of the gall bladder and bile duct, and the pleural, pericardial and/or peritoneal cavities may contain straw-colored or blood-stained fluid. The brain and meninges can be congested, edematous or hemorrhagic. Animals that die peracutely may have few or poorly developed lesions.

In animals with chronic African swine fever, the carcass may be emaciated. Other possible post-mortem lesions include focal areas of skin necrosis, skin ulcers, consolidated lobules in the lung, caseous pneumonia, nonseptic fibrinous pericarditis, pleural adhesions, generalized lymphadenopathy and swollen joints. Some lesions may result from secondary infections.

Aborted fetuses can be anasarcous and have a mottled liver. They may have petechiae or ecchymoses in the skin and myocardium. Petechiae can also be found in the placenta.

DIAGNOSTIC TESTS

African swine fever can be diagnosed by virus isolation. This virus can be detected in blood from live animals or tissues (especially spleen, kidney, tonsils and lymph nodes) collected at necropsy. ASFV is not found in aborted fetuses; in cases of abortion, a blood sample should be collected from the dam. Cell types used for virus isolation include pig leukocyte or bone marrow cultures, porcine alveolar macrophages and blood monocyte cultures. One recent study used MARC-145 (African green monkey kidney) cells. ASFV-infected cells may be detected by their ability to induce hemadsorption of pig erythrocytes to their surfaces. A few non-hemadsorbing isolates can be missed with this test; most of these viruses are avirulent, but some do produce acute, symptomatic disease. PCR or immunofluorescence can also be used to detect the virus, and PCR can be used to confirm its identity.

PCR is often used to detect ASFV nucleic acids in clinical samples. It can be employed with putrefied samples, which are unsuitable for virus isolation and antigen detection, as well as with fresh tissues or blood. One study reported that, after death, the levels of viral DNA were highest in the spleen, and persisted longest in this tissue. There is also a published report describing the use of PCR with tonsil scrapings from live, experimentally infected animals, as well as blood or nasal swabs. Isothermal amplification methods are also in development.

ASFV antigens may be found in tissue smears or cryostat sections, as well as in buffy coat samples, using ELISAs or immunofluorescence. These tests are best employed as herd tests, and in conjunction with other assays. Antigens are easiest to detect in acute cases; these tests are less sensitive in subacutely or chronically infected animals. A hemadsorption "autorosette" test can also be used to detect ASFV directly in peripheral blood leukocytes; however, this test has mostly been replaced by PCR, which is easier to evaluate.

Serology may be useful, particularly in endemic regions. Pigs with acute disease often die before developing antibodies; however, antibodies to ASFV persist for long periods in animals that survive. Many serological tests have been developed for the diagnosis of African swine fever, but only a few have been standardized for routine use in diagnostic laboratories. Currently used tests include ELISAs, immunoblotting and indirect fluorescent antibody (IFA) tests. The ELISA is prescribed for international trade, and is generally confirmed by immunoblotting (although IFA can also be used).

TREATMENT

There is no treatment for African swine fever, other than supportive care.

CONTROL

Disease reporting

A quick response is vital for containing outbreaks in ASFV-free regions. Veterinarians who encounter or suspect African swine fever should follow their national and/or local guidelines for disease reporting. In the U.S., state or federal veterinary authorities should be informed immediately.

Prevention

In the past, heat treatment was used to inactivate viruses in pig swill (scraps fed to pigs) and prevent the entry of ASFV into areas free of this disease. Due to the risk that this and other viruses may not be completely inactivated (for example, if parts of the swill do not reach the target temperature), feeding swill to pigs has now been completely forbidden in some countries.

Some areas that experienced ASFV outbreaks successfully eradicated the virus by the slaughter of infected and in-contact animals, safe carcass disposal, sanitation, disinfection, movement controls and quarantines, and the prevention of contact with wild suids and infected ticks. However, the length and complexity of eradication campaigns differed with the local conditions. On the Iberian Peninsula, for example, ASFV had become established in wild boars and *Ornithodoros erraticus* ticks, and complete eradication took decades. Pigpens with infected ticks were destroyed or isolated as part of this campaign. Current regulations in the EU allow pig farms to be restocked as soon as 40 days after cleaning and disinfection, if an African swine fever outbreak occurs in the absence of vectors; however, the minimum quarantine is 6 years if vectors are thought to be involved in transmission.

Ornithodoros ticks apparently did not become chronically infected during outbreaks in South America, and this (together with the absence of virus in wildlife or feral pigs) simplified eradication.

Eradication of ASFV from some wild reservoirs in Africa, such as warthogs, appears unlikely. However, compartments where African swine fever is controlled and barriers prevent contact with wild reservoirs have been established in some regions. No vaccine is currently available.

MORBIDITY AND MORTALITY

In domesticated pigs, the morbidity rate can approach 100% in naïve herds; however, viruses may take days or several weeks to spread through the herd. The mortality rate depends on the virulence of the isolate, and can range from < 5% to 100%. Highly virulent isolates can cause nearly 100% mortality in pigs of all ages. Less virulent isolates are more likely to be fatal in pigs with a concurrent disease, pregnant animals and young animals. Mortality also tends to be high when ASFV is introduced into new regions, with an increased incidence of subacute and subclinical cases once it becomes endemic. In subacute disease, the mortality rate ranges from 30% to 70%, and may differ between age groups. In some situations, rates can be as high as 70-80% in young pigs but less than 20% in older animals.

AVIAN INFLUENZA

Fowl Plague, Grippe Aviaire

IMPORTANCE

Avian influenza viruses are highly contagious, extremely variable viruses that are widespread in birds. Wild birds in aquatic habitats are thought to be their natural reservoir hosts, but domesticated poultry and other birds can also be infected. Most viruses cause only mild disease in poultry, and are called low pathogenic avian influenza (LPAI) viruses. Highly pathogenic avian influenza (HPAI) viruses can develop from certain LPAI viruses, usually while they are circulating in poultry flocks. HPAI viruses can kill up to 90-100% of the flock, and cause epidemics that may spread rapidly, devastate the poultry industry and result in severe trade restrictions. In poultry, the presence of LPAI viruses capable of evolving into HPAI viruses can also affect international trade.

Avian influenza viruses can occasionally affect mammals, including humans, usually after close contact with infected poultry. While infections in people are often limited to conjunctivitis or mild respiratory disease, some viruses can cause severe illness. In particular, Asian lineage H5N1 HPAI viruses have caused rare but life-threatening infections, now

totaling nearly 850 laboratory-confirmed cases since 1997, and H7N9 LPAI viruses have caused more than 600 serious human illnesses in China since 2013. Avian influenza viruses can also infect other species of mammals, sometimes causing severe or fatal disease. In rare cases, avian influenza viruses can become adapted to circulate in a mammalian species. During the last century, such viruses have caused or contributed to at least three pandemics in humans, contributed to the diversity of swine influenza viruses in pigs, and also produced one of the two canine influenza viruses now circulating among dogs.

ETIOLOGY

Avian influenza results from infection by viruses belonging to the species *influenza A virus*, genus *influenzavirus A* and family Orthomyxoviridae. These viruses are also called type A influenza viruses. Influenza A viruses are classified into subtypes based on two surface proteins, the hemagglutinin (HA) and neuraminidase (NA). A virus that has a type 1 HA and type 2 NA, for example, would have the subtype H1N2. At least 16 hemagglutinins (H1 to H16), and 9 neuraminidases (N1 to N9) have been found in viruses from birds, while two additional HA and NA types have been identified, to date, only in bats. Some hemagglutinins, such as H14 and H15, seem to be uncommon, or perhaps are maintained in wild bird species or locations that are not usually sampled.

Avian influenza viruses are classified as either low pathogenic (also called low pathogenicity) avian influenza viruses or highly pathogenic (high pathogenicity) avian influenza viruses. A virus is defined as HPAI or LPAI by its ability to cause severe disease in intravenously inoculated young chickens in the laboratory, or by its possession of certain genetic features that have been associated with high virulence in HPAI viruses (i.e., the sequence at the HA cleavage site). HPAI viruses usually cause severe disease in chicken and turkey flocks, while LPAI infections are generally much milder in all avian species. With rare exceptions, HPAI viruses found in nature have always contained the H5 or H7 hemagglutinin. Two exceptions were H10 viruses that technically fit the HPAI definition if they were injected directly into the bloodstream of chickens, but caused only mild illness in birds that became infected by the respiratory (intranasal) route. Another H10 virus also fit the HPAI definition; however, this virus affected the kidneys and had a high mortality rate in intranasally inoculated young chickens. In the laboratory, the insertion of genetic sequences from HPAI viruses into non-H7, non-H5 viruses has created some viruses that are pathogenic only after intravenous inoculation, and other viruses (containing H2, H4, H8 or H14) that were highly virulent after both intravenous and intranasal inoculation. Recently, an H4N2 virus with a genetic signature characteristic of HPAI viruses was isolated from a flock of naturally infected quail. It was a LPAI virus, with low virulence when inoculated into chickens.

In rare cases, an H5 or H7 virus has a genetic signature that classifies it as an HPAI virus, but causes only mild illness in poultry. Such viruses may have been isolated when they were evolving to become more virulent. Their presence triggers the same regulatory responses as fully virulent HPAI viruses.

Antigenic shift and drift in influenza A viruses

The viral HA, and to a lesser extent the NA, are major targets for the immune response, and there is ordinarily little or no cross-protection between different HA or NA types. Influenza A viruses are very diverse, and two viruses that share a subtype may be only distantly related. The high variability is the result of two processes, mutation and genetic reassortment. Mutations cause gradual changes in the HA and NA proteins of the virus, a process called 'antigenic drift.' Once these proteins have changed enough, immune responses against the former HA and NA may no longer be protective.

Genetic reassortment can cause more rapid changes. The influenza A genome consists of 8 individual gene segments, and when two different viruses infect the same cell, gene segments from both viruses may be packaged into a single, novel virion. This can occur whenever two influenza viruses replicate in the same cell, whether the viruses are adapted to the same host species (e.g., two different avian influenza viruses) or originally came from different hosts (for instance, an avian influenza virus and a swine influenza virus). An important aspect of reassortment is that it can generate viruses containing either a new HA, a new NA, or both. Such abrupt changes, called 'antigenic shifts,' may be sufficient for the novel virus to completely evade existing immunity. After a subtype has become established in a species and has circulated for a time, antigenic shifts and drift can produce numerous viral variants.

Avian influenza virus lineages

There are two well-recognized lineages of avian influenza viruses, Eurasian and North American. As implied by the names, Eurasian lineage viruses primarily circulate among birds in Eurasia, and North American lineage viruses in the Americas. The amount of reassortment between these lineages seems to differ between regions, with very few reassortant viruses detected in some areas or wild bird populations, but significant reassortment where there is overlap between migratory flyways, such as in Alaska and Iceland. Viruses in wild birds (or portions of viruses) are more likely to be transferred between hemispheres in the latter regions. Avian influenza virus surveillance in Central and South America has been limited, but the viruses detected include a unique South American sublineage (or lineage) as well as viruses closely related to the North American lineage. The viruses in New Zealand and Australia might be geographically isolated to some extent, although there is also evidence of mixing with viruses from other areas.

Transfer of influenza viruses between species

Although influenza A viruses are adapted to circulate in a particular host or hosts, they can occasionally infect other species. In most cases, the virus cannot be transmitted efficiently between members of that species, and soon disappears. On rare occasions, however, a virus continues to circulate in the new host, either "whole" or after reassorting with another influenza virus. Some influenza A viruses have become adapted to circulate in pigs (swine influenza viruses), horses (equine influenza viruses), humans (human influenza A viruses) and dogs (canine influenza viruses). The ancestors of these viruses are thought to have originated in birds, either in the distant past or more recently. Further information about virus transmission between species can be found in the 'Influenza' factsheet.

SPECIES AFFECTED

Wild birds

The vast majority of LPAI viruses are maintained in asymptomatic wild birds, particularly birds in wetlands and other aquatic habitats, which are thought to be their natural reservoir hosts. Some species may maintain viruses long-term, while others might be spillover hosts. Infections are particularly common among members of the order Anseriformes (waterfowl, such as ducks, geese and swans) and two families within the order Charadriiformes, the Laridae (gulls and terns) and Scolopacidae (shorebirds). However, infections may be uncommon in some members of these orders. Within the Laridae, viruses tend to occur more often in gulls than terns. The prevalence of infection among wading birds (waders) is reported to be high in some areas, but low in others. Aquatic species belonging to other orders occasionally have high infection rates, and might also be involved in the epidemiology of this disease. For instance, infections among seabirds seem to be particularly common in murres (*Uria* spp.).

The most common influenza subtypes in wild birds may differ between species and regions, and can change over time. Migrating birds, which can fly long distances, may exchange viruses with other populations at staging, stopover or wintering sites. Virus diversity seems to be particularly high among charadriform birds. A few avian influenza subtypes seem to have a limited host range. Examples include H13 and H16 viruses, which have mainly been found in gulls and terns, and H14 viruses, which have been detected rarely and only in a few species.(i.e., in a few ducks, sea ducks and a herring gull). Such viruses may rarely (or never) be transferred to poultry.

LPAI viruses can also infect wild birds that live on land (terrestrial birds), such as raptors and passerines, but under ordinary conditions, infections seem to be uncommon in these species, and they are not thought to be important reservoirs.

Higher infection rates are occasionally reported in individual species, and in a study from Vietnam, viruses were particularly common in some terrestrial birds that forage in flocks, with an especially high prevalence in Japanese White-eyes (*Zosterops japonicus*). Similarly, a recent study from Central and West Africa detected influenza virus RNA in an unusually high percentage of passerine birds.

HPAI viruses are not usually found in wild birds, although they may be isolated transiently near outbreaks in poultry. Exceptions include the Asian lineage H5N1 viruses and some of their reassortants (e.g., H5N8 viruses), which have been found repeatedly in wild birds, an H5N3 virus isolated from an outbreak among terns in the 1960s, an H7N1 virus that was isolated from a sick wild siskin, *Carduelis spinus*, and an H5N2 virus found in a few asymptomatic wild ducks and geese in Africa.

Domesticated birds and mammals

When LPAI viruses from wild birds are transferred to poultry, the viruses may circulate inefficiently and die out; become adapted to the new host and continue to circulate as LPAI viruses; or if they contain H5 or H7, they may evolve into HPAI viruses. Once a virus has adapted to poultry, it rarely re-establishes itself in wild birds. HPAI and LPAI viruses have been found in many domesticated birds, including gallinaceous poultry and game birds, ducks, geese, ratites, pigeons and cage birds; however, some species seem to be more resistant to infection and/or illness than others. For example, there are few reports of infections in psittacine birds, and pigeons appear to be relatively resistant to infection compared to poultry.

Avian influenza virus infections have been detected occasionally in numerous species of mammals. Some of these species include cats, dogs, pigs, horses, donkeys, mink, and various wild and captive wild mammals. Ferrets can be infected experimentally with many viruses.

Important viral lineages and susceptible species

Poultry can be infected by many different LPAI and HPAI viruses, belonging to multiple subtypes, but three viral lineages are currently of particular concern. Some of these viruses have also been reported in mammals.

Host range of the Asian lineage H5N1 avian influenza viruses and reassortants including H5N8

The A/goose/Guangdong/1996 lineage ('Asian lineage') of H5N1 HPAI viruses first emerged among poultry in China in the late 1990s, and has become widespread and very diverse. Some variants of H5N1 differ in their virulence for mammals and/or birds. HPAI H5N2, H5N5, H5N6 and H5N8 viruses, resulting from reassortment between Asian lineage H5N1 viruses and other avian influenza viruses, have been reported among poultry in Asia. H5N8 viruses became widespread among birds in Asia and Europe in 2014. They reached

North America in late 2014, and have reassorted with North American lineage viruses to produce unique variants of other subtypes such as H5N1 and H5N2.

Whether wild birds can maintain Asian lineage H5 viruses for long periods (or indefinitely), or are repeatedly infected from poultry, is still controversial. However, the evidence that wild birds can transfer H5N1 HPAI viruses and some of their reassortants (e.g., H5N8) to new geographic regions now appears strong.

Asian lineage H5N1 HPAI viruses seem to have an unusually wide host range. These viruses can infect a wide variety of wild birds belonging to many different orders, including the Anseriformes and Charadriiformes. Both clinical cases and asymptomatic infections have been described. These viruses can also infect many species of mammals, and their full host range is probably not yet known. They have been found in pigs, cats, dogs, donkeys, tigers (*Panthera tigris*), leopards (*Panthera pardus*), clouded leopards (*Neofelis nebulos*), lions (*Panthera leo*), Asiatic golden cats (*Catopuma temminckii*), stone martens (*Mustela foina*), raccoon dogs (*Nyctereutes procyonoides*), palm civets (*Chrotogale owstoni*), plateau pikas (*Ochotona curzoniae*) and a wild mink (*Mustela vison*). Serological evidence of infection or exposure has also been reported in horses and raccoons. Experimental infections have been established in cats, dogs, foxes, pigs, ferrets, laboratory rodents, cynomolgus macaques (*Macaca fascicularis*) and rabbits. Cattle could be experimentally infected with viruses isolated from cats, but studies in Egypt detected no antibodies to H5N1 viruses in cattle, buffalo, sheep or goats, suggesting that these species are not normally infected.

Some Asian lineage H5 reassortants, such as an H5N2 virus isolated recently from a dog with respiratory signs, may be able to cause illness in mammals. This H5N2 virus could be transmitted from experimentally infected dogs to dogs, chickens and cats. There have been no reports of illnesses caused by Asian lineage H5N8 viruses in mammals, as of November 2015, although seropositive dogs were detected on some infected farms in Asia. Initial laboratory experiments in ferrets and mice reported low to moderate virulence in these species, suggesting that the currently circulating H5N8 viruses may be less pathogenic for mammals than some H5N1 isolates. In another study, virus replication was inefficient in experimentally infected dogs, which developed no clinical signs. Cats were more likely to become infected, and had mild and transient signs. Asian lineage H5N6 viruses have not, to date, been isolated from apparently healthy pigs.

Host range of Eurasian H9N2 (LPAI) avian influenza viruses

A Eurasian lineage of H9N2 (LPAI) viruses is currently widespread among poultry in some areas, and has become very diverse, with numerous reassortants, including some that share internal genes with H5N1 viruses. H9N2 viruses have been detected in wild birds including some terrestrial species.

H9N2 viruses have been found occasionally in pigs, and might sometimes cause clinical signs in this species. They have also been detected in dogs, and by serology in cats, and infections can be reproduced experimentally in both dogs and cats, although virus replication may be limited. Serological evidence of infection was found in performing macaques in Bangladesh, and in wild plateau pikas in China. Pikas could be infected experimentally. H9N2 variants may differ in their ability to replicate in mammals and/or cause disease.

Host range of the zoonotic H7N9 avian influenza viruses

An H7N9 LPAI virus, which has recently caused serious human outbreaks in China, circulates there in poultry. This virus acquired some of its genes from H9N2 viruses. It has diversified considerably since its introduction, and regionally distinct lineages now exist.

Among birds, infections have mainly been found in poultry (and in environmental samples from poultry markets, farms and similar sites), although this virus or its nucleic acids were also detected in two pigeons, an asymptomatic tree sparrow, and wild waterfowl. Whether wild birds play any role in spreading this virus is uncertain. Experimental infections have been established in Japanese quail (*Coturnix coturnix japonica*), several species of ducks, Embden geese, pigeons, zebra finches (*Taeniopygia guttata*), society finches (*Lonchura striata domestica*), house sparrows (*Passer domesticus*) and parakeets (*Melopsittacus undulates*), but pigeons and Pekin ducks were resistant to infection (requiring high doses), and only chickens and quail transmitted this virus efficiently to other birds. Nevertheless, some of these birds (including passerine birds and parakeets), shed high titers in oropharyngeal secretions, and may be capable of infecting humans.

There have been no reports of illnesses in mammals, as of November 2015, and no evidence of H7N9 infections was found among stray dogs living near live poultry markets. In experimental studies, isolates from humans could infect miniature pigs, ferrets, laboratory mice and cynomolgus macaques. At present, there have been no reports of infected pigs in China, and one serological survey reported little or no evidence of exposure in this species.

H7N7 LPAI viruses that resemble these H7N9 viruses in some of their genes have also been identified among poultry in China, and might have the potential to infect mammals.

Other avian influenza viruses reported in mammals

Infections caused by other avian influenza viruses are reported sporadically in mammals. In addition to H5N1 and Eurasian H9N2 viruses, diverse subtypes (e.g., H4, H5N2, H5N6, H6N6, H7, H10N5 and H11N2) have been isolated occasionally from pigs, especially in Asia, and antibodies to avian H3 viruses have also been found. While many infections with avian influenza viruses are transient, some established swine influenza viruses are wholly of avian origin or contain avian-origin gene segments. (The Swine Influenza factsheet has additional information about these viruses.) One avian H3N8 virus affected horses in China for a short time, starting in 1989, but did not persist long term. An H10N4 virus was responsible for an epidemic in farmed mink in Europe, and an H9N2 virus was recently isolated from this species in Asia. Experimental infections with H3N8, H4N6, H5N3, H7N7, H8N4, H9N2 and H11N4 avian influenza viruses have been established in mink.

Cats have been infected experimentally with some LPAI viruses (H1N9, H6N4, and H7N3) from waterfowl, as well as with an H7N7 HPAI virus isolated from a fatal human illness. An H6N1 virus was isolated from a dog coinfected with canine distemper virus, and dogs were also infected experimentally with an H6N1 LPAI virus. In addition, serological evidence of infection with H10N8 viruses has been reported in dogs. Domesticated guinea pigs in South America had antibodies to H5 influenza viruses.

Few studies have investigated wild animals; however, antibodies to H4 and H10 viruses were found in raccoons in the U.S. (in addition to antibodies to H1 and H3 viruses, which could also originate from mammals), and antibodies to H3N8 viruses, possibly of avian origin, were reported in Japan. Raccoons could be infected experimentally with an avian H4N8 virus, striped skunks (*Mephitis mephitis*) with H4N6 and H3N8 viruses, and cottontail rabbits with an H4N6 virus. A number of influenza viruses (H3N3, H3N8, H7N7, H4N5, H4N6 and H10N7), closely related to avian viruses, have been isolated from seals. Similarly, H1N3, H13N2 and H13N9 viruses, most likely of avian origin, have been isolated from whales. Antibodies to various subtypes, some maintained only in birds, have also been detected in seals, and in some cases, in sea lions, walruses (*Odobenus rosmarus*) or porpoises.

Laboratory mice (*Mus musculus*) and ferrets serve as models for mammalian infections with influenza viruses, including avian influenza viruses. Most laboratory mice have a defective gene (Mx1), which increases their susceptibility to influenza viruses compared to their wild-type progenitors. However, one recent study suggested that wild *Mus musculus* mice may also be susceptible to experimental inoculation with certain LPAI viruses. Wild house mice (*Mus musculus*) at the site of an H5N8 avian influenza outbreak in poultry had serological evidence of infection with influenza A viruses (either avian or mammalian), but confirmatory testing and identification of the serotype could not be done due to the low sample volumes, and the virus could not be detected directly. Some other studies have found no evidence for influenza viruses in wild mice.

Zoonotic potential

The two most commonly reported avian influenza viruses from human clinical cases have been the Asian lineage H5N1 HPAI viruses, and recently, H7N9 LPAI viruses in China. There have been no reported human infections caused by

Asian lineage H5N8 viruses, although four infections with H5N6 viruses have been reported in China since 2014. Illnesses caused by other subtypes have also been reported sporadically, with documented clinical cases caused by H9N2 (Eurasian lineage), H6N1 and multiple H7 and H10 avian influenza viruses. Whether these infections are truly less common than subtypes such as H5N1 is unclear: viruses that tend to cause milder illnesses (e.g., H9N2 viruses) are less likely to be identified than those causing severe disease. Serological surveys in some highly exposed populations suggest the possibility of low level exposure to HA types found in birds, including H4, H5, H6, H7, H9, H10, H11 and H12. Human volunteers were also infected with some subtypes (e.g., H4N8, H10N7 and H6N1), and sometimes developed mild respiratory signs and other influenza symptoms. Adaptation to humans is possible, though rare, and some previous human pandemics were caused by partially or wholly avian viruses.

GEOGRAPHIC DISTRIBUTION

LPAI viruses are cosmopolitan in wild birds, although the specific viruses differ between regions. These viruses are often absent from commercial poultry in developed nations, but they may be present in other domesticated birds. Eurasian lineage H9N2 viruses are currently widespread among poultry in parts of Asia and the Middle East. They have been detected in wild birds in Europe, where they also caused a few outbreaks in poultry flocks, and were isolated from game birds. The zoonotic H7N9 LPAI viruses causing outbreaks in mainland China have not been reported from other regions, with the exception of imported cases in travelers.

HPAI viruses are eradicated from all domesticated birds, whenever possible, and developed countries are usually HPAI-free. Asian lineage H5N1 HPAI viruses are currently considered to be endemic among poultry in a few nations in Asia and the Middle East, with outbreaks occurring at times in other countries in the Eastern Hemisphere. These H5N1 viruses can also be found in wild birds in Eurasia, but have not been detected in the Americas, Australia or New Zealand, as of 2015. Asian lineage HPAI H5N8 viruses were widely detected in Asia and Europe in 2014, and reached North America (the Pacific Northwest region) in late 2014. In North America, these viruses have reassorted with North American lineage viruses to generate unique viruses of other subtypes such as H5N1 and H5N2 (e.g., containing HA from the H5N8 virus and NA from a North American LPAI virus). Whether the H5N8 viruses or any of these reassortants will persist in the Americas is still uncertain. Worldwide eradication of the Asian lineage H5 viruses is not expected in the near future.

TRANSMISSION

Avian influenza viruses are shed in the feces and respiratory secretions of birds, although the relative amount of virus can vary with the specific virus, host species and other factors. The feces contain large amounts of virus in aquatic birds such as waterfowl, and the fecal-oral route is thought to predominate in wild bird reservoirs. Fecal-cloacal transmission might also be possible, but respiratory transmission is ordinarily thought to play little or no role. However, there are some exceptions. Some viruses that have adapted to gallinaceous poultry, such as recent isolates of Asian lineage H5N1 HPAI viruses, can be found in higher quantities in respiratory secretions than the feces, even in wild waterfowl. There are also reports of a few LPAI viruses found mainly in respiratory swabs from wild waterfowl, and respiratory spread might be important in some wild terrestrial birds.

Once an avian influenza virus has entered a poultry flock, it can spread on the farm by both the fecal-oral route and aerosols, due to the close proximity of the birds. Fomites can be important in transmission, and flies may act as mechanical vectors. The possibility of wind-borne transmission of HPAI viruses between farms was suggested by one study, but has not been conclusively demonstrated. Avian influenza viruses have also been found in the yolk and albumen of eggs from chickens, turkeys and quail infected with HPAI viruses. Although infected eggs are unlikely to hatch, broken eggs could transmit the virus to other chicks in the incubator. It might be possible for LPAI viruses to be shed in eggs, but the current evidence suggests this is very rare, if it occurs at all.

How long birds remain contagious differs between avian species, and with the severity of the infection (chickens and turkeys infected with HPAI viruses die very soon after infection). Most chickens usually excrete LPAI viruses for a week, and a minority of the flock for up to two weeks, but individual birds of some species, including waterfowl, can shed some LPAI or HPAI viruses for a few weeks in the laboratory.

Transmission of avian influenza viruses to mammals

People and other mammals are usually infected with avian influenza viruses during close contact with infected birds or their tissues, although indirect contact via fomites or other means is also thought to be possible. Respiratory transmission is likely to be an important route of exposure, and the eye may also act as an entry point. A few H5N1 HPAI virus infections in animals, and rare cases in humans, have been linked to the ingestion of raw tissues from infected birds. Housecats in an animal shelter might have become infected from contaminated avian feces, ingested while grooming. Feeding experiments provide evidence that H5N1 viruses can enter the body by the oral route in cats, pigs, ferrets, mice, hamsters and foxes, and transmission has been confirmed in cats by direct inoculation of the virus into the gastrointestinal tract. In humans, the strongest evidence for oral transmission is that two people became infected with an Asian lineage H5N1 virus after eating uncooked duck blood. There are other human cases where ingestion probably occurred, but additional routes of exposure also existed.

A ferret model suggested that some viruses might be transmitted to the fetus, when there is high viremia during systemic infections. Viral antigens and nucleic acids were also found in the fetus of a woman who died of an Asian lineage H5N1 infection. Transplacental transmission seems much less likely with influenza viruses that replicate only in the respiratory tract.

Host-to-host transmission of avian influenza viruses in mammals

Infected animals and people shed avian influenza viruses in respiratory secretions. Fecal shedding has been reported occasionally, although its significance is still uncertain. Some avian influenza viruses that have been detected in feces include Asian lineage H5N1 HPAI viruses in humans and experimentally infected cats and foxes; H7N9 viruses in humans; and Eurasian H9N2 viruses in experimentally infected dogs. Most studies used PCR, and the presence of live influenza viruses in feces was confirmed by virus isolation in only rare instances. The source of these viruses is still uncertain, and could be swallowed respiratory fluids, but Asian lineage HPAI H5N1 viruses seem to be able to replicate in human intestinal tissues. There are also reports of Asian lineage H5N1 HPAI viruses in the urine of some mammals.

Sustained transmission of avian influenza viruses is a rare event in mammals, but limited host-to-host transmission has caused clusters of infections or outbreaks in animals (e.g., in mink and horses). While most infected people do not seem to transmit avian viruses to others, including family members, Asian lineage H5N1 HPAI viruses are capable of person-to-person transmission in rare instances, and one H7N7 HPAI virus was found in a few family members of poultry workers in the Netherlands. Likewise, the H7N9 virus in China does not appear to spread readily between people, but human-to-human transmission was suspected in a few family clusters and one case of suspected nosocomial transmission in a hospital. Close, unprotected contact, seems to be necessary to transmit any of these viruses. Sometimes person-to-person transmission can be difficult to distinguish from exposure to a common source of the virus (e.g., on fomites).

Animal-to-animal transmission of Asian lineage H5N1 HPAI viruses was reported among tigers in one outbreak at a zoo, and experimentally between cats. However, asymptomatic, naturally infected cats appeared to excrete these viruses only sporadically, and there was no evidence for animal-to-animal transmission. In another study, there was no evidence for H5N1 virus transmission between small numbers of experimentally infected dogs and cats. One experiment indicated that H5N1 viruses are not transmitted between pigs, but recent evidence from Indonesia suggested that limited pig-to-pig transmission occurred within infected herds. Some authors have also speculated about the possibility of virus transmission between mammals and birds in wild ecosystems,

based on evidence from Qinghai Lake, China, where H5N1 viruses related to those previously found in wild plateau pikas were isolated from dead migratory birds in 2009-2010, although this clade had not been found in wild aquatic birds at this location in 2007. However, there was no serological evidence of exposure to H5 viruses in a recent study of plateau pikas in this area, despite evidence of exposure to H9 viruses.

Survival of influenza viruses in the environment

Fecal-oral transmission of avian influenza viruses in birds may be facilitated by prolonged survival in some environments. The persistence of these viruses can be influenced by many factors such as the initial amount of virus; temperature and exposure to sunlight; the presence of organic material; pH and salinity (viruses in water); the relative humidity (on solid surfaces or in feces); and in some studies, by the viral strain. Avian influenza viruses survive best in the environment at low temperatures, and some studies suggest that they are more persistent in fresh or brackish water than salt water. Some viruses may survive for several weeks to several months or more in distilled water or sterilized environmental water, especially under cold conditions. However, the presence of natural microbial flora may considerably reduce their survival in water, and at some temperatures, viruses may remain viable for only a few days (or less, in some environments) to a few weeks. Other physical, chemical or biological factors in natural aquatic environments may also influence persistence. Freeze-thaw cycles might help inactivate influenza viruses in cold climates.

In feces, some anecdotal field observations stated that LPAI viruses can survive for at least 44 or 105 days, but the conditions were not specified. Under controlled laboratory conditions, LPAI or HPAI virus persistence in feces ranged from < 1 day to 7 days at temperatures of 15-35°C (59-95°F), depending on the moisture content of the feces, protection from sunlight and other factors. At 4°C (39°F), some viruses survived for at least 30-40 days in two studies, but they remained viable for times ranging from less than 4 days to 13 days in two recent reports. On various solid surfaces and protected from sunlight, viruses were reported to persist for at least 20 days and up to 32 days at 15-30°C (59-86°F); and for at least 2 weeks at 4°C if the relative humidity was low; but also for less than 2 days on porous surfaces (fabric or egg trays) or less than 6 days on nonporous surfaces at room temperature. Survival was longer on feathers than other objects in two reports: at least 6 days at room temperature in one study, and 15 days at 20°C (68°F) and 160 days at 4°C in another report. Some viruses persisted for up to 13 days in soil (4°C), for more than 50 days (20°C) or 6 months (4°C) in poultry meat (pH 7), and for 15 days in allantoic fluid held at 37°C (99°F). Exposure to direct sunlight greatly reduced virus survival. Environmental sampling in Cambodia suggested that virus persistence in tropical environments might be brief: although RNA from Asian lineage H5N1 HPAI viruses was found in many samples including dust, mud, soil, straw and water, virus isolation was only successful from one water puddle.

DISINFECTION

Influenza A viruses are susceptible to a wide variety of disinfectants including sodium hypochlorite, 60% to 95% ethanol, quaternary ammonium compounds, aldehydes (glutaraldehyde, formaldehyde), phenols, acids, povidone-iodine and other agents. Influenza A viruses can also be inactivated by heat of 56-60°C (133-140°F) for a minimum of 60 minutes (or higher temperatures for shorter periods), as well as by ionizing radiation or extremes of pH (pH 1-3 or pH 10-14).

INFECTIONS IN ANIMALS

INCUBATION PERIOD

The incubation period in poultry can be a few hours to a few days in individual birds, and up to 2 weeks in the flock. A 21-day incubation period, which takes into account the transmission dynamics of the virus, is used for an avian population in the context of disease control. The incubation period for avian influenza viruses in mammals is also thought to be short, and might be as little as 1-2 days in some cases.

CLINICAL SIGNS

Low pathogenic avian influenza

LPAI viruses usually cause subclinical infections or mild illnesses in poultry and other birds. Decreased egg production, misshapen eggs, decreased fertility or hatchability of the eggs, respiratory signs (sneezing, coughing, ocular and nasal discharge, swollen infraorbital sinuses), lethargy, decreased feed and water consumption, or somewhat increased flock mortality rates may be seen in chickens and turkeys. Illnesses exacerbated by factors such as concurrent infections or young age can be more severe. Viruses with higher virulence might also exist. One unusual H10 virus isolated from waterfowl affected the kidneys and had a 50% mortality rate in some intranasally inoculated chickens.

Some gallinaceous game birds (e.g., quail, pheasants, guinea fowl, partridges) infected with LPAI viruses have been asymptomatic, while others had clinical signs including lethargy, respiratory signs such as sinusitis, conjunctivitis, decreased egg production and diarrhea. One study reported neurological signs and elevated mortality in guinea fowl (*Numida meleagris*) infected with an H7N1 virus. High mortality has been seen in young ostriches in some outbreaks; however, a virus isolated from one outbreak caused only green diarrhea in experimentally infected young birds. Domesticated waterfowl (e.g., ducks and geese) are often infected subclinically, although there may be mild signs such as sinusitis.

Wild birds infected with LPAI viruses usually have few or no obvious clinical signs, even during some epidemics among young birds at breeding colonies. However, subtle effects (e.g., decreased weight gain, behavioral effects or transient increases in body temperature) have been described in some cases.

The H9N2 viruses currently circulating among poultry in the Eastern Hemisphere appear to be relatively virulent, and may cause significant respiratory signs and malaise in chickens, including experimentally infected birds that are not co-infected with other pathogens. Both broilers and layers can be affected by these viruses. Although quail are usually mildly affected by most other LPAI viruses, clinical signs were reported in some H9N2 outbreaks and experimentally infected birds. One H9N2 virus caused severe clinical signs in experimentally infected quail, and mild signs in jungle fowl, while house sparrows developed respiratory signs, and crows (*Corvus splendens*) had mild or no signs. The zoonotic H7N9 LPAI viruses in China have caused only mild or asymptomatic infections in poultry and experimentally infected birds including poultry, parakeets and most songbirds. One house sparrow became ill with lethargy and loose droppings and died during this experiment, and one zebra finch died without clinical signs, but these deaths might not have been caused by the virus.

HPAI viruses in birds

HPAI viruses usually cause severe illness in chickens and turkeys, and few birds in infected flocks survive. Marked depression, decreased feed and water intake, and other systemic, respiratory and/ or neurological signs are often seen, but no signs are pathognomonic, and sudden death can also occur. Commonly reported signs include coughing, sneezing, sinusitis, blood-tinged oral and nasal discharges, ecchymoses on the shanks and feet, edema and cyanosis of the unfeathered skin on the head, comb and wattle (and snood in turkeys), and diarrhea. Egg production drops or ceases, and depigmented, deformed and shell-less eggs may be produced. Because a virus can be defined as highly pathogenic based on its genetic composition alone, HPAI viruses may rarely be found in chicken or turkey flocks that have mild signs consistent with low pathogenic avian influenza.

HPAI virus infections can be asymptomatic, mild or severe in other birds, including gallinaceous birds other than chickens and turkeys. Nonspecific clinical signs (e.g., anorexia, lethargy), neurological signs, diarrhea and sudden death have been reported in gallinaceous game birds, but milder or minimal signs were seen in some flocks. Domesticated waterfowl tend to be mildly affected, but respiratory signs (e.g., sinusitis), diarrhea, corneal opacity, occasional cases with neurological signs, and increased mortality may be seen, and some Asian lineage H5N1 HPAI viruses can cause severe acute disease with neurological signs and high mortality rates. Pigeons are also thought to be relatively resistant to illness, although there have been reports of sporadic deaths and rare outbreaks, with clinical signs that included neurological signs, greenish diarrhea and sudden death. Some pigeons that were experimentally infected with H5N1 viruses remained asymptomatic, while others became moderately to severely ill.

There is limited information about avian influenza viruses in ostriches, but HPAI viruses may not necessarily be more pathogenic than LPAI viruses in this species. The clinical signs tend to be mild in adult ostriches, and more severe in young birds less than 6 months of age, which can develop nonspecific signs (e.g., depression), dyspnea; green urine, diarrhea or hemorrhagic diarrhea, with increased mortality. Elevated mortality reported in some outbreaks in ostriches, pigeons and other relatively resistant birds might be caused by concurrent infections and other complications.

Studies in experimentally infected wild birds and observations in captive and wild birds suggest that some species can be severely affected by Asian lineage H5N1 HPAI viruses, while others may have much milder signs or shed viruses asymptomatically. During one H5N1 outbreak at a wildlife rescue center, some birds died without preceding clinical signs, while others developed anorexia, extreme lethargy, dark green diarrhea, respiratory distress and/or neurological signs, with death often occurring within 1-2 days. Some species at the facility did not seem to be affected. Neurological signs, varying from mild to severe, have been documented in a number of experimentally infected wild birds including some species of ducks, geese, gulls, house finches and budgerigars, as well as in naturally or experimentally infected raptors. Respiratory and nonspecific signs were reported in experimentally infected common reed buntings (*Emberiza schoeniclus*). Other experimentally infected birds, such as zebra finches and brown-eared bulbuls (*Hypsipetes amaurotis*), had high mortality rates, but only nonspecific signs of depression and anorexia, or sudden death. Starlings, pale thrushes (*Turdus pallidus*) and some species of ducks were mildly affected or unaffected, while house sparrows developed severe clinical signs in one study, and remained asymptomatic in another.

Asian lineage H5N8 viruses have also been associated with wild bird die-offs in some countries, and these viruses and/or their reassortants have been detected in wild birds including sick, dead and apparently healthy waterfowl, and sick or dead birds in several other orders including raptors. In some cases, the virus appeared to have affected the brain and the kidneys. Experimental infections with one H5N8 isolate were asymptomatic in mallards, and either fatal or asymptomatic in Baikal teal (*Anas formosa*).

Information about the effects of other HPAI viruses on wild birds is limited. Wild waterfowl infected with most viruses seem to be resistant to clinical signs, but an H5N3

HPAI virus caused high mortality among South African terns in the 1960s. A wild siskin naturally infected with an H7N1 HPAI virus was ill, and the same virus caused conjunctivitis, apathy and anorexia, with a high mortality rate, in captive canaries (*Serinus canarius*) that had been exposed to this bird.

Mammals infected with Asian lineage H5N1 viruses

Asian lineage H5N1 HPAI viruses have caused fatal disease, as well as milder illnesses or asymptomatic infections, in mammals. A few clinical cases have been described, at most, in each species. Both symptomatic and subclinical infections have been reported in felids. One cat had a fever, depression, dyspnea, convulsions and ataxia, and a few infected housecats were found dead. One of the latter cats was apparently well up to 24 hours before its death. Fatal illnesses with conjunctivitis and severe respiratory signs were described in experimentally infected cats. Asymptomatic infections were reported in housecats in an animal shelter that had been accidentally exposed to a sick, H5N1-infected swan. Some captive tigers and leopards died with clinical signs of respiratory distress, serosanguineous nasal discharge, high fever and neurological signs. In another outbreak, captive lions, tigers, leopards and Asiatic golden cats were lethargic and had decreased appetites (without respiratory signs) for 5-7 days, but recovered.

A dog that had eaten infected poultry developed a high fever, with panting and lethargy, and died the following day. However, serological and virological evidence of infection has also been found in stray dogs in China during routine surveillance. Most experimentally infected dogs remained asymptomatic or had relatively mild signs such as fever (which was transient in some studies), anorexia, conjunctivitis and/ or diarrhea. More severe respiratory signs (cough, labored breathing), with one fatal infection, were reported only in dogs inoculated directly into the trachea. A study that infected both dogs and cats found that the cats were more susceptible and developed severe clinical signs, while the dogs were more likely to have few or no signs despite shedding virus.

Experimental infections, as well as reports of infected herds, suggest that H5N1 HPAI virus-infected pigs usually remain asymptomatic or have only mild signs (e.g., mild respiratory disease and anorexia). Fever, respiratory and/or neurological signs, as well as sudden death, have been reported in a handful of cases in other species. One H5N1 virus was isolated from donkeys during a respiratory disease outbreak in Egypt, and a subsequent investigation detected antibodies to these viruses in healthy donkeys and horses in that country. The role of the H5N1 virus in this outbreak was unclear, as the affected donkeys responded well to antibiotics. Fatal respiratory disease, and possibly diarrhea, was reported in H5N1 virus-infected raccoon dogs, while captive palm civets had neurological signs, with evidence of interstitial pneumonia, encephalitis and hepatitis at necropsy, and a wild stone marten was found with neurological signs.

Mammals infected with other subtypes

Infections with influenza A viruses, apparently of avian origin, have been associated with outbreaks of pneumonia or mass mortality in seals. The clinical signs in some outbreaks included weakness, incoordination, dyspnea and subcutaneous emphysema of the neck. A white or bloody nasal discharge was seen in some animals. Experimental infections with these viruses were milder or asymptomatic, suggesting that co-infections may have increased the severity of the illness. An influenza virus was also isolated from a diseased pilot whale, which had nonspecific signs including extreme emaciation, difficulty maneuvering and sloughing skin. Whether this virus was the cause of the disease or an incidental finding is uncertain. Other viruses were isolated from whales that had been hunted, and were not linked with illness.

There are only a few reports of naturally acquired or experimental infections in other mammals, except in animal models for human disease (ferrets and mice). An H10N4 virus caused respiratory signs (sneezing, coughing, and nasal and ocular discharges) and elevated mortality in mink during an outbreak in Europe. An H9N2 virus outbreak among mink in China was characterized by mild respiratory signs, with no reported deaths. Respiratory signs were seen in a dog infected with an Asian lineage H5N2 HPAI virus in China, and this virus caused mild respiratory signs in experimentally infected dogs. One cat exposed to these dogs developed respiratory signs and conjunctivitis, but 4 other cats seroconverted without clinical signs. One study reported no clinical signs and inefficient virus replication in dogs that were experimentally infected with an Asian lineage H5N8 virus, while cats had mild and transient signs, including fever and marginal weight loss.

Coughing, sneezing and nasal discharge were reported in dogs inoculated with a Eurasian H9N2 virus, and 13 H9N2 viruses were isolated from sick and healthy dogs in a study from China. Some of the sick dogs in the latter study had clinical signs that could be consistent with influenza virus infections, but other infected dogs had signs likely to be unrelated. Dogs and cats experimentally infected with an H9N2 virus remained asymptomatic, although virus replication was detected, especially in cats. Few or no clinical signs were seen in cats inoculated with an H7N7 HPAI virus isolated from a fatal human case, cats inoculated with several LPAI viruses from waterfowl, or raccoons experimentally infected with an H4N8 virus.

No natural infections with the zoonotic H7N9 LPAI viruses in China have been reported, as of November 2015, and experimental inoculation of this virus resulted in fever alone in cynomolgus macaques and asymptomatic infections in miniature pigs.

POST MORTEM LESIONS

Low pathogenic avian influenza in birds

Poultry infected with LPAI viruses may exhibit rhinitis, sinusitis, congestion and inflammation in the trachea, but lower respiratory tract lesions such as pneumonia usually occur only in birds with secondary bacterial infections. Lesions (e.g., hemorrhagic ovary, involuted and degenerated ova) may also be observed in the reproductive tract of laying hens, and the presence of yolk in the abdominal cavity can cause air sacculitis and peritonitis. A small number of birds may have signs of acute renal failure and visceral urate deposition.

Highly pathogenic avian influenza in birds

The lesions in chickens and turkeys are highly variable and resemble those found in other systemic avian diseases. Classically, they include edema and cyanosis of the head, wattle and comb; excess fluid (which may be blood-stained) in the nares and oral cavity; edema and diffuse subcutaneous hemorrhages on the feet and shanks; and petechiae on the viscera and sometimes in the muscles. There may also be other abnormalities, including hemorrhages and/or congestion in various internal organs including the lungs, as well as severe airsacculitis and peritonitis (caused by yolk from ruptured ova). However, the gross lesions in some outbreaks may not fit the classical pattern, and birds that die peracutely may have few or no lesions.

Variable lesions have also been reported in other gallinaceous birds. Necrotic lesions in the pancreas (multiple foci of parenchymal discoloration) are common in quail and partridges infected with some HPAI viruses. There may also be splenomegaly with parenchymal mottling, renal lesions, hemorrhages in internal organs and skeletal muscles, and pulmonary lesions (consolidation, edema, congestion and hemorrhages). However, some lesions seen in chickens and turkeys, such as cyanosis and hemorrhagic lesions in unfeathered skin, may not be as prominent in other gallinaceous birds.

In ostriches infected with avian influenza viruses, the gross lesions are usually hepatitis and peritonitis, with other secondary lesions. Petechial hemorrhages, pancreatic lesions (e.g., multifocal hemorrhagic necrosis), pulmonary congestion and edema, and additional gross lesions have been reported in other species of birds infected with HPAI viruses.

Avian H5N1 influenza viruses in mammals

Asian lineage H5N1 HPAI viruses can cause systemic lesions as well as pulmonary lesions in some animals. Gross lesions reported in some cats and other felids included pulmonary consolidation and/or edema, pneumonia; hemorrhagic lesions in various internal organs; and in some cases, other lesions such as multifocal hepatic necrosis, hemorrhagic pancreatitis, or cerebral, renal and splenic congestion. Bloody nasal discharge, severe pulmonary congestion and edema, and congestion of the spleen, kidney and liver were reported in a naturally infected dog. Pulmonary lesions including interstitial pneumonia have been noted in some experimentally infected pigs, while others had mild to minimal gross lesions.

DIAGNOSTIC TESTS

Avian influenza viruses can be detected in oropharyngeal, tracheal and/or cloacal swabs from live birds, with differing recovery rates from each site depending on the virus, species of bird and other factors. Very small (pediatric) swabs can be valuable in small birds, but feces can be substituted if cloacal samples are not practical (e.g., cannot be collected without harming the bird). A recent study, which examined experimentally infected birds, suggested that immature feathers may also be a useful sample. Samples from internal organs (e.g., trachea, lungs, air sacs, intestine, spleen, kidney, brain, liver and heart) are also tested in dead birds suspected of having HPAI. Diagnostic tests should be validated for the species of bird, and some tests that are useful in chickens and turkeys may be less reliable in other avian species.

Virus isolation can be performed in all species, and can be useful for virus characterization. Avian influenza viruses are isolated in embryonated eggs, and can be identified as influenza A viruses with agar gel immunodiffusion (AGID), antigen-detection ELISAs or other immunoassays, or by a molecular test such as RT-PCR. They can be subtyped with specific antisera in hemagglutination and neuraminidase inhibition tests, by RT-PCR, or by sequence analysis of the viral HA and NA genes. Genetic tests to identify characteristic patterns in the HA (at its cleavage site) and/or virulence tests in young chickens are used to distinguish LPAI viruses from HPAI viruses.

RT-PCR assays can detect influenza viruses directly in clinical samples, and real-time RT-PCR is the diagnostic method of choice in many laboratories. Viral antigens can be detected with ELISAs including rapid tests. Currently, the World Organization for Animal Health (OIE) recommends that antigen detection tests be used to identify avian influenza only in flocks and not in individual birds.

Serology can be valuable for surveillance and demonstrating freedom from infection, but it is not very useful in diagnosing HPAI infections in highly susceptible birds, as they usually die before developing antibodies. Serological tests used in poultry include AGID, hemagglutination inhibition (HI) and ELISAs. AGID tests and ELISAs to detect conserved influenza virus proteins can recognize all avian influenza subtypes, but HI tests are subtype specific and may miss some infections. Cross-reactivity between influenza viruses can be an issue in serological tests. Tests that can distinguish infected from vaccinated birds (DIVA tests) should be used in surveillance when vaccination is part of a control program.

TREATMENT

There is no specific treatment for influenza virus infections in animals. Poultry flocks infected with HPAI viruses are depopulated (this is generally mandatory in HPAI-free countries), while the disposition of infected LPAI flocks may differ, depending on the specific virus and the country.

CONTROL

Disease reporting

A quick response is vital for containing avian influenza outbreaks, and in some cases, for minimizing the risk of zoonotic transmission. In addition to national notification requirements, HPAI viruses and LPAI viruses that contain H5 or H7 must be reported to the OIE by member nations. Veterinarians who encounter or suspect a reportable disease should follow their country-specific guidelines for informing the proper authorities (state or federal veterinary authorities in the U.S. for diseases in animals). Unusual mortality among wild birds should also be reported (e.g., to state, tribal or federal natural resource agencies in the U.S.)

Prevention

The risk of introducing a virus to poultry or other birds can be reduced by good biosecurity and hygiene, which includes preventing any contact with other domesticated or wild birds, mechanical vectors and fomites including water sources. All-in/ all-out flock management is helpful in poultry flocks, and birds should not be returned to the farm from live bird markets or other slaughter channels. To help prevent reassortment between human and avian influenza viruses, people are encouraged to avoid contact with birds while suffering flu symptoms.

Avian influenza vaccines may include both inactivated whole virus vaccines and newer recombinant vectored vaccines. Most vaccines are produced for chickens, although they may be validated for use in turkeys, and their effectiveness can differ in other species. In addition to suppressing clinical signs, some vaccines are capable of increasing resistance to infection, and decreasing virus excretion and transmission. However, clinical protection is not necessarily correlated with reduced virus shedding, and some birds can become infected even in the best case scenario. Thus, vaccination can mask infections if good surveillance programs are not used simultaneously. Vaccination can also place selection pressures on influenza viruses, which may encourage the emergence of vaccine-resistant isolates. In different countries, vaccines may be used routinely to protect poultry flocks, as an adjunct control measure during an outbreak, or to protect valuable species such as zoo birds from highly virulent viruses such as H5N1. Vaccination in the U.S. is restricted and requires the approval of the state veterinarian, and in the case of H5 and H7 vaccines, USDA approval.

During outbreaks, HPAI viruses are normally eradicated by depopulation of infected flocks, combined with other measures such as movement controls, quarantines and perhaps vaccination. Insect and rodent control, disposal of contaminated material, and thorough cleaning and disinfection are also important.

For mammals, prevention involves avoiding close contact with infected birds or their tissues. Keeping susceptible animals indoors may be helpful during outbreaks.

MORBIDITY AND MORTALITY

Birds

Exposure to influenza viruses and shedding patterns among wild birds are complex and likely to reflect their exposure to different habitats, as well as gregariousness and other social factors, and pre-existing immunity. Reported infection rates with LPAI viruses range from < 1% to more than 40%, and seroprevalence rates from < 1% to greater than 95%, typically with much higher rates in birds from aquatic environments than terrestrial species. Some studies have reported that infection rates are higher in young birds than adults (e.g., young egrets and herons at breeding colonies or young ducks). LPAI virus prevalence can also be higher during certain seasons, such as in late summer staging areas before migration, when bird densities are high and young "hatch year" birds have not yet developed immunity. Currently, surveillance suggests that carriage of H5N1 HPAI viruses in wild bird populations without unusual mortality events is rare.

The prevalence of influenza viruses in poultry differs between nations, but commercial poultry in developed countries are often free of both LPAI and HPAI viruses. Even in these regions, LPAI viruses may be present in backyard flocks, live poultry markets and similar sources. HPAI outbreaks are uncommon under ordinary conditions, while LPAI outbreaks tend to occur more often. However, the continued presence of Asian lineage H5 HPAI viruses in poultry elevates the risk of outbreaks throughout the world. These H5N1 viruses tend to reemerge during colder seasons in endemic areas.

Avian influenza differs in severity, depending on the species of bird as well as the virus. LPAI viruses usually cause mild illnesses or asymptomatic infections in birds, including chickens and ducks, but outbreaks can be more severe when there are concurrent infections or other exacerbating factors. High mortality is occasionally seen in young ostriches infected with either LPAI or HPAI viruses, although adult birds seem to be only mildly affected by both.

HPAI viruses usually cause high and rapidly escalating mortality in chicken and turkey flocks, with cumulative morbidity and mortality rates that may approach 90-100%. Any survivors are usually in poor condition and do not begin laying again for several weeks. Morbidity and mortality rates

can sometimes approach 100% in other domesticated and wild birds, but susceptibility can vary greatly, and certain species such as waterfowl tend not to be severely affected. Some Asian lineage H5N1 viruses cause severe illness even in waterfowl, and the introduction of these viruses may be heralded by unusual deaths among wild birds (e.g., swans in Europe and recently crows in Pakistan). Thousands of wild birds were killed in some outbreaks, such as one at Qinghai Lake, China in 2005. Wild bird deaths have also been associated with some Asian lineage H5 reassortants, such as H5N8 viruses, in Asia.

Mammals

Pigs seem to be infected fairly regularly by avian influenza viruses from birds, often with only minor consequences even when the virus belongs to the Asian lineage of H5N1 HPAI viruses. Low levels of exposure have been reported for H5N1, H9N2 and other subtypes in some endemic areas, with seroprevalence to these viruses typically ranging from < 1% to 5% and occasionally higher, and virus detection rates of < 1% to 7.5% in pigs during H5N1 outbreaks among poultry. Some studies reporting higher seroprevalence to H5N1 viruses examined pigs in poor neighborhoods where they are fed dead bird carcasses and other organic remains, and in one Egyptian study, 8 of 11 positive samples came from a single herd.

H5N1 HPAI virus infections reported in housecats and large zoo felids ranged from asymptomatic to fatal, while experimentally infected cats exhibited severe disease with high mortality. No seropositive cats were found in parts of Austria and Germany where these viruses had been found in wild birds, but low titers were detected in 8% of 25 cats in Egypt, and 73% of 11 cats in an unpublished study from Thailand. Recently, a survey of more than 900 healthy cats in northeastern China reported that approximately 2% had antibodies to H5N1 viruses, using the HI test, but no sera reacted in a confirmatory microneutralization assay. Another large survey, which examined 700 stray cats, found that a very small number of sera (3 cats) reacted to H5N1 viruses in both serological assays, and larger numbers of cats (18) had antibodies to H9N2 viruses. Several avian influenza viruses have been reported in dogs, although in some cases, there may be little information about the consequences of infection. While there is one report of a fatal H5N1 HPAI case in a dog, experimental infections have been mild or symptomatic in this species, except when the inoculation method bypassed normal upper respiratory defense mechanisms. Surveys reported antibodies to H5N1 viruses in 25% of dogs during outbreaks in Thailand, 4% of 25 dogs in Egypt (low titers), and 1% of stray dogs in live markets and on poultry farms in China, with virological confirmation of infection from 2 dogs in China by PCR. Eurasian lineage H9N2 viruses have also been isolated from dogs, and surveys in China reported seroprevalence rates to these viruses that ranged from < 5% (with evidence of infection in 0.4% of dogs by RT-PCR) to 20-45% in various populations of dogs. Unpublished work found serological evidence of exposure to H10N8 viruses in few feral dogs living near poultry markets, but whether this virus can affect dogs is not known.

The effects of Asian lineage H5N1 HPAI viruses on equids are still uncertain, but some surveys from Egypt reported that approximately 25% of donkeys and horses were seropositive. Fatal infections with these viruses have also been reported occasionally in other species such as raccoon dogs, palm civets and mink, but little more is known. An outbreak caused by a avian H10N4 virus in 1984 affected 33 mink farms in Sweden, with a morbidity rate of nearly 100% and mortality rate of 3%. However, an H9N2 outbreak among mink in China was reported to be mild, with no elevated mortality. The prevalence of this virus in mink is currently uncertain; however, mink on some other Chinese farms were also seropositive. The severity of influenza in mink is thought to be influenced by co-infections and other factors.

INFECTIONS IN HUMANS

INCUBATION PERIOD

Most zoonotic infections caused by Asian lineage H5N1 HPAI viruses seem to become apparent within approximately 5 days, although the incubation period for some cases may be as long as 8 and possibly 17 days. Estimates of the mean incubation period for the zoonotic H7N9 viruses have varied from 3 days (in two analyses, which considered large numbers of cases) to 5-6 days, with a range of 1-13 days.

CLINICAL SIGNS

Asian lineage H5N1 HPAI viruses

Most infections with Asian lineage H5N1 HPAI viruses have been severe. The initial signs are often a high fever and upper respiratory signs resembling human seasonal influenza, but some patients may also have mucosal bleeding, or gastrointestinal signs such as diarrhea, vomiting and abdominal pain. Respiratory signs are not always present at diagnosis; two patients from Vietnam had acute encephalitis without symptoms to indicate respiratory involvement. Similarly, a patient from Thailand initially exhibited only fever and diarrhea. Lower respiratory signs (e.g., chest pain, dyspnea, tachypnea) often develop soon after the onset of the illness. Respiratory secretions and sputum are sometimes blood-tinged. Most patients deteriorate rapidly, and serious complications including heart failure, kidney disease, encephalitis and multiorgan dysfunction are common in the later stages. Milder cases have been reported occasionally, particularly among children.

Three infections with Asian lineage H5N6 HPAI viruses in older adults were also severe, with fever and severe respiratory signs in at least two patients. One of these cases was fatal; the other patient required mechanical ventilation but recovered after treatment with oseltamivir and antibiotics (details of the third case have not been published). A child infected with an H5N6 virus had a mild illness with prompt recovery.

Eurasian lineage H9N2 LPAI viruses

Most illnesses caused by H9N2 viruses have been reported in children and infants. These cases were usually mild and very similar to human influenza, with upper respiratory signs, fever, and in some cases, gastrointestinal signs (mainly vomiting and abdominal pain) and mild dehydration. All of these patients, including a 3-month-old infant with acute lymphoblastic lymphoma, made an uneventful recovery. Acute, influenza-like upper respiratory signs were also reported in two adults, a 35-year-old woman and a 75-year-old man. Severe lower respiratory disease, which developed into respiratory failure, was seen in a 47-year-old woman, who had chronic graft vs. host disease and bronchiolitis obliterans after a bone marrow transplant, and was receiving immunosuppressive therapy. She survived after treatment with antiviral drugs, antibiotics for pneumonia, and supportive care, but required long-term oxygen supplementation on discharge.

Zoonotic H7N9 LPAI viruses in China, 2013-2014

Most clinical cases caused by H7N9 viruses in China have been serious, to date. The most common symptoms were fever and coughing, but a significant number of patients also had dyspnea and/or hemoptysis, and severe pneumonia (frequently complicated by acute respiratory distress syndrome and multiorgan dysfunction) developed in most laboratory-confirmed cases. A minority of patients had diarrhea and vomiting, but nasal congestion and rhinorrhea were not common initial signs. Conjunctivitis (which is a common sign with some other avian influenza viruses) and encephalitis were uncommon. In most cases, patients deteriorated rapidly after the initial signs. Concurrent bacterial infections were identified in some patients, and may have contributed to the clinical picture.

A few uncomplicated cases were characterized by mild upper respiratory signs or fever alone, especially in children. At least one asymptomatic infection has been reported in an adult.

Other avian influenza viruses

Mild illnesses, with conjunctivitis and/or upper respiratory signs, have been reported in a number of people infected with various H7 LPAI or HPAI viruses and an H10N7 virus. One H7N7 HPAI virus, which caused only mild illnesses in most people, resulted in fatal acute respiratory distress syndrome and other complications in one otherwise healthy person. His initial symptoms included a persistent high fever and headache, but no signs of respiratory disease. The virus isolated from this case had accumulated a significant number of mutations, while viruses from most other infected individuals had not, and it also caused severe illness in experimentally infected ferrets and mice. Severe illness (pneumonia) was reported in a person infected with an LPAI H7N2 virus; however, he had serious underlying medical conditions, including HIV infection and infection with *Mycobacterium avium* complex. This patient was hospitalized but recovered without antiviral treatment. A 20-year-old woman infected with an H6N1 virus in China developed a persistent high fever and cough, progressing to shortness of breath, with radiological evidence of lower respiratory tract disease. She made an uneventful recovery after treatment with oseltamivir and antibiotics. Severe lower respiratory tract disease, progressing in some cases to multiple organ failure and septic shock, was reported in three people with H10N8 infections in China. Two cases were fatal, one in a 73-year-old patient who had underlying health conditions, and another in a 75-year old. The third patient, who was 55 years of age, recovered after mechanical ventilation and treatment with various drugs including oseltamivir. The other two patients also received oseltamivir.

DIAGNOSTIC TESTS

Avian influenza viruses may be detected in samples from the upper and/or lower respiratory tract, depending on the site of the infection. RT-PCR is usually the primary test for Asian lineage H5N1 HPAI viruses. RT-PCR assays have also been published for the H7N9 influenza viruses causing outbreaks in China. Virus isolation can be performed, but it is slower. Antiviral resistance can be evaluated with phenotypic tests or gene-based testing to detect molecular markers of resistance, but is available in a limited number of laboratories, and takes several days to perform. Testing for novel influenza viruses is generally performed by state, regional or national public health laboratories, and in some cases by reference laboratories capable of handling dangerous human pathogens such as H5N1 HPAI viruses.

During routine influenza diagnosis, testing that identifies the presence of influenza A, but does not detect the hemagglutinins in common human influenza viruses, might indicate a novel, possibly zoonotic, virus. Commercial rapid diagnostic test kits used for seasonal human influenza virus infections may not detect avian influenza viruses.

Serology is used for epidemiological studies, and occasionally for retrospective diagnosis of a case. The microneutralization assay is considered to be the most reliable test for detecting antibodies to avian influenza viruses in humans, although other serological tests (e.g. hemagglutination inhibition) have also been used. No seroconversion occurred with some avian influenza viruses, even in virologically confirmed cases. Seroconversion might also vary with the severity of the illness (and the test): although adults with severe illnesses caused by the H7N9 virus in China seroconverted, titers were low or absent in a few mild cases in children.

TREATMENT

Treatment for avian influenza may vary, depending on the severity of the case. In addition to symptomatic treatment, it can include various drugs, including antibiotics to treat or prevent secondary bacterial pneumonia, and antivirals. Two groups of antiviral drugs – the adamantanes (amantadine, rimantadine), and neuraminidase inhibitors (zanamivir, oseltamivir, peramivir and laninamivir) – are effective against some influenza A viruses, but some of these drugs (peramivir and laninamivir) are not licensed in all countries. Antiviral drugs are most effective if they are started within the first 48 hours after the clinical signs begin, although they may also be used in severe or high risk cases first seen after this time. Oseltamivir appears to increase the chance of survival in patients infected with Asian lineage H5N1 and H7N9 viruses, particularly if it is given early. Side effects including gastrointestinal and CNS effects are possible, particularly with some drugs.

Antiviral resistance can develop rapidly in influenza viruses, and may even emerge during treatment. At present, Asian lineage H5N1 HPAI viruses are usually sensitive to oseltamivir, and they are often (though not always) resistant to adamantanes. Although resistance to zanamivir and oseltamivir has been reported, it is currently uncommon. Likewise, the H7N9 LPAI viruses are often sensitive to oseltamivir, and all of the H7N9 isolates from humans have contained a mutation suggesting resistance to adamantanes. Oseltamivir-resistant viruses of H7N9 viruses have also been described. One recent study documented low levels of resistance to neuraminidase inhibitors among avian influenza viruses in wild birds.

CONTROL

Protective measures for zoonotic avian influenza viruses include controlling the source of the virus (e.g., eradicating HPAI viruses, closing infected poultry markets); avoiding contact with sick animals, animals known to be infected, and their environments; employing good sanitation and hygiene (e.g., hand washing); and using personal protective equipment (PPE) where appropriate. While the recommended PPE can vary with the situation and risk of illness, it may include respiratory and eye protection such as respirators and goggles, as well as protective clothing including gloves. The hands should be washed with soap and water before eating, drinking, smoking, or rubbing the eyes.

Because HPAI viruses have been found in meat and/or eggs from several avian species careful food handling practices are important when working with raw poultry or wild game bird products in endemic areas, and all poultry products should be completely cooked before eating. Sanitary precautions and cooking methods recommended to destroy *Salmonella* and other poultry pathogens in meat are sufficient to kill avian influenza viruses, and eggs should be cooked until the whites and yolks are both firm. Wild birds should be observed from a distance, as they may be infected with some viruses, and hunters should not handle or eat sick game. H5N1 vaccines for humans have been developed in the event of an epidemic, but are not in routine use.

More detailed recommendations for specific groups at risk of exposure (e.g., people who cull infected birds, field biologists, and hunters) have been published by some national agencies, including the CDC, the Department of the Interior and U.S. Geological Survey National Wildlife Health Center in the U.S., and international agencies such as the World Health Organization. In some cases, recommendations may include antiviral prophylaxis (e.g., for people who cull birds infected with Asian lineage H5N1 HPAI viruses) and/ or vaccination for human influenza to reduce the risk of reassortment between human and animal influenza viruses. People who become ill should inform their physician of any exposure to avian influenza viruses.

MORBIDITY AND MORTALITY

H5N1 avian influenza

Between 1997 and September 2015, there were nearly 850 laboratory-confirmed human infections with Asian lineage H5N1 viruses, which generally occurred as the result of close contact with poultry. Illnesses caused by H5N1 viruses have been rare, overall; however, these viruses have been found in poultry (including small backyard flocks) for over a decade, resulting in high levels of human exposure. Increased numbers of human infections have been noted recently in Egypt, possibly due to the prevalence of certain viral strains. Most patients with illnesses caused by H5N1 viruses have been young and had no predisposing conditions. The case fatality rate for all laboratory confirmed cases reported to WHO has consistently been about 59-60% in the last few years. Likewise, a summary of confirmed, probable and suspected H5N1 cases documented worldwide between 2006 and 2010 found that 56% of these cases were fatal. However, the case fatality rate differs between countries and groups of patients. It is lower in young children than adults, and in patients with milder symptoms at the time of diagnosis. One study found that rhinorrhea was linked to improved survival, possibly because it was indicative of milder cases or upper respiratory disease. Conversely, delays in antiviral (oseltamivir) treatment were associated with a worse prognosis. The case fatality rate seems to be particularly low in Egypt, where 28% of confirmed, suspect and probable cases were fatal between 2006 and 2010, and the median age of patients was 6 years. Their young age, which tends to be associated with early diagnosis, as well as treatment-related factors and the virulence of the circulating viruses might be factors in the relatively high survival rate.

Antibodies to H5N1 viruses have been reported in some poultry-exposed populations that have no history of severe H5N1 disease, fueling speculation on the likelihood of

asymptomatic or mild infections. Most studies have reported seroprevalence rates of 0% to 5%, with a few reporting higher levels, and a meta-analysis of studies published before 2012 suggests that the overall seroprevalence is approximately 1-2% or less. Factors such as cross-reactivity with human influenza viruses in serological assays, or poor seroconversion to some avian viruses, might influence estimates of exposure, and the true prevalence of mild cases is still uncertain and controversial. Rare, laboratory confirmed, asymptomatic or mild cases have also been recognized. Rapid treatment with antiviral drugs might have been a factor in some of these cases; however, one child had only upper respiratory signs and made an uncomplicated recovery after antibiotic treatment alone. Prospective studies from Nigeria and rural Thailand documented rare instances of seroconversion to H5 avian influenza viruses, but were unable to find virological evidence of any avian influenza viruses during influenza-like illnesses. The occurrence of milder cases would be expected to lower the case fatality rate. However, it is possible that some severe cases have also been missed or attributed to other diseases; thus, the net effect of any undiagnosed cases is uncertain.

Three illnesses caused by Asian lineage H5N6 viruses in patients aged 49 years or older were severe; however, one infection in a child was mild. One of the two published cases in older adults was fatal; the other person recovered with intensive treatment.

H7N9 avian influenza

Approximately 680 laboratory-confirmed clinical cases, with at least 275 fatalities, have been caused by LPAI H7N9 viruses in China (or in travelers to China), as of September 2015. They mainly occurred in three waves to date, the first consisting of approximately 130 cases between February and May 2013, the second from October 2013 to May 2014, and the third beginning in Fall 2015, with sporadic cases reported between outbreaks. This H7N9 virus is circulating subclinically in poultry, and human illnesses have mainly been associated with live bird poultry markets, although infected farms have also resulted in at least one human illness. During the first wave, culling of live birds in wholesale markets, and closure of markets with cleaning and disinfection, were associated with declines in the number of human cases. However, many live markets were not closed, or re-opened after being closed for a short period. Significant environmental contamination with H7N9 viruses has since been reported in some new poultry slaughter and processing plants, which have replaced live bird markets or serve as an alternative in some areas.

Many of the clinical cases have occurred in older patients. During the first wave, 55% of the patients were older than 59 years. Elderly men were overrepresented in urban areas, particularly in locations where their traditional family roles result in increased exposure to retail live poultry, but men were not affected significantly more often than women in rural regions. Most reported cases in adults (including young and middle-aged adults) have been serious, while many cases in children were mild. Some cases may have been mitigated by prompt treatment with oseltamivir, but other mild cases occurred in people admitted to the hospital for observation alone, or were identified only after the person had recovered. Analyses of cases to October, 2014 reported case fatality rates in hospitalized, laboratory confirmed patients of approximately 36% to 48% during the first two waves, with the risk of death among hospitalized patients increasing significantly with age. Concurrent diseases or predisposing causes have been reported in a significant number of patients (e.g., 45% of cases in the first wave), although serious cases and fatalities also occurred in previously healthy individuals. Delayed treatment with antiviral drugs was also suggested as a possible factor in the high case fatality rate.

The likelihood of additional, undiagnosed mild or asymptomatic infections is still being assessed. In the majority of cases, there was no virological evidence of exposure among patient contacts who developed influenza-like signs. Some of the known mild cases were identified through national virological sampling of people with influenza-like illnesses. However, these samples are collected from people who visit primary care centers with influenza-like illnesses, and some cases could have been missed. Some initial serological studies found no H7N9 reactivity among poultry market workers, healthcare staff, patient contacts and other populations. However, several surveys have now detected antibody titers to H7N9 viruses in up to 17% of poultry workers or live bird market workers, with two studies documenting recent increases in seroprevalence. These studies report that seroprevalence rates are low (≤ 1%) in the general population, with one survey also documenting low seroprevalence in veterinarians. (2%). Although cross-reactivity with other H7 viruses that may circulate in poultry is possible, these surveys suggest that mild or asymptomatic infections may have occurred among poultry workers. As a result, some authors have suggested that the overall case fatality rate in all symptomatic cases might be as low as < 1% to 3%, if milder cases are also accounted for; however, such estimates currently have a high degree of uncertainty.

H9N2 avian influenza viruses

Clinical cases caused by Eurasian lineage H9N2 viruses have mainly been reported in children. Most cases, including an infection in an immunocompromised infant, have been mild, and were followed by uneventful recovery. Severe illness was reported in an adult with serious underlying medical conditions. Many serological studies have found antibodies to H9N2 viruses in < 1% to 5% of poultry-exposed groups in endemic regions; however, a few studies have reported higher seroprevalence rates, including 9% of agricultural workers in Bulgaria, 11% of poultry workers and 23% of live bird market workers in China, and 48% of poultry workers in Pakistan.

A review and meta-analysis of the literature, which included exposure to all H9N2 viruses worldwide in both Eastern and Western Hemispheres, reported a median seroprevalence of 5%, using the HI test. For microneutralization assays, the median seroprevalence rate was 3% (range < 1% to 9%) if the cutoffs employed by the authors of each study were used, and 0.3% (range 0.1% to 1.4%) if these cutoffs were adjusted to those recommended by the World Health Organization. A prospective study of adults with poultry exposure in rural Thailand reported rare instances of seroconversion to H9 viruses, but the two people who seroconverted did not report being ill, and no avian influenza viruses were detected in other people who had influenza-like illnesses.

Other avian influenza viruses

With the exception of the H7N9 viruses in China, most reported infections with H7 viruses in healthy people have been mild, whether they were caused by an LPAI or HPAI virus; however, one H7N7 HPAI virus caused a fatal illness in a healthy person, while affecting others only mildly. Mild signs were reported in poultry workers infected with an H10N7 virus in Australia, but H10N8 viruses caused fatal infections in two elderly patients in China and a serious illness in a 55-year-old. A young woman infected with an H6N1 virus in China had evidence of lower respiratory tract complications, but recovered with treatment. The possibility of other, unrecognized infections may be suggested by the occurrence of antibodies to various subtypes, generally at a low prevalence, in people who are exposed to poultry or waterfowl. Susceptibility (and/or seroconversion) might differ between viruses: 3.8% of poultry workers seroconverted during an H7N3 LPAI outbreak in Italy in 2003, but no seropositive individuals were identified in serum samples collected during H7N1 epidemics from 1999-2002. Rare seroconversion to H6, H7 and H12 viruses was reported in prospective studies of adults with poultry exposure in Cambodia and rural Thailand, but no clinical cases were identified.

BLUETONGUE

Sore Muzzle, Pseudo Foot-and-Mouth Disease, Muzzle Disease, Malarial Catarrhal Fever, Epizootic Catarrh, Beksiekte

IMPORTANCE

Bluetongue is a viral disease of ruminants transmitted by midges in the genus *Culicoides*. Bluetongue virus is very diverse: there are more than two dozen serotypes, and viruses can reassort to form new variants. This virus is endemic in a broad, worldwide band of tropical and subtropical regions from approximately 35°S to 40°N; however, outbreaks also occur outside this area, and it may persist long-term if the climate and vectors are suitable. While overwintering in regions with cold winters is unusual, bluetongue virus recently demonstrated the ability to survive from year to year in central and northern Europe.

Bluetongue virus can replicate in many species of ruminants, often asymptomatically. Clinical cases tend to occur mainly in sheep, but cattle, goats, South American camelids, wild or zoo ruminants, farmed cervids and some carnivores are occasionally affected. Cases range in severity from mild to rapidly fatal, and animals that survive may be debilitated. Additional economic costs result from reproductive losses, damaged wool and decreased milk production. Control of this vector-borne disease is difficult, except by vaccination. The existence of multiple serotypes complicates control, as immunity to one serotype may not be cross-protective against others.

ETIOLOGY

Bluetongue results from infection by bluetongue virus, a member of the genus *Orbivirus* and family Reoviridae. At least 26 serotypes have been identified worldwide. A few bluetongue viruses have additional names (e.g., Toggenburg orbivirus for the prototype strain of serotype 25). Isolates differ in virulence, and some strains seem to cause few clinical signs. Like some other viruses such as influenza virus, bluetongue viruses can reassort and recombine to produce new variants.

Bluetongue viruses are closely related to the viruses in the epizootic hemorrhagic disease (EHD) serogroup, a factor that can influence the development and/or selection of some diagnostic tests.

SPECIES AFFECTED

Bluetongue virus can infect many domesticated and wild ruminants including sheep, goats, cattle, water buffalo, African buffalo (*Syncerus caffer*), bison (*Bison* spp.*)*, various cervids, wild relatives of sheep and goats, wildebeest

(*Connochaetes* spp.) and other species. Both domesticated ruminants (especially cattle) and wild ruminants can be maintenance hosts. Infections are often subclinical. The virus can also infect camelids, and antibodies have been detected in some nonruminant wildlife including African elephant (*Loxodonta africana*), black and white rhinoceros (*Diceros bicornis* and *Ceratotherium simum*) and giraffe (*Giraffa camelopardalis*) in Africa, and collared peccaries (*Pecari tajacu*) in South America.

Among domesticated animals, clinical cases mainly occur in sheep; however, cattle, goats, yaks (*Bos grunniens*), llamas and alpacas were also affected in some outbreaks. In North America, cases of bluetongue have been documented in wild white-tailed deer (*Odocoileus virginianus*), pronghorn (*Antilocapra americana*) and bighorn sheep (*Ovis canadensis*), and captive Reeve's muntjac (*Muntiacus reevesi*) and greater kudu (*Tragelaphus cupensis*). There are no published reports of outbreaks among wild ruminants in Africa or Europe; however, clinical cases were reported in some zoo animals during serotype 8 outbreaks in Europe. Affected species included North American bison (*Bison bison)*, European bison/wisents (*Bison bonasus*), yaks, musk ox (*Ovibos moschatus*), Alpine ibex (*Capra ibex*), Siberian ibex (*Capra sibirica*) mouflon (*Ovis aries musimon*), blackbuck (*Antilope cervicapra*), fallow deer (*Dama dama*) and a Bactrian camel (*Camelus bactrianus*).

Accumulating evidence suggests that carnivores can also be infected by bluetongue virus. Antibodies to this virus have been detected in dogs, cats, cheetahs (*Acinonyx jubutus*), lions (*Panthera leo*), wild dogs (*Lycaon pictus*), jackals (*Canis* spp.) spotted hyenas (*Crocuta crocuta*) and large-spotted genets (*Genetta maculata*). Clinical signs have been reported in pregnant dogs infected by serotype 11, and nonpregnant Eurasian lynx (*Lynx lynx*) infected by serotype 8.

Zoonotic potential

Bluetongue virus is not zoonotic.

GEOGRAPHIC DISTRIBUTION

Bluetongue virus can be found worldwide within tropical and subtropical climates from approximately 35° S to 40° N, and in some areas outside this region (e.g., in parts of California). Endemic areas exist in Africa, Europe, the Middle East, North and South America and Asia, as well as on numerous islands (e.g., Australia, the South Pacific, the Caribbean). Multiple serotypes can be found in many regions.

Outbreaks can occur outside endemic areas, but in most cases, the virus does not persist once cold weather kills the *Culicoides* vectors. Unusually, a serotype 8 virus overwintered for multiple years in central and northern Europe.

TRANSMISSION

Bluetongue virus is mainly transmitted by biting midges in the genus *Culicoides,* which are biological vectors. These midges can fly short distances of 1-2 km, but they can be blown much farther by wind. Some species known to be effective vectors include *Culicoides sonorensis* in the United States; *C. brevitarsis* in Australia and parts of Asia; *C. imicola* in Africa, the Middle East, southern Europe and parts of Asia; *C. bolitinos* in some cooler regions of Africa; and *C. insignis* in the Caribbean, Central and South America and parts of the U.S. Additional species (e.g., members of the *C. obsoletus-dewulfi* complex in northern Europe) may be important locally. Other biting arthropods such as sheep keds (*Melophagus ovinus*), cattle lice (*Haematopinus eurysternus*), ticks and mosquitoes might be capable of transmitting the virus mechanically, but their role, if any, is thought to be minor. Bluetongue virus can also be spread mechanically on surgical equipment and needles. Some field strains and attenuated vaccine strains can infect the fetus *in utero*. Some of these animals can be born infected, and may introduce the virus to new areas if the dam is transported. Bluetongue virus can overwinter in some cold regions, by unknown mechanisms.

Bluetongue virus can persist in the blood of some animals for relatively long periods, facilitating transmission to *Culicoides*. Live virus has been isolated from some cattle for as long as 5 to 9 weeks, and viral RNA has been found much longer. Prolonged viremia has also been reported in other species, such as red deer (*Cervus elaphus*). However, animals eventually clear the virus, and there is no evidence that they remain persistently infected, even when infected *in utero*. Serotype 25 (Toggenburg orbivirus) in goats might be an exception. In one report, serotype 25 viral RNA was found for at least 2 years in individual animals, and the blood of some goats was infectious at 12-19 months.

At least some bluetongue strains (including members of serotypes 1, 8 and 26) can be transmitted directly between ruminants in close contact. This is a newly recognized route, and is generally thought to be of little epidemiological significance compared to transmission by midges. Serotypes 25 and/or 26 might be exceptions, as these viruses do not seem to replicate readily in some *Culicoides* vectors or in cell lines derived from these midges. The mechanisms of contact transmission are still uncertain. Suggestions have included shared feed and water troughs, contamination of wounds with blood during fighting among red deer, and contact with infected placentas in a case in cattle. Oral transmission of bluetongue virus has been demonstrated in colostrum, and experimentally via cultured viruses or urine from an experimentally infected sheep. Serotype 26 nucleic acids were found at low levels in nasal and ocular secretions of goats, and this virus was isolated from ocular swabs. Bluetongue virus can also be shed in semen.

How bluetongue virus infects carnivores is still uncertain. Seropositive dogs, cats and wild carnivores in Africa were thought to have eaten tissues from infected animals, and Eurasian lynx in a zoo had been fed ruminant fetuses and stillborn animals from outbreak areas. However, seropositive dogs in Morocco had not been fed raw diets, suggesting that they were infected by *Culicoides*. Bites from midges were also thought to have been responsible for some clinical cases among pregnant dogs in the U.S., although other routes (e.g., infection via semen or a contaminated semen extender) could not be entirely ruled out. Other dogs became infected when they accidentally received a bluetongue virus-contaminated vaccine. Transplacental transmission has been demonstrated in dogs, at least for serotype 11.

DISINFECTION

Disinfectants reported to be effective against bluetongue virus include sodium hypochlorite and 3% sodium hydroxide. Sodium hypochlorite, iodine (potassium tetraglicine triiodide) and a quaternary ammonium disinfectant (didecyldimethylammonium chloride) could inactivate another orbivirus, African horse sickness virus, and may also be active against bluetongue.

INCUBATION PERIOD

The incubation period is estimated to be approximately a week, with a range of 2-10 days.

CLINICAL SIGNS

Clinical cases of bluetongue occur mainly in sheep, while subclinical infections seem to predominate in most other species.

Sheep

Sheep infected with bluetongue virus may remain asymptomatic, or become mildly to severely ill. Common clinical signs include fever and depression; serous to mucopurulent nasal discharge, which may crust around the nostrils; and hyperemia of the muzzle, oral and nasal mucous membranes, conjunctiva and coronary band of the hooves. The muzzle, periocular region and face often become edematous; in some cases the swelling may also involve the ear and/or submandibular region, and occasionally even extends as far as the axillae. The lips and tongue may be very swollen in some animals; the tongue is occasionally cyanotic in severe cases, and may protrude from the mouth. Petechiae and ecchymoses can also develop on the muzzle, oral mucous membranes and coronary band. The oral lesions, which often include erosions and ulcerations, can result in drooling, soreness during eating, or anorexia. Involvement of the coronary bands leads to lameness, with hot and painful hooves; sloughing of the hooves is possible. The udder and teats may also have lesions, and muscle damage can result in torticollis. Some sheep with bluetongue develop pulmonary edema and die rapidly, with clinical signs of dyspnea.

Pregnant ewes can abort or give birth to lambs that are stillborn or have CNS lesions, retinal lesions and/or skeletal malformations. CNS lesions can result in neurological signs or "dummy" lambs that cannot nurse or follow the ewe. The specific syndromes vary with the stage of gestation, and lambs infected later in the pregnancy can be born normal.

Deaths are often the result of pulmonary edema in acute cases, or secondary bacterial complications and exhaustion when the course is more prolonged. In animals that survive, sequelae may include general loss of condition and hoof deformities. Some surviving sheep have abnormal wool growth, or lose some or all of their wool a few weeks after the illness, and poor quality semen has been reported transiently in rams. Mildly affected sheep usually recover rapidly.

Wild relatives of sheep and goats

Some bighorn sheep in North America or European mouflon affected by serotype 8 outbreaks in Europe had clinical signs resembling classical bluetongue in sheep, while other animals died suddenly without preceding signs. Hemorrhages were also reported. Nasal discharge and sudden death were seen in Alpine ibex in European zoos during the serotype 8 outbreaks. A Siberian ibex developed swelling of the head and neck, but survived.

Cattle and goats

Infections in cattle and goats are usually subclinical in endemic areas. These species are more likely to be affected when a naïve population is first exposed to bluetongue virus, such as during recent serotype 8 outbreaks in Europe. Clinical cases resemble the disease in sheep, but tend to be milder. Reported signs in cattle include inappetence, lethargy, facial edema, submandibular edema, oral inflammation with vesicles or ulcers in the mouth, excess salivation, nasal discharge, an elevated respiratory rate, edema of the distal limbs, and hyperemia of the coronary band with lameness. The muzzle of some cattle was reported to have a "burned" cracked appearance. Body temperature was sometimes normal. Cattle can also develop various skin lesions including vesicular and ulcerative dermatitis, periocular dermatitis, necrotic lesions, sloughing of affected skin and photodermatitis. In some cases, the skin may develop thick folds and cracks, particularly around the withers and neck. Udder and teat lesions, such as erythema, ulcers, cracking and necrotic lesions, have been reported in both cattle and goats, and milk production can be decreased. In some goats, a high fever and drop in milk production were reported to be the only sign. Abortions and stillbirths have been reported in both species, and congenital abnormalities including CNS lesions have been observed in newborn

calves. Temporary sterility may be seen in bulls. Deaths are possible, but uncommon.

Camelids

Only a few cases have been described in llamas and alpacas. Several fulminant, fatal infections were characterized by brief (< 24 hour) histories of severe respiratory distress, with recumbency or reluctance to rise, followed rapidly by death. Additional signs in some of these animals included coughing, foaming at the mouth, abnormal lung sounds, abortion, paresis and disorientation. Some reports described isolated cases; in others, a few additional llamas also had dyspnea, or were reported to have developed respiratory signs but recovered. In two studies, small numbers of experimentally infected llamas or alpacas had only mild signs (anorexia, mild conjunctivitis, periods of recumbency/signs of discomfort, low grade lung sounds) or remained asymptomatic.

Sudden death was reported in one Bactrian camel at a European zoo during serotype 8 outbreaks. Three dromedary camels experimentally infected with a serotype 1 virus remained asymptomatic.

Yaks, bison and musk ox

During serotype 8 outbreaks in Europe, some yaks, North American bison and European bison in zoos developed clinical signs resembling the illness in sheep. Corneal edema as well as conjunctivitis was reported in all three species, and some yaks had udder erythema with papules and crusts. Dyspnea occurred in some yaks and European bison, and sudden death was reported in all three species. Fever, lethargy, conjunctivitis and abortion were seen in a musk ox during this outbreak. North American bison inoculated with a serotype 11 isolate remained asymptomatic.

Cervids

While subclinical infections appear to be common in some species of cervids, a number of bluetongue cases have been reported in white-tailed deer. Syndromes reported in naturally- or experimentally-infected white-tailed deer include nonspecific signs such as fever, severe depression, anorexia and loss of normal fear responses, as well as signs similar to classical bluetongue in sheep. Some animals had severe respiratory distress, and others developed hemorrhagic signs including multifocal hemorrhages in the skin and mucosa, severe bloody diarrhea, or excessive bleeding and hematoma formation at venipuncture sites. Peracute disease characterized by head and neck edema, or acute cases mainly characterized by hemorrhages throughout the body, predominated in some epidemics, and were often fatal, Rumen and hoof lesions have been reported in white-tailed deer from areas where the disease was endemic. Lameness can persist after other signs have resolved. Syndromes reported in free-ranging pronghorn antelope in the U.S. include sudden death after the animals were disturbed, or a more prolonged illness (1-6 days), with signs of anorexia, decreased activity, recumbency and reluctance to move. Two pronghorn inoculated with a serotype 8 virus became depressed and inappetent, with labored breathing, and were able to stand only with extreme difficulty. Both cases were fatal

There is limited information other cervids. Although fatal illness associated with bluetongue infection has been reported in wild mule deer (*Odocoileus hemionus*) in the U.S., fever of a few days' duration was the only sign in experimentally infected black-tailed deer (*Odocoileus hemionus columbianus*). There are no reports of outbreaks or clinical cases among wild cervids in Europe, despite evidence of widespread exposure, particularly among red deer. Fallow deer and blackbuck (*Antilope cervicapra*) became ill during serotype 8 outbreaks at European zoos. The clinical signs in fallow deer included oral ulcers, excess salivation, difficulty eating and lameness in some animals, and sudden death in others. Sudden death was reported in blackbuck. Experimentally infected red deer (*Cervus elaphus*) and North American elk (*Cervus elaphus canadensis*), which are closely related, remained asymptomatic or only had mild clinical signs consisting of transient fever, mild conjunctivitis and diarrhea with small amounts of blood and mucus.

Carnivores

Bluetongue virus can cause abortions, sometimes accompanied by fatal illness, in dogs. Serotype 11 was involved in all cases to date. Four experimentally infected pregnant dogs died 5-10 days after aborting, or were euthanized with dyspnea. Some naturally infected dogs also died after an abortion, with respiratory distress and signs of heart failure in some cases. One dog was found dead after apparent recovery from a caesarean section the previous day. Other dogs aborted, but did not become ill. A few nonpregnant dogs inoculated with serotype 1 or 11 viruses remained well. The existence of healthy seropositive dogs in some endemic regions also suggests that some infections are asymptomatic.

Lethargy was the only clinical sign reported in 2 bluetongue virus-infected Eurasian lynx. One of these animals died after 2 days with a virologically confirmed infection. The other animal died several months later, and had only serological evidence of exposure at this time.

POST MORTEM LESIONS

In addition to the external lesions seen in living animals, such as facial edema and coronary band lesions, sheep may have hyperemia, hemorrhages, erosions and/or ulcers in the mucosa of the gastrointestinal tract from the mouth to the forestomachs, particularly where mechanical abrasion occurs (e.g., the buccal surface of the cheek and the mucosa of the esophageal groove and omasal fold). The heart may contain petechiae, ecchymoses and necrotic foci; in bluetongue, focal necrosis is particularly common in the papillary muscle of

the left ventricle. Subintimal hemorrhage at the base of the pulmonary artery is also characteristic. Pulmonary edema, which may be accompanied by pleural and pericardial effusion, is a common cause of death in fatal cases, and may be a prominent finding. Hyperemia, hemorrhages and/or edema may also be detected in other internal organs. In addition, the skeletal muscles may have focal hemorrhages or necrosis, and the intermuscular fascial planes may be expanded by edema fluid. Lesions in fetuses and newborn lambs can include cavitating lesions in the brain, hydranencephaly, porencephaly, retinal dysplasia and skeletal abnormalities.

Similar signs may be seen in other species. Pulmonary edema was the most prominent finding in llamas, alpacas, and experimentally infected pregnant dogs. Widespread petechial to ecchymotic hemorrhages were common in some animals, including some white-tailed deer. A Eurasian lynx that died with virologically confirmed bluetongue virus infection had gross lesions of petechial hemorrhages, subcutaneous hematomas, anemia and lung congestion with edema. A second lynx that died several months later was emaciated, with anemia, enlarged and gelatinous lymph nodes, petechial hemorrhages and pneumonia.

DIAGNOSTIC TESTS

Bluetongue virus can be found in blood from living animals, and in spleen, lymph node or bone marrow samples collected at necropsy. Reverse transcriptase-polymerase chain reaction (RT-PCR) tests are widely used to identify viral RNA in clinical samples, and can also identify the serotype. Bluetongue virus can be isolated in embryonated chicken eggs or various mammalian or insect cell lines (e.g., KC [*Culicoides variipennis*] cells). Animal inoculation in sheep or suckling mice is not usually employed, except where cell culture facilities are unavailable; however, it is reported to be more sensitive than isolation in cell culture. Blood samples for virus isolation should be collected as early as possible after infection. Bluetongue viruses are usually identified (i.e., to the bluetongue serogroup level) by RT-PCR. Immunofluorescence/immunoperoxidase staining, or group-specific antigen-capture ELISAs may also be used. Viruses can be serotyped by RT-PCR, gene sequencing or virus neutralization tests. Serotyping by virus neutralization can be difficult to interpret, as some serotypes cross-react in this assay.

Serology can be used to identify animals that have been infected or exposed to bluetongue virus. Antibodies typically appear 7 to 14 days after infection and are usually persistent. ELISAs are often used, but agar gel immunodiffusion (AGID) or virus neutralization can also be employed. AGID cannot reliably distinguish whether the animal was infected by bluetongue virus or epizootic hemorrhagic disease (EHD) virus; however, monoclonal antibody-based competitive ELISAs can distinguish antibodies to these two viruses. An indirect ELISA can detect antibodies to bluetongue virus in bulk milk samples. Complement fixation has largely been replaced by other tests, although it may still be used in some countries.

TREATMENT

No specific treatment is available, other than supportive care.

CONTROL

Disease reporting

Bluetongue is difficult to control once it has been transmitted to its vectors, and infections should be reported quickly in countries where this virus is not endemic. Reporting requirements in endemic areas may vary, depending on factors such as the existence of a control program. Appropriate sources (e.g., state authorities in the U.S.) should be consulted for the most current information.

Prevention

Bluetongue is mainly controlled by vaccination. Vaccines should be matched to the viral serotype; protection against other serotypes can be limited or nonexistent. Both attenuated and killed vaccines are currently made (although not necessarily sold in all regions), and multivalent vaccines are available. Attenuated vaccines are considered to be more effective than killed vaccines; however, midges may transmit these vaccine strains to unvaccinated animals during the vector season. Such vaccine strains could reassort with field strains, although how often this happens is currently unclear. Attenuated vaccine strains can also cause fetal malformations in pregnant ewes, and in some cases, may be able to cause systemic disease in highly susceptible animals.

Surveillance of sentinel animals may detect bluetongue viruses before outbreaks occur, and allow vaccination campaigns or other controls to be implemented early. Movement controls for infected animals (including pregnant, seropositive animals) may help limit virus introduction into new areas. Measures to reduce exposure to the *Culicoides* vectors may also be helpful during outbreaks or in endemic regions, although they are unlikely to be effective as the sole control measure. Such measures can include avoidance of environments where midges are more prevalent (e.g., low-lying, damp pastures), stabling animals from dusk to dawn, and/or the use of insecticides or insect repellents (e.g., insecticide-impregnated nets in stables) to help protect groups of animals. Effective vector control is challenging, due to factors such as the extensive breeding sites and large populations of *Culicoides*, and there are also environmental concerns with widespread use of pesticides. Some species of *Culicoides* are now known to enter barns and stables, especially late in the season when temperatures are becoming colder. Direct contact transmission is thought to have only a minor role in most outbreaks; however,

disinfection and other infection control measures might be considered in some situations.

MORBIDITY AND MORTALITY

Bluetongue is a seasonal disease in many areas, due to fluctuations in vector populations caused by cold temperatures or other factors such as rainfall. In regions where multiple serotypes circulate, the dominant serotypes may differ between years. Seroprevalence rates vary widely in endemic regions, ranging from 1% to more than 80% in domesticated and wild ruminants such as sheep, goats, cattle and cervids, as well as in some other species such as camels. In Europe, red deer seem to be the most important wildlife species; during serotype 8 outbreaks, more than half the red deer surveyed in some areas were seropositive. Some studies in endemic areas have not detected antibodies in South American camelids; however, 14% of these animals were seropositive during serotype 8 outbreaks in Germany, with rates varying from < 1% to 43% in different parts of the country. Infections in carnivores are still poorly understood, but antibodies were found in 21% of dogs sampled in an endemic region of Morocco, as well as in some dogs, cats and wild carnivores in Africa. A few seropositive dogs have been reported in the U.S.

Sheep are usually the most severely affected species, and in endemic regions, they are often the only domesticated animal with obvious clinical signs. Morbidity rates in sheep range from < 5% to 50-75% (or higher), and are usually at their highest when the virus is first introduced. The case fatality rate is typically < 30%, but can reach 50-90% in highly susceptible populations. Once a virus has become endemic, morbidity may decrease to low levels (e.g., 1-2%), with very few deaths. Outbreaks are uncommon where a virus circulates year-round. Other species such as cattle and goats can also be affected when a bluetongue virus is introduced into a naïve population. Many cattle became ill during recent serotype 8 outbreaks in Europe. Generally, cases in cattle and goats are milder than in sheep, and the mortality rate is lower. However, the case fatality rate was reported to be 26% in some goats infected with serotype 8 in Germany. Few cases have been documented in llamas and alpacas, and they were generally fatal. Among wildlife, whitetail deer and pronghorn antelope can be severely affected, with morbidity rates reported to be as high as 100% and case fatality rates up to 80-90%. Disease severity can also be influenced by factors such as the virus strain, host factors (e.g., immunity, general health, genetic factors, age and possibly breed) and environmental stressors.

BOVINE SPONGIFORM ENCEPHALOPATHY

Mad Cow Disease, BSE

IMPORTANCE

Bovine spongiform encephalopathy (BSE) is a fatal neurodegenerative disease, caused by a prion, that mainly affects cattle. Other ruminant species, cats, non-human primates and humans are occasionally affected; this disease is called feline spongiform encephalopathy (FSE) in cats, and variant Creutzfeldt-Jakob disease (vCJD) in people. BSE is a relatively new disease that was first reported in the United Kingdom in the 1980s. It is spread by ingestion; animals or humans become infected when they eat prion-containing tissues from an infected animal. Cooking and standard disinfection procedures do not destroy this agent. Infected animals or people do not become ill for years; however, the disease is always progressive and fatal once the symptoms develop.

The origins of BSE are unknown; however, the recycling of ruminant proteins in ruminant feed amplified this prion and caused an explosive epidemic in the U.K in the 1980s and 1990s. This epidemic peaked in 1992, with almost 1,000 new cases diagnosed each week. Although cases continue to be detected, control measures have greatly decreased their prevalence; fewer than 15 bovine cases were reported annually in the U.K. during 2009-2011. BSE also spread to many European countries, North America, parts of Asia, and possibly other areas of the world. The presence of BSE in a country can result in trade sanctions, as well as increased public concern about meat safety. Many nations, including the U.S., conduct control and surveillance programs. Many countries have also passed new regulations to prevent BSE-containing tissues from entering human or animal food supplies.

As a result of increased surveillance, BSE prions that differ from the prion causing 'classical' BSE have been identified at very low levels in cattle populations. Currently, it is thought that these "atypical" prions may represent a spontaneous form of prion disease. Some experiments suggest that an atypical prion might have given rise to the BSE epizootic when it was amplified in cattle feed.

ETIOLOGY

BSE is a member of the transmissible spongiform encephalopathies (TSEs), a group of neurodegenerative disorders caused by unconventional disease agents. These agents are resistant to the treatments that ordinarily destroy bacteria, spores, viruses, and fungi. They are generally thought to be prions, although a minority opinion suggests that TSEs may be caused by virinos or retroviruses. Prions are infectious proteins that appear to replicate by converting a normal cellular protein into copies of the prion. The cellular protein, which is called PrP^c, is found on the surface of neurons. Pathogenic isoforms of PrP^c are designated PrP^{res}; PrP^{Sc} or PrP^{TSE} are other names for this protein. Prions that cause different diseases (e.g. BSE or scrapie) are considered to be different strains of PrP^{res}.

In addition to the 'classical' BSE prion, at least two atypical BSE prions can be found in cattle. One has higher molecular mass fragments than classical BSE and is called 'H-type' BSE or H-BSE; the other has a lower molecular mass and is called 'L-type' BSE or L-BSE. Some authors call the disease caused by the latter organism 'bovine amyloidotic spongiform encephalopathy (BASE).' Atypical BSE prions are thought to represent additional strains of BSE. Currently, the most likely hypothesis is that these prions arise spontaneously in cattle, similarly to some prion diseases in other species (e.g., spontaneous Creutzfeldt-Jakob disease in humans). Atypical L-BSE has been reported to change to a classical BSE phenotype on transmission to inbred mice or to some transgenic mice. Similarly, H-BSE developed features of classical BSE in some wild type mice. This has led to the suggestion that one of these prions may have originally given rise to the BSE epidemic after amplification through the food chain.

SPECIES AFFECTED

BSE mainly occurs in cattle, but the host range of this prion is unusually broad compared to most prions. BSE has been reported from exotic ruminants in zoos; affected species include nyala (*Tragelaphus angasi*), kudu (*Tragelaphus strepsiceros*), gemsbok (*Oryx gazella*), eland (*Taurotragus oryx*), Arabian oryx (*Oryx leucoryx*), scimitar-horned oryx (*Oryx dammah*), ankole cattle, and bison (*Bison bison*). Rare field cases have been documented in goats, and experimental infections have been reported in both sheep and goats. European red deer (*Cervus elaphus elaphus*) are susceptible to oral exposure at a high dose, as well as to intracerebral inoculation, and develop neurological signs. BSE prions have also caused disease in various felids including housecats, cheetahs (*Acinonyx jubatus*), pumas (*Felis concolor*), ocelots (*Felis pardalis*), tigers (*Panthera tigris*), and Asian golden cats (*Catopuma temminckii*). (See the feline spongiform encephalopathy factsheet for details on infections in felids.) Two lemurs at a French zoo were apparently infected in contaminated feed. In addition, the BSE agent has been experimentally transmitted to mink, mice, marmosets, squirrel monkeys (*Saimiri sciureus*) and cynomolgus macaques (*Macaca fascicularis*). Pigs could be infected by the intracranial, intravenous, and intraperitoneal routes, but short-term feeding trials did not cause disease. One study reported that sea bream

(*Sparus aurata*) might be susceptible to infection, although they did not develop clinical signs.

L-BSE can infect cynomolgus macaques by intracerebral inoculation. It has also been transmitted to lemurs by the oral route, with the development of neurological signs. L-BSE and H-BSE can infect mice by intracerebral inoculation.

Zoonotic potential

Humans occasionally develop variant Creutzfeldt-Jakob disease following ingestion of prion-containing tissues from an infected animal.

GEOGRAPHIC DISTRIBUTION

Cases of BSE have been reported in indigenous cattle in most European countries, Canada, the U.S., Israel, and Japan. This disease was seen in imported cattle in the Falkland Islands and Oman. Some countries including Iceland, Australia, and New Zealand appear to be free of BSE. The presence or absence of this disease cannot be determined in countries without adequate surveillance programs. Atypical BSE prions have been reported in Europe, the U.S., Canada, and Japan, as the result of surveillance programs for BSE. They are also likely to exist in other countries.

TRANSMISSION

BSE is usually transmitted when an animal or human ingests tissues containing the BSE prion. Young animals may be particularly susceptible to infection; some studies suggest that most cattle become infected with BSE during the first six months of life. The prions are thought to replicate initially in the Peyer's patches of the ileum, then are transported via the peripheral nerves to the central nervous system (CNS). In cattle, prions can accumulate in the brain as early as 24 months after infection. The risks of transmission from various tissues are still incompletely understood; however, the highest prion concentration occurs in the CNS and ileum. In naturally infected cattle, BSE prions have been found mainly in the brain, spinal cord, retina, and distal ileum, but more sensitive techniques have recently detected this agent in the dorsal root ganglia, peripheral nerves (including the optic, facial and sciatic nerves), and adrenal glands. In experimentally infected cattle, it has been reported from the CNS, dorsal root ganglia, trigeminal ganglion, thoracic ganglia, some peripheral nerves, distal ileum (particularly in the Peyer's patches), jejunum, ileocecal junction, cecum, colon, myenteric plexus of the intestines, adrenal glands, tonsils, and bone marrow. In one animal, immunostaining detected prions in the macrophages of the subiliac lymph nodes but not other lymph nodes tested. In this animal, very weak immunostaining was also detected in the renal tubular epithelial cells, the thymus, and the islets of Langerhans. Using a very sensitive system (transgenic mouse bioassay), infectivity was recently detected in the tongue and nasal

mucosa of cattle in the terminal stages of the disease, although no prions could be found by immunoblotting or the protein misfolding cyclic amplification (PMCA) method. Unpublished data suggested that BSE prions might occur in the lymphoid tissues of nictitating membranes, but no evidence to confirm this has been published.

In some tissues, the quantity of prions may be low or the incidence rare, and the risk of transmission is uncertain. Some tissues may contain prions only in the late stages of the disease. For example, the accumulation of these agents in the peripheral nerves and adrenal gland seems to coincide with or follow prion accumulation in the CNS. Classical BSE has not been found in muscle, except in one sample tested by mouse bioassay, where infectivity was thought to be associated with the endings of the sciatic nerve. However, meat could become contaminated with CNS tissues during slaughter or processing. For this reason, high-risk slaughter and processing techniques have been banned in many nations (see 'Prevention'). Epidemiological evidence and transmission studies suggest that BSE is not transmitted in milk, semen, or embryos.

There is no evidence that BSE is transmitted horizontally between cattle; however, there is an unexplained increase in the risk of BSE among the offspring of infected animals. In one study, the risk that a calf would develop BSE appeared to be higher when the dam was in the later stages of infection (i.e., nearer to the onset of clinical signs). These observations have led to speculation that vertical transmission might be possible. If it occurs, vertical transmission seems to be rare, and the route is unknown. One model suggested that the cumulative risk of BSE transmission from dam to offspring is about 2%; however, the confidence interval included zero.

BSE transmission in experimentally infected sheep resembles transmission in cattle, but the prions are more widely disseminated in the body, and additional routes of transmission may occur. In sheep inoculated orally, BSE prions are readily found in many lymphoid tissues including the spleen, lymph nodes, and gut-associated lymphoid tissue (GALT), as well as in the CNS. Blood-borne transmission has been demonstrated in this species. Transmission from two ewes to their lambs occurred in an experimental flock; it is not known whether this event took place *in utero* or soon after birth.

Atypical BSE

In cattle, some studies report that the tissue distribution of atypical L-BSE and H-BSE seems to resemble that of classical BSE, with prions detected mainly in the CNS. (There are, however, some differences in the pattern of distribution within the brain.) H-BSE and L-BSE have also been found in peripheral nerves and sensory receptors (muscle spindles) and the trigeminal ganglion in some studies, and L-BSE was detected in the adrenal gland. In a recently published study,

PrP^{res} was reported to occur in the muscles of L-BSE infected cattle by immunostaining, and infectivity was found in muscle homogenates using a transgenic mouse bioassay.

Very little is known about the potential for vertical transmission. One calf born to a cow in the late stages of infection with L-BSE did not have any evidence of infection.

Transmission to humans and iatrogenic spread

In humans, variant Creutzfeldt-Jakob disease usually results from the ingestion of BSE prions. Based on studies in humanized transgenic mice, some authors have suggested that BSE isolates from sheep and goats might be more readily transmitted to humans than isolates from cattle. Iatrogenic transmission has also been seen. Probable person-to-person spread was reported in several patients who received blood transfusions from asymptomatically infected individuals. There is also potential for transmission by routes such as transplantation or the use of prion-contaminated equipment during surgeries. Prions can be found in the brain, spinal cord, dorsal root ganglia, trigeminal ganglia, retina, optic nerves, and lymphoid tissues of humans with vCJD. Although prions are particularly common in the spleen, tonsils, appendix and other gut-associated lymphoid tissues (GALT), they can also be found in lymph nodes throughout the body. Prions have been found in the appendix as early as two years before the onset of clinical disease. They have not been demonstrated in human blood, but this may be due to the insensitivity of the assays used to detect these agents. Person-to-person transmission of vCJD does not occur during casual contact.

Origins of the BSE epidemic

The origins of BSE are not well understood. This disease was first reported in the 1980s, but it was probably present in cattle since the 1970s or earlier. The two most popular hypotheses are that BSE originated as a spontaneous PrP^c mutation in cattle, or that it came from a mutated scrapie prion that contaminated ruminant feed. Other sources suggest that BSE might have originated from a wildlife population or a human TSE agent. Once the BSE agent entered cattle populations, it was amplified by recycling tissues from infected cattle into ruminant feed supplements, mainly as meat-and-bone meal (MBM). MBM is a rendered concentrate derived from animal offal and carcasses. Rendering cannot completely inactivate prions, but the epidemic may have been facilitated by changes in rendering practices that allowed more prions to survive.

Banning ruminant tissues from ruminant feed has significantly reduced the number of new cases of BSE, but cases have been reported in cattle born after these regulations came into effect ("born-after-the-ban" cases). These cases might be caused by the use of imported feed components produced under inadequate quality controls, illegal feeding of ruminant proteins, or cross-contamination of cattle feed with swine or poultry feed. Theoretical possibilities include inadequate heating of bone meal or tallow used in concentrates and milk replacers, horizontal transmission, or environmental reservoirs. Current diagnostic techniques are not sensitive enough to detect very low levels of prions, and there is little information on prion survival in the environment; however, hamster-adapted scrapie prions have been shown to survive in the soil for at least three years.

DISINFECTION

Prions can differ in their resistance to inactivation, and one study found that BSE prions from cattle were more resistant than prions from human spontaneous Creutzfeldt-Jakob disease (CJD), mouse-passaged BSE prions, or hamster prions.

Decontamination of prion-contaminated tissues, surfaces, and environments is difficult. These agents are highly resistant to most disinfectants (including formalin), heat, ultraviolet radiation, and ionizing radiation, particularly when they are protected in organic material or preserved with aldehyde fixatives, or when the prion titer is high. Prions can bind tightly to some surfaces, including stainless steel and plastic, without losing infectivity. Prions bound to metal seem to be highly resistant to decontamination. Few effective decontamination techniques have been published. A 1-2 N sodium hydroxide solution, or a sodium hypochlorite solution containing 2% available chlorine, has traditionally been recommended for equipment and surfaces. Surfaces should be treated for more than 1 hour at 20°C (68°F). Overnight disinfection is recommended for equipment. Cleaning before disinfection removes organic material that may protect prions. In experiments, milder treatments including a phenolic disinfectant, an alkaline cleaner (KOH with detergents), and an enzymatic cleaner combined with vaporized hydrogen peroxide were shown to inactivate scrapie prions. The alkaline cleaner and phenolic disinfectant were also effective against BSE and vCJD prions. New commercial decontaminants have been developed for prions. In one experiment, the most effective commercial reagents, using a rodent prion on stainless steel wires, were those that contained proteolytic agents. One of these solutions was prepared in an 2 M NaOH alkali carrier, which may have contributed to its effectiveness. A commercial alkali/detergent reagent was unable to completely decontaminate the wires.

Physical inactivation of prions can be carried out by porous load autoclaving at 134-138°C (273-280°F) for 18 minutes at 30 lb/in², but residual infectivity has been demonstrated in some studies. Autoclaving items in water is more effective than autoclaving without immersion. Dry heat is less effective; hamster-adapted scrapie prions can survive dry heat at temperatures as high as 360°C (680°F) for an hour. A combination of chemical and physical decontamination can be more effective than either procedure alone; chemical disinfection should be carried out first, then the items should be rinsed and autoclaved. Anecdotal evidence suggests that decontamination of contaminated facilities is very difficult.

Even the harshest combination of chemical and physical disinfection is not guaranteed to destroy all prions. In experiments, a stainless-steel wire remained infectious after cleaning with sodium hydroxide and autoclaving. Surgical instruments that have undergone repeated cycles of cleaning and disinfection have transmitted the sporadic (genetic) form of CJD iatrogenically. For this reason, disposable equipment and instruments may be recommended instead of disinfection during some medical procedures.

INFECTIONS IN ANIMALS

INCUBATION PERIOD

The incubation period for classical BSE is estimated to be 2 to 8 years in cattle. The peak incidence of disease occurs in four to five year old animals. Atypical BSE is usually detected in cattle that are at least eight years of age. Some research suggests that the incubation period might be shorter for atypical L-BSE than classical BSE; however, this is based on comparisons in intracerebrally inoculated cattle and bovinized transgenic mice.

The incubation period in experimentally infected sheep varies with the animal's age and genetic susceptibility, and the route of exposure and dose. In genetically susceptible sheep, the incubation period was 21 to 38 months for animals inoculated orally at six months of age, and 18 to 24 months in lambs inoculated orally at two weeks of age. In genetically resistant (ARR/ARR) sheep, the incubation period was approximately 3 to 5 years.

One European red deer challenged by the oral route developed clinical signs after approximately 4 years, 9 months, while four other deer were still healthy more than 5 years after challenge. In experimentally infected macaques inoculated orally, the incubation period was 3.6 to 5 years.

CLINICAL SIGNS

Cattle with classical BSE

Bovine spongiform encephalopathy is a neurological disease that usually has an insidious onset in cattle. The clinical signs may include gait abnormalities (particularly hindlimb ataxia), hyperresponsiveness to stimuli, tremors, and behavioral changes such as aggression, nervousness or apprehension, changes in temperament, and even frenzy. The combination of behavioral changes, hyperreactivity to stimuli, and gait abnormalities is highly suggestive of BSE, but some animals exhibit only one category of neurological signs. Pacing, a modified gait in which the legs move in lateral pairs, occurred in 25% of the cattle with BSE in one study, and may be suggestive of this disease. Intense pruritus is not usually seen in cattle, but some animals may lick or rub persistently.

Nonspecific signs include loss of condition, weight loss, teeth grinding (possibly due to visceral pain or neurological disease), and decreased milk production. Decreased rumination, bradycardia, and altered heart rhythms have also been reported. The signs of BSE usually worsen gradually over a few weeks to six months, but rare cases can develop acutely and progress rapidly. Rapid, acute onset neurological disease seems to be particularly common in exotic ruminants in zoos. Once clinical signs appear, BSE is always progressive and fatal. The final stages are characterized by recumbency, coma, and death.

Cattle with atypical BSE

The features of atypical BSE in cattle are still incompletely understood. Most atypical strains have been found in asymptomatic cattle during routine surveillance, in fallen stock ('downer' cattle), or at emergency slaughter. However, H-BSE associated with neurological signs was reported in a 19-year-old zebu bull (Bos indicus) at a zoo. Experiments (all using intracerebrally inoculated cattle) have reported varying clinical signs, with some researchers concluding that L-BSE can be distinguished clinically from classical BSE, and others reporting that the spectrum of clinical signs overlaps to a greater or lesser extent between all forms of BSE.

In Friesian and Alpine brown cattle, one group of researchers reported that an Italian isolate of L-BSE mainly causes a form characterized by inactivity, mental dullness, and muscle atrophy, which could be distinguished from classical BSE. The early clinical signs included muscle fasciculations, a dull coat, decreased alertness, low carriage of the head, and mild kyphosis. These signs progressed to muscle atrophy, which began in the gluteal region and progressed to involve other areas, with relative sparing of forelimb muscles. Although a "downer" cow was reported in this study, other animals did not develop ataxia or difficulty rising. However, sudden falls were seen. The animals in this study were reported to be hyperresponsive to tactile facial stimuli, but not to light or sound. In this experiment, the same breeds inoculated with classical BSE prions developed behavioral changes including aggressiveness, bellowing and head shaking, as well as postural abnormalities and hyperresponsiveness to stimuli.

Another group reported that, in Holstein-Friesian cattle inoculated with German isolates of H-BSE and L-BSE, the first signs were weight loss and loss of condition. Animals tended to separate from the herd and carried their head low. However, these cattle were hyperresponsive to acoustic and visual stimuli as well as tactile facial stimuli, similarly to cattle with classical BSE. Ataxia and difficulty rising were also reported in this experiment. These researchers concluded that, although the initial signs appear to be more nonspecific and subtle in atypical BSE, the differences are not sufficient to unambiguously distinguish these forms from classical BSE.

Another experiment used Danish Holstein/Aberdeen Angus crosses inoculated with an Italian L-BSE strain and an H-BSE strain. Both "dull" and "nervous" forms of the illness were reported in this study. Behavioral, sensory, and motor signs were all seen, and cattle infected with H-BSE and L-BSE had similar clinical signs. Low head carriage and separation from the herd did not occur consistently, and most of the animals had no signs of dullness. Instead, many animals became hyperreactive to external stimuli including tactile and facial stimuli. No cattle developed tremors. In this study, the cattle tended to develop dysmetria and have difficulty in rising, early in the course of the disease, but none progressed to permanent recumbency (unlike animals with classical BSE that develop ataxia).

A study that used a Japanese L-BSE isolate in Holstein cattle reported decreased activity, hyperresponsiveness to stimuli, ataxia mainly of the hindlegs, difficulty rising, and little aggression.

Sheep with classical BSE

Various neurological signs have been reported in experimentally infected sheep. In one study, Cheviot sheep mainly developed ataxia with minimal pruritus, and died in a few days to a week. In indigenous French breeds, the signs included ataxia and intense pruritus with loss of fleece. These animals deteriorated slowly and died in approximately three months. A third study mainly used ARQ homozygous Suffolk and Romney sheep, but also included a few individuals of other breeds, and reported that the clinical signs were similar in all animals. Pruritus was detected in all clinically affected sheep in this study (however, it should be noted that this sign was also reported in 29% of the sheep that did not have evidence of BSE at slaughter). Other signs in some animals included behavioral changes, teeth grinding, movement abnormalities including tremor and ataxia, hyperresponsiveness to auditory stimuli or decreased menace response in a few animals, and weight loss and loss of body condition. Altered behavior combined with ataxia and pruritus was detected in 40% of these sheep. The course of the illness lasted 16 to 20 weeks before animals were culled due to the progression of neurological signs.

Goats with classical BSE

The few BSE cases that have been reported in naturally infected goats were discovered during routine surveillance at slaughter. One goat was reported to be a scrapie suspect. Neurological signs have been reported in experimentally infected animals. In one study, the disease was characterized by ataxia and tremors, and progressed rapidly in intracerebrally inoculated goats; however, the signs in orally inoculated goats were mainly lethargy and weight loss, which progressed to recumbency over three weeks. Ataxia was not seen in orally inoculated goats, and neither intracerebrally nor orally inoculated goats had signs of pruritus. In another study, intracerebrally inoculated Saanen goats developed abnormalities in movement (e.g., ataxia, tremors, postural

deficits, and especially hypermetria) and hyperresponsiveness to stimuli. Over the course of the experiment, sniffing and nibbling of the animal handlers and instruments changed to aversive behavior, including head tossing or shaking, or kicking, and these signs became more pronounced with time. One goat carried its head low when undisturbed and was inappetent. Other signs in some animals included pruritus, an absent menace response, teeth grinding, and weight loss.

POST MORTEM LESIONS

Gross lesions are not found in BSE, with the exception of nonspecific signs, such as emaciation or wasting. The histopathologic lesions are confined to the CNS. Neuronal vacuolation and non-inflammatory spongiform changes in the gray matter are characteristic of the disease in cattle. These lesions are usually but not always bilaterally symmetrical. Amyloid plaques are not typical of classical BSE or infection with H-BSE, but are associated with L-BSE prions. Similar spongiform changes occur in experimentally infected sheep and macaques.

DIAGNOSTIC TESTS

There is no live animal test for BSE. This disease is usually diagnosed by detecting prions (PrP^{res}) in the CNS. Accumulations of prions can be found in unfixed brain extracts by immunoblotting, and in fixed brains by immunohistochemistry. In addition, several rapid diagnostic tests based on enzyme-linked immunosorbent assays (ELISAs), automated immunoblotting (Western blotting) and lateral flow devices (LFD) are available. Rapid tests allow large numbers of samples to be screened, and are often used in surveillance and slaughter testing. Positive samples in rapid tests are traditionally confirmed with more specific assays such as immunohistochemistry or immunoblotting. However, the OIE now states that confirmation of positive results with a second rapid test is acceptable under some circumstances. Preferred test combinations, which are not in danger of producing false positives by the use of shared reagents, are listed on the OIE website. Two rapid tests can only be used to confirm a BSE case; a negative result on the confirmatory test is not adequate to rule out BSE, and should be investigated with other assays. A diagnosis of BSE may also be confirmed by finding characteristic prion fibrils called scrapie-associated fibrils (SAF) with electron microscopy in brain extracts. Some of these tests can be used on frozen or autolyzed brains. Techniques used diagnostically to detect prions are relatively insensitive compared to assays for other types of pathogens; prions cannot usually be detected in the brain until 3 to 6 months before the onset of disease.

Atypical prions can be detected with the same tests, including rapid tests, in animals infected with H-BSE or L-BSE. A complete evaluation of the rapid tests has not been done for these prions. The distribution patterns of H-BSE and L-BSE in the brain differ somewhat from that of classical BSE, as well as from each other; however, all three prions can be detected in the obex. Atypical prions can be differentiated from classical BSE prions by their biochemical properties, for example by immunoblotting. H-BSE has higher molecular mass fragments than classical BSE. It also reacts with a monoclonal antibody to an N-terminal epitope that is not found in classical BSE after proteinase K cleavage. L-BSE has a lower molecular mass than classical BSE prions. Its glycosylation pattern differs from classical BSE, and it has an unusual deposition pattern characterized by amyloid plaques.

Histological examination of the brain can be very helpful in diagnosis, but some animals in early stages of infection have few or no spongiform changes. In addition, BSE can be detected by transmission studies in mice; however, an incubation period of several months makes this technique impractical for routine diagnosis. Serology is not useful for diagnosis, as antibodies are not made against the BSE agent.

TREATMENT

There is no treatment for BSE. Suspect animals are usually euthanized for testing.

CONTROL

Disease reporting

Veterinarians who encounter or suspect BSE should follow their national and/or local guidelines for disease reporting. In the U.S., state or federal veterinary authorities should be informed immediately.

Prevention

Some nations conduct active surveillance of cattle at slaughter (using rapid tests) to detect cases of BSE. Active surveillance for BSE has been conducted in the E.U. since 2001; however, the age limits have increased since the programs began. As of 2011, cattle that must be tested (with rapid tests) in most E.U. member states include animals over the age of 48 months that die, undergo emergency slaughter, are killed for reasons other than human consumption, or display certain abnormalities at ante-mortem inspection. Healthy cattle over the age of 72 months and intended for human consumption must also be tested. Lower age limits apply to cattle from some other areas. Japan has unusually strict requirements. At one time, the Japan government required all cattle to be tested for BSE. Since 2005, only cattle that are 21 months of age or older must be tested; however, there has been public resistance to relaxing testing requirements, and local authorities have continued to test all slaughtered cattle regardless of age. Some countries may also conduct BSE surveillance in small ruminants.

Some countries with a low incidence of disease, including the U.S., test only a percentage of cattle at slaughter. In the

U.S., surveillance is targeted particularly at high risk cattle such as nonambulatory animals and those with neurological disease. These animals cannot be used in human food, and the carcass is held until testing is complete. The U.S. also conducts passive surveillance for BSE. When an infected animal is identified, the affected herd is quarantined, and the source of the infection is investigated. Due to the increased risk of BSE in the offspring of infected cattle, they are usually traced and euthanized.

BSE can be prevented by not feeding ruminant tissues that may contain prions to susceptible species. Complete avoidance is generally necessary, as cooking or rendering cannot completely inactivate prions. Many nations have now banned the use of either ruminant or mammalian proteins, with certain exceptions such as milk and blood, in livestock feed. The specific bans, and protein sources prohibited, vary with the country. In some countries, bans also apply to other animal feeds, or even to fertilizer. The latter measures can help prevent cross-contamination and accidental exposure of cattle to BSE prions. Preventing prions from re-entering the ruminant food chain can interrupt transmission and control BSE epidemics; however, due to the long incubation period, the number of BSE cases may not decline for some time. In addition, countries may place trade bans on the importation of live cattle and certain ruminant proteins from affected countries.

BSE suspects are usually euthanized for testing. These carcasses cannot be used as food and must be destroyed. In the U.K., BSE carcasses are rendered at 133°C (3 bar pressure) for at least 20 minutes.

MORBIDITY AND MORTALITY

Classical BSE is seen most often in four to five year old cattle, particularly dairy animals. This disease is always fatal once the symptoms appear. The prevalence of BSE varies widely. At one time, the estimated prevalence in various countries ranged from more than 100 cases per million cattle to fewer than two cases per million. The latter are defined as World Organization for Animal Health (OIE) 'minimal risk' countries for BSE. Control measures have greatly decreased the prevalence in the most severely affected nations since that time.

BSE epidemics were reported in several European countries. The first outbreak occurred in the U.K., where more than 180,000 cases have been confirmed since the 1980s. The U.K. epidemic peaked in 1992, with nearly 1,000 new cases confirmed each week. At the time, the annual incidence in affected herds was approximately 2-3%. As a result of control measures (particularly feed bans), the incidence declined to approximately 5-10 new cases per week in 2004. This number continued to drop, with the annual incidence decreasing to 99 confirmed cases in 2006, 35 cases in 2008, and 7 to 11 cases each year between 2009 and 2011. The peak of the epidemic curve occurred later in countries where feed bans were established more recently. In the U.S., only four cases of BSE have been reported. One case occurred in an animal imported from Canada. Three additional cases have been reported in indigenous cattle; one was caused by the H-form of atypical BSE. The most recent case (April 2012) was infected by an L-BSE prion.

As of 2012, approximately 60 cases of L-BSE or H-BSE have been identified worldwide as a result of surveillance for classical BSE. The incidence of atypical BSE appears to be much lower than classical BSE. Its prevalence among cattle in France and Germany may be as low as 1 case per 3 million adult cattle. Nearly all L-BSE and H-BSE prions have been detected in cattle over the age of 8 years, with the exception of an L-BSE prion reported from a 23-month old steer in Japan.

Cases of BSE are very rarely reported in goats. Infections have not been seen in sheep or deer other than experimentally infected animals. Surveillance conducted in Europe suggests that the prevalence of BSE is very low in sheep, if it occurs at all. Estimates of the maximum proportion of sheep TSE cases that could be BSE range from 0.7% to 5%. Experimentally infected sheep that are genetically resistant to scrapie seem to have some resistance to BSE, but are not immune to infection or disease.

INFECTIONS IN HUMANS

INCUBATION PERIOD

The incubation period for vCJD is difficult to establish with certainty; however, the average incubation period is estimated to be 11 to 12 years, and incubation periods up to 16 years have been reported. In three cases transmitted in blood transfusions, the incubation period was 6 to 8.5 years. For comparison, some other human prion diseases have similar median incubation periods, but have been reported up to 40 years after exposure.

CLINICAL SIGNS

The symptoms of vCJD are broadly similar to the sporadic (genetic) form of CJD, but usually appear in younger patients. The median age of onset is 26 years (range 12 to 74 years). The first signs are usually psychiatric symptoms, such as anxiety, depression, insomnia, social withdrawal, and/or persistent painful sensory symptoms. In most patients, frank neurological signs such as gait disturbances, ataxia, incoordination, memory loss, slurring of speech, and tremor appear a few months later; however, neurological signs coincide with or precede psychiatric symptoms in a minority of patients. Cognitive function gradually deteriorates. Chorea, dystonia, myoclonus, visual disturbances, and dementia typically develop late in the course of disease. Most patients die in six months to two years.

DIAGNOSTIC TESTS

A tentative diagnosis can be made before death by the history, clinical signs, and cortical atrophy on magnetic resonance imaging (MRI) of the brain. The electroencephalogram (EEG) is sometimes normal during the early stages of disease, but later develops characteristic abnormalities. A definitive diagnosis can be made if the abnormal prion protein is found in tonsil biopsies by immunoblot (Western blot) or immunohistochemistry. In other cases, the diagnosis is made by microscopic examination of brain tissue, usually at necropsy. Numerous amyloid plaques surrounded by vacuoles are found in vCJD; such plaques are seen in only 5-10% of cases of sporadic (genetic) CJD. Large amounts of prion protein can be found around the plaques by immunohistochemistry.

TREATMENT

No treatment is available, other than supportive care.

CONTROL

Variant Creutzfeldt-Jakob disease can usually be avoided by not eating tissues from BSE-infected cattle. Active surveillance of cattle at slaughter (using rapid tests) to detect cases of BSE, performed in some nations, can help decrease the risk to humans. Tissues that have a high risk of transmitting BSE have been banned from human food in many countries. In the U.S., prohibited tissues include the brain, skull, eyes, trigeminal ganglia, dorsal root ganglia, spinal cord, and most of the vertebrae from cattle 30 months of age and older. The tonsils and distal ileum from all cattle are also banned. In the E.U., banned tissues include the skull (including the brain and eyes but not the mandible) and spinal cord in cattle over 12 months of age, and the spinal column in cattle over 30 months of age. The tonsils, entire intestines, and mesentery are not allowed from any cattle. Slaughter and processing techniques that have a high risk of contaminating muscle tissues with CNS have been prohibited in many countries, including the U.S.

Person-to-person transmission of vCJD can be reduced by the use of disposable surgical instruments in high risk surgeries, when this disease is suspected. Because prions can be found in the tonsils, some authors also suggest that disposable equipment always be used during tonsillectomies, in countries with a significant risk of this disease. Transmission in blood cannot be completely prevented with current techniques; however, many countries do not allow people who have spent time in the U.K. and/or other European countries to be blood donors. Some countries have taken other measures, such as universal leucodepletion of blood, to reduce the risk of vCJD. Prion filters have been developed to reduce infectivity in plasma, but are still being evaluated and are not in wide use. Some countries import fresh frozen plasma from low-risk countries for patients without dietary exposure to BSE (e.g., patients born after 1996 in the U.K.).

Although laboratory or abattoir-related cases have not been reported, veterinarians and laboratory workers should always take precautions when conducting necropsies on BSE suspects or handling tissues; BSL-3 is the recommended level of protection. Standard precautions include the use of protective clothing and the avoidance of penetrating injuries, contamination of abraded skin, and ingestion. A negative pressure laminar flow hood should be used for tissue manipulations whenever possible. Because prions may be able to survive in the environment for years and are difficult to disinfect, precautions should be taken to avoid contamination of surfaces and equipment. Disposable plastic-coated paper sheets can be used to protect tables and other surfaces. Disposable instruments and work clothing can also be used. No vaccine is available.

MORBIDITY AND MORTALITY

The prevalence of vCJD is unknown. Most cases have been seen in people who lived in either the U.K. or France during the peak of the BSE epidemic. As of April 2012, 176 cases of vCJD had been reported in the U.K. The incidence peaked in 2000, when 28 cases were diagnosed, and gradually fell to five cases per year in 2005. Between 2006 and 2011, two to five cases were reported each year. As of April 2012, 25 cases had been reported from France, as well as four from the Republic of Ireland, five from Spain, three each from the United States and the Netherlands, and two from Canada, Portugal, and Italy. Japan, Saudi Arabia, and Taiwan have each reported one case. To date, all cases of vCJD in the U.S. seem to have been acquired in other countries. The number of people who are infected but asymptomatic is unknown. Based on the pattern of infection in the U.K, some sources suggest that, at most, 70 additional cases can be expected; however, surveillance conducted on appendectomy samples in the U.K. suggested a prevalence of 237 cases per million population, with 95% confidence intervals of 49-692. Another study, based on samples from tonsils, estimated a prevalence of 1 case per 10,000 population.

Variant Creutzfeldt-Jakob disease is usually seen in young patients. The reason is unknown, but it is possible that children and adolescents are more susceptible to infection than adults. The median age of onset is 26 years for vCJD (range 12 to 74 years); in contrast, it is 65 years (range 15 to 94 years) in the sporadic (genetic) form of Creutzfeldt-Jakob disease. People who are homozygous for methionine at codon 129 in the PrPC protein have an increased risk of developing vCJD. All clinical cases have occurred in people with this genotype. One infection was reported in a person who was heterozygous for methionine/valine at this codon, but did not develop vCJD symptoms. This person became infected in a blood transfusion and died of unrelated causes after five years. It is not known whether people with resistant genotypes (valine/valine or methionine/ valine) are completely resistant to the development of disease, or simply have a longer incubation period. Once the symptoms of vCJD develop, this disease is always fatal.

As of 2012, no human infections have been reported with atypical BSE prions, but these prions are also likely to be of zoonotic concern. In particular, L-BSE seems to be more virulent than classical BSE in intracerebrally inoculated macaques and humanized transgenic mice, with a shorter incubation period and more rapid progression. There is currently no evidence that this is the case for H-BSE; however, H-BSE (like L-BSE) is capable of changing to resemble classical BSE in transgenic mice.

CANINE INFLUENZA

IMPORTANCE

Influenza is a viral disease that has long been known to affect birds and some mammals, but was only recently recognized in dogs. Each influenza virus is maintained in one or more related host species; however, host specificity is not absolute. A virus may occasionally infect other animals, or on rare occasions, become adapted to a new species. No influenza viruses were known to circulate in dogs until 2004-2006, when a virus caused outbreaks of severe and often fatal respiratory disease among racing greyhounds in the U.S. This virus was acquired from horses, and probably entered greyhound populations several years before these outbreaks. Although it has spread to other dogs since this time, the illness in these animals has been more typical of influenza. The most common syndrome is a relatively mild upper respiratory disease with a persistent cough. Pneumonia is possible, generally as the result of secondary infection with bacteria or mycoplasma, but uncommon. At present, infections tend to be seen mainly in animal shelters, kennels, dog day care facilities, or other sites where groups of susceptible dogs are in close contact. This virus does not seem to have spread widely in other pets, and it has not yet been reported outside North America.

A second canine influenza virus was recognized in 2007, when a different virus caused an outbreak of severe respiratory disease in South Korea. This virus seems to have been acquired from birds, and may have entered canine populations around 2005. It was subsequently reported in China and Thailand, and can affect cats as well as dogs. Many reported clinical cases from Asia have been severe, but antibodies have been found in significant numbers of healthy dogs and cats there, suggesting that some animals have milder illnesses. This virus entered North America in 2015. While large numbers of cases have been reported among dogs in the U.S., there have been few deaths, as of November 2015, and most cases appear to be mild.

Other influenza viruses can also affect dogs, without persisting in canine populations. Equine influenza viruses have caused a few small outbreaks, and there are occasionally reports of infections or clinical cases caused by viruses adapted to birds or humans.

ETIOLOGY

Canine influenza viruses belong to the species *influenza A virus*, genus *Influenzavirus A*, and family Orthomyxoviridae. Other influenza A viruses circulate in birds (avian influenza viruses), horses and other equids (equine influenza viruses), pigs (swine influenza viruses) or people (human influenza A viruses). Influenza A viruses are classified into subtypes based on two surface proteins, the hemagglutinin (HA) and neuraminidase (NA). The subtype designation consists of the HA and NA found in that virus (e.g., H1N2). While at least 16 types of hemagglutinins (H1 to H16), and 9 neuraminidases (N1 to N9) are known to exist in birds, and two additional HA and NA types occur in bats, only a few avian subtypes (and no bat subtypes) have adapted to circulate in other mammals.

Influenza A viruses are extremely variable, and two viruses that share a subtype may be only distantly related. Nevertheless, all influenza A viruses (except possibly the bat viruses) are similar enough that they can 'reassort,' exchanging gene segments to produce progeny containing elements of both parental viruses – regardless of their original host specificity or subtype. Influenza A viruses can also infect species other than the hosts in which they normally circulate, and on rare occasions, they may adapt to circulate in a new host. [The 'Influenza' factsheet contains a more extensive description of these processes.] Dogs have acquired two influenza viruses since 1999, an H3N8 virus that came from horses, and an H3N2 virus that came from birds. The North American H3N8 canine influenza virus seems to have jumped directly from horses to dogs, probably in the late 1990s or early 2000s. It is most closely related to the 'Florida lineage' of H3N8 equine influenza viruses, which emerged in the early 1990s. The H3N8 canine influenza virus is maintained in dog populations, and has diverged considerably from equine influenza viruses. It no longer seems to be capable of replicating efficiently in horses. The H3N2 canine influenza virus seems to have originated in birds. It is reported to contain gene segments that may have come from several different avian influenza viruses. There is some evidence for its presence among dogs in South Korea as early as 2005, and in China in 2006.

Other influenza A viruses are also found sporadically in dogs, but are not maintained in canine populations, and are not considered to be canine influenza viruses. They include H3N8 equine influenza viruses, which have caused a few isolated outbreaks in dogs exposed to infected horses, and human influenza viruses including the 2009 pandemic H1N1 influenza virus. An H3N1 virus, which seems to be the result of reassortment between the H3N2 canine influenza virus and the 2009 pandemic H1N1 virus, was recently isolated from a dog with respiratory signs in Korea. A naturally co-infected dog, infected with the latter two 'parental' viruses, has been described. A few dogs have also been affected by some viruses found in birds, such as the Asian lineage H5N1 highly pathogenic avian influenza (HPAI) viruses, an H5N2 HPAI virus that is closely related to this virus, and H9N2 viruses. Reassortments might occur between avian and canine influenza viruses. One recent analysis suggested that one canine H3N2 isolate may have acquired a gene from an avian H5N1 HPAI virus.

SPECIES AFFECTED

As of 2015, the H3N8 canine influenza virus has only been reported in dogs. Its ability to replicate in horses appears to be greatly reduced, with low or absent virus shedding, and inefficient transmission from experimentally infected horses to naïve horses. One study reported that horses were not infected when kept in close contact with experimentally infected dogs. In laboratory studies, the H3N8 canine influenza virus was not transmitted readily to chickens, turkeys or ducks.

The H3N2 canine influenza virus has caused clinical cases in dogs and cats, and antibodies to this virus have been found in both species. Dogs and cats can be infected by contact with experimentally infected dogs, and cats can transmit the virus to other cats. Ferrets can become infected after direct inoculation of the virus in the laboratory, but they seem to be less susceptible: ferrets did not become infected after exposure to experimentally infected dogs, and ferret-to-ferret transmission was limited. Guinea pigs are also susceptible to experimental infection, but there was no evidence for virus replication or shedding in experimentally inoculated chickens, ducks, mice or pigs.

GEOGRAPHIC DISTRIBUTION

The H3N8 canine influenza virus has been detected, at least sporadically, in most states in the U.S. The distribution of this virus is patchy; in some cases, it caused an outbreak or was detected serologically in an area, but later disappeared. There is no evidence that it currently circulates outside the U.S. As of November 2015, the H3N2 canine influenza virus has been confirmed in Korea, China, Thailand and North America (the U.S.). A serological study found no evidence of its presence in Japan.

Infections with viruses not adapted to dogs can occur wherever these viruses are endemic. Human influenza viruses occur worldwide, and H3N8 equine influenza viruses are widely distributed. Avian influenza viruses are also widely distributed, although different viruses can circulate in different areas.

TRANSMISSION

In mammals, influenza viruses are usually transmitted in droplets and aerosols created by coughing and sneezing, and by contact with nasal discharges, either directly or on fomites. Close contact and closed environments favor transmission. The H3N8 and H3N2 canine influenza viruses are both found in respiratory secretions, as is typical of mammalian influenza viruses. Fecal shedding has not been reported for either virus.

The H3N8 canine influenza virus can be detected in the respiratory secretions of both symptomatic and subclinically infected dogs. Overall, virus titers seem to be low, and the H3N8 canine influenza virus does not appear to spread rapidly in the community. However, transmission can occur more efficiently where groups of susceptible dogs are in close contact (e.g., in a kennel). The H3N2 canine influenza virus might be transmitted more efficiently. In addition, treatment with glucocorticoids (prednisolone) was reported to prolong the shedding of the latter virus; in one experiment, the H3N2 canine influenza virus could be detected in the nasal secretions of some treated dogs for as long as 13 days, compared to 8 days in the controls. Experimentally infected cats can shed the H3N2 canine influenza virus, and transmission between cats was reported to be rapid during one outbreak at an one animal shelter in South Korea.

Dogs infected with other influenza viruses (i.e., those not adapted to dogs) may or may not transmit them to others in close contact. There seems to be no significant dog-to-dog transmission of H3N8 equine influenza viruses.

There is no specific information on the persistence of canine influenza viruses in the environment; however, it is likely to be similar to other mammalian influenza viruses. Human influenza A viruses seem to remain viable for less than 24-48 hours on most surfaces, with recovery from porous surfaces sometimes lasting less than 8-12 hours. Nevertheless, some data indicate that they might survive longer on some fomites or in some conditions. Low temperatures and protection from sunlight enhance virus survival. Swine influenza viruses and avian influenza viruses can persist in feces from < 1 day to 2 weeks or longer, depending on environmental factors including desiccation. Avian influenza viruses and human influenza A viruses may be found for weeks or months in some types of water (e.g., distilled), although they might be inactivated faster in aquatic environments that contain normal microbial flora.

DISINFECTION

Influenza A viruses are susceptible to a wide variety of disinfectants including sodium hypochlorite, 60% to 95% ethanol, quaternary ammonium compounds, aldehydes (glutaraldehyde, formaldehyde), phenols, acids, povidone-iodine and other agents. Common household agents including 1% bleach, 10% malt vinegar or 0.01-0.1% dishwashing liquid (washing up liquid), as well as antimicrobial wipes,

were found to destroy the viability of human influenza viruses, although hot water alone (55°C; 131°F) did not eliminate these viruses rapidly. Influenza A viruses can also be inactivated by heat of 56-60°C (133-140°F) for a minimum of 60 minutes (or higher temperatures for shorter periods), as well as by ionizing radiation or extremes of pH (pH 1-3 or pH 10-14).

INCUBATION PERIOD

The incubation period for H3N8 canine influenza is thought to be one to 5 days, with most cases appearing in 2 to 3 days.

Fever has been reported as soon as one to 3 days in dogs inoculated with the H3N2 canine influenza virus, with respiratory signs developing 2 to 8 days after inoculation. In experimentally infected cats, clinical signs first appeared after 2 to 7 days.

CLINICAL SIGNS

Canine influenza (H3N8)

The most common presentation in H3N8 canine influenza is a mild illness that resembles infectious tracheobronchitis (kennel cough) or other upper respiratory diseases. An initial (usually low grade) fever may be followed by a persistent cough, which tends to be nonproductive and dry (in cases not complicated by co-infections), but may also be soft and moist. The cough can last for up to 3 weeks regardless of treatment. Other common clinical signs include nasal discharge, sneezing, ocular discharge, lethargy and anorexia. The nasal discharge can start clear but may quickly become mucopurulent. Purulent discharges seem to resolve with antibiotics, suggesting the involvement of secondary bacterial infections. Some dogs have only a low fever, without respiratory signs, and asymptomatic seroconversion has been reported.

More severely affected dogs exhibit a high fever with an increased respiratory rate and other signs of pneumonia or bronchopneumonia. Severe lung involvement seems to occur mainly in cases with secondary bacterial or mycoplasmal infections. During the initial outbreaks among racing greyhounds, some dogs were found dead peracutely with evidence of hemorrhages in the respiratory tract. This syndrome does not seem to be prominent in pets.

Experimentally infected horses had mild clinical signs compared to horses inoculated with equine influenza viruses, or remained asymptomatic.

Canine influenza (H3N2)

Clinical cases reported in dogs have been characterized by fever (which may be low) and respiratory signs including nasal discharge, sneezing, coughing and anorexia. The nasal discharge was described as copious in one report. Dogs affected in early reports from South Korea and China were severely ill, and although few cases were reported, a number of them were fatal. Affected dogs developed mild to severe respiratory signs during two outbreaks at animal shelters in South Korea, with significant numbers of deaths. Similar respiratory signs were described during a recent outbreak at a veterinary hospital in Thailand. The severity of the clinical signs was not described in this report, but no deaths are mentioned. Some of these dogs were ill for as long as 7-10 days. In Asia, some dogs without a history of severe respiratory disease are seropositive, suggesting that subclinical infections may also occur. There are currently no published articles describing the outbreaks in the U.S.; however, informal reports suggest that most cases have been characterized by relatively mild upper respiratory signs, with few deaths.

The H3N2 canine influenza virus also seems to cause illness in cats. This virus has been found in cats during outbreaks of respiratory disease among dogs and cats at two animal shelters in South Korea. The clinical signs in the cats included coughing, dyspnea, tachypnea and lethargy, and a significant number of infections were fatal. Co-infections might have played some role in at least one of these outbreaks, as *Bordetella bronchiseptica* was also found in at least one cat. Cats that were experimentally infected with the H3N2 canine influenza virus had elevated temperatures, lethargy and respiratory signs including coughing, sneezing, ocular and nasal discharge, conjunctivitis and abdominal breathing. Antibodies to the H3N2 canine influenza virus have also been reported in apparently healthy cats.

Although ferrets were not very susceptible to this virus, some experimentally infected animals developed clinical signs. Sneezing was seen most often, and some animals were lethargic and anorectic. Experimentally infected guinea pigs remained asymptomatic, but developed lung lesions.

Other influenza viruses in dogs

In the U.K., an H3N8 equine influenza virus caused a limited outbreak among foxhounds in 2002. The disease was characterized by coughing, lethargy and weakness, sometimes progressing to loss of consciousness, and was diagnosed as bronchointerstitial pneumonia. One dog died and several were euthanized. Clinical signs in dogs infected with H3N8 equine influenza viruses in Australia included anorexia, depression, slight nasal discharge, and in some cases, a cough that persisted for several weeks. All of these dogs recovered. Dogs that were experimentally infected with H3N8 equine influenza viruses remained asymptomatic or had very mild clinical signs (e.g., periodic anorexia and sneezing).

An H3N1 virus, which appears to be a reassortant between the canine H3N2 virus and the human 2009 pandemic H1N1 virus, was isolated from a dog with respiratory signs in Korea. Dogs inoculated with this virus remained asymptomatic and had only mild lung lesions.

There are only a few descriptions of human influenza virus infections in dogs. Some viruses, such as the 2009 pandemic H1N1 virus, are capable of causing severe respiratory signs, with radiological evidence of pneumonia, but milder signs have also been reported, and several studies have detected antibodies to human influenza viruses in healthy dogs that had no history of severe respiratory illness. Natural or experimental avian influenza virus infections in dogs have, likewise, ranged from asymptomatic or mild (e.g., transient fever, conjunctivitis or mild respiratory signs) to severe illnesses with respiratory signs, fever, and in some cases, systemic signs such as diarrhea. As with human influenza viruses, antibodies to various avian influenza viruses have been detected in healthy dogs in some locations (e.g., China). Additional details are available in the 'Influenza' factsheet.

POST MORTEM LESIONS

Canine influenza (H3N8)

Fatal H3N8 canine influenza cases in racing greyhounds were often characterized by hemorrhages in the lungs, mediastinum and pleural cavity. The lungs also exhibited signs of severe pneumonia, and were dark red to black. Fibrinous pleuritis was seen in some cases. In other dogs, fatal cases seem to be characterized mainly by suppurative secondary bacterial pneumonia, and hemorrhagic pneumonia does not appear to be common. Bronchitis and tracheitis were the only significant lesions in 5 shelter dogs that were euthanized primarily for a chronic cough unresponsive to antibiotics.

Based on studies in experimentally infected dogs, the early lesions are thought to be tracheitis and bronchitis, with some extension to the bronchioles. Variable lower respiratory tract lesions may be seen, especially later in the illness, and may include petechiae, areas of consolidation and other lesions consistent with viral pneumonia.

Canine influenza (H3N2)

Severe hemorrhagic, cranioventral bronchointerstitial pneumonia was reported in most fatal cases of canine H3N2 influenza in naturally infected dogs from Asia; however, only partial necropsies were available and only for a limited number of cases. Experimentally infected dogs also had signs of pneumonia with multifocal to coalescing reddish consolidation, edema and hemorrhages in the lungs. No lesions were found outside the respiratory tract.

During one outbreak of severe respiratory disease in cats, the lesions included severe bronchopneumonia with consolidation in large areas of the lung, and pulmonary edema in some cats. Some cats were coinfected with other respiratory pathogens.

Some experimentally infected ferrets and guinea pigs had areas of consolidation in the lungs.

DIAGNOSTIC TESTS

Canine influenza (H3N8)

Serology and reverse transcription polymerase chain reaction (RT-PCR) assays are the most reliable methods for detecting H3N8 canine influenza. Hemagglutination inhibition is considered the serological test of choice. Virus neutralization (microneutralization test) can also be done, but this test is usually too cumbersome for routine use. Antibodies usually develop 7-10 days after infection and continue to rise to high levels around 14 days. Although acute and convalescent titers are ideal, many dogs do not have pre-existing titers to this virus, and a single sample collected more than 7 days after the onset of clinical signs may be useful.

RT-PCR is the most reliable method to detect the virus directly, due to its sensitivity. Nasal swabs are the preferred sample from live dogs, and were more likely to yield virus than nasopharyngeal swabs in experimentally infected dogs. Lung tissue samples are collected at necropsy. Virus isolation may also be done, but it is unlikely to be successful in a dog that has had clinical signs for more than 3 days. The H3N8 canine influenza virus has been isolated in both embryonated eggs and cell cultures (MDCK cells); some viruses have been recovered in only eggs or cells, while others can be isolated in both systems. Both virus isolation and RT-PCR can fail to detect the virus in infected dogs if the samples are collected too late.

Antigen-capture ELISA tests do not seem to be reliable in individual dogs, probably because virus shedding is low, and the timing of sample collection is not always optimal. A recent study suggested that the sensitivity of these tests is much lower than RT-PCR and lower than virus isolation, and false positives were also common. However, they may be useful during investigations of outbreaks at kennels or other facilities housing groups of dogs.

Canine influenza (H3N2)

Little has been published about diagnostic testing for H3N2 canine influenza, but virus isolation and RT-PCR were used in some outbreaks. Respiratory samples (e.g., nasal swabs) are collected. Serological tests may also be helpful, and at least one test is now available in the U.S. It should be noted that the H3N8 and H3N2 canine influenza viruses differ significantly; RT-PCR and serological tests used to detect the H3N8 canine influenza virus will not detect infections with the H3N2 virus.

TREATMENT

Treatment is supportive, and often includes antibiotics to control secondary bacterial infections. Although antiviral drugs (e.g., neuraminidase inhibitors) are sometimes used in cases of human influenza, these drugs have not been tested in canine influenza. They are most useful during the first 48 hours after the onset of clinical signs, and in many cases, this period is likely to have passed by the time the dog is seen by a veterinarian. The risk that viruses might become resistant to these drugs is also a concern.

CONTROL

Disease reporting

Official reporting requirements for canine influenza differ between areas, and this disease is currently reportable in some U.S. states, but not others. However, information about outbreaks is often disseminated even in locations with no formal requirement to report this disease.

Prevention

Vaccines for canine influenza are available in some areas. A licensed vaccine for the H3N8 canine influenza virus is commercially available in the U.S. An H3N2 canine influenza virus has been approved in South Korea. The degree of cross-protection between these viruses, if any, is currently unclear.

Influenza viruses usually spread most readily when susceptible animals are in close contact. Infection control measures are similar to those used for other contagious respiratory diseases, and include isolation of infected animals; cleaning and disinfection of cages, bowls and other fomites; and hygiene measures including hand washing. Clothing can be cleaned by washing it with detergent at normal laundry temperatures.

Veterinarians should be alert to announcements of canine influenza outbreaks in an area. Clients should also be advised to consult a veterinarian if their dog develops signs of a respiratory illness, and should be questioned about potential exposures to other dogs (e.g., recent boarding). When outbreaks occur at establishments, quarantines and the isolation of infected animals can reduce virus dissemination to the community and within the facility.

MORBIDITY AND MORTALITY

In mammals, the severity of influenza can differ with the virus, and is also influenced by host factors such as immunity, age and concurrent diseases. Uncomplicated infections with influenza viruses adapted to that host tend to be associated with high morbidity rates, low mortality rates and rapid recovery. More severe disease and higher mortality rates may be seen in young, old or debilitated animals. Secondary bacterial infections can exacerbate the clinical signs, prolong recovery and result in complications such as pneumonia. Infections with viruses not adapted to that host vary widely in severity; some viruses typically cause asymptomatic infections and mild illnesses, while others tend to cause severe disease.

Canine influenza (H3N8)

Although H3N8 canine influenza was first reported in racing greyhounds, all breeds are now considered to be susceptible. The greatest risk of infection is among dogs that reside in kennels or are exposed to transient groups of dogs, as in animal shelters or dog day care facilities. In some facilities, more than 40% of the dogs may be seropositive. Infected dogs from these high risk populations may introduce the virus into new areas. Currently, the H3N8 canine influenza virus does not appear to be common among household pets in the U.S., with studies reporting seroprevalence rates less than 5%. In some areas, exposure rates have been low even in pets that participate in some types of gatherings (e.g., flyball tournaments). One study suggested that canine influenza is rare, if it exists at all, in Canada. In the province of Ontario, a survey found antibodies to the H3N8 virus in only one of 225 dogs in 2006. This dog was a greyhound that had come from a racetrack in Florida, and may have been infected there. More recently, no seropositive dogs were found among Canadian and U.S. dogs that participated in the 2010 Iditarod race.

During outbreaks among fully susceptible dogs in close contact (e.g., in kennels), the infection rate may approach 100%, and clinical signs in 60-80% of the dogs is not unusual. Most dogs are expected to develop the less severe form of the disease and recover; however, a more severe form with pneumonia occurs in a minority. The overall mortality rate is thought to be 1-5%, although some sources suggest that it might be as high as 8%. Secondary bacterial infections appear to contribute significantly to these deaths. Higher case fatality rates have been reported in small groups of greyhounds. At one Florida greyhound racetrack, the case fatality rate was 36%. More severe illness would also be expected in debilitated animals.

Canine influenza (H3N2)

Illnesses caused by the H3N2 canine influenza virus have been reported from veterinary hospitals, kennels and animal shelters in South Korea, China and Thailand, and recently, from dogs in the U.S. There is no known breed predilection; cases have been described in various species of dogs, as well as cats. Many of the reported clinical cases from Asia have been severe. In the initial report from Korea, only one of the 5 dogs seen at 3 veterinary clinics survived. Similarly, 2 of 4 cases in pet dogs diagnosed in China were fatal. During one explosive, severe outbreak at a Korean animal shelter, approximately 200 dogs and 50 cats showed signs of respiratory disease. The morbidity rate in this outbreak was 100% in cats, while the case fatality rate was 25% in affected dogs, and 40% in cats. It is possible that other pathogens also contributed to this outbreak. At least one cat that died was co-infected with *Bordetella bronchiseptica*. During another outbreak in a South Korean animal shelter, the morbidity and mortality rates were reported to be 77% and 23%, respectively, in dogs, and 47% and 22%, respectively, in cats. Currently, signs among dogs in the U.S. generally appear to be mild, and the case fatality rate is reported to be low; news reports indicated that there were

approximately 8 confirmed deaths due to this virus, in more than 1500 cases as of May, 2015.

Studies from Asia have reported antibodies to the H3N2 canine influenza virus among cats and dogs with or without respiratory signs. One study found that 3.5% of serum samples collected from dogs in South Korea between 2005 and 2009 were seropositive. Approximately 3% of pet cats and cats in colonies in South Korea also had antibodies to this virus, Studies from China have reported seroprevalence rates ranging from 3.5% to 33% in dogs, and 1% to 10% in cats. Some of these studies reported relatively high seroprevalence rates among stray dogs in animal shelters (20%), dogs raised for food (12%), and dogs living on poultry farms and near poultry markets (5-14% or 16-33%, depending on the assay); however, one study also reported antibodies in 33% of pet dogs. While cross-reactivity with other influenza viruses can complicate serological studies, some of these studies reported a pattern of reactivity that is higher to the H3N2 canine influenza virus than to H3 influenza viruses from other species.

PUBLIC HEALTH

There are no reports of human infections with canine influenza viruses, although such infections are theoretically possible. As a precaution, physicians, veterinarians and others have been asked to report any cases of human influenza that seem to be linked to exposure to canine influenza. As a general practice, it is prudent for immunocompromised people, the elderly, young children and pregnant women to avoid contact with animals that are ill.

CLASSICAL SWINE FEVER

Hog Cholera, Swine Fever, European Swine Fever, Peste du Porc, Colera Porcina, Virusschweinepest

IMPORTANCE

Classical swine fever (CSF) is a highly contagious and economically significant viral disease of pigs. The severity of the illness varies with the strain of the virus, the age of the pig, and the immune status of the herd. Acute infections, which are caused by highly virulent isolates and have a high mortality rate in naïve herds, are likely to be diagnosed rapidly. However, infections with less virulent isolates can be more difficult to recognize, particularly in older pigs. The range of clinical signs and similarity to other diseases can make classical swine fever challenging to diagnose.

Although classical swine fever was once widespread, many countries have eradicated this disease from domesticated swine. Reintroduction of the virus can be devastating. In 1997-1998, an outbreak in the Netherlands spread to involve more than 400 herds and cost $2.3 billion to eradicate. Approximately 12 million pigs were killed, some in eradication efforts but most for welfare reasons associated with the epidemic. Other European counties have also experienced outbreaks, and the ongoing presence of the virus among wild boar presents a risk of reintroduction to domesticated swine. North America is also at risk for the reintroduction of classical swine fever, which is still endemic in South and Central America.

ETIOLOGY

Classical swine fever (hog cholera) results from infection by classical swine fever virus (CSFV), a member of the genus *Pestivirus* and family Flaviviridae. There is only one serotype but several genotypes and subgenotypes. CSFV is closely related to pestiviruses found in ruminants, and some of the latter viruses can cause serological reactions in pigs that may be mistaken for CSF.

SPECIES AFFECTED

CSFV appears to be capable of infecting most or all members of the pig family (Suidae). Clinical cases occur in domesticated pigs and Eurasian wild boar. CSFV has been detected in a white-lipped peccary *(Tayassu pecari)*, and experimental infections have been established in common warthogs *(Phacochoerus africanus)*, bush pigs *(Potamochoerus larvatus)* and collared peccaries *(Tayassu tajacu)*.

Experimental infections without clinical signs have been reported in cattle, sheep, goats and deer, but there is no evidence that these species become infected in nature. Strains of CSFV can also be adapted to passage in rabbits.

Zoonotic potential

There is no evidence that CSFV infects humans.

GEOGRAPHIC DISTRIBUTION

Classical swine fever is endemic in parts of Asia, parts of South and Central America, and on some Caribbean islands. CSFV has been eradicated from a number of countries, including the U.S., Canada, New Zealand, Australia, Iceland and Japan. It is also absent from the domesticated pig populations of most of western and central Europe, although it is still present among wild boar in some regions. The status of classical swine fever in some areas of Africa may be uncertain, due to limited or no surveillance; as of 2014, it was reported to the World Organization for Animal Health (OIE) as endemic in Madagascar, suspected in Equatorial Guinea in 2013, and either absent or eradicated in other reporting countries.

TRANSMISSION

Pigs are mainly thought to become infected by the oral or oronasal routes. CSFV may also enter the body via other mucus membranes (including genital transmission in semen),

the conjunctiva and skin abrasions. It can be shed in oronasal and ocular secretions, urine, feces and semen; one study reported that pigs infected with strains of low virulence excreted the virus mainly in oronasal secretions. Shedding can begin before the onset of clinical signs. Because CSFV can persist in blood and tissues after death, it is readily spread by feeding uncooked swill that contains tissues from infected pigs. Aerosol transmission has been demonstrated experimentally with some strains. It is most likely to occur between mechanically ventilated buildings in close proximity, when there are large concentrations of animals. Piglets and wild boar infected before birth or shortly thereafter (i.e., on the day of birth in one experiment) may become persistently infected without developing an antibody response to CSFV. These animals can shed the virus continuously or intermittently for months.

CSFV can be spread on fomites, and may be transmitted on live mechanical vectors such as insects. Estimates of its persistence in the environment differ, and are influenced by the initial concentration of virus and the presence of organic matter. Some studies suggest that CSFV is inactivated on some fomites, in feces (or slurry) and in urine within a few days to 2 weeks at room temperature (e.g., 20°C). Others describe survival at 4-5°C for 1-3 months when protected by material such as pig slurry. One study reported that this virus also persisted in pig slurry for at least 70 days at 17°C. CSFV can remain infectious for nearly three months in refrigerated meat and for more than four years in frozen meat. In this proteinaceous environment, it does not appear to be inactivated by smoking or salt curing. Reported virus survival times in cured and smoked meats vary with the technique, and range from 17 days to more than 180 days.

DISINFECTION

CSFV can be inactivated with sodium hypochlorite, phenolic compounds, detergents, organic solvents, quaternary ammonium compounds and aldehydes (formaldehyde, glutaraldehyde). It is also sensitive to drying, heat and ultraviolet light. This virus is reported to be destroyed by heating for a minute or less at 90-100°C or 5 minutes at 70°C. In meat, CSFV is susceptible to a temperature of 65.5°C or higher, maintained for 30 minutes. It is stable at pH 5-10, but inactivated by pH ≤ 3 or pH > 10.

INCUBATION PERIOD

The incubation period can range from 2 to 15 days, and is often 3-7 days in acute cases. Under field conditions, the disease may not become evident in a herd for 2 to 4 weeks or longer.

CLINICAL SIGNS

The clinical signs vary with the strain of CSFV, and the age and susceptibility of the pigs. While highly virulent strains were prevalent in the past, most outbreaks are now caused by moderately virulent strains, and the clinical signs are often less severe and distinctive.

Highly virulent strains of CSFV tend to cause acute, severe illness in naïve herds. Common clinical signs in the acute form include a high fever, huddling, weakness, drowsiness, anorexia and conjunctivitis, which can cause severe crusting of the eyelids. Constipation, with the passage of hard fecal pellets, is typically followed by, or intermittent with, watery diarrhea. Pigs may be incoordinated or exhibit an unsteady, weaving or staggering gait, which often progresses to posterior paresis. Some pigs may vomit yellow, bile-containing fluid, or develop respiratory signs. The skin can become hyperemic, and may develop hemorrhages (especially on the abdomen, inner thighs, ears) or a purple cyanotic discoloration, which tends to be seen on the snout, ears and tail. Severe leukopenia is a common laboratory abnormality. Pigs with acute classical swine fever often die within 1-3 weeks, and convulsions may occur in the terminal stages. The subacute form is similar; however, the signs are less severe, the course is prolonged, and the mortality rate lower. Blotching of the ears has been described in both subacute and chronic cases.

Chronic disease tends to be seen with less virulent strains or in partially immune herds, and may affect only a few animals. In the initial stages, it can resemble the other forms, with signs such as anorexia, depression, elevated temperature, leukopenia, and periods of constipation and/or diarrhea. Affected pigs usually improve after several weeks, but after a period where they may appear relatively normal, these signs can recur. Additional signs include wasting or stunted growth, alopecia and skin lesions, and immunosuppression may lead to concurrent infections. The clinical signs can wax and wane for weeks to months, and the outcome is often fatal.

Poor reproductive performance may be the only sign in some breeding herds infected with less virulent strains. Sows in these herds may abort or give birth to stillborn, mummified, malformed, weak or dead piglets. Some piglets may be born with a congenital tremor or congenital malformations of the visceral organs and central nervous system. Others can be persistently infected but asymptomatic at birth. These piglets become ill after several months, with signs of "late onset" disease such as inappetence, depression, stunted growth, dermatitis, diarrhea, conjunctivitis, ataxia or posterior paresis. Although congenitally infected pigs can survive for 2 months or more, all typically die within a year.

Clinical signs in wild boar appear to be similar to the signs in domesticated pigs. Experimentally infected bushpigs also became ill and some cases were severe, with fever, anemia, prolonged clotting times upon blood collection, diarrhea and conjunctivitis. Most experimentally infected warthogs in the same study did not develop clinical signs, despite virological and serological evidence of infection. One warthog had moderate to severe diarrhea. Short-term fever and nonspecific signs were reported in collared peccaries inoculated with CSFV.

POST MORTEM LESIONS

The lesions of classical swine fever are highly variable. During outbreaks, the likelihood of observing the characteristic necropsy lesions is better if four or five pigs are examined. In acute disease, the most common lesion is hemorrhage. The skin may be discolored purple and the lymph nodes may be swollen and hemorrhagic. Petechial or ecchymotic hemorrhages can often be seen on serosal and mucosal surfaces, particularly on the kidney, urinary bladder, epicardium, epiglottis, larynx, trachea, intestines, subcutaneous tissues and spleen. In the intestines, the lesions may include hemorrhagic lesions in the stomach, mild to moderate catarrhal enteritis in the small intestine, and button ulcers in the colon. Straw-colored fluid may be found in the peritoneal and thoracic cavities and the pericardial sac. Severe tonsillitis, sometimes with necrotic foci, is common. Splenic infarcts (raised, dark, wedge-shaped lesions) are seen only occasionally with the currently circulating strains of CSFV, but are highly suspicious of this disease if detected. The lungs may be congested and hemorrhagic, and encephalitis may be noted in the brain. In some acute cases, lesions may be absent or inconspicuous.

The lesions of chronic disease are less severe and may be complicated by secondary infections. Necrotic foci or "button" ulcers may be found in the intestinal mucosa, epiglottis and larynx. Button ulcers in the intestine may be followed by diffuse, diphteroid-necrotizing enteritis. In growing pigs that have survived for more than a month, bone lesions can also occur at the costochondral junction of the ribs and the growth plates of the long bones.

In congenitally infected piglets, common lesions include cerebellar hypoplasia, thymic atrophy, ascites, and deformities of the head and legs. Edema and petechial hemorrhages may be seen in the skin and internal organs.

DIAGNOSTIC TESTS

CSFV can be detected in blood or tonsil swabs collected from live animals, or in tissue samples (tonsils, pharyngeal and mesenteric lymph nodes, spleen, kidneys, distal ileum) taken at necropsy. Samples from live animals should be collected when they are febrile. Reverse transcriptase polymerase chain reaction (RT-PCR) tests, which detect viral nucleic acids, are often used for diagnosis. Loop-mediated isothermal amplification (RT-LAMP) assays have also been published. Identification to the genotype or subgenotype level, using nucleic acid-based tests, can be useful in epidemiology. CSFV antigens can be detected with direct immunofluorescence (FAT or FATST) or ELISAs. ELISAs are only considered suitable as herd tests. In addition, CSFV can be isolated in several cell lines including pig kidney (e.g. PK–15) cells, with virus identification by direct immunofluorescence, immunoperoxidase staining or RT-PCR.

Ruminant pestiviruses (e.g., bovine virus diarrhea virus and border disease virus) can occasionally infect pigs. Serum neutralization tests, or immunoperoxidase procedures that use monoclonal antibodies, can differentiate CSFV from these viruses. They can also be distinguished with genetic methods such as RT-PCR.

Serology can be useful for diagnosis and surveillance. Antibodies develop relatively late (after 2 to 3 weeks) in most animals, but persist lifelong. However, piglets (including wild boar) infected before or immediately after birth may be immunotolerant and negative on serology. The most commonly used tests are virus neutralization (e.g., the fluorescent antibody virus neutralization [FAVN] and neutralizing peroxidase-linked assay [NPLA] tests) and various ELISAs. Assays that use monoclonal antibodies can distinguish antibodies to CSFV from responses to ruminant pestiviruses. The definitive test is the comparative neutralization test.

Companion ELISAs are also available for use with marker vaccines. At present, these tests are considered suitable as herd tests, but are not reliable in individual animals.

TREATMENT

There is no treatment for classical swine fever, other than supportive care.

CONTROL

Disease reporting

A quick response is vital for containing outbreaks in CSFV-free regions. Veterinarians who encounter or suspect classical swine fever should follow their national and/or local guidelines for disease reporting. In the U.S., state or federal veterinary authorities should be informed immediately.

Prevention

In countries where classical swine fever is endemic, this disease may be excluded from a herd by buying animals from CSFV-free herds, quarantining the new stock for 4 months and testing the animals before allowing them to contact the rest of the herd. Vaccines are also used to protect animals from clinical signs, and may be employed to reduce the prevalence of infections during an eradication program. Both modified live and subunit (marker) vaccines are manufactured.

Outbreaks in CSFV-free regions are generally eradicated by slaughter of confirmed cases and contact animals, cleaning and disinfection of infected premises, safe carcass disposal, movement controls/quarantines and surveillance. Pre-emptive slaughter of animals on nearby farms and/or emergency vaccination may also be employed. Because the currently circulating viruses are often less readily detected by clinical signs, some countries conduct routine virological surveillance for CSFV, such as periodic sampling of tonsils from dead pigs.

Controlling endemic infections in wild populations is difficult. Oral vaccination is used in wild boar in Europe. Contact between domesticated herds and wild pigs should be avoided.

MORBIDITY AND MORTALITY

The severity of classical swine fever is influenced by the viral strain, the age and immune status of the pigs, and other factors such as the animals' general health and viral dose. Highly virulent strains of CSFV, which were prevalent at one time, cause outbreaks with morbidity and mortality rates that can approach 100%. However, most outbreaks are now caused by moderately virulent strains, and less virulent strains also circulate. Some strains of low virulence have caused only 20% mortality in experimentally infected pigs. Case fatality rates also differ with the form of the disease, and are very high in the acute form, but lower in subacute cases. Mortality tends to be lower in adult pigs, compared to young animals, especially with less virulent strains.

CONTAGIOUS BOVINE PLEUROPNEUMONIA

IMPORTANCE

Contagious bovine pleuropneumonia (CBPP) is one of the most important infectious diseases of cattle in Africa. Naïve herds can experience losses up to 80%, and many cattle that survive remain chronic carriers. These carriers may suffer from recurrent low-grade fever, loss of condition, and respiratory signs upon exercise, and might introduce the causative agent into uninfected herds. Although contagious bovine pleuropneumonia was once found worldwide, it was eradicated from most continents, including North America, by the mid-20th century. Its incidence also began to decline in Africa by the 1970s. During the late 1980s and 1990s, however, this disease increased in prevalence in endemic areas. It also re-emerged in some African and European countries that had been CBPP-free, in some cases for 25 years or more. Eradication was successful in Europe, with the most recent case reported in 1999. However, contagious bovine pleuropneumonia remains a serious concern in Africa, where the end of widespread combined rinderpest/CBPP vaccination programs (after rinderpest eradication) may have contributed to its resurgence.

ETIOLOGY

Contagious bovine pleuropneumonia is caused by *Mycoplasma mycoides* subsp. *mycoides*, a member of the

Mycoplasma mycoides cluster in the family Mycoplasmataceae. This organism was previously specified as the small-colony (SC) type of this organism; however, *Mycoplasma mycoides* subsp. *mycoides* large colony type no longer exists (these organisms are now considered to belong to *M. mycoides* subsp. *capri*). Nevertheless, many sources continue to use the full designation *Mycoplasma mycoides* subsp. *mycoides* SC. *M. mycoides* SC can be grouped into at least two major lineages (African and European), or into at least 3 or 4 genetic groups. Strains can differ in virulence.

Zoonotic potential

There is no evidence that humans are infected by *M. mycoides* SC.

SPECIES AFFECTED

Cattle (*Bos taurus* and *Bos indicus*) and Asian buffalo (*Bubalus bubalis*) are the primary hosts for *M. mycoides* SC. Clinical cases have also been reported in yak (*Poephagus grunniens/Bos grunniens*) and captive bison (*Bison bison*). Sheep and goats can be infected, although they are not thought to be important in the epidemiology of CBPP. White-tailed deer (*Odocoileus virginianus*) have been infected experimentally. There is little published surveillance for *M. mycoides* SC in wildlife, with the exception of two studies conducted before 1970, which reported that African wildlife were unlikely to be infected.

GEOGRAPHIC DISTRIBUTION

Contagious bovine pleuropneumonia is endemic in parts of Africa. Sporadic outbreaks have been reported in the Middle East, and are probably caused by cattle imported from Africa. There is limited information about Asian countries in the most recent reports to the World Organization for Animal Health (OIE), although some countries have indicated that they are CBPP-free. *M. mycoides* SC is not currently endemic in Europe or the Western Hemisphere.

TRANSMISSION

M. mycoides SC is mainly transmitted from animal to animal in respiratory aerosols. This organism also occurs in saliva, urine, fetal membranes and uterine discharges. Close, repeated contact is generally thought to be necessary for transmission; however, *M. mycoides* SC might be spread over longer distances (up to 200 meters) if the climatic conditions are favorable. Carrier animals, including subclinically infected cattle, can retain viable organisms in encapsulated lung lesions (sequestra) for several months or more (one source indicates up to two years). These animals are thought to be capable of shedding organisms, particularly when stressed. Transplacental transmission is also possible.

Although there are a few anecdotal reports of transmission on fomites, mycoplasmas do not survive for more than a few days in the environment and indirect transmission is thought to be unimportant in the epidemiology of this disease.

DISINFECTION

Mycoplasma spp. are generally short-lived, fragile organisms in the environment. If disinfection is needed, they are reported to be susceptible to many disinfectants including 1% sodium hypochlorite, 70% ethanol, phenolic disinfectants, iodophores, formaldehyde, glutaraldehyde, and peracedic acid.

INCUBATION PERIOD

The incubation period for contagious bovine pleuropneumonia can be 3 weeks to 6 months, with most cases becoming apparent in 3-8 weeks. After experimental inoculation of large doses into the trachea, the clinical signs appeared in 2 to 3 weeks.

CLINICAL SIGNS

A few cattle with CBPP may die peracutely with no clinical signs other than fever. Acute cases in cattle are characterized by nonspecific signs of fever, loss of appetite, depression and a drop in milk production, followed by respiratory signs, which may include coughing, purulent or mucoid nasal discharges, and rapid respiration. Clinical signs can differ in severity between outbreaks, but some cases progress rapidly to dyspnea. Respiration can be painful, and animals may react intensely if pressed between the ribs. Severely affected cattle may stand with their head and neck extended and forelegs apart, breathing through the mouth. The throat and dewlap sometimes swell. Epistaxis and diarrhea have also been reported, and pregnant animals may abort or give birth to stillborn calves. Severely affected cattle often die, typically within three weeks. Animals that recover are frequently weak and emaciated, and may remain chronically infected. Subclinical infections also occur.

In calves up to six months of age, the primary sign may be polyarthritis, especially of the carpal and tarsal joints, often without respiratory signs. The affected joints may be so painful that the animal is very reluctant to bend them.

Chronic CBPP is characterized by recurrent low-grade fever, loss of condition, and respiratory signs that may be apparent only when the animal is exercised. Many cattle eventually recover fully, although the lung lesions can take a long time to heal.

The effects of *M. mycoides* SC on small ruminants are still unclear. There have been reports of its isolation from sheep with mastitis and goats with respiratory disease. Other agents, including other mycoplasmas, were also detected in some outbreaks, but not others. Experimentally infected sheep remained asymptomatic, although some animals had a slight cough, and slight lesions of interstitial pneumonia (evident only microscopically) were found in the lungs. In another study, goats in close contact with experimentally infected cattle did not become infected. One of two experimentally infected white-tailed deer developed a fever and died with severe respiratory lesions; the second deer remained healthy.

POST MORTEM LESIONS

The lesions of CBPP are often unilateral. In acute disease, large amounts of straw-colored fluid may be present in the thoracic cavity and pericardial sac. The lymph nodes of the chest are enlarged and edematous, and may contain petechiae and small necrotic foci. The lungs are consolidated and typically marbled; areas of different color (pale pink, red and dark red) may be separated by a network of pale bands. Extensive fibrin accumulation can be found on the pleural surfaces and within the interlobular septa, causing enlargement of the septa. The fibrin is replaced by fibrous connective tissue over time. Fluid is not usually seen in chronic cases, but pleural adhesions are common. Necrotic lung tissue becomes encapsulated, forming pulmonary sequestra that may contain viable organisms. These sequestra are 2 cm to 25 cm in diameter and are surrounded by a fibrous connective tissue capsule up to 1 cm thick. The necrotic tissue in the sequestrum is odorless and can retain its lobular structure as it shrinks and dries, although it may later liquefy. Sequestra deep in the lung may not be seen, but can be palpated. Sequestra can be found even in recovered animals. Lesions considered to be typical of CBPP, such as marbling of lung tissue and the presence of sequestra, have been absent in some confirmed cases.

In calves with poly-arthritis, affected joints are filled with fluid and abundant fibrin. Infarcts, appearing as chronic fibrotic foci, may be found in the kidneys of these animals.

A fatal case in an experimentally infected deer was characterized by pneumonia with secondary hemorrhages; however, marbling, sequestra, fibrinous adhesions and excessive pleural fluid were absent.

DIAGNOSTIC TESTS

In live animals, a definitive diagnosis can be made by detecting M. mycoides SC in nasal swabs or discharges, bronchoalveolar lavage or transtracheal wash fluid, pleural fluid, or synovial fluid from swollen joints. At necropsy, the organism is most likely to be found in lung lesions, pleural fluid and regional lymph nodes of the respiratory tract. Ideally, lung samples should be collected at the interface between diseased and normal tissue. Recent European isolates have sometimes been recovered from the lungs of animals without typical CBPP lesions. Isolation from blood or the kidneys may also be successful. Members of the Mycoplasma mycoides cluster cross-react in serological tests and share biochemical and antigenic similarities, complicating the identification of CBPP unless genetic tests such as polymerase chain reaction (PCR) assays are used.

A definitive diagnosis can be made by recovering M. mycoides SC from infected animals. Isolation may not be successful after antibiotics have been used, and cultures from sequestra in chronic cases are often negative. Culture can be performed on standard mycoplasma media. This organism is usually identified by PCR, although biochemistry and serological methods (growth inhibition, immunofluorescence, dot immunobinding on a membrane filter [MF-dot] test, agar gel immunodiffusion) can also be employed and were used more frequently in the past. Biochemical tests are unable to unequivocally identify the members of the M. mycoides cluster, and serological identification is hampered by cross-reactivity. There have been reports of unusual field isolates (e.g., M375 from Botswana) that were more fastidious than expected and had altered colony morphology, unique polymorphisms following immunoblotting, and altered properties in growth-inhibition and biochemical tests.

PCR assays are more likely to be successful than culture, and can be used to identify M. mycoides SC directly in clinical samples. At least one isothermal loop-mediated amplification method has also been published. Various antigen detection tests (e.g., immunofluorescence/immunohistochemistry, antigen-capture ELISA, agar gel immunodiffusion, interface precipitin test, lateral flow assay) have been described or used in diagnosis.

Serology is generally employed at the herd level (i.e., in screening and eradication programs), rather than as a diagnostic test in individual animals. Animals may not develop measurable titers in the early stages of CBPP, and few animals with chronic disease are seropositive. Serological tests include complement fixation (CF), ELISA, immunoblotting (generally as a confirmatory test for CF or ELISA), and a rapid slide agglutination test (SAT). The SAT is relatively insensitive and can only identify animals in the acute stage of disease. Other mycoplasmas, particularly other members of the M. mycoides cluster, can result in false positive reactions in serological assays.

TREATMENT

Tetracyclines, macrolides and fluoroquinolones are reported to be useful in treatment, but individual drugs may differ in their effects. Complete elimination of mycoplasmas is reported to be rare. The degree of risk from treated animals is still uncertain; however, treatment is controversial, and some countries do not permit antibiotics to be used. Antibiotics are reported to be ineffective in chronic cases.

CONTROL

Disease reporting

A quick response is vital for containing outbreaks in regions free of contagious bovine pleuropneumonia. Veterinarians who encounter or suspect this disease should follow their national and/or local guidelines for disease reporting. In the U.S., state or federal veterinary authorities should be informed immediately.

Prevention

CBPP is most likely to be introduced in an infected animal or embryo, as the organism does not survive for long periods on fomites. Quarantines and serological testing of imported animals are helpful. Outbreaks are eradicated with quarantines, movement controls, slaughter of infected and in-contact animals, and cleaning and disinfection.

Vaccines are used to control CBPP in endemic areas. On-farm quarantine of CBPP suspects (both clinically affected and carrier animals) and contact animals is helpful in controlling the spread of disease.

MORBIDITY AND MORTALITY

The morbidity and mortality rates for CBPP are highly variable. In a naïve herd, the outcome varies from complete recovery of all animals to the death of the majority. Morbidity increases with close confinement, due to the increase in transmission, and infection rates can be as high as 50-80% in some situations. The mortality rate ranges from 10% to 80%, although mortality greater than 50% is reported to be uncommon. The severity of the illness can also be affected by the virulence of the strain, and secondary factors in the animal, such as nutrition and parasitism. There may be breed-related differences in susceptibility.

African and recent European isolates may differ in virulence. When they are first introduced into a naïve herd, African isolates usually cause acute disease, severe clinical signs and high mortality. Once the disease has become established, the mortality rate falls and the number of animals with chronic disease rises. Much milder illnesses were reported during the recent outbreaks in Europe, and affected animals usually developed subacute or chronic disease. The morbidity rate was generally low (for example, less than 5% in one Italian herd), and few animals died. The decreased severity of CBPP in Europe might also be related to animal husbandry and the availability of antibiotics and anti-inflammatory drugs.

CONTAGIOUS CAPRINE PLEUROPNEUMONIA

Pleuropneumonie, Contagieuse Caprine, Bou-frida, Abunini

IMPORTANCE

Contagious caprine pleuropneumonia (CCPP) is one of the most severe diseases of goats. This disease, which affects the respiratory tract, is extremely contagious and frequently fatal; in some naïve flocks, the morbidity and mortality rates may reach 100%. CCPP causes major economic losses in Africa, Asia and the Middle East, where it is endemic. Definitive diagnosis can be difficult, as the causative agent is one of the most fastidious mycoplasmas and can be missed during routine bacteriological analysis. CCPP is now known to also affect some species of exotic ungulates. This has raised concerns for zoos and for the conservation of some endangered species exposed to goats.

ETIOLOGY

Contagious caprine pleuropneumonia is caused by *Mycoplasma capricolum* subsp. *capripneumoniae* (formerly *Mycoplasma* biotype F-38), a member of the family Mycoplasmataceae. Epidemiological studies of this organism are still limited; however, genetic analyses have grouped *M. capripneumoniae* isolates into two major clusters representing two evolutionary lines of the organism, five lineages which correspond to geographic regions, or six genotypes (A to F).

M. capripneumoniae belongs to a closely related group of mycoplasmas called the *Mycoplasma mycoides* cluster. Another organism in this group, *M. mycoides* subsp. *capri* (a species now containing both *M. mycoides* subsp. *capri* and the former *M. mycoides* subsp. *mycoides* large-colony type) can cause a disease that resembles CCPP but may have extrapulmonary signs and lesions. Some texts consider *M. mycoides* subsp. *capri* to be a minor cause of contagious caprine pleuropneumonia; however, the World Organization for Animal Health (OIE) defines CCPP as only the disease caused by *M. capricolum* subsp. *capripneumoniae*.

SPECIES AFFECTED

Goats are the primary hosts for *M. capripneumoniae,* and the only domesticated animals proven to be affected by this organism. At present, the significance of infections in sheep is uncertain; however, at least two papers have reported the occurrence of *M. capripneumoniae* in healthy or sick sheep. There is also a possibility that this organism might have been involved in an outbreak of acute respiratory disease among goats and sheep in Ethiopia in 2002. *M. capripneumoniae* has caused clinical cases in some wild ungulates including wild

C

goats (*Capra aegagrus*), Nubian ibex (*Capra ibex nubiana*), Laristan mouflon (*Ovis orientalis laristanica*), gerenuk (*Litocranius walleri*), sand gazelles (*Gazella subgutturosa marica*), Arabian oryx (*Oryx leucoryx*), and Tibetan antelope (*Pantholops hodgsonii*).

Zoonotic potential

There is no evidence that humans are infected by *M. capripneumoniae*.

GEOGRAPHIC DISTRIBUTION

Contagious caprine pleuropneumonia can be found in many countries in Africa, Asia) and the Middle East. *M. capripneumoniae* is difficult to isolate from clinical material, and its presence has not been confirmed in all affected countries. In some cases, reports of its occurrence are based on clinical signs alone.

TRANSMISSION

Contagious caprine pleuropneumonia is highly contagious. This disease is transmitted during close contact, by the inhalation of respiratory droplets. Chronic carriers may exist, but this remains unproven. Some outbreaks have occurred in endemic areas when apparently healthy goats were introduced into flocks, and in one experiment, a goat developed clinical CCPP nearly three months after contact with infected goats and a month after all other animals had recovered. However, one study that followed a large flock of experimentally infected goats for up to 105 days did not find any chronic carriers.

DISINFECTION

Mycoplasma spp. are generally short-lived, fragile organisms in the environment. If disinfection is needed, they are reported to be susceptible to a number of agents including 1% sodium hypochlorite, 70% ethanol, phenolic disinfectants, iodophores, formaldehyde, glutaraldehyde, and peracetic acid.

INCUBATION PERIOD

The incubation period is commonly 6 to 10 days, but is reported to range from 2 days to 4 weeks.

CLINICAL SIGNS

Contagious caprine pleuropneumonia is strictly a respiratory disease. Peracute, acute and chronic forms may be seen in endemic areas. Peracutely affected goats can die within 1 to 3 days with minimal clinical signs. In acute disease, the initial signs are a very high fever (41-43°C; 106-109°F) lethargy and anorexia, followed by coughing and labored respiration. The cough is frequent, violent and productive. In the final stages of disease, the goat may not be able to move, and stands with its front legs wide apart, and its neck stiff and extended. Saliva can drip continuously from the mouth, and the animal may grunt or bleat in pain. Frothy nasal discharge

and stringy saliva may be seen terminally. Pregnant goats can abort. Acutely affected goats generally die within 7 to 10 days. Subacute or chronic cases tend to be milder, with coughing mainly following activity. Chronic CCPP is characterized by a chronic cough, nasal discharge and debilitation.

Clinical signs in wild or captive wild ungulates have been similar to cases in goats.

POST MORTEM LESIONS

The lesions of contagious caprine pleuropneumonia are limited to the respiratory system. Acute disease is characterized by unilateral or bilateral pneumonia and serofibrinous pleuritis with straw-colored fluid in the thorax. On cut surface, the lung is granular with copious straw-colored exudate. Pea-sized, yellow nodules may be found in the lungs; these nodules are surrounded by areas of congestion. Varying degrees of lung consolidation or necrosis can be seen, and the regional (bronchial) lymph nodes are enlarged. Some long-term survivors have chronic pleuropneumonia or chronic pleuritis, with encapsulation of acute lesions and numerous adhesions to the chest wall. The interlobular septa are not usually thickened in domesticated goats.

Wild ruminants with CCPP have similar lesions; however, thickening of the interlobular septa has been reported in some animals.

DIAGNOSTIC TESTS

A definitive diagnosis can be made by detecting *M. capripneumoniae* in lung tissue, exudate from lung lesions, pleural fluid or regional lymph nodes at necropsy. Samples should be taken from active lung lesions, ideally from the interface between consolidated and unconsolidated areas. Although morphology does not provide definitive identification, *M. capripneumoniae* has a branching, filamentous structure in exudates, impression smears or tissue sections examined under the microscope. Other caprine mycoplasmas usually appear as short filamentous organisms or coccobacilli. *M. capripneumoniae* and other members of the *M. mycoides* cluster cross-react in serological tests and share biochemical and antigenic similarities, making specific identification of this organism difficult and time-consuming unless genetic tests such as polymerase chain reaction (PCR) assays are used.

M. capripneumoniae is one of the most fastidious mycoplasmas, and must be isolated on mycoplasma media such as 'viande foie goat' (VFG), modified Hayflick's or modified Newing's tryptose. Colonies or other evidence of growth (i.e., faint turbidity in broth) may appear in 5-15 days. PCR is generally used for identification of the culture, although biochemical tests and serological assays (growth inhibition, immunofluorescence) can also be employed and were used more frequently in the past. Biochemical tests are unable to unequivocally identify the members of the *M.*

mycoides cluster, and serological identification is hampered by cross-reactivity. Because *M. capripneumoniae* is so fastidious and cultures can be overgrown with other mycoplasmas, it may not be isolated from clinical samples, particularly if the sample has not been conserved adequately. This organism has not been found in lesions from animals with chronic disease.

PCR is more likely to be successful than culture, and can be used to identify *M. capripneumoniae* directly in tissue samples or pleural fluid. Isothermal amplification methods (loop-mediated isothermal amplification, recombinase polymerase amplification) have been reported in the literature. *M. capripneumoniae* antigens can be detected in tissue samples by immunostaining or gel immunoprecipitin tests, and a latex agglutination test to detect antigens has been described in the literature. Cross-reactions can be an issue in antigen detection tests.

Serological tests to detect antibodies to *M. capripneumoniae* include complement fixation, latex agglutination (which can identify early IgM antibodies), and competitive enzyme linked immunosorbent assays (ELISA). Animals with acute CCPP rarely develop measurable titers before death; antibodies usually become detectable 7-9 days after the first clinical signs. Whenever possible, paired serum samples should be collected 3-8 weeks apart. Serological tests are generally used on a herd basis and not for individual diagnosis. These tests do not identify all reactors, and cross-reactivity is an issue. A more specific competitive binding ELISA, described in 2014, was reported not to cross-react with other *Mycoplasma* found in goats.

TREATMENT

Some antibiotics, such as tetracyclines, fluoroquinolones (e.g., danofloxacin) and the macrolide family, can be effective if given early. Complete elimination of mycoplasma is reported to be rare, and treated animals may be potential carriers. The degree of risk from treated animals spreading *M. capripneumoniae* is still uncertain.

CONTROL

Disease reporting

A quick response is vital for containing outbreaks in regions free of contagious caprine pleuropneumonia. Veterinarians who encounter or suspect this disease should follow their national and/or local guidelines for disease reporting. In the U.S., state or federal veterinary authorities should be informed immediately.

Prevention

Contagious caprine pleuropneumonia is most likely to enter a country in infected animals, due to the poor survival of mycoplasmal organisms in the environment. It is uncertain whether long-term subclinical carriers exist; however, some outbreaks in endemic areas have occurred when apparently healthy goats were introduced into flocks. Outbreaks can be eradicated with quarantines, movement controls, slaughter of infected and exposed animals, and cleaning and disinfection of the premises. Some countries have included vaccination in their eradication procedures.

In endemic areas, care should be taken when introducing new animals into the flock. Flock testing, slaughter, and on-site quarantine may be helpful in controlling the spread of disease. Vaccines help prevent disease in some countries.

Vaccination has also been helpful in ending some outbreaks among captive wild animals. In addition, antibiotic treatment and reductions in animal density (to decrease contact between animals) were sometimes employed. In endemic areas, exotic ungulates that may be susceptible should be kept from contact with goats. Fencing may be helpful; however, there is one report of transmission from sick sand gazelle to an Arabian oryx in the adjacent enclosure, when the animals were separated by a double mesh fence. *Mycoplasma* screening may be considered before animals are released into a zoo or other site, but *M. capripneumoniae* infections can be difficult to detect.

MORBIDITY AND MORTALITY

Contagious caprine pleuropneumonia is a highly contagious disease in naïve animals. Exposure to *M. capripneumoniae* appears to be common among goats in some endemic regions. In some herds, most animals may be seropositive. One recent study, which used a new, more specific, monoclonal antibody-based cELISA, found that the seroprevalence among goats with respiratory signs ranged from < 5% to 44% in some parts of Asia. During outbreaks, the morbidity rate can be as high as 100% and the mortality rate up to 70-100%. These rates can be influenced by previous exposure, and by the amount of contact between animals (close contact facilitates transmission).

High morbidity and mortality rates have also been reported in some exotic ungulates. During an outbreak among captive wild ungulates in 2007, the morbidity and mortality rates were 100% and 82%, respectively, in wild goats, and 93% and 58% in Nubian ibex. During a later outbreak, 34% mortality occurred in one enclosure of sand gazelle. A CCPP outbreak among wild Tibetan antelope resulted in thousands of deaths and the estimated loss of 16% of the population, although it is possible that some deaths were due to other causes.

CONTAGIOUS EQUINE METRITIS

IMPORTANCE

Contagious equine metritis (CEM) is a highly communicable venereal disease of horses, caused by the bacterium *Taylorella equigenitalis*. This disease can spread widely from a single asymptomatic carrier, particularly a stallion. Infected horses do not become systemically ill or die, but reproductive success is reduced. Additional economic impacts include the cost of pre-breeding tests and treatment in endemic areas, as well as screening before importation into CEM-free countries.

Excluding *T. equigenitalis* from a country can be challenging. Control programs have significantly reduced the incidence of this disease in Thoroughbreds, which were severely affected by outbreaks in the 1970s; however, it also occurs in other breeds, and identifying carriers can be difficult. *T. equigenitalis* is fastidious and can be difficult to culture, and serological tests are useful only in mares and for short periods. In addition, some recent strains circulate with only mild clinical signs. In the U.S., an outbreak in 2008-2010 may have resulted from the importation of an infected horse 8 years earlier. Similarly, *T. equigenitalis* appears to have circulated for some time before the 2011 outbreak in South Africa, although the country was thought to be CEM-free. Thus, contagious equine metritis should be a diagnostic consideration even where this organism is thought to be absent.

ETIOLOGY

Contagious equine metritis is caused by *Taylorella equigenitalis*, a fastidious microaerophilic gram-negative coccobacillus in the family Alcaligenaceae. Only one serotype is known; however, there are two biotypes, one sensitive and the other resistant to streptomycin. Streptomycin-resistant strains were common in the past, but most of the currently circulating strains are streptomycin-sensitive. *T. equigenitalis* strains can differ significantly in virulence.

The closely related organism *Taylorella asinigenitalis* seems to be associated mainly with donkeys. *T. asinigenitalis* can cause clinical signs in some experimentally infected (horse) mares; however, no symptomatic infections have been reported in naturally infected equids, as of 2015, and this organism is currently considered to be nonpathogenic. At present, its major significance is that it must be distinguished from *T. equigenitalis* during diagnostic testing.

SPECIES AFFECTED

Horses appear to be the only natural hosts for *T. equigenitalis*, although donkeys have been infected under experimental conditions. Attempts to infect cattle, pigs, sheep and cats were unsuccessful, but some laboratory rodents could be infected for relatively short periods by intrauterine inoculation.

Donkeys are thought to be the major hosts for *T. asinigenitalis*, but this organism has also been isolated from a small number of mares and a few stallions. Most of these horses appear to have been infected during contact with donkey jacks, especially during breeding.

Zoonotic potential

There is no evidence that *T. equigenitalis* infects humans.

GEOGRAPHIC DISTRIBUTION

The geographic distribution of *T. equigenitalis* is difficult to estimate accurately. This organism has been detected at times in Europe, North and South America, Africa and Asia and on some islands. In some countries, it may be absent or rare in some breeds of horses (e.g., Thoroughbreds) due to control programs, but present in others. Some nations reported to have eradicated contagious equine metritis include certain European countries, the U.S., Canada, Australia and Japan.

T. asinigenitalis has been detected in North America (the U.S.) and Europe (e.g., France, Sweden, Italy), and probably exists in other areas.

TRANSMISSION

T. equigenitalis is transmitted mainly during mating. It can also be spread by infected semen during artificial insemination (AI) or introduced to the genital tract on fomites. The risk of infection appears to be lower in mares bred by AI than natural service, and one study reported that the antibiotics in semen extenders significantly decreased infection rates. Transmission risks associated with embryo transfer are incompletely understood.

Stallions are the most common source of the infection. In untreated stallions, *T. equigenitalis* can persist for months or years on the reproductive tract, where it may be detected in the urethral fossa and its associated sinus, the distal urethra, the exterior of the penis and prepuce, and occasionally in the pre-ejaculatory fluid. Up to 20-25% of mares can also carry *T. equigenitalis* after they recover from acute disease. The vast majority of carrier mares maintain *T. equigenitalis* on the clitoris, particularly in the clitoral sinuses and fossa, but a few carry it in the uterus. Carriage is typically shorter in mares than stallions (often a few weeks to months); however, there have been cases where mares carried the organism for organism for years. Foals born to infected mares can also maintain *T. equigenitalis* on the external genitalia, and may become long-term asymptomatic carriers.

There is no evidence that *T. equigenitalis* survives long-term in a free-living form in the environment. However, this organism has been reported to persist, at least for short periods, in some free-living amoebae (e.g., *Acanthamoeba castellanii*).

DISINFECTION

T. equigenitalis is susceptible to most common disinfectants, including chlorhexidine, ionic and nonionic detergents, and sodium hypochlorite (400 parts per million).

INCUBATION PERIOD

The incubation period is 2 to 14 days; most infections become apparent 10 to 14 days after breeding.

CLINICAL SIGNS

Infected stallions display no clinical signs. Mares can develop metritis and become temporarily infertile, although they have no systemic signs. Some of these infections are subclinical; the only sign may be a return to estrus after a shortened estrus cycle. In other cases, a mucopurulent, grayish-white vaginal discharge develops a week or two after breeding; in severe cases, the discharge is copious. Mixed bacterial infections may result in a gray to yellow exudate. Variable degrees of endometritis, cervicitis and vaginitis can sometimes be found if the reproductive tract is examined with a speculum. Infertility usually lasts a few weeks, with the discharge often disappearing in a few days to two weeks. Long-term effects on reproduction have not been reported; however, some mares can carry *T. equigenitalis* for a time. Carriers are usually asymptomatic, although a few mares many have an intermittent vaginal discharge.

Most infected mares do not conceive. Those that do usually give birth to a normal full-term foal, which may carry the organism asymptomatically. Some infected mares have an intermittent vaginal discharge during the pregnancy, while others do not. Abortions also occur, but appear to be rare.

T. asinigenitalis has not been reported to cause disease in donkeys or horses under natural conditions; however, some experimentally infected mares developed cervicitis and metritis, with vaginal and cervical discharges. These mares had a shortened estrus cycle and failed to conceive. The clinical signs were milder than in mares infected with *T. equigenitalis*.

POST MORTEM LESIONS

The most severe lesions are usually found in the uterus. The endometrial folds may be swollen and edematous, and a mucopurulent exudate may be apparent. Edema, hyperemia and a mucopurulent exudate may be seen on the cervix. Salpingitis and vaginitis also occur. The lesions are most apparent approximately 14 days after infection, then gradually decrease in severity over the next few weeks. They are not pathognomonic for contagious equine metritis.

DIAGNOSTIC TESTS

Microscopic examination of the uterine discharge may reveal numerous gram-negative coccobacilli or bacilli (present individually or arranged end-to-end) and large numbers of inflammatory cells. *T. equigenitalis* is often pleomorphic and may exhibit bipolar staining.

Contagious equine metritis can be diagnosed by isolation of the causative organism from the genital tract, or with polymerase chain reaction (PCR) assays. Samples collected from mares include vaginal discharges from clinical cases; or swabs of the clitoral fossa and its sinuses from suspected carriers, with the addition of cervical and endometrial swabs if the animal is not pregnant. If possible, carrier mares should be cultured during estrus, particularly during the first part of the cycle. In stallions, swabs are taken from the urethral fossa and sinus, distal urethra, and external surface of the penis and the prepuce. The pre-ejaculatory fluid may also be sampled. For optimal success, carriers should be sampled on more than one occasion, at intervals of 7 days or more. No systemic antibiotics should be used for at least 7 days, or topical antibiotics for 21 days, before a sample is taken for culture. If an infected mare conceives, *T. equigenitalis* may also be found on the placenta, on the genital tract of some normal foals, and in multiple sites in aborted fetuses. The fragility of the organism dictates special transport conditions (e.g., transport in Amies medium) and rapid transfer to the laboratory.

PCR (where available) can be used directly on clinical samples, and some assays can distinguish *T. equigenitalis* from *T. asinigenitalis*. Culture should be performed by a laboratory experienced in isolating *T. equigenitalis*; this organism is fastidious and difficult to grow. It can be isolated on chocolate (heated blood) agar. Additives (e.g., Timoney's medium) are often incorporated to suppress the growth of commensal organisms, which may otherwise prevent its recovery. Some media take advantage of the resistance of certain *T. equigenitalis* strains to streptomycin; however, streptomycin-sensitive biotypes are now more common, and isolation should not rely solely on such media. Colonies usually become visible in 3-6 days, although they may rarely take up to 2 weeks to appear. *T. equigenitalis* colonies can be identified by PCR, biochemical tests, identification with immunological techniques and molecular genotyping (e.g., 16S rRNA gene analysis). Immunological methods for identification can include slide agglutination, latex agglutination and immunostaining. Rare cross-reactions with *Mannheimia haemolytica* have been reported in some tests. *T. equigenitalis* and *T. asinigenitalis* react identically in biochemical tests, and cross-react in some serological assays. Tests that could distinguish these two organisms in published reports have been based on PCR, 16S rRNA sequencing, loop-mediated isothermal amplification methods, MLST and indirect immunofluorescence. *T. equigenitalis* can be genotyped for epidemiological purposes with molecular tests such as pulsed-field gel electrophoresis (PFGE). A multilocus sequence typing (MLST) scheme was described recently.

Because carrier stallions can have few organisms, cultures from these animals may be unsuccessful. For this reason, stallions may be bred to test mares and these mares tested for *T. equigenitalis*.

Serology is unreliable as a diagnostic tool, but it may be helpful as an adjunct screening test. Serological tests include complement fixation, rapid plate agglutination, enzyme-linked immunosorbent assay (ELISA), passive hemagglutination and agar-gel immunodiffusion. Antibodies can be found in acutely infected mares beginning 7 days after infection; however, in some animals, they may be undetectable for up to 2 to 3 weeks. Antibodies persist for up to 6 to 10 weeks after the primary infection, then disappear. Complement fixation can detect infected mares 21-45 days after they have been bred to a suspected carrier stallion, but this test becomes unreliable thereafter. Carrier mares may or may not be seropositive. Stallions do not produce detectable antibodies to *T. equigenitalis*.

TREATMENT

In carriers, *T. equigenitalis* may be cleared by washing the external genitalia with disinfectants (e.g., chlorhexidine), combined with local antimicrobial treatments such as nitrofurazone, silver sulfadiazine or gentamicin ointment. Particular care should be taken in the washing of the clitoral fossa and sinuses. Systemic antibiotics might also be recommended in some animals. Treatment may need to be repeated in some cases in both mares and stallions, and the optimal length of treatment is undefined. Surgical excision of the clitoral sinuses (which can be difficult to expose for topical treatment) may eliminate the organism in mares that do not respond to treatment, but this is uncommon and it is rarely used. Some mares can also clear the infection on their own; however, this is unpredictable and may take several months or more in some cases. Acutely infected mares may or may not be treated with antibiotics; it is unclear whether treated mares eliminate the organism more rapidly.

Similar treatments could eliminate *T. asinigenitalis* from donkeys and horses in one study.

CONTROL

Disease reporting

Veterinarians who encounter or suspect contagious equine metritis should follow their national and/or local guidelines for disease reporting. In the U.S., state or federal veterinary authorities should be informed immediately.

Prevention

In countries free from contagious equine metritis, horses are screened for *T. equigenitalis* during importation. Infected animals must be treated and test negative before they are released into the community. The fastidious nature of the organism complicates its detection.

Where this disease is present, it is controlled by breeding only from stallions and mares that have been tested for the organism and are known not to be carriers. Control programs have generally been based on the UK's Horserace Betting Levy Board's Code of Practice (www.hblb.org.uk/codes.htm), which is reviewed and updated annually. Samples are generally taken from all stallions at the beginning of the breeding season, and from mares according to the risk that they carry this organism. Mares with clinical signs, including those that return to estrus prematurely, should be investigated. Good hygiene, decontamination of potential fomites, and sanitation during breeding are also important. While fomites associated with breeding are the primary risk, other objects, such as sponges used to groom multiple horses, might also transfer the organism. There is no vaccine.

T. equigenitalis has been eradicated from some countries by surveillance/ testing, quarantine of infected animals, treatment and a moratorium on breeding from infected animals.

MORBIDITY AND MORTALITY

The transmission rate during natural service varies between animals and over time, but it can be very high in some instances. In some cases, nearly every mare mated to an infected stallion will become infected. Approximately 30-40% of infected mares are estimated develop clinical signs. Most mares recover without incident, but some continue to carry *T. equigenitalis*, usually asymptomatically. Fatal infections have not been seen.

Immunity after an infection is not complete, and mares can be infected repeatedly during a short period of time. The first infection is usually the most severe; infertility and clinical signs are less likely to occur during later bouts of the disease, and some mares conceive.

DOURINE

Covering Disease, Morbo Coitale Maligno, Slapsiekte, El Dourin, Mal de Coit, Beschalseuche, Sluchnaya Bolyezn Lappessa Dirressa

IMPORTANCE

Dourine is a serious, often chronic, venereal disease of horses and other equids. This protozoal infection can result in neurological signs and emaciation, and the case fatality rate is high. No vaccine is available, and the long-term efficacy of treatment is uncertain.

ETIOLOGY

Dourine is caused by the protozoan parasite *Trypanosoma equiperdum* (subgenus *Trypanozoon*, Salivarian section). It is very closely related to the causative agents of African trypanosomiasis (*Trypanosoma brucei*, and surra (*T evansi*), and whether it should be considered a distinct species is controversial. Strains of *T. equiperdum* appear to differ in pathogenicity.

SPECIES AFFECTED

Dourine mainly affects horses, donkeys and mules. These species appear to be the only natural reservoirs for *T. equiperdum*. Zebras have tested positive by serology, but there is no conclusive evidence of infection.

Naturally occurring infections or clinical cases have not been reported in other species. It is difficult to infect healthy laboratory animals directly with isolates from equids, but mice immunosuppressed with glucocorticoids were more susceptible, and some rabbits were infected by intratesticular inoculation. Sheep, goats, dogs, rabbits, rats and mice can be infected with mouse-adapted strains, and may develop clinical signs. However, ruminants do not seem to be susceptible to isolates from equids, and a recent attempt to inoculate dogs with samples from horses also failed.

Zoonotic potential

There is no evidence that *T. equiperdum* can infect humans.

GEOGRAPHIC DISTRIBUTION

Dourine was once widespread, but it has been eradicated from many countries. Diagnosing dourine can be difficult, especially where other trypanosomes are also present, and the current distribution of this organism is unclear. Between 1995 and 2015, published papers and reports to the World Organization for Animal Health (OIE) suggested that this disease is endemic in parts of Africa and Asia. *T. equiperdum* is also reported to exist in South America, although there is little or no recent information from this region. In addition, dourine may occur in some areas where testing is not done.

TRANSMISSION

Unlike other trypanosomal infections, dourine is transmitted almost exclusively during breeding. Transmission from stallions to mares is more common, but mares can also transmit the disease to stallions. *T. equiperdum* can be found in the vaginal secretions of infected mares and the seminal fluid, mucous exudate of the penis, and sheath of stallions. Periodically, the parasites disappear from the genital tract and the animal becomes noninfectious for weeks to months. Noninfectious periods are more common late in the disease. Male donkeys can be asymptomatic carriers. (Note: While mules are usually sterile, they have functional reproductive organs and can become infected with *T. equiperdum* if they

are allowed to mate.). There is currently no evidence that arthropod vectors play any role in transmission.

Rarely, infected mares have been reported to pass the infection to their foals, possibly before birth or through the milk. Trypanosomes have been detected in the mammary secretions of some infected animals. Infections are also thought to occur through mucous membranes such as the conjunctiva. Sexually immature animals that become infected can transmit the organism when they mature.

T. equiperdum is reported to be unable to survive for long outside a living organism. The related organism *T. brucei* remained viable for up to 6 days in blood under some carefully controlled laboratory conditions.

DISINFECTION

There is limited need for disinfectants, due to the fragility of trypanosomes in the environment, and no studies have examined the disinfectant susceptibility of *T. equiperdum* directly. The closely related organism *T. brucei* can be inactivated by various agents including 0.05% sodium hypochlorite, 70% ethanol, 2% TriGene™, 0.1% hand soap, 2% formaldehyde and 0.05% glutaraldehyde. The temperature reported to kill 100% of trypomastigotes is 50°C.

INCUBATION PERIOD

The incubation period is a few weeks to several years.

CLINICAL SIGNS

The initial lesions of dourine often involve the genitalia. Mares typically develop a mucopurulent vaginal discharge, and the vulva becomes edematous. Vulvitis, vaginitis with polyuria, and signs of discomfort may be seen. There may also be raised and thickened semitransparent patches on the vaginal mucosa. Some mares may abort. Stallions develop edema of the prepuce and glans penis, and can have a mucopurulent discharge from the urethra. Paraphimosis is possible. Genital edema can disappear and reappear in both stallions and mares; each time it resolves, the extent of the permanently thickened, indurated tissue becomes greater. Vesicles or ulcers may also be detected; when they heal, these ulcers can leave permanent white scars called leukodermic patches. In addition, the genital region, perineum and udder may become depigmented. In some horses, edema can spread to involve the ventral abdomen and perineum, including the scrotum in stallions and mammary gland in mares. A serum-like or cloudy, whitish mammary secretion may be noted. Some horses in Italy had severe swelling of the ventral abdominal and legs (especially the hindlegs) without genital involvement, most likely because the genital lesions had resolved.

Edematous patches called "silver dollar plaques" (up to 10 cm diameter and 1 cm thick) may appear on the skin, particularly over the ribs. These cutaneous plaques usually last for 3 to 7 days and are considered pathognomonic for the disease, although they have been reported occasionally with *T. evansi.* They do not occur with all *T. equiperdum* strains. Horses in Italy were reported to have smaller, variable wheals and plaques, which lasted for hours to days, and waxed and waned in different parts of the body. Pustular dermatitis was also described in this outbreak.

Neurological signs can develop soon after the genital edema, or weeks to months later. Restlessness and weight shifting from one leg to another is often followed by progressive weakness, stiffness, lameness (especially in the hindlegs) incoordination and, eventually, paralysis. Facial paralysis, which is generally unilateral, may be seen in some animals, and ptosis of the lower lip is common. During outbreaks in Italy, the neurological signs were not accompanied by sensory dysfunction.

Conjunctivitis and keratitis are common in some reports, and ocular disease may sometimes be the first sign of dourine. Anemia is common, and intermittent fever may be found. In addition, dourine results in progressive loss of condition, predisposing animals to other diseases. Affected animals can become emaciated, although the appetite remains good. Overall, the course of the disease ranges from a chronic, relatively mild condition that persists for years to a more acute illness that often lasts only 1-2 months, and in rare cases, can progress to the end stage in as little as a week. The clinical signs can develop over weeks or months. They frequently wax and wane; relapses may be precipitated by stress. This can occur several times before the animal either dies or experiences an apparent recovery. Whether animals can recover permanently is controversial. Subclinical infections have also been described.

POST MORTEM LESIONS

Cachexia and genital edema are often seen at necropsy. In stallions, the scrotum, sheath and testicular tunica may be thickened and infiltrated. The testes may be embedded in sclerotic tissue and may not be recognizable. In mares, a gelatinous infiltrate may thicken the vulva, vaginal mucosa, uterus, bladder and mammary glands. In one case, the uterine mucosa was reported to be congested with widespread hemorrhages. There may also be swelling of the ventral abdomen and the legs, and gelatinous exudates can often be found under the skin. One report described pustular dermatitis, with histological lesions consisting of severe inflammation and vacuolar degeneration of the skin, and exudates consisting of cellular detritus (mainly eosinophils) and free protozoa. Chronic lymphadenitis may also be apparent. The perineural connective tissue can be infiltrated with edematous fluid, and the spinal cord may be surrounded by a serous infiltrate. A soft, pulpy or discolored spinal cord may be noted, particularly in the lumbar or sacral regions.

DIAGNOSTIC TESTS

Dourine is usually diagnosed by serology combined with clinical signs, supported by evidence from histopathology and epidemiological evidence of non-insect-mediated transmission. The complement fixation (CF) test is the prescribed test for international trade, and has been used successfully in eradication programs. However, no serological test is specific for dourine, as cross-reactions occur with Old World trypanosomes, especially *T. brucei* and *T. evansi.* In addition, uninfected animals, particularly donkeys and mules, often have inconsistent or nonspecific reactions (false positives) in the CF test, due to anticomplementary effects in equid serum. Indirect fluorescent antibody tests may help to resolve these cases. A chemiluminescent immunoblot assay for *T. equiperdum* has been described in the literature, and is also reported to resolve false positives. Other serologic tests that have been employed include ELISAs, radioimmunoassay, counter immunoelectrophoresis, agar gel immunodiffusion (AGID) and card agglutination. Immunostaining has been used to detect trypanosomes in tissues.

Dourine can also be diagnosed by identification of the parasite; however, the organisms are extremely difficult to find, and *T. equiperdum* cannot be distinguished microscopically from *T. evansi.* A small number of trypanosomes may be present in the lymph, edematous fluids of the external genitalia, vaginal or preputial washings or scrapings (collected soon after infection), mammary gland exudates or fluid content of plaques. The organisms are more likely to be detected soon after the edema or plaques first appear, and they only occur for a few days in plaques. Repeated sampling may be helpful. On rare occasions, *T. equiperdum* can be found in thick blood films; however, it is present very transiently in the blood, and is usually undetectable. The success rate can be improved by concentration techniques such as capillary tube centrifugation or mini anion exchange centrifugation. PCR assays have also been used in diagnosis (with exudates or tissue samples) and are more sensitive than culture; however, they identify the parasite only to the level of the subgenus *Trypanozoon. T. evansi* is also a member of this subgenus, and currently there is no genetic technique that can distinguish these two organisms.

TREATMENT

Treatment may be possible in endemic areas; however, it is still uncertain whether trypanosomal drugs can completely eliminate this parasite. In some areas, relapses are reported to be common after drug treatment. One recent study found that bis (aminoethylthio) 4-melaminophenylarsine dihydrochloride (cymelarsan) was effective in a small number of acutely or chronically infected horses, and relapses were not observed up to a year after treatment. Further evaluation of this drug is still required.

CONTROL

Disease reporting

Veterinarians who encounter or suspect dourine should follow their national and/or local guidelines for disease reporting. In the U.S., state or federal veterinary authorities should be informed immediately.

Prevention

To prevent dourine from being introduced into a herd or dourine-free region, new animals should be quarantined and tested by serology. When this disease is found in an area, quarantines and the cessation of breeding can prevent transmission while infected animals are identified. Dourine can be eradicated from a herd, using serology to identify infected equids. Infected animals are typically euthanized. While *T. equiperdum* does not survival for long in the environment, good hygiene and sanitation are nevertheless advisable at assisted matings to avoid any potential for fomite-mediated transmission. No vaccine is available.

Stallions have sometimes been castrated in an attempt to prevent disease transmission; however, geldings can still transmit the disease if they display copulatory behavior.

MORBIDITY AND MORTALITY

The severity and duration of dourine may vary with the virulence of the strain and the health of the horse (e.g., nutritional status, concurrent illnesses) and existence of stressors that may precipitate a relapse. While some animals progress to the end stage of the disease within 1-2 months, experimentally infected horses have survived up to 10 years. More severe disease is usually seen in improved breeds of horses, while donkeys, mules and native ponies tend to be more resistant. Subclinical infections have also been described.

The mortality rate in untreated cases is estimated to be 50-70%. However, apparent recoveries have been questioned by some, in view of the long course of the disease and the waxing and waning symptoms. Some authors feel that nearly all cases are eventually fatal.

EBOLAVIRUS AND MARBURGVIRUS INFECTIONS

Ebola and Marburg Virus Disease, Ebola and Marburg Hemorrhagic Fever, African Hemorrhagic Fever

IMPORTANCE

Ebolaviruses and marburgviruses are incompletely understood pathogens that cause severe, often fatal, illnesses in humans and non-human primates. These diseases have been known as Ebola and Marburg hemorrhagic fevers, respectively, after the most dramatic symptoms in severe cases. The names "Ebola virus disease" or Marburg virus disease" are now preferred by the World Health Organization (WHO) and some other groups.

Most species of ebolaviruses and the only known species of marburgvirus occur in Africa. Current evidence suggests that the reservoir hosts are probably bats, while other animals and people are incidental hosts. Humans seem to become infected with marburgviruses mainly in caves or mines harboring bats, while ebolavirus infections are often associated with handling tissues from infected nonhuman primates and other species. Once a virus has entered human populations, it can spread from person to person. Some epidemics have affected hundreds of people, particularly when nosocomial spread occurs from inadequate medical supplies or barrier nursing procedures, or when outbreaks are not recognized for long periods. An outbreak of unprecedented size in West Africa began in December 2013, and was first recognized in March 2013. It is being spread in some densely populated urban regions, and has affected thousands of people to date. Although the mortality rate has varied between outbreaks, some ebolaviruses or marburgviruses have killed up to 90% of those who become infected. Treatment options are limited, and with the exception of experimental treatments, consist of supportive care alone. Epizootics in gorillas and chimpanzees are equally serious, and may threaten the survival of these species in the wild. Other wild mammals including duikers also seem to be killed during outbreaks.

One species, *Reston ebolavirus*, has been reported outside Africa, in the Philippines and China. This virus does not seem to affect humans, although some people may seroconvert. However, it can cause fatal illness in some species of nonhuman primates. Between 1989 and 1996, *Reston ebolavirus* was isolated repeatedly at primate quarantine facilities in the U.S. and Italy; in all but one instance, infected monkeys had been imported from a single facility in the Philippines. The source of the virus was never found, but

D

E

infected monkeys do not seem to have been exported since this facility was closed in 1997. In 2008, however, *Reston ebolavirus* was discovered in pigs during an unusually severe outbreak of porcine reproductive and respiratory syndrome (PRRS) in the Philippines. This virus was also found in pigs with PRRS in China. Based on experimental studies, *Reston ebolavirus* alone does not seem to cause any illness in pigs, although its effect during co-infection with other pathogens has not yet been evaluated. Accumulating evidence suggests that ebolaviruses or their relatives may also occur in other locations, although the clinical significance of these viruses for humans and domesticated animals is uncertain.

ETIOLOGY

Ebola and Marburg hemorrhagic fever are caused by members of the genera *Ebolavirus* and *Marburgvirus,* respectively, in the family Filoviridae. The names of these viruses have undergone several taxonomic changes since they were first discovered, including new changes officially accepted in 2013. Currently, the genus *Ebolavirus* contains five recognized viral species: *Zaire ebolavirus, Sudan ebolavirus, Taï Forest ebolavirus* (formerly *Cote d'Ivoire ebolavirus*), *Reston ebolavirus* and *Bundibugyo ebolavirus*. The common name for the single virus in each of these species is Ebola virus (formerly Zaire ebolavirus), Sudan virus (formerly Sudan ebolavirus), Tai Forest virus (formerly Cote d'Ivoire ebolavirus), Reston virus (formerly Reston ebolavirus) and Bundibugyo virus. *Marburgvirus* contains a single species, *Marburg marburgvirus* (formerly *Lake Victoria marburgvirus*), and two individual viruses, Marburg virus and Ravn virus, within this species.

A third genus, *Cuevavirus*, (species *Lloviu cuevavirus;* Lloviu virus) has been proposed for a filovirus found during an outbreak of viral pneumonia among Schreiber's bats (*Miniopterus schreibersii*) in Europe. Very little is known about Lloviu virus. To date, it has not been isolated in culture, or found in other species.

[Note: because the distinctions between terms such as 'Ebola virus,' 'ebolaviruses,' '*Zaire ebolavirus*' and the recently used common name 'Zaire ebolavirus' can be confusing, specific viruses are identified by species name rather than common name in this factsheet.]

SPECIES AFFECTED

Reservoir hosts

Bats are thought to be the reservoir hosts for filoviruses, and appear to carry these viruses asymptomatically. Antibodies to ebolaviruses and/or viral RNA have been found in a number of bat species in Africa, with a high seroprevalence in several species of fruit bat. All studies to date have examined bats for *Zaire ebolavirus* or *Reston ebolavirus*, although the other ebolaviruses are probably also maintained in these animals. Outside Africa, antibodies to *Reston ebolavirus* were found in a species of fruit bat (*Rousettus amplexicaudatus*) in the Philippines. The cave-dwelling Egyptian fruit bat (*Rousettus aegyptiacus*) seems to be the primary host for *Marburg marburgvirus*, although evidence of infection has been found in other fruit bats and insectivorous bats. *Marburg marburgvirus* is the only filovirus, to date, that has actually been isolated from the tissues of bats in the wild. Surveillance among wildlife is incomplete, and it is possible that other reservoir or amplifying hosts also exist. In 1998, *Zaire ebolavirus* RNA was found in six mice (*Mus setulosus* and *Praomys* sp) and a shrew (*Sylvisorex ollula*), and these species were proposed as possible reservoir hosts. However, the results have not been confirmed by other groups, and virus isolation was unsuccessful. Domesticated pigs have also been suggested as possible amplifying and/or maintenance hosts for some viruses.

African filoviruses

The African filoviruses (all filoviruses except *Reston ebolavirus*) can cause severe illness in nonhuman primates and some other animals. African ebolaviruses and *Marburg marburgvirus* are typically lethal in experimentally infected nonhuman primates. In Africa, ebolavirus outbreaks have been linked to reports of dead and dying gorillas (*Gorilla gorilla*), chimpanzees (*Pan troglodytes*), mandrills (*Mandrillus* sp.), guenon (*Cercopithecus* sp.) and other nonhuman primates, as well as duikers (a species of forest antelope, *Cephalophus dorsalis*), bush pigs (red river hog, *Potamochoerus porcus*), brush-tailed porcupines (*Atherurus africanus*) and other animals. While there is no formal evidence for a causative role in some species, attempts to isolate ebolaviruses or detect viral RNA were successful in the carcasses of chimpanzees, gorillas and duikers. Antibodies to filoviruses have been reported in nonhuman primates including mandrills, drills (*Mandrillus* sp.), baboons (*Papio* sp.), colobus monkeys (*Colobus badius*), guenon, chimpanzees and gorillas.

There have been no reports of illnesses or unusual deaths among domesticated animals during ebolavirus outbreaks in Africa. One study detected antibodies in dogs, but did not find virological evidence of infection at the time the study was conducted. What these antibodies indicate is currently uncertain, as 1) some filoviruses are cross-reactive in serological tests, and 2) the dogs could have either been infected with ebolaviruses or exposed without productive infection. One pet dog exposed to its *Zaire ebolavirus*-infected owner in the U.S. did not become infected. Older serological studies sometimes reported antibodies in guinea pigs, some livestock, and even chickens in Africa, but they used a serological test (IFA) that is no longer considered to be reliable. Viruses were not found during very limited sampling of live cattle, sheep, goats and pigs during outbreaks. Some animal species (e.g., sheep and goats) were described as "completely insensitive" to the effects of the virus when inoculated with large amounts of live ebolaviruses for the production of hyperimmune serum in Russian studies, but whether this indicates asymptomatic infection or complete absence of virus replication seems to be uncertain. Pigs have been infected experimentally with *Zaire ebolavirus* and developed respiratory signs. Various laboratory rodents are used as models for human disease; however, the viruses used have been artificially adapted to replicate at high levels in these animals.

Reston ebolavirus

Other than bats, *Reston ebolavirus* has been found in nature only in nonhuman primates (e.g., cynomolgus macaques, *Macaca fascicularis*), which become ill, and domesticated pigs. Whether *Reston ebolavirus* can be maintained long term in swine populations is not known. In one study, this virus caused severe clinical signs in cynomolgus monkeys, but minimal or no signs in African green monkeys inoculated intraperitoneally with the same virus, despite evidence of viremia in the latter species.

Zoonotic potential

Zaire ebolavirus, Sudan ebolavirus, Bundibugyo ebolavirus and *Tai Forest ebolavirus* can cause severe illness in humans, although Tai Forest virus infections have rarely been documented. *Reston ebolavirus* does not seem to be pathogenic for humans, but people may seroconvert after exposure to infected nonhuman primates or pigs.

GEOGRAPHIC DISTRIBUTION

Zaire ebolavirus, Sudan ebolavirus, Tai Forest ebolavirus and *Bundibugyo ebolavirus* are endemic in parts of Africa south of the Sahara desert. Human illnesses caused by these viruses have been reported mainly in central and western Africa, and have typically been associated with rain forests. While outbreaks have been documented in a limited number of countries, serological surveys, as well as the distribution of bat species known to be infected, suggest that some viruses may be more widespread.

Marburg marburgvirus has been found in bats, nonhuman primates and/or humans from eastern Africa to the far western edge of the Congo. The human illness seems to be most prevalent in eastern Africa, although one outbreak was documented in Angola (western Africa). A case reported from South Africa was most likely acquired in Zimbabwe. Imported human cases have been seen sporadically in other areas, including Europe and North America. In recent decades, such cases have mainly been reported among travelers returning from Africa, but a large Marburg hemorrhagic fever outbreak occurred in Germany and Yugoslavia in 1967, among laboratory workers who had been exposed to tissues from imported African green (vervet) monkeys (*Cercopithecus aethiops*).

Reston ebolavirus occurs in the Philippines, and has also been reported in PRRS virus-infected pigs from a 2008 outbreak in China. This or other filoviruses might also exist in other locations. Antibodies to filoviruses have been detected

in several species of fruit bats in China and Bangladesh, and 18% of healthy Bornean orangutans (*Pongo pygmaeus*) in rehabilitation facilities were seropositive on Kalimantan Island, Indonesia. Outbreaks among imported, nonhuman primates in the United States and Italy were eradicated.

TRANSMISSION

How filoviruses are transmitted between bats, or transmitted from bats to other animals, is still uncertain. Although these viruses can be found in bat tissues and blood, they typically seem to be absent from secretions or excretions such as oral fluids, urine and feces (although virus was found in the feces of one experimentally infected bat), and attempts to inoculate bats by exposing respiratory and oral mucus membranes to virus were unsuccessful. It is possible that virus shedding in secretions and excretions occurs intermittently, at very low levels and/or under certain physiological conditions. There is some evidence that transmission might occur when bats give birth. Seasonal changes in the prevalence of *Marburg marburgvirus* RNA were reported in older juvenile Egyptian fruit bats, with peaks during the twice-yearly birthing seasons. These peaks seem to coincide with a higher risk of human infection. Pregnant fruit bats are also more likely to be seropositive than nonpregnant females.

Filoviruses emerge periodically in nonhuman primates or people after infection from an outside source. Most *Marburg marburgvirus* infections in humans have been associated with transmission within caves, probably from infected bats, although some people were infected by exposure to nonhuman primate tissues in the laboratory. Some ebolaviruses might also be acquired directly from bats; however, humans often become ill after handling the carcasses of animals found in the forest, especially nonhuman primates and duikers. Blood, secretions and excretions, and tissues from these animals may contain infectious virus. Filoviruses have been reported to survive for some time in blood and tissues at room temperature, and can be transmitted on fomites, particularly those contaminated by blood. Survival is prolonged when viruses are kept at 4°C. In incidental hosts, filoviruses are thought to enter the body mainly through mucous membranes and broken skin. Arthropod-borne transmission is theoretically possible, but most authors suggest it is unlikely.

Once ebolaviruses or marburgviruses have infected humans, they can spread from person to person. Viruses are thought to occur in secretions and excretions only after the onset of fever. Blood can contain large amounts of virus, contaminating the environment if patients hemorrhage. These viruses are also found in many secretions and excretions that are not visibly contaminated with blood, including saliva, tears, breast milk, semen and feces. Urine may be a source of virus, but *Zaire ebolavirus* was absent from patients' urine during one outbreak. Aerosol and/or respiratory droplet transmission between nonhuman primates is still controversial: it has

E

been implicated in some experimentally infected nonhuman primates, but alternative explanations may be possible, and virus did not seem to spread readily between cages in other studies. While people might theoretically become infected by this route, aerosols do not seem to be important during human outbreaks. Filoviruses disappear from blood and most tissues after the acute stage of the disease. They may, however, persist for a time in some "immune privileged" body sites, such as the testes and possibly the anterior chamber of the eye. In one patient, *Marburg marburgvirus* was apparently transmitted sexually, 13 weeks after the onset of disease. *Zaire ebolavirus* was isolated from the semen of another convalescent patient up to 82 days after the onset of clinical signs, and detected by RT-PCR for as long as 91 days. This virus was also recovered from the breast milk of a convalescing patient, 15 days after the onset of disease (after the virus had been cleared from the blood), and transmission to a nursing child may be possible. How efficiently filoviruses can spread by casual contact during the early stages of the illness is still uncertain, but the risk is currently thought to be low except during close contact:

The extent of transmission between nonhuman primates during outbreaks in the wild is controversial; however, current evidence suggests that these viruses are not spread efficiently, and nonhuman primates are unlikely to act as maintenance hosts. Virus spread is likely to depend on the extent of interactions between members of the population, as well as the infectivity of body fluids and carcasses. Most other species (e.g., duikers) have not been examined, but the role of domesticated pigs is under investigation. Young pigs (3-6 months of age) inoculated with either *Zaire ebolavirus* or *Reston ebolavirus* shed these viruses in nasal and oral fluids, and evidence of infection was also found sometimes in blood, rectal swabs and various tissues. Pigs infected with *Zaire ebolavirus* transmitted this virus to pigs in close contact, as well as to cynomolgus macaques housed in the same room but not in direct contact with the pigs. In pigs infected with *Reston ebolavirus*, the virus had disappeared from blood and tissues by one month after infection. Whether sustained transmission of ebolaviruses can occur in swine populations has not yet been determined.

DISINFECTION

Ebolaviruses and marburgviruses are both reported to be susceptible to sodium hypochlorite, glutaraldehyde, β-propiolactone, 3% acetic acid (pH 2.5), formaldehyde and paraformaldehyde. Recommended dilutions of sodium hypochlorite may vary with the use. Calcium hypochlorite, peracetic acid, methyl alcohol, ether, sodium deoxycholate and some other agents have also been tested against ebolaviruses, and found to be effective. In addition, filoviruses can be inactivated by ultraviolet light, gamma irradiation, heating to 60°C (140°F) for 60 minutes or boiling for 5-20 minutes.

INFECTIONS IN ANIMALS

INCUBATION PERIOD

Experimental inoculation of nonhuman primates with filoviruses often results in clinical signs after 3-5 days, although the incubation period was reported to be as long as 16 days in some animals. Pigs developed a fever 4 days after inoculation with *Zaire ebolavirus*.

CLINICAL SIGNS

Nonhuman primates are severely affected by filoviruses. Wild chimpanzees and gorillas are often found dead. Clinical signs observed in dying wild animals (of various species) during ebolavirus outbreaks have included vomiting, diarrhea, hair loss and emaciation, as well as bleeding from the nostrils. Whether all of these signs are associated with filovirus infections or some were caused by other diseases is uncertain. During the 1989 *Reston ebolavirus* outbreak in Virginia, the clinical signs in cynomolgus monkeys included anorexia, swollen eyelids, increased lacrimation, nasal discharge, coughing and splenomegaly. Fever, subcutaneous hemorrhages, epistaxis and/or bloody diarrhea were less common. These animals were also infected with simian hemorrhagic fever virus; thus, the contributions of each virus to the signs were uncertain. The most common clinical signs at the infected exporting facility were respiratory signs and diarrhea, while hemorrhages occurred but were rare (1% of animals). However, these signs were reported in both infected and uninfected animals, and some cynomolgus monkeys that died with *Reston ebolavirus* infection had no apparent signs before death.

Nonhuman primates that are experimentally infected with filoviruses may develop fever, anorexia, vomiting, diarrhea, dyspnea, splenomegaly and weight loss. A skin rash is common, although it can be absent in some species, or in animals inoculated by certain routes. Hemorrhagic signs may include petechiae, bleeding into the gastrointestinal tract, or bleeding from puncture wounds and mucous membranes. Shock and hypothermia are soon followed by death. African species of ebolaviruses are usually more pathogenic than *Reston ebolavirus*: the clinical signs are more severe, hemorrhages are more common and the mortality rate is higher.

Piglets (approximately 5-6 weeks of age) inoculated with *Zaire ebolavirus* developed a fever and respiratory signs, which progressed to dyspnea, anorexia and lethargy, while less severe respiratory signs occurred in slightly younger piglets inoculated with the same virus. Guinea pigs infected with unpassaged filoviruses from primates may have a fever and weight loss, but recover. In this species, severe illness is only seen in animals infected with serially passaged virus adapted to guinea pigs. No clinical signs have been reported in infected wild bats, and experimentally infected bats remain asymptomatic.

Reston ebolavirus does not seem to causes any illness in experimentally inoculated pigs. However, this virus has been detected in pigs with porcine reproductive and respiratory syndrome in both the Philippines and China, and whether it can exacerbate other illnesses or predispose animals to other infections is unknown. The PRRS outbreak in the Philippines and China were unusually severe, but consistent with other outbreaks caused by atypical PRRS viruses. Some of the pigs in the Philippines were also infected with porcine circovirus type 2.

POST MORTEM LESIONS

Hemorrhagic signs (especially petechiae and ecchymoses) may be found in various internal organs, the skin and mucous membranes. The liver, spleen, lymph nodes, adrenal glands and some other organs may be enlarged and/or congested and friable. The liver may be severely reticulated and discolored. Some species have a maculopapular rash. Microscopic lesions include focal to widespread hepatocyte necrosis, necrosis of the zona glomerulosa of the adrenal cortex; signs of lymphoid depletion (with apoptosis and necrosis) in lymphoid tissues including lymph nodes and the white pulp of the spleen, and fibrin deposition or fibrin thrombi in various organs.

The gross lesions in young pigs experimentally infected with *Zaire ebolavirus* were pulmonary consolidation and enlargement of the lung-associated lymph nodes, which were sometimes mildly hemorrhagic. Microscopically, the lung lesions were identified as bronchointerstitial pneumonia. The right atrium was hemorrhagic in some animals, although the cause of this lesion was uncertain. Mild lung and lymph node lesions were reported in some asymptomatic piglets infected with *Reston ebolavirus,* but it was not certain if they could be attributed to this virus.

DIAGNOSTIC TESTS

Filovirus infections can be diagnosed by detecting antigens with an antigen-capture ELISA or immunostaining, and by detecting viral RNA with RT-PCR. Ebolaviruses and marburgviruses can be isolated in many cell lines, particularly Vero cells (viruses from pigs may not show cytopathic effect until the 2nd or 3rd passage). Electron microscopy can identify virus particles, which have a distinctive, filamentous pleomorphic, appearance, in tissues. In primates, filoviruses occur in high concentrations in the liver, spleen, lungs, lymph nodes and skin. Liver, spleen, muscle and skin have been taken from wild animal carcasses in good condition for surveillance. RT-PCR can sometimes detect ebolavirus RNA in the bones of decomposed carcasses. Virus isolation is more difficult: unpublished data suggests that carcasses decomposing in the African forests may contain infectious virus for only 3 to 4 days after death. In bats, filoviruses or their nucleic acids

have been found in tissues such as the liver and spleen, and sometimes in the blood.

Serological tests that may be used to detect antibodies to filoviruses include ELISAs, indirect immunofluorescence (IFA) and immunoblotting, but neutralization tests are unreliable. Cross-reactions can occur, particularly between different species of ebolaviruses. The IFA test is thought to be prone to nonspecific reactions, and is uncommonly used at present.

TREATMENT

Because most filovirus infections are serious and often fatal in both humans and nonhuman primates, infected animals are usually euthanized.

CONTROL

Disease reporting

Animals that may be infected with ebolaviruses or marburgviruses must be reported immediately, to protect humans who may be exposed and aid in controlling the outbreak.

Prevention

Quarantine of nonhuman primates during importation protects humans and healthy nonhuman primates from exposure to filoviruses. To prevent the exportation of *Reston ebolavirus*, the government of the Philippines has banned wild-caught monkeys from export and established a quarantine period for captive-bred primates. During outbreaks, suspects and exposed animals should be isolated, and euthanized after confirmation of the disease. Strict infection control procedures are necessary to prevent virus transmission on fomites. Prevention of human exposure during diagnosis and eradication activities is vital, as humans are severely affected by most filoviruses.

Measures to prevent infection of swine with *Reston ebolavirus* in endemic areas have not yet been established, but normal biosecurity measures should be helpful. Pigs should not be allowed to contact bats or nonhuman primates.

Very little is known at present about the susceptibility of other species. As a precaution, some animals in the U.S. (e.g., pets in the home of an ebolavirus-infected human) may be quarantined and monitored similarly to exposed humans. The disposition of exposed animals may differ in other countries.

MORBIDITY AND MORTALITY

In Africa, high mortality rates have been reported in some animal populations, including nonhuman primates and duikers, during some human ebolavirus epidemics. Outbreaks in wild animals can occur suddenly, and may cause widespread mortality on one area while having little or no impact on other regions. The effect on local populations can be severe. Gorilla and duiker numbers fell an estimated 50% in one preserve, while chimpanzee populations decreased by 88% during another outbreak. One study estimated 90-95% mortality (5000 animals) in a population of gorillas. Experimental inoculation of gorillas or chimpanzees is not done, but mortality can be very high in other nonhuman primates inoculated with African filoviruses. Nevertheless, antibodies have also been reported in some wild primates or wild-born captive primate populations, suggesting that some animals can recover or are resistant to disease. (However, reactivity to nonpathogenic filoviruses is difficult to rule out as the cause of these antibodies.)

Reston ebolavirus has a case fatality rate greater than 80% in experimentally infected cynomolgus macaques. Infected monkeys at quarantine facilities were euthanized once the outbreaks were recognized, and the cumulative case fatality rate is unknown; however, 82% of the animals with Reston virus antigens in the blood at the infected export facility died. The overall mortality rate was also higher at this facility, compared to similar facilities in the Philippines. The source of the infection for the monkeys was not found, but imported primates from the Philippines were virus-free after the infected export facility was closed in 1997. However, *Reston ebolavirus* was detected in domesticated pigs in the Philippines in 2008, during an investigation of a PRRS outbreak. Seroprevalence to *Reston ebolavirus* was high (approximately 70%) among pigs on affected farms, but no antibodies were found in pigs from an area unaffected by illness. The illness was reported to be severe in sick pigs infected with both viruses in the Philippines and China, but pigs inoculated experimentally with *Reston ebolavirus* alone remained asymptomatic. In pigs, *Zaire ebolavirus* infections have currently been described only in experimentally infected animals less than 2 months of age. The illness seems to be more severe in older piglets than one-month-old animals, which all survived in one experiment.

INFECTIONS IN HUMANS

INCUBATION PERIOD

The precise incubation period for filovirus infections is difficult to determine, as the time of exposure is uncertain or not described in most cases. Some estimates indicate a potential range of 2 to 21 days, with symptoms usually appearing in 4 to 10 days. The initial signs occurred after 3 to 13 days in a limited number of cases where the time of exposure was known. Estimates of the mean incubation period during outbreaks have ranged from 6 to 13 days, and sometimes differ even for the same outbreak.

CLINICAL SIGNS

Marburg marburgvirus, Zaire ebolavirus, Sudan ebolavirus and *Bundibugyo ebolavirus* appear to cause similar diseases, although the severity of the illness and most prevalent syndromes might differ with the virus. Published information for clinical signs during outbreaks is limited; however, the initial symptoms have been described as nonspecific and flu-like, with a high fever, chills, headache, severe malaise and muscle aches or generalized pain, followed by abdominal pain, nausea, vomiting and diarrhea. A nonpruritic, erythematous, maculopapular rash, which may develop fine scaling, can appear on the face, torso and extremities. Dysphagia, pharyngitis, and conjunctivitis or conjunctival congestion are reported to be common. One clinical summary described a grayish exudate in the pharynx, sometimes with tapioca-like whitish-clear granules on the soft palate. Other mucosal lesions, such as glossitis, gingivitis, and cold-sore like lesions, have been mentioned. Debilitation is often rapid, and generalized pain may be seen. Pregnant women may abort. Common changes in laboratory parameters include leukopenia (at the early stage) and thrombocytopenia, as well as elevated liver enzymes. Some patients are reported to experience a brief remission before deteriorating, while some may recover without developing more severe signs.

After a few days, patients can develop other symptoms including neurological signs, dyspnea, and signs of increased vascular permeability, especially conjunctival injection and edema. Mild to severe bleeding tendencies may also be seen. In mild cases, this can be limited to bruising, bleeding of the gums, epistaxis, petechiae and/or mild oozing from venipuncture sites. While frank hemorrhaging is reported to be uncommon, it can occur, especially from the gastrointestinal tract. Other serious signs include metabolic disturbances, severe dehydration, diffuse coagulopathy, shock and multi-organ failure. Although many patients die, some begin to recover after a week or two. During convalescence, which can be slow, reported complications have included joint pain, uveitis, deafness, orchitis, recurrent hepatitis, transverse myelitis, pericarditis and mental dysfunction (e.g., psychosis). Secondary infections can also occur at this stage, and skin in the area of the rash often sloughs.

It should be noted that descriptions of the syndromes caused by filoviruses are generally limited to severe cases seen in hospitals, and milder cases might not have been observed. In rare, documented mild cases caused by *Marburg marburgvirus*, nonspecific symptoms and slight signs of purpura were reported in an adult, and fever, diarrhea, vomiting and splenomegaly in an infant. Neither patient was reported to be seriously ill. Evidence for asymptomatic seroconversion has also been documented rarely in ebolavirus and marburgvirus infected patients.

Unlike other filoviruses, *Reston ebolavirus* does not seem to be pathogenic for humans. Asymptomatic seroconversion can be seen.

DIAGNOSTIC TESTS

Ebola or Marburg hemorrhagic fever can be diagnosed by detecting antigens with an antigen-capture ELISA or immunostaining, and by detecting viral RNA by RT-PCR. Reverse transcription loop-mediated isothermal amplification methods have been described. Virus isolation can also be used (though available in limited locations) and electron microscopy may be helpful. In humans, filoviruses are most reliably detected in the blood (including serum) during the acute-stage of the disease, but they may also be found in oral fluids and in some cases in urine, breast milk, semen, anterior eye fluid and other body fluids, and in many tissues including the skin. Skin biopsies may be collected at post-mortem. Serological assays include ELISA tests, IFA and immunoblotting, but neutralization tests are unreliable. ELISA tests are used most often, while IFA is thought to be prone to nonspecific reactivity. Because the consequences of misdiagnosis (including false positive diagnosis) are severe, multiple techniques are used to confirm the infection whenever possible.

TREATMENT

Standard treatment currently consists of supportive therapy, including maintenance of blood volume and electrolyte balance, as well as analgesics and standard nursing care.

No specific treatment has been demonstrated yet to be safe and effective in humans; however, experimental drugs, vaccines and monoclonal antibodies to filoviruses have been tested in animals, with varying degrees of success in nonhuman primates. These experimental treatments are diverse, and may be aimed at inhibiting virus replication and/or entry into cells, treating clotting abnormalities or sepsis, or boosting immune responses. Most experimental treatments have been tested very early in the incubation period, but some were promising when started up to 2 days after exposure, or even after early clinical signs (e.g., mild elevation in temperature) developed. A few drugs have advanced to human phase I clinical trials, which are the initial tests to determine whether agents appear to be safe for human use. When supplies are available, some experimental treatments have been used in humans on a compassionate basis.

CONTROL

Disease reporting

International health regulations require that nations report acute hemorrhagic fever syndromes immediately to WHO, without waiting for the causative agent to be identified. Suspected human cases of Ebola or Marburg hemorrhagic fever should be reported immediately to the nation's public health service, to prevent transmission and aid in case management and diagnosis. In the U.S., cases are reported to public health departments and to CDC's Special Pathogens Branch.

Prevention

In Africa, ebolavirus infections are often linked to exposure to wild animal tissues during butchering. Because the full host range may not be known, all sick and dead wild animals should be avoided (including for use as food). To prevent infection from animals that might be infected but have not yet developed obvious clinical signs, good personal hygiene should be used when handling and preparing meat, and the meat should be thoroughly cooked. Surveillance for deaths and illness in wild animals may provide an early warning to prevent human epidemics, but such deaths have not been seen in all human outbreaks.

Marburg marburgvirus infections have been linked to exposure to caves, mines and cave-dwelling bats, but the means of transmission from bats to humans is still unknown. If contact is unavoidable (e.g., occupational exposure), personal protective equipment and good hygiene should be used. Some caves have been closed after human cases were recognized.

Human epidemics have been successfully stopped in the past by tracing infected individuals, and isolating patients in facilities with barrier nursing procedures and strict infection control measures. Healthcare workers should use the personal protective equipment currently recommended by experts (e.g., gloves, gowns, masks, eye protection and other equipment) to prevent exposure to blood and body fluids. Burial practices should avoid all contact with the body or fomites. During convalescence, the possibility of exposure during breastfeeding or sexual intercourse should be considered. Ebolaviruses have been found in milk 15 days after the onset of illness (although the maximum period of shedding is unknown), and in semen for much longer. Sexual abstinence has been recommended for at least three months after recovery.

Reston ebolavirus is not known to affect humans. As a precaution, tissues from infected animals should not be eaten or handled. Good hygiene and appropriate personal protective equipment should be used if these animals or their tissues must be handled.

MORBIDITY AND MORTALITY

Illnesses caused by filoviruses have occurred as isolated cases, small clusters of cases, or large outbreaks which may affect hundreds of people. The 2013-2014 outbreak is unusual in its scale, having affected thousands. Some outbreaks seem to originate with a single person, while multiple transmission events have been reported in others. High risk activities include butchering wild animals and visiting caves and mines. Outbreaks can be propagated by transmission to family members and other close contacts through nosocomial transmission, unsafe self-treatment at home, funeral practices and other routes. Healthcare workers are at high risk, as hospital supplies are limited in some areas where filoviral diseases occur, and barrier nursing practices may be inadequate. Other factors that help propagate the disease include poor availability of healthcare, reluctance to see a medical practitioner, and difficulty in distinguishing some cases from other serious illnesses, particularly in the early stages. As a result, some outbreaks have been identified months after they began. Delayed identification, together with the introduction of the virus into urban areas, and socioeconomic factors (e.g., poverty and healthcare-associated risk factors), are thought to have fueled the 2014-2015 outbreak in West Africa.

Outbreaks of Ebola hemorrhagic fever are reported periodically in Africa. The number of reported outbreaks has increased, due either to a higher incidence or better recognition of the disease. Marburg hemorrhagic fever was only recently recognized as a serious and recurring problem in humans. This disease was initially recognized in 1967, during an outbreak in laboratory workers exposed to infected primate tissues. Only 6 cases were described during the following 3 decades, 3 cases in travelers to Africa and three in their contacts. In 1998, however, this virus caused an epidemic affecting hundreds of people in the Democratic Republic of the Congo (DRC). This outbreak was associated with a mine where infected bats were later discovered. Several different viral strains were isolated during the epidemic, suggesting that the virus had been introduced repeatedly into the population via infected miners. This outbreak also uncovered a pattern of hemorrhagic disease in the mine dating to 1987 or earlier, and one survivor of an earlier outbreak was found to have antibodies to this virus. In 2004-2005, another large outbreak was reported in Angola, where *Marburg marburgvirus* was not thought to exist. Unlike the previous outbreak, it seems to have originated with a single person, and was propagated by person-to-person transmission. Several additional cases have been reported since that time, in miners or travelers who visited caves.

Case fatality rates are usually high for African filoviruses, and the prognosis is poor in patients who become severely ill. *Zaire ebolavirus* is thought to be the most pathogenic virus, with case fatality rates from outbreaks in Africa ranging from 44% to 88%. *Sudan ebolavirus* appears to be less virulent, with a case fatality rate estimated to be 41-65%, (or 26-54%, depending on the cases included). However, higher mortality rates have been reported in small numbers of *Sudan ebolavirus*-infected individuals who were not treated. The reported case fatality rate was 36% in the initial outbreak caused by *Bundibugyo ebolavirus*. It varies widely in Marburg hemorrhagic fever, from 22-23% during the 1967 laboratory-associated outbreak in Europe, to 83% (56% in laboratory-confirmed cases) during the outbreak in DRC, and 88% in Angola. It is not known whether higher mortality rates are associated with more virulent filoviruses (or strains of these viruses), higher doses of virus, concurrent malnutrition and disease, or the availability and quality of healthcare. Only a limited number of cases have been treated in Western countries with advanced healthcare facilities.

The incidence of mild or asymptomatic infections is still uncertain. Asymptomatic infections have been documented in rare cases, and the possibility of such infections is also suggested by reports of antibodies and cell-mediated immune responses to filoviruses in people who have no history of Ebola or Marburg hemorrhagic disease. Seroprevalence rates tend to be higher in groups that have more contact with wild animals or live in rural forest ecosystems. However, illnesses without hemorrhages might have been misdiagnosed as other diseases such as malaria, which can also be severe. Cross-reactivity with other viruses may also be a problem in serological tests. In particular, there may be undiscovered filoviruses in Africa (and other locations) that are less pathogenic or nonpathogenic for humans.

Seroconversion to *Reston virus* does not seem to be common. In the Philippines, seroprevalence rates ranged between 1% and 4% (overall 2%) in people who had been exposed to either nonhuman primates or infected pigs. All of the primate-exposed positive samples came from people associated with the single export facility known to have housed infected animals.

EASTERN, WESTERN AND VENEZUELAN EQUINE ENCEPHALOMYELITIS

Sleeping Sickness

Eastern Equine Encephalomyelitis (EEE), Eastern Equine Encephalitis, Eastern Encephalitis

Western Equine Encephalomyelitis (WEE), Western Equine Encephalitis

Venezuelan Equine Encephalomyelitis (VEE), Peste Loca, Venezuelan Equine Encephalitis, Venezuelan Encephalitis, Venezuelan Equine Fever

IMPORTANCE

Eastern equine encephalomyelitis (EEE), Western equine encephalomyelitis (WEE), and Venezuelan equine encephalomyelitis (VEE) viruses are mosquito-borne pathogens that can cause nonspecific illnesses and encephalitis in equids (horses, mules, burros, donkeys and zebras) and humans in the Americas. Some of these viruses also affect birds and occasionally other mammals. No specific treatment is available, and depending on the virus, host and form of the disease, the case fatality rate may be as high as 90%. Epidemic VEE viruses are also potential bioterrorist weapons.

ETIOLOGY

Eastern, Western and Venezuelan equine encephalomyelitis result from infection by the respectively named viruses in the genus *Alphavirus,* family Togaviridae. In the human literature, the disease is usually called eastern, Western or Venezuelan equine encephalitis.

Eastern equine encephalomyelitis virus

Until recently, Eastern equine encephalomyelitis virus (EEEV) contained four genetic lineages. Lineage I was considered to be the North American variant of EEEV, while lineages II, III and IV were the South American variants. The latter three lineages have now become a new viral species, Madariaga virus. Unless otherwise specified, "EEEV" in this factsheet refers to all viruses formerly classified under this name, rather than lineage I viruses alone.

The North American EEEV seems to be more virulent than Madariaga virus in people, and under some conditions, it is also more pathogenic in experimentally infected nonhuman primates (e.g., marmosets), sparrows and rodents. Comparative studies in horses have not been published, but severe illness has been reported in this species in both North and South America.

Western equine encephalomyelitis viruses

The Western equine encephalomyelitis virus complex contains Western equine encephalomyelitis virus (WEEV) and several closely related alphaviruses including Sindbis virus, Whataroa virus, Fort Morgan virus (and variants Stone Lakes virus and Buggy Creek virus), aura virus, and highlands J virus.. WEEV is the most important virus in this complex in the Western Hemisphere, although highlands J virus and Fort Morgan virus can affect some birds. Sindbis virus and Whataroa virus cause a febrile illness with polyarthritis in humans, but occur only in the Eastern Hemisphere, and are not discussed in this factsheet. Aura virus, found in South America, has not been linked to any illness in humans or animals.

Venezuelan equine encephalomyelitis viruses

The Venezuelan equine encephalomyelitis complex contains a number of viruses, which have been classified into 6 viral subtypes, I to VI, with subtype I further subdivided into five antigenic variants or serovars, AB to F. The currently recognized viral species in this complex are Venezuelan equine encephalomyelitis virus (VEEV), which contains variants AB, C, D and E in subtype I (i.e., variants I-AB, I-C, I-D and I-E), Mosso das Pedras virus (variant I-F), Everglades virus (subtype II), Mucambo virus (subtype III variants A, C and D), Tonate virus (subtype III variant B), Pixuna virus (subtype IV), Cabassou virus (subtype V) and Rio Negro virus (subtype VI). One isolate of Tonate virus, which was detected in the U.S. Rocky Mountains region in the 1970s, is also called Bijou Bridge virus. VEE complex viruses are sometimes referred to

by their subtype and variant designation, rather than their species name.

VEE complex viruses are divided into epidemic (or epizootic) and enzootic (or endemic) groups, based on their epidemiological characteristics. All viruses except VEEV variants I-AB and I-C are considered to be enzootic. Enzootic VEE viruses occur in limited geographic areas, where they are maintained in cycles involving wild animals. They are not amplified in equids, and do not usually cause disease in these animals. In contrast, epidemic VEE viruses are detected only sporadically, are amplified in equids, and can cause extensive epidemics affecting both equids and humans. The origins of epidemic VEE viruses are uncertain, as I-AB and I-C viruses do not seem to be maintained in natural cycles between outbreaks. Some evidence suggests that they may arise when mutations in enzootic VEE viruses allow efficient amplification in horses, and die out once the epidemic ends.

One enzootic I-E virus strain, which has been detected in Mexico since the 1990s, differs from other enzootic viruses in that it affects horses. This virus has caused extensive outbreaks in Mexico, although it has not spread further. Like other enzootic VEE viruses, it is not thought to be amplified in equids.

SPECIES AFFECTED

Eastern equine encephalomyelitis

Passerine birds are thought to be the principal reservoir hosts for North American EEEV in natural cycles, but small mammals (e.g., rodents) might also amplify the virus. The primary reservoir hosts for Madariaga virus (South American EEEV) are still uncertain, but small mammals might play a more prominent role. Some experiments have suggested that reptiles (especially snakes) might help maintain EEEV over the winter. Domesticated mammals including equids are not important in virus amplification.

Most infections in passerine birds appear to be asymptomatic, although a few species become ill after experimental inoculation. Clinical cases have been reported in some non-passerine birds including chukar partridges, pheasants, turkeys, ratites (emus, ostriches), psittacine birds, pigeons (*Columba livia*), house sparrows (*Passer domesticus*), egrets, glossy ibises (*Plegadis falcinellus*), whooping cranes (*Grus americana*) and African penguins (*Spheniscus demersus*). Among mammals, EEV mainly causes disease in horses and other equids, but clinical cases have also been reported in sheep, cattle, dogs, South American camelids (llamas and alpacas), pigs, deer and a captive harbor seal (*Phoca vitulina*), as well as in some experimentally infected rodents and nonhuman primates. Some other species susceptible to infection, without reported disease to date, include goats, moose (*Alces alces*), certain rodents, bats, reptiles and amphibians.

Western equine encephalomyelitis

Passerine birds are the usual reservoir hosts for WEEV, but this virus may also cycle in blacktail jackrabbit (*Lepus califomicus*) populations. Reptiles have been proposed as possible overwintering hosts. Domesticated mammals including equids are not important in virus amplification.

WEEV causes disease in equids and some species of birds such as emus, turkeys, pheasants and chukar partridges. Other species reported to be susceptible to infection (usually asymptomatic) include cattle; various small mammals including squirrels, other rodents and snowshoe hares (*Lepus americanus*); opossums; and snakes, tortoises and frogs.

Other WEE complex viruses

Highlands J virus mainly seems to infect wild birds. Although this virus is not known to be a significant cause of illness in mammals, it was isolated from the brain of at least one horse with encephalitis. It can also cause disease in experimentally infected young chickens and partridges, and turkeys of various ages.

Fort Morgan virus occurs in cliff swallows (*Petrochelidon pyrrhonota*) and house sparrows, and can affect house sparrow nestlings. It is not known to infect other species.

Venezuelan equine encephalomyelitis

Wild rodents are thought to be the usual reservoir hosts for enzootic VEE viruses, but birds may be involved in a few cycles (e.g., the Bayou Bridge variant of Tonate virus). Although rodent reservoir hosts in endemic areas seem to be unaffected, other wild and laboratory (or pet) rodents can become ill. Mice and hamsters are generally more susceptible than guinea pigs. Enzootic VEE viruses can also infect opossums (*Didelphis marsupialis*), bats and various other mammals including dogs. They are not known to cause any illness in equids, other domesticated livestock, dogs or cats, with the exception of one Mexican I-E variant, which is pathogenic for equids. Horses do not seem to be efficient amplifying hosts for any enzootic VEE viruses, including this variant.

Epidemic VEE viruses mainly affect equids and are also amplified in these animals. These viruses can infect wild and laboratory rodents, and cause severe disease in some species (including guinea pigs, mice and hamsters); however, there is no evidence that they are maintained in rodents or other animals between epidemics. Infections have also been reported in other mammals (e.g., pigs, cattle, goats, sheep, dogs, rabbits) and some birds, but most infections appear to be subclinical.

Zoonotic potential

Human illnesses have been reported after infection with EEEV, Madariaga virus, WEEV, epidemic VEE viruses and most enzootic VEE viruses. EEEV in North America is generally thought to be more virulent for humans than Madariaga virus in South America; however, both viruses can cause severe illness. Highlands J virus and Fort Morgan virus do not appear to affect people.

Humans infected with epidemic strains of VEEV can develop viremia sufficient to infect mosquitoes, but are not thought to be important in the epidemiology of this disease. People do not appear to transmit EEEV or WEEV to mosquitoes.

GEOGRAPHIC DISTRIBUTION

All EEE and VEE complex viruses and most WEE complex viruses occur only in the Western Hemisphere. WEEV has been isolated from western North America, including Canada, and as far south as Argentina. Highlands J virus circulates in the eastern U.S., while Fort Morgan virus (with its variants) is widespread in North America.

EEEV has been detected in eastern Canada, all U.S. states east of the Mississippi, and some additional states such as Arkansas, Minnesota, South Dakota and Texas. This virus is usually associated with swamps and marshes, and its distribution is not homogeneous: it is particularly common along the Gulf coast from Texas to Florida, along the Atlantic coast, and in some midwestern states around the Great Lakes. Madariaga virus occurs in parts of Central and South America, especially along the Gulf coast.

Enzootic VEE viruses have varying distributions in parts of Mexico, South and Central America. They are absent from Canada and most of the U.S.; however, Everglades virus (subtype II) occurs in Florida, and Tonate virus (variant III-B) was detected in Colorado and South Dakota in the 1970s. Enzootic VEEV I-E viruses pathogenic for equids have been detected only in Mexico; I-E viruses currently found in other parts of Latin America do not seem affect these animals.

Epidemics caused by epidemic VEE viruses (VEEV I-AB and I-C) tend to occur in northern South America, but also affect other parts of South and Central America. Some outbreaks have spread into North America.

TRANSMISSION

Eastern equine encephalomyelitis

In North America, EEEV is normally maintained in wild bird populations. *Culiseta melanura,* a mosquito that preferentially feeds on birds, is the most important vector in this sylvatic cycle. Other, mosquito species that feed on both birds and mammals ("bridge vectors") may transmit EEEV to humans and domesticated mammals; however, recent evidence suggests that *C. melanura* may also play a direct, and perhaps significant, role. *Culex* spp. might be the main vectors for Madariaga virus (EEEV lineages II-IV) in South American sylvatic cycles. Other arthropods including chicken lice, chicken mites (Dermanyssidae) and assassin bugs can be infected with EEEV, and chicken mites can transmit the virus experimentally. How EEEV survives the winter in cold climates is still uncertain, but several mechanisms, including persistence in reptiles, prolonged persistence in birds, vertical transmission in mosquitoes, and periodic reintroduction by migrating birds have been suggested.

When birds are in close contact, EEEV can sometimes spread by methods not involving arthropods. This has been documented in captive game birds (e.g., pheasants), which can be infected by the oral route. The presence of large amounts of virus on the feathers of these birds suggests that transmission might occur by pecking, feather picking or preening. Cannibalism could also play a role. Emus can shed large amounts of virus in rectal and oral secretions, and in regurgitated material.

Horses, humans and other mammals are generally considered to be incidental (dead end) hosts for EEEV, but some horses develop a transient viremia sufficient to infect mosquitoes, and horse to horse transmission has been demonstrated by this route in the laboratory.

Western equine encephalomyelitis
WEEV is normally maintained in wild bird populations, and *Culex tarsalis* appears to be the most important vector for this virus in North America. WEEV can also be transmitted by other mosquitoes, especially some members of the genus *Aedes*. A sylvatic cycle between the mosquito *Aedes melanimon* and blacktail jackrabbits (*Lepus califomicus*) has also been reported, probably after they become infected from the bird/mosquito cycle. Overwintering mechanisms for WEEV are uncertain, but similar mechanisms as for EEEV have been proposed.

Horses and humans infected with WEEV do not develop significant viremia, and are true dead-end hosts. This virus can cross the placenta in humans, and congenitally infected infants have been reported.

Other WEEV complex viruses
Highlands J virus is transmitted by *Culiseta melanura* mosquitoes, but the main vector for Fort Morgan virus is the cimicid swallow bug (*Oeciacus vicarius*), an ectoparasite of swallows.

Venezuelan equine encephalomyelitis
Enzootic VEE viruses are mainly thought to cycle between mosquitoes in the genus *Culex* and wild small mammals, especially rodents. In the North American Rocky Mountains, the cycle for Tonate virus (Bijou Bridge virus) was reported to involve birds and the swallow bug *Oeciacus vicarius*. Equids do not amplify enzootic VEE viruses.

Horses are the main amplifiers for epidemic VEE viruses. Other mammals do not seem to be epidemiologically significant in transmission, although sufficient viremia to infect mosquitoes has been reported in humans, and occasionally in other species (e.g., cattle, pigs, dogs). Many species of mosquitoes can transmit epidemic VEEV, and efficient vectors

have been described in the genera *Aedes, Anopheles, Culex, Mansonia, Psorophora* and *Deinocerites*. Blackflies could be important mechanical vectors for epidemic strains during some outbreaks. Mites are also capable of transmitting these viruses mechanically. Ticks including *Amblyomma cajennense* and *Hyalomma truncatum* can be infected by both enzootic and epidemic VEEV strains, although their role in nature (if any) is unclear. Horses can shed epidemic VEEV in body fluids, and some authorities suggest that these viruses might be spread occasionally by direct contact or via aerosols. However, there are no reports of direct transmission between horses, or from horses to humans, in nature.

Most people are infected by exposure to VEEV-infected arthropods, but cases have also been documented after laboratory accidents or exposure to aerosolized debris from the cages of infected laboratory rodents. Person-to-person transmission has never been reported, although VEEV has been detected in pharyngeal secretions and horizontal transmission is theoretically possible. VEEV can cross the placenta in pregnant women.

VEEV is reported to persist for a time in the environment, in dried blood and exudates. In a recent experiment, inactivation of 90% of an epizootic strain of VEEV on a glass surface took approximately 98 hours at room temperature (20-25ºC) in the dark. Whether viruses in the environment would infect animals or humans this long is uncertain, as the researchers used various procedures such as sonication to recover as much bound virus from the glass as possible. The persistence of EEV and WEEV in the environment is unknown, but EEEV has been isolated from feather quills for up to 6 days.

DISINFECTION
As enveloped viruses, alphaviruses are likely to be susceptible to many common disinfectants including 1% sodium hypochlorite, 70% ethanol, quaternary ammonium compounds, phenolic disinfectants, 2% glutaraldehyde and formaldehyde. EEEV is known to be inactivated by exposure to 50% ethanol for 1 hour. Alphaviruses are susceptible to moist or dry heat, and to drying or ultraviolet light. Togaviruses have been inactivated by heat of 65°C for 15 minutes.

INFECTIONS IN ANIMALS

INCUBATION PERIOD
The incubation period for WEE or EEE in horses is 5-14 days. The initial signs of VEE can occur 1-5 days after infection, although neurological signs usually appear around day 5.

CLINICAL SIGNS

Eastern and western equine encephalomyelitis complex viruses in equids

Eastern and western equine encephalomyelitis are very similar in horses, although the course of EEE may be shorter. Some animals may have asymptomatic infections or mild cases without neurological signs; however, in classic cases of encephalitis, an initial prodrome characterized by nonspecific signs (e.g., fever, anorexia and depression) is followed by neurological signs that may include altered mentation, hypersensitivity to stimuli, involuntary muscle movements, impaired vision, behavioral changes (e.g., aimless wandering, head pressing, circling), an inability to swallow, ataxia, paresis, paralysis and/or convulsions. Periods of excitement or intense pruritus have been reported, and laterally recumbent animals sometimes have a characteristic paddling motion. In addition, some animals may develop diarrhea or constipation, or have significant weight loss. Some affected horses die within a few days, particularly when infected with EEEV. Horses that recover from encephalitis have a high incidence of residual deficits.

Other WEEV complex viruses in equids

Highlands J virus has been linked rarely with encephalitis in horses. Fort Morgan virus is not known to affect mammals.

Venezuelan equine encephalomyelitis in equids

Infections with epidemic VEE viruses may be asymptomatic, mild or resemble clinical EEE and WEE. In symptomatic horses, a febrile prodrome with depression, tachycardia, and inappetence is sometimes followed by neurological signs indicative of encephalitis. Some animals also have diarrhea and colic. Death can occur within hours after the onset of neurological signs; after a protracted illness accompanied by dehydration and extreme weight loss; or in animals without signs of encephalitis. Sudden death has also been reported. Animals that recover may have permanent neurological signs.

Enzootic VEE viruses usually infect equids subclinically or cause only mild, nonspecific clinical signs. However, an I-E strain found in Mexico can cause severe illness with encephalitis and high mortality.

Equine encephalomyelitis viruses in other mammals

Neurological signs caused by EEEV have been reported in various animals including llamas, alpacas, deer, sheep, cattle, dogs, pigs and a harbor seal. In one published report, all affected dogs were young (≤ 6 months of age), and the clinical signs included fever and diarrhea as well as signs of encephalitis. The clinical signs in these dogs progressed rapidly to recumbency, seizures and other CNS signs within 24-36 hours, and all affected dogs died or were euthanized. During outbreaks in pigs, the illness was most severe in nursing piglets, with reported signs including fever, lethargy, frank CNS signs and high mortality in some outbreaks. Emaciation, dyspnea and excessive salivation, as well as neurological signs, were documented in white-tailed deer (*Odocoileus virginianus*). A young sheep remained alert and maintained a good appetite until it was euthanized, despite fever and neurological involvement that progressed from front limb incoordination to forelimb and hindlimb paralysis with muscle fasciculation and paddling. Seizures were the main sign in a harbor seal, together with anorexia and lethargy; the latter signs may also have been related to molting.

Deaths have been reported in various mammals including rabbits, goats, dogs and sheep during some VEE epidemics; however, laboratory experiments suggest that illnesses in most of these species are unusual. Fatal infections have been documented in experimentally infected rabbits; however, goats, sheep and dogs inoculated with epidemic VEE viruses had few or no clinical signs (although some dogs infected via mosquitoes developed leukopenia and lymphopenia in addition to fever). Susceptible rodents can develop nonspecific signs (e.g., lethargy, anorexia, weight loss) and/or neurological signs after inoculation, and nonspecific febrile illness has been reported in nonhuman primates.

Western and Eastern equine encephalomyelitis viruses in birds

WEEV and EEEV infections are asymptomatic in many birds; however, EEE outbreaks have been reported in several avian species, with syndromes ranging from neurological signs to hemorrhagic enteritis. Clinical signs reported in pheasants included fever, depression, weakness and profuse diarrhea, in addition to neurological signs such as incoordination, circling, tremors, and partial or complete paralysis of the legs. Chukar partridges infected with EEEV were dull and listless, typically found with ruffled feathers, sitting on their hocks with the beak on the ground, while lethargy, ataxia and paresis of the legs and neck were reported in whooping cranes. In a colony of African penguins, early signs of anorexia, mild lethargy and intermittent vomiting, were followed by persistent regurgitation, ataxia, seizures, and diarrhea that was mild in most birds but voluminous in a few. Most penguins recovered, but subtle, intermittent ataxia persisted in some birds. Hemorrhagic enteritis, with signs of depression, diarrhea (which may contain varying amounts of blood) and regurgitation, has been reported in ratites. The onset of disease is usually rapid in these birds, and the mortality rate high. EEEV can also cause depression, decreased egg production and death in turkeys. Although adult chickens are usually unaffected, experimentally infected, 2-week-old chickens developed severe depression, followed by abdominal distention and growth retardation. Some of these chickens died. In addition, EEEV has been isolated from psittacine birds with viral serositis.

WEE has been linked less often with disease in birds. WEEV-infected emus can be mildly to severely affected, with clinical signs that may include anorexia, lethargy, weight loss, watery diarrhea or hemorrhagic enteritis, neurological signs and sudden death. Turkeys can experience a drop in egg production and poor egg quality.

Highlands J virus has caused death in experimentally infected young chickens, turkeys and partridges, and nonspecific signs of illness and decreased egg production in adult turkeys. Fort Morgan virus can cause encephalitis and hepatitis in house sparrow nestlings, but is not known to affect other species.

POST MORTEM LESIONS

The gross lesions of equine encephalitis are usually nonspecific. Equids with VEE may have no lesions in the CNS or there may be extensive necrosis with hemorrhages. Necrotic foci are sometimes seen in the pancreas, liver and heart, but in general, the extracranial lesions are too variable to be diagnostically useful. Congestion of the brain and meninges has been found in some cases of EEE and WEE, and antemortem trauma can result in ecchymotic hemorrhages with any of the encephalomyelitis viruses. Piglets experimentally infected with EEEV had multifocal necrosis and inflammation in the myocardium, in addition to encephalitis. Most birds affected by EEE or WEE have encephalitis, but hemorrhagic enteritis with multiple petechiae on the viscera has been reported in some species, including EEEV-infected emus.

Microscopic analysis of the brain tissue is often diagnostic. The typical lesion is severe inflammation of the gray matter; neuronal degeneration, infiltration by inflammatory cells, gliosis, perivascular cuffing and hemorrhages may be seen. WEE, EEE and VEE sometimes differ in the location and pattern of the lesions in the brain.

DIAGNOSTIC TESTS

Eastern and Western equine encephalomyelitis

In equids, EEE and WEE can be diagnosed by serology, particularly the presence of antibodies in an IgM antibody-capture ELISA, or a 4-fold rise in titer in the plaque reduction neutralization (PRN) test. Unlike in humans, cerebrospinal fluid (CSF) is not considered more reliable for detecting EEEV-specific IgM than serum. Hemagglutination inhibition (HI) and complement fixation tests can also detect antibodies to WEEV and EEEV, but cross-reactions are more of an issue than with the PRN test. In addition, complement fixing antibodies tend to appear late and do not persist, making this assay less useful for diagnosis. A presumptive diagnosis may be obtained with a high titer in a single sample from an unvaccinated horse, particularly when a combination of serological tests is used. Because viremia usually occurs early in the infection (before the

onset of neurological signs), blood is unlikely to contain EEEV in affected horses. This virus may be isolated from the brain after death, as the amount of virus in this tissue is often high, but it can disappear if the illness is prolonged. It can also be found sometimes in extracranial tissues such as the liver or spleen. Virus isolation is rarely successful in WEEV-infected horses. A number of vertebrate and mosquito cell lines can be used to isolate EEEV and WEEV viruses, including primary chicken or duck embryo fibroblasts, African green monkey kidney (Vero) cells, rabbit kidney (RK–13) cells, and baby hamster kidney (BHK–21) cells, as well as embryonating chicken eggs. If necessary, these viruses may also be recovered in newborn mice or newly hatched chicks. North American EEEV can only be distinguished from Madariaga virus with specialized tests not typically available in diagnostic laboratories. Tests that can be used to detect EEEV or WEEV antigens and nucleic acids in tissues, particularly the brain, include immunohistochemistry and reverse transcription PCR (RT-PCR).

Similar tests can be used to diagnose EEEV infections in other mammals. This virus has been isolated from the brain of some animals, including dogs, after death. Clinical EEE or WEE is relatively difficult to diagnose in birds. Avian infections have usually been diagnosed by virus isolation, but serology, immunohistochemistry to detect viral antigens in the brain, or RT-PCR may also be helpful.

Venezuelan equine encephalomyelitis

VEE can be diagnosed by virus isolation or serology. Epidemic strains of VEEV can often be recovered from the blood during the early, febrile stage of disease, but equids are usually no longer viremic once they develop neurological signs. In this situation, it may be helpful to collect blood for virus isolation from other febrile equids found nearby. VEEV is sometimes isolated from the brain at necropsy, but it may no longer be present in many symptomatic cases. This virus has been found occasionally in other tissues, such as the pancreas. Systems that have been used for virus isolation include Vero, RK–13, BHK–21 and other cell lines; duck or chicken embryo fibroblasts; and guinea pigs, mice or 1-4 day-old hamsters. VEE subtypes and variants can be identified at reference laboratories with tests such as immunofluorescence, differential PRN tests and nucleic acid sequencing. RT-PCR assays have been published.

Serological tests that have been used to detect infected horses include virus neutralization (PRN), IgM capture ELISAs, complement fixation and hemagglutination inhibition. Because antibodies develop early, some horses with encephalitis may not have a fourfold increase in paired IgG titers. Paired serum samples taken from febrile herdmates may be helpful in this situation. Antibodies from vaccination, and cross-reactivity with enzootic VEE viruses (which do not usually cause disease in horses), complicate serological diagnosis.

E

TREATMENT

There is no specific treatment for WEE, EEE or VEE other than supportive care.

CONTROL

Disease reporting

EEE, WEE and VEE viruses are usually reportable in North America, although the specific requirements can differ with the disease and location. In addition to detecting the incursion of epidemic VEEV, which is exotic to the U.S. and Canada, reporting allows endemic diseases to be recognized when populations of infected mosquitoes threaten domesticated animals. In addition, animal cases are a warning that humans may be at risk from mosquito-borne transmission.

Prevention

Vaccination is the main method of protecting equids from EEE, WEE and VEE. Because equids are the primary amplifiers for epidemic VEEV, vaccination and movement controls on these animals are also important in controlling outbreaks. Some susceptible species of birds may be vaccinated for EEE, and the efficacy of vaccination has been tested in experimentally infected pigs. Preventing transmission from mosquitoes is difficult, but methods that have been suggested include housing animals in screened barns, particularly during the hours of high mosquito activity, and the use of mosquito repellents and fans. Mosquito abatement measures may also be implemented.

MORBIDITY AND MORTALITY

Eastern and Western equine encephalomyelitis

EEE and WEE tend to occur during summer and fall in temperate areas, but can be seen year-round in tropical regions. In temperate areas, these outbreaks usually end when infected mosquitoes are killed by freezes, and do not continue the following spring. Before vaccines were developed, EEE and WEE outbreaks of varying severity occurred regularly in the U.S. and Canada. Some epidemics were extensive: one WEE outbreak in 1937-38 affected more than 350,000 horses and mules in North America, and a 1947 EEE outbreak killed an estimated 12,000 horses in Louisiana. Since vaccines became available, the incidence of both diseases has decreased significantly. Relatively few cases of WEE have been reported recently, although EEE outbreaks may still be seen, particularly in unvaccinated horses or in the southern U.S., where the long mosquito season may outlast the duration of immunity from vaccination. EEE and WEE have been documented less often in South America; however, one EEE (Madariaga virus) outbreak in 2008-2009 affected more than 200 horses in Brazil, with a case fatality rate of 73%.

EEE is a life-threatening disease in equids, with a case fatality rate as high as 90% in horses with encephalitis.

Many surviving animals have severe residual neurological signs. Asymptomatic infections have been recognized in serological studies, but their incidence is uncertain. Although such infections are thought to be uncommon, a recent study from Canada (Quebec) found that approximately 7-9% of unvaccinated horses had antibodies to EEEV. WEE is more likely to be asymptomatic or mild in horses than EEE; the case fatality rate is usually 20-30%, although 50% of sick animals died during one severe outbreak in 1930.

EEE can also cause significant morbidity and mortality in some other mammals and birds. All clinical cases in dogs were fatal in one report, and case fatality rates as high as 89% have been reported in alpacas and llamas. In pigs, high mortality was reported only in nursing piglets. Reported case fatality rates range from 5% to 75% in EEEV-infected pheasants, while the morbidity rate in emus was 76% during one outbreak, and the case fatality rate was 87%. High mortality has also been reported in EEEV-infected whooping cranes and glossy ibises. In a penguin colony, the prevalence of infection was 64%, and 93% of clinically affected birds recovered with intensive supportive care. Symptomatic infections have been reported less often in WEEV-infected birds; however, the morbidity rate in eight flocks of WEEV-infected emus ranged from 15% to 50%, and approximately 9% of the birds died.

Venezuelan equine encephalomyelitis

Epidemic VEE viruses arise sporadically, but can cause epidemics that may last for several years. Up to 90% of susceptible equids may be infected, with morbidity rates ranging from 10-40% in some areas to 50-100% in others. Case fatality rates in horses are estimated to be 38-90%.

Most enzootic VEE viruses do not cause serious disease or deaths in horses, but some I-E strains in Mexico have caused limited outbreaks of encephalitis. During some of the initial outbreaks in the 1990s, the case fatality rates were 30-50%.

INFECTIONS IN HUMANS

INCUBATION PERIOD

Although sources vary, the incubation period is estimated to be 1 to 7 days for VEE, 2-10 days for WEE and 4-10 days for EEE.

CLINICAL SIGNS

Eastern equine encephalomyelitis

EEE usually begins abruptly, with fever, chills, myalgia, arthralgia and abdominal pain, which may be severe enough to mimic an acute abdominal emergency. This prodrome is often but not always followed within a few days by neurological signs suggestive of encephalitis, which may include headache, irritability, focal neurological deficits, neck stiffness, confusion, somnolence or stupor, disorientation, tremors, seizures and paralysis. Some cases progress to coma. Vomiting and diarrhea may also be seen, and children sometimes develop generalized edema, facial edema or periorbital edema. The illness may be biphasic in some cases, with apparent recovery from the prodromal illness before the onset of encephalitis. Infants can develop encephalitis without other symptoms. The mortality rate for EEE encephalitis is high, and permanent brain damage, often severe, occurs in many survivors. However, people who do not develop neurological signs usually recover completely after an illness of 1 to 2 weeks. Subclinical infections also occur.

Western equine encephalomyelitis

WEE resembles EEE, but tends to be milder in most age groups. As with EEE, the initial signs are nonspecific and resemble other febrile illnesses (e.g., fever, chills, headache, vomiting, myalgia), and occasionally include respiratory signs. This prodrome may be followed by neurological signs such as restlessness, irritability, tremor and signs of focal meningeal irritation - or, infrequently, by more severe neurological signs that resemble EEE. CNS signs are more likely to occur in children, especially infants under a year of age, and are uncommon in healthy adults. Patients who recover from encephalitis can have fatigue, headaches, irritability or tremors for up to two years. Infants may have severe, lasting CNS deficits, but permanent sequelae in older children (≥ 1 year) are usually limited to persistent seizures if there were convulsions during the illness. Most adults recover completely, although permanent neurological damage is possible.

Venezuelan equine encephalomyelitis

In humans, VEE is usually an acute, often mild, systemic illness. The symptoms caused by endemic and epidemic strains are similar. The initial signs are nonspecific and may include fever, chills, generalized malaise, severe headache, photophobia and myalgia particularly in the legs and lumbosacral region. Coughing, sore throat, nausea, vomiting and diarrhea may also be seen. A macular rash and arthralgia in the wrists and ankles were reported in some epidemics. Mild to severe neurological signs can be seen in a small percentage of affected children, and to a lesser extent in adults over the age of 50 years, but in few healthy adults (e.g., less than 1% of symptomatic young adults). VEE usually resolves within 1 to 2 weeks, with acute symptoms subsiding after 4 to 6 days, and deaths are rare.

In pregnant women, VEE can affect the fetus; fetal encephalitis, placental damage, abortion/ stillbirth or severe congenital neurological anomalies may be seen.

DIAGNOSTIC TESTS

Eastern, Western and Venezuelan equine encephalitis are often diagnosed by serology in humans. A definitive diagnosis can be made by serology if 1) specific IgM is found in cerebrospinal fluid (CSF), 2) there is greater than a fourfold

increase between paired titers in other serological tests, or 3) conversion from IgM to IgG is seen. A single high antibody titer may be used for presumptive identification.

In some circumstances, VEEV, WEEV or EEEV can be detected directly with virus isolation, tests to detect viral antigens or RT-PCR. VEEV may be found in blood or throat swabs, mainly during the early febrile stage of the disease, and in CSF. EEEV and WEEV can be hard to find in living patients, but EEEV can sometimes be found in the blood during the prodromal stage of the illness, and WEEV or EEEV may be detected in the CSF of patients with CNS signs. Throat swabs are occasionally positive. At autopsy, encephalitic viruses may be found in the brain, and possibly in other tissues.

TREATMENT

Treatment consists of supportive care. Mechanical ventilation, as well as other measures, may be necessary in some cases. The efficacy of antiviral drugs is currently unknown.

CONTROL

Measures to prevent mosquito bites, including the use of repellants and protective clothing (e.g., long pants and long-sleeved shirts) can reduce the risk of infection. Outdoor exposure should be limited at times when mosquitoes are active, especially during outbreaks. Mosquito abatement programs such as habitat modification (e.g. the removal of standing water sources around the home) and/or the application of larvicides or adulticides may reduce the risk of human infection. Improved irrigation management has decreased vector populations in California, where a primary mosquito vector for WEEV is associated with irrigation systems.

During VEE epidemics, controlling these viruses in horses can help prevent human infections. Even when equids are not important in the epidemiology of a disease (i.e., EEE or WEE), cases in horses can provide an early warning for human disease. Surveillance programs in birds (including sentinel chickens) are also helpful in predicting EEE outbreaks.

Precautions should be taken to prevent exposure to body fluids when performing necropsies on horses. Containment level 3 is required for work with EEEV, WEEV or VEEV in the laboratory. Investigational VEEV and EEEV vaccines may be available for people at high risk of infection, but have limited availability, and are not without side effects.

MORBIDITY AND MORTALITY

Eastern equine encephalomyelitis

In North America, the annual incidence of EEE varies from 0 to 36 cases, with an average of 5-10 cases per year in the U.S. since the 1960s. Approximately 4-5% of people who become infected with this virus are thought to develop EEE, but studies from the 1950s and 60s suggested that few people may be exposed. Clinical cases of encephalitis occur most often in people over 55 years of age and children younger than 15. Estimates of the case fatality rate vary from 30% to 75% (survival has improved in recent years), and permanent neurological deficits can occur in survivors. Only 10% of patients are estimated to recover fully, and many survivors with severe impairment die within a few years. Permanent neurological damage and death are particularly common in children.

Clinical cases caused by Madariaga virus are infrequently reported in Latin America. During a recent outbreak in Panama, there were no deaths among 13 confirmed clinical cases, although one person with suspected EEE died. Some affected people were, however, hospitalized with severe neurological signs, and sequelae were common in these cases. Antibodies to EEEV were detected in 3% of healthy people living nearby.

Western equine encephalomyelitis

WEE was relatively common in North America at one time. Between 1955 and 1984, an average of 34 confirmed cases were reported annually in the U.S., with a range of 0 to 172. Extensive epidemics were also seen at times, with more than 3000 cases in the U.S. and Canada in 1941, and 375 confirmed cases and nine deaths reported in California in 1952. However, clinical cases have rarely been reported in North America in recent decades. The reason for this decline is uncertain; however, it does not appear to be due to reduced virus virulence. Some studies suggest that seroprevalence in healthy people has also diminished (e.g., from 34% in 1960 to < 3% in the 1990s). WEE is uncommonly reported in Central and South America, but some cases might be attributed to other diseases common in tropical regions.

WEE is usually much milder than EEE in symptomatic cases; the overall case fatality rate is estimated to be 3-4%, although it was as high as 8-15% during a severe epidemic in 1941. Adults tend to be mildly affected or remain asymptomatic, but cases can be more severe in children and the elderly. Approximately 5-30% of young patients, and 56% of infants under a month of age, have permanent neurological damage. Except in infants (≤ 1 year), this damage mainly consists of persistent seizures.

Venezuelan equine encephalomyelitis

VEE can be widespread in human populations during epidemics, and more than 10% of the population in an area may be affected. During these outbreaks, cases usually begin weeks after the first illnesses are noted in horses. Serological studies suggest that enzootic VEE viruses might also cause significant numbers of clinical cases in Latin America; however, they may be misdiagnosed as other diseases such as dengue.

Most infections with epidemic or enzootic VEE viruses are mild or asymptomatic, with an overall case fatality rate estimated to be ≤ 1% in healthy adults. Very young or elderly patients are more likely to develop severe disease. Mild to severe neurological signs may occur in 4-15% of symptomatic VEE cases, mainly in children. In these patients, estimates of the case fatality rate range from 10% to 35%, with the highest rates in children. The prognosis is considered to be excellent in patients who recover.

FOOT AND MOUTH DISEASE

Fiebre Aftosa

IMPORTANCE

Foot and mouth disease (FMD) is a highly contagious viral disease that primarily affects cloven-hooved livestock and wildlife. Although adult animals generally recover, the morbidity rate is very high in naïve populations, and significant pain and distress occur in some species. Sequelae may include decreased milk yield, permanent hoof damage and chronic mastitis. High mortality rates can sometimes occur in young animals or in some wildlife populations. Foot and mouth disease was once found worldwide; however, it has been eradicated from some regions including all of North America and western Europe. Where it is endemic, this disease is a major constraint to the international livestock trade. Unless strict precautions are followed, FMD can be readily re-introduced into disease-free regions via animals or animal products. Once introduced, the virus can spread rapidly, particularly if livestock densities are high or detection is delayed. Outbreaks can severely disrupt livestock production, result in embargoes by trade partners, and require significant resources to control. Direct and indirect economic losses equivalent to several billion US dollars are not uncommon. Since the 1990s, a number of outbreaks have occurred in FMD-free countries. Some, such as the 2001 outbreak in the U.K., were devastating.

ETIOLOGY

The foot and mouth disease virus (FMDV) is a member of the genus *Aphthovirus* in the family Picornaviridae. There are seven major viral serotypes: O, A, C, SAT 1, SAT 2, SAT 3 and Asia 1. Serotype O is the most common serotype worldwide. It is responsible for a pan-Asian epidemic that began in 1990 and has affected many countries throughout the world. Other serotypes also cause serious outbreaks; however, serotype C is uncommon and has not been reported since 2004.

Some FMDV serotypes are more variable than others, but collectively, they contain more than 60 strains. New strains occasionally arise. While most strains affect all susceptible host species, some have a more restricted host range (e.g., the serotype O Cathay strain, which only affects pigs). Immunity to one FMDV serotype does not protect an animal from other serotypes. Protection from other strains within a serotype varies with their antigenic similarity.

SPECIES AFFECTED

FMDV mainly affects members of the order Artiodactyla (cloven-hooved mammals). Most species in this order are thought to be susceptible to some degree. Important livestock hosts include cattle, pigs, sheep, goats, water buffalo and yaks. Cattle are important maintenance hosts in most areas, but a few viruses are adapted to pigs, and some isolates might circulate in water buffalo. It is uncertain whether small ruminants can maintain FMDV for long periods if cattle are absent. Other susceptible species include ranched or farmed cervids such as reindeer (*Rangifer tarandus*), deer and elk (*Cervus elaphus nelsoni*). Llamas and alpacas can be infected experimentally, and infections in alpacas were suspected during one outbreak, although there are currently no confirmed cases from the field. Experiments suggest that Bactrian camels (*Camelus bactrianus*) can develop FMD, but dromedary camels (*Camelus dromedarius*) have little or no susceptibility to this virus.

FMDV has also been reported in at least 70 species of wild (or captive wild) artiodactyls including African buffalo (*Syncerus caffer*), bison (*Bison* spp.), moose (*Alces alces*), chamois (*Rupicapra rupicapra*), giraffes (*Giraffa camelopardalis*), wildebeest (*Connochaetes gnou*), blackbuck (*Antilopa cervicapra*), warthogs (*Phacochoerus aethiopicus*), kudu (*Tragelaphus strepsicornis*), impala (*Aepyceros melampus*), and several species of deer, antelopes and gazelles. African buffalo are important maintenance hosts for FMDV in Africa. They are mainly thought to maintain the SAT serotypes, although antibodies to other serotypes have been found in buffalo populations. Other species of wildlife do not seem to be able to maintain FMD viruses, and are usually infected when viruses spread from livestock or buffalo.

FMDV can also infect a few animals that are not members of the Artiodactyla, such as hedgehogs (both *Erinaceus europaeus* and *Atelerix prurei*), bears, armadillos, kangaroos, nutrias (*Myocastor coypus*), and capybaras (*Hydrochaerus hydrochaeris*).

Several clinical cases have been reported in captive Asian elephants (*Elephas maximus*), but there are few reports of FMDV in African elephants *(Loxodonta africana)*, and the latter species is not considered susceptible under natural conditions in southern Africa. Laboratory animal models include guinea pigs, rats and mice, but these animals are not thought to be important in transmitting FMDV in the field. Early reports suggested that transmission occurred between cattle and European hedgehogs (*Erinaceus europaeus*), but there is no evidence that this species has helped to propagate FMDV in the last 50 years.

GEOGRAPHIC DISTRIBUTION

Foot and mouth disease is endemic in parts of Asia, Africa, the Middle East and South America. While serotypes O and A are widely distributed, SAT viruses occur mainly in Africa (with periodic incursions into the Middle East) and Asia 1 is currently found only in Asia. North and Central America, New Zealand, Australia, Greenland, Iceland and western Europe are free of FMDV. Western Europe was affected by some recent outbreaks (eradication was successful), but FMD has not been reported in North America for more than 60 years. The last U.S. outbreak occurred in 1929, while Canada and Mexico have been FMD-free since 1952-1953.

TRANSMISSION

FMDV can be found in all secretions and excretions from acutely infected animals, including expired air, saliva, milk, urine, feces and semen, as well as in the fluid from FMD-associated vesicles, and in amniotic fluid and aborted fetuses in sheep. The amount of virus shed by each route can be influenced by the host species and viral strain. Pigs produce large amounts of aerosolized virus, and the presence of large herds of infected swine may increase the risk of airborne spread. Peak virus production usually occurs around the time vesicles rupture and most clinical signs appear. However, some animals can shed FMDV for up to four days before the onset of clinical signs. The virus can enter the body by inhalation, ingestion or through skin abrasions and mucous membranes. Susceptibility to each route of entry can differ between species. Cattle are particularly susceptible to aerosolized virus, while pigs require much higher doses to be infected by this route. Sexual transmission could be a significant route of spread for the SAT type viruses in African buffalo populations. In sheep, FMDV has been shown to cross the placenta and infect the fetus.

Mechanical transmission by fomites and living (e.g., animal) vectors is important for this virus. Airborne transmission can occur under favorable climatic conditions, with some viruses potentially spreading long distances, particularly over water. In 1981, one viral strain apparently traveled more than 250 km (155 miles) from Brittany, France to the Isle of Wight, U.K. However, aerosolized FMD viruses are rarely thought to travel more than 10 km (approx. 6 miles) over land. There is limited information on the survival of FMDV in the environment, but most studies suggest that it remains viable, on average, for three months or less. In very cold climates, survival up to six months may be possible. Virus stability increases at lower temperatures; in cell culture medium at 4°C (39°F), this virus can remain viable for up to a year. The presence of organic material, as

E

F

well as protection from sunlight, also promote longer survival. Reported survival times in the laboratory were more than 3 months on bran and hay, approximately 2 months on wool at 4°C (with significantly decreased survival at 18°C [64°F]), and 2 to 3 months in bovine feces. FMDV is sensitive to pH, and it is inactivated at pH below 6.0 or above 9.0. This virus can persist in meat and other animal products when the pH remains above 6.0, but it is inactivated by acidification of muscles during rigor mortis. Because acidification does not occur to this extent in the bones and glands, FMDV may persist in these tissues.

Humans as vectors for FMDV

People can act as mechanical vectors for FMDV, by carrying the virus on clothing or skin. The virus might also be carried for a time in the nasal passages, although several studies suggest prolonged carriage is unlikely. In one early study, nasal carriage was reported for up to 28 hours but less than 48 hours after contact with animals. In two recent studies, people did not transmit serotype O viruses to pigs or sheep when personal hygiene and biosecurity protocols were followed, and no virus could be detected in nasal secretions 12 hours after contact with the animals. In another recent study, FMDV nucleic acids (serotypes O or Asia 1) were found in only one person tested 16-22 hours after exposure to infected animals, and live virus could not be isolated from this sample. Because factors such as sub-optimal facility sanitation or poor compliance with personal hygiene and biosecurity protocols could also influence transmission to animals, these studies might not apply directly to the situation in the field.

Carriers

FMDV carriers are defined as animals in which either viral nucleic acids or live virus can be found for more than 28 days after infection. Animals can become carriers whether or not they had clinical signs. In most species, FMDV can be found only in esophageal-pharyngeal fluid, and not in other secretions or excretions (e.g., oral or nasal swabs); however, virus isolation was recently reported from the nasal fluid of experimentally infected water buffalo for as long as 70 days. Nonreplicating virus has also been found in the lymph nodes of ruminants for up to 38 days. The epidemiological significance of livestock FMDV carriers is uncertain and controversial. Although there are anecdotal reports of apparent transmission from these animals in the field, and esophageal-pharyngeal fluid is infectious if it is injected directly into an animal, all attempts to demonstrate transmission between domesticated livestock in close contact during controlled experiments have failed. The only successful experiments were those that involved African buffalo carrying SAT viruses, which transmitted the virus to other buffalo and sporadically to cattle. Some authors have speculated that sexual transmission might have been involved in this case, as FMDV can be found in semen and all successful experiments included both bulls and cows.

How long an animal can remain a carrier varies with the species. Most cattle carry FMDV for six months or less, but some animals can remain persistently infected for up to 3.5 years. The virus or its nucleic acids have been found for up to 12 months in sheep (although most seem to be carriers for only 1 to 5 months), up to 4 months in goats, for a year in water buffalo, and up to 8 months in yaks (*Bos grunniens*). Individual African buffalo can be carriers for at least five years, and the virus persisted in one herd of African buffalo for at least 24 years. Camelids do not seem to become carriers. Pigs are not thought to become carriers, although there have been a few reports documenting the presence of viral nucleic acids after 28 days. One study suggested this might have been an artifact caused by slow degradation of this DNA. Persistent infections have been reported in some experimentally infected wildlife including fallow (*Dama dama*) and sika deer (*Cervus nippon*), kudu and red deer (*Cervus elaphus*). Some deer could carry FMDV for up to 2.5 months. In one early study, experimentally infected brown rats (*Rattus norvegicus*) were carriers for 4 months.

DISINFECTION

Various disinfectants including sodium hydroxide, sodium carbonate, citric acid and Virkon-S® are effective against FMDV. Iodophores, quaternary ammonium compounds, hypochlorite and phenols are reported to be less effective, especially in the presence of organic matter. The disinfectant concentration and time needed can differ with the surface type (e.g., porous vs nonporous surfaces) and other factors.

INCUBATION PERIOD

The incubation period for FMD can vary with the species of animal, the dose of virus, the viral strain and the route of inoculation. It is reported to be one to 12 days in sheep, with most infections appearing in 2-8 days; 2 to 14 days in cattle; and usually 2 days or more in pigs (with some experiments reporting clinical signs in as little as 18-24 hours). Other reported incubation periods are 4 days in wild boar, 2 days in feral pigs, 2-3 days in elk, 2-14 days in Bactrian camels, and possibly up to 21 days in water buffalo infected by direct contact.

CLINICAL SIGNS

While there is some variability in the clinical signs between species, FMD is typically an acute febrile illness with vesicles (blisters) localized on the feet, in and around the mouth, and on the mammary gland. Vesicles occur occasionally at other locations including the vulva, prepuce, or pressure points on the legs and other sites. The vesicles usually rupture rapidly, becoming erosions. Pain and discomfort from the lesions leads to clinical signs such as depression, anorexia, excessive salivation, lameness and reluctance to move or rise. Lesions on the coronary band may cause growth arrest lines on the hoof. In severe cases, the hooves or footpads may be sloughed.

Reproductive losses are possible, particularly in sheep and goats. Deaths are uncommon except in young animals, which may die from multifocal myocarditis or starvation. Most adults recover in 2 to 3 weeks, although secondary infections may slow recovery. Possible complications include temporary or permanent decreases in milk production, hoof malformations, chronic lameness or mastitis, weight loss and loss of condition.

Cattle

Cattle with FMD, especially the highly productive breeds found in developed countries, often have severe clinical signs. They usually become febrile and develop lesions on the tongue, dental pad, gums, soft palate, nostrils and/or muzzle. The vesicles on the tongue often coalesce, rupture quickly, and are highly painful, and the animal becomes reluctant to eat. Profuse salivation and nasal discharge are common in this species; the nasal discharge is mucoid at first, but becomes mucopurulent. Affected animals become lethargic, may lose condition rapidly, and may have gradual or sudden, severe decreases in milk production. In some cases, milk may not be produced again until the next lactation, or milk yield may be lower indefinitely. Hoof lesions, with accompanying signs of pain, occur in the area of the coronary band and interdigital space. Young calves may die of heart failure without developing vesicles. In areas where cattle are intensively vaccinated, the entry of FMD into the herd can sometimes cause swelling of tongue and severe clinical signs that resemble an allergic disease.

In addition to other complications such as mastitis or hoof malformations, some cattle that recover from FMD are reported to develop heat-intolerance syndrome (HIS; also called 'hairy panters'). This poorly understood syndrome is characterized by abnormal hair growth (with failure of normal seasonal shedding), pronounced panting with elevated body temperature and pulse rate during hot weather, and failure to thrive. Some affected animals are reported to have low body weight, severely reduced milk production and reproductive disturbances. Animals with HIS do not appear to recover. The pathogenesis of this syndrome is not known, and a definitive link with FMD has not been established, but endocrine disturbances were suspected by some early investigators.

Water buffalo

Both mouth and foot lesions can occur in water buffalo, but the clinical signs are reported to be milder than in cattle, and lesions may heal more rapidly. Some studies reported that mouth lesions were smaller than in cattle, with scant fluid. In one study, foot lesions were more likely to occur on the bulb of the heel than in the interdigital space.

Pigs

Pigs, usually develop the most severe lesions on their feet. In this species, the first signs of FMD may be lameness and blanching of the skin around the coronary bands. Vesicles then develop on the coronary band and heel, and in the interdigital space. The lesions may become so painful that pigs crawl rather than walk. The horns of the digits are sometimes sloughed. Mouth lesions are usually small and less apparent than in cattle, and drooling is rare. However, vesicles are sometimes found on the snout or udder, as well as on the hock or elbows if the pigs are housed on rough concrete floors. Affected pigs may also have a decreased appetite, become lethargic and huddle together. Fever may be seen, but the temperature elevation can be short or inconsistent. In some cases, the temperature is near normal or even below normal. Young pigs up to 14 weeks of age may die suddenly from heart failure; piglets less than 8 weeks of age are particularly susceptible.

Lesions may be less apparent in feral pigs than domesticated pigs, in part due to their thicker skin and long, coarse hair.

Sheep and goats

Although severe cases can occur, FMD tends to be mild in sheep and goats. A significant number of infected animals may be asymptomatic or have lesions only at one site. Common signs in small ruminants are fever and mild to severe lameness of one or more legs. Vesicles occur on the feet, as in other species, but they may rupture and be hidden by foot lesions from other causes. Mouth lesions are often not noticeable or severe, and generally appear as shallow erosions. Vesicles may also be noted on the teats, and rarely on the vulva or prepuce. Milk production may drop, and rams can be reluctant to mate. Significant numbers of ewes abort in some outbreaks. Young lambs and kids may die due to heart failure (vesicles may be absent) or from emaciation. The clinical signs in young animals can include fever, tachycardia and marked abdominal respiration, as well as collapse. In some cases, large numbers of lambs may fall down dead when stressed.

Camelids

Experimentally infected llamas and alpacas are generally reported to have only mild clinical signs, or to remain asymptomatic, although some reviews indicate that severe infections can also occur. Mild signs were reported in alpacas during one FMD outbreak in Peru, but the virus could not be isolated and these cases are unconfirmed. There are no reports of natural infections in llamas.

Two experimentally infected Bactrian camels developed moderate to severe clinical signs, with hindleg lesions including swelling and exudation of the footpad, but no oral lesions. However, mouth lesions and salivation, as well as severe footpad lesions and skin sloughing at the carpal and tarsal joints, the chest and knee pads were reported from Bactrian camels during outbreaks in the former Soviet Union. Detachment of the soles of the feet has been noted in several reports. Dromedary camels do not seem to be susceptible to FMD.

F

Wildlife

The clinical signs in wildlife resemble those in domesticated livestock, with vesicles and erosions particularly on the feet and in the mouth. More severe lesions occur where there is frequent mechanical trauma, e.g. on the feet and snout of suids or the carpal joints of warthogs. Loss of horns has also been seen. Bears developed vesicles on the footpads, as well as nasal and oral lesions. The severity of the illness varies; subclinical infections or mild disease are common in some species, while others are more likely to become severely ill. Infections with SAT-type viruses in African buffalo are often subclinical, although small mouth and/or foot lesions have been reported. However, severe outbreaks have been documented in wild populations of some species such as mountain gazelles (*Gazella gazelle*), impala and saiga antelope (*Saiga tatarica*), and high mortality or severe clinical signs has been reported in some captive wildlife species (see Weaver et al., 2013 for a detailed review). Young animals can die suddenly of myocarditis.

POST MORTEM LESIONS

The characteristic lesions of foot and mouth disease are single or multiple, fluid-filled vesicles or bullae; however, these lesions are transient and may not be observed. The earliest lesions can appear as small pale areas or vesicles, while ruptured vesicles become red, eroded areas or ulcers. Erosions may be covered with a gray fibrinous coating, and a demarcation line of newly developing epithelium may be noted. Loss of vesicular fluid through the epidermis can lead to the development of "dry" lesions, which appear necrotic rather than vesicular. Among domesticated animals, dry lesions are particularly common in the oral cavity of pigs.

The location and prominence of FMD lesions can differ with the species (see 'Clinical Signs'); however, common sites for lesions include the oral cavity and snout/ muzzle; the heel, coronary band and feet; the teats or udder; pressure points of the legs; the ruminal pillars (in ruminants); and the prepuce or vulva. Coronitis may be seen on the hooves, and the hooves or claws may be sloughed in severe cases. Involvement of the pancreas, as well as heart failure and emaciation, were reported in mountain gazelles. The pancreas was also severely affected in experimentally infected pronghorn (*Antilocapra americana*). In young animals, cardiac degeneration and necrosis can result in irregular gray or yellow lesions, including streaking, in the myocardium; these lesions are sometimes called "tiger heart" lesions. Piglets can have histological evidence of myocarditis without gross lesions in the heart. Signs of septicemia, abomasitis and enteritis, as well as myocarditis, have been reported in lambs.

Only nonspecific gross lesions were described in infected fetuses from experimentally infected sheep. They included petechial hemorrhages in the skin, subcutaneous edema, ascites with blood-tinged peritoneal fluids and epicardial petechiae. Vesicles were not found, and the placenta did not appear to be affected. Some infected fetuses had no gross lesions. In another study, infected fetuses were generally autolyzed.

DIAGNOSTIC TESTS

Testing for foot-and-mouth disease varies with the stage of the disease and purpose of the test. In acutely infected animals, FMDV, its antigens or nucleic acids can be found in a variety of samples including vesicular fluid, epithelial tissue, nasal and oral secretions, esophageal-pharyngeal fluids, blood and milk, and in tissue samples such as myocardium collected at necropsy. (The OIE- recommended samples at this stage are epithelium from unruptured or freshly ruptured vesicles, or vesicular fluid. In cases with no vesicles, the OIE recommends blood [serum] and esophageal-pharyngeal fluid samples, taken by probang cup from ruminants, or as throat swabs from pigs.) Carrier animals can only be identified by collecting esophageal-pharyngeal fluids for virus isolation and/ or the detection of nucleic acids. Repeated sampling may be necessary to identify a carrier, as the amount of virus is often low and fluctuates.

Viral antigens are usually identified with enzyme-linked immunosorbent assays (ELISAs), and nucleic acids by reverse transcription polymerase chain reaction (RT-PCR). Other commercial tests to detect antigens, such as lateral flow devices, may be available in some countries. Virus isolation can be performed in primary bovine thyroid cells, primary pig, calf or lamb kidney cells, or BHK-21 or IB-RS-2 cell lines. The virus is generally identified with ELISAs or RT-PCR; however, complement fixation is still in use in some countries or for some purposes. If necessary, unweaned mice can be used to isolate FMDV. Nucleotide sequence analysis can identify viral strains.

Serological tests can be used in surveillance, to certify animals for export, to confirm suspected cases during an outbreak, to monitor immunity from vaccination, and in matching vaccines to field strains. Test cutoff values can differ with the purpose of the test. Some serological tests detect antibodies to the viral structural (e.g., capsid) proteins. They include ELISAs and virus neutralization tests, and are serotype specific. Because FMDV vaccines also induce antibodies to structural proteins, these tests can only be used in unvaccinated animals. Other serological tests (e.g., some ELISAs and the enzyme-linked immuno-electrotransfer blot) detect antibodies to FMDV nonstructural proteins (NSPs), which are expressed only during virus replication. NSP tests are not serotype specific, and can be used in both vaccinated and unvaccinated animals. However, they are less sensitive and may not detect cases with limited virus replication, including some vaccinated animals that become infected. Due to such limitations, serological tests that detect antibodies to NSPs are generally used as herd tests.

TREATMENT

There is no specific treatment for FMD, other than supportive care. Treatment is likely to be allowed only in countries or regions where FMD is endemic.

CONTROL

Disease reporting

A quick response is vital for containing outbreaks in FMD-free regions. Veterinarians who encounter or suspect this disease should follow their national and/or local guidelines for disease reporting. In the U.S., state or federal veterinary authorities should be informed immediately of any suspected vesicular disease.

Prevention

Import regulations help prevent FMDV from being introduced from endemic regions in infected animals or contaminated foodstuffs fed to animals. Waste food (swill) fed to swine is a particular concern. Heat-treatment can kill FMDV and reduces the risk of an outbreak; however, some countries have completely banned swill feeding, due to difficulty in ensuring that adequate heat-treatment protocols are followed. Protocols for the inactivation of FMDV in various animal products such as milk products, meat, hides and wool have been published by the OIE. Global FMD control programs have recently been established to reduce virus circulation and the incidence of this disease.

Measures taken to control an FMD outbreak include quarantines and movement restrictions, euthanasia of affected and exposed animals, and cleaning and disinfection of affected premises, equipment and vehicles. Additional actions may include euthanasia of animals at risk of being infected and/or vaccination. Infected carcasses must be disposed of safely by incineration, rendering, burial or other techniques. Rodents and other vectors may be killed to prevent them from mechanically disseminating the virus. People who have been exposed to FMDV may be asked to avoid contact with susceptible animals for a period of time, in addition to decontaminating clothing and other fomites. Good biosecurity measures should be practiced on uninfected farms to prevent entry of the virus.

Vaccination may be used to reduce the spread of FMDV or protect specific animals (e.g. those in zoological collections) during some outbreaks. The decision to use vaccination is complex, and varies with the scientific, economic, political and societal factors specific to the outbreak. Vaccines are also used in endemic regions to protect animals from illness. FMDV vaccines only protect animals from the serotype(s) contained in the vaccine. For adequate protection, the vaccine strains must also be well matched with the field strain.

Wildlife transmission may need to be considered in some locations. One important issue is the persistence of FMDV in wild African buffalo, which may make eradication unfeasible in some areas. In southern Africa, transmission from African buffalo has been controlled by separating wildlife reserves from domesticated livestock with fences, and by vaccination of livestock. However, wildlife fencing may not be practical in some areas, and there are also some disadvantages to its use. Another issue is the protection of highly susceptible wildlife species from FMDV. Vaccination of livestock was reported to decrease outbreaks in some populations, such as saiga antelope.

MORBIDITY AND MORTALITY

Morbidity from FMD varies with the animal's species, breed and pre-existing immunity, as well as the dose of virus and other factors. The morbidity rate can approach 100% in naïve cattle or swine herds, but some FMD viruses can disappear from a sheep flock after infecting a relatively low percentage of the animals. The pattern of disease is influenced by the epidemiological situation. When more than one virus circulates in a region, there may be periodic outbreaks, due to the lack of protection between serotypes and the limited cross-protection between some strains. When there is only a single serotype in a region, the virus may cause only mild clinical signs, with cases seen mainly in young animals as they lose their protection from maternal antibodies. Adult livestock do not usually die from FMD (the case fatality rate is approximately 1-5% for most strains), but deaths can occur in young animals. In lambs, reported mortality rates range from 5% to 94%. Mortality has also been reported to reach 80% in some groups of calves, and 100% in suckling piglets (with lower rates in older piglets). The percentage of FMDV-infected animals that become carriers, with or without vaccination, is still uncertain. Estimates vary widely, with experimental and field studies reporting carrier rates ranging from less than 5% to more than 50% under different conditions.

Most infections in wildlife species appear to be similar to those in domesticated animals; however, some species or populations may be more severely affected. Approximately 2000 mountain gazelles, representing at least half of the population on the reserve, died from FMD during an outbreak in Israel. During a second outbreak, an estimated 10-15% of the population was affected, and the case fatality rate was greater than 50%. Likewise, the case fatality rate was as high as 75% in experimentally infected saiga antelope, and some outbreaks resulted in the death of an estimated 10% of the wild population. Livestock (or African buffalo) seem to be the source of the virus in wildlife outbreaks, and FMDV does not seem to persist long-term except in African buffalo. Some modeling studies suggest that sustained wildlife outbreaks might be theoretically possible, depending on animal density and other factors.

F

PUBLIC HEALTH

Foot and mouth disease is not considered to be a public health problem, as infections seem to be very rare and their consequences mild. In the past, many people who worked with FMDV in vaccine laboratories or other locations developed antibodies to this virus, but there were few clinical cases. One laboratory reported only 2 cases in more than 50 years, and a large FMD vaccine manufacturer documented 3 cases among its workers. It may be that exposure to extremely large amounts of virus or a predisposing condition is necessary for infection.

Between 1921 and 1969, reports of more than 40 laboratory-confirmed cases of FMD in humans were published. The symptoms included vesicular lesions and influenza-like symptoms, and the disease was generally mild, short-lived and self-limiting. Broken skin was a recognized route of entry for some human cases, with the initial lesions developing at the inoculation site. There is also a report that three veterinarians deliberately infected themselves in 1934, by drinking virus-contaminated, unpasteurized milk for three days. Person-to-person transmission has never been reported; however, vesicles from affected people do contain virus.

[Note: Foot-and-mouth disease is not related to hand, foot and mouth disease, a condition seen only in humans.]

GLANDERS

Farcy, Malleus, Droes

IMPORTANCE

Glanders is a serious zoonotic bacterial disease that primarily affects horses, mules and donkeys. Some animals die acutely within a few weeks. Others become chronically infected, and can spread the disease for years before succumbing. Glanders also occurs occasionally in other mammals, including carnivores that eat meat from infected animals. Although cases in humans are uncommon, they can be life threatening and painful. Without antibiotic treatment, the case fatality rate may be as high as 95%.

Glanders was a worldwide problem in equids for several centuries, but this disease was eradicated from most countries by the mid-1900s. Outbreaks are now uncommon and reported from limited geographic areas. In non-endemic regions, cases may be seen in people who work with the causative organism, *Burkholderia mallei,* in secure laboratories. An infection was reported in a U.S. researcher in 2000. Glanders is also considered to be a serious bioterrorist threat: *B. mallei* has been weaponized and tested against humans, and it was also used as a biological weapon against military horses in past wars.

ETIOLOGY

Glanders results from infection by *Burkholderia mallei*, a Gram negative rod in the family Burkholderiaceae. This organism was formerly known as *Pseudomonas mallei*. It is closely related to and appears to have evolved from the agent of melioidosis, *Burkholderia pseudomallei*.

SPECIES AFFECTED

The major hosts for *B. mallei* are horses, mules and donkeys. Most other domesticated mammals can be infected experimentally (pigs and cattle were reported to be resistant), and naturally occurring clinical cases have been reported in some species. Members of the cat family seem to be particularly susceptible, with cases documented in domesticated cats, tigers, lions, leopards and other felids. Deaths have also been reported in other carnivores that ate glanderous meat, including dogs, bears, wolves, jackals and hyenas, and clinical cases were described in dromedary camels. Hamsters and guinea pigs are susceptible to glanders after experimental inoculation, but mice do not become ill unless the dose of organisms is high, and laboratory rats are resistant to infection. Wild rodents (e.g., field mice and voles) can also be infected experimentally. Birds are highly resistant.

Zoonotic potential

B. mallei affects humans.

GEOGRAPHIC DISTRIBUTION

Glanders is thought to be endemic in parts of the Middle East, Asia, Africa and Central and South America. This disease has sometimes reemerged in countries where it appeared to be absent or was limited to small foci of infection (e.g., India in 2006). It has been eradicated from western Europe, Canada, the U.S., Australia, Japan and some other countries, and it was never endemic in New Zealand. The geographic distribution of *B. mallei* can be difficult to determine precisely, as cross-reactions with *B. pseudomallei* interfere with serological surveys.

TRANSMISSION

Glanders is mainly transmitted by contact with infected horses, mules and donkeys, most often via their respiratory secretions and exudates from skin lesions. Chronically or subclinically infected equids can shed *B. mallei* intermittently or constantly. This organism can enter the body by contamination of skin abrasions and mucous membranes, or inhalation in aerosols. Equids often become infected when they ingest *B. mallei* in contaminated food or water, and carnivores when they eat contaminated meat. There are reports of venereal transmission from stallions to mares, and vertical transmission from the dam.

B. mallei is readily spread on fomites including harnesses, grooming tools, and food and water troughs. Flies might act as mechanical vectors. Although this organism is inactivated by heat and sunlight, its survival is prolonged in wet or humid environments. It was reported to survive for up to 6 weeks in some infected stables, and one early report suggested that it might remain viable in room temperature water for up to 100 days. Under most conditions, however, it is not thought likely to survive in the environment for more than 2 weeks.

Humans can be infected by contact with sick animals, contaminated fomites, tissues or bacterial cultures. The organism is thought to enter the body through wounds and abrasions in the skin, and by ingestion or inhalation. Transmission through unbroken skin has been reported, but not proven (minor breaks in the skin could also explain these cases). Most laboratory-acquired infections have occurred during routine handling and processing of cultures or samples, rather than after injuries or accidents. Rare cases of person-to-person transmission have been reported in family members who nursed sick individuals. Two cases were thought to have been sexually transmitted.

DISINFECTION

B. mallei is susceptible to many common disinfectants including 1% sodium hypochlorite, 70% ethanol, 2% glutaraldehyde, iodine, benzalkonium chloride, mercuric chloride in alcohol and potassium permanganate. It is less susceptible to phenolic disinfectants. This organism can be destroyed by heating to 55°C (131°F) for 10 minutes, or exposure to ultraviolet irradiation. In the environment, *B. mallei* is susceptible to drying and sunlight.

INFECTIONS IN ANIMALS

INCUBATION PERIOD

The incubation period in equids is reported to range from a few days to many months, but many cases become apparent in 2-6 weeks. Infections can be latent for varying periods. Experimental infections can result in fever after a day or two, and other clinical signs after 3 days. Less is known about the incubation period in other species; however, some cats developed clinical signs 8-14 days after eating infected meat.

CLINICAL SIGNS

Horses, donkeys and mules

In equids, glanders is traditionally categorized into nasal, pulmonary and cutaneous forms, based on the most commonly affected sites.

In the nasal form, deep ulcers and nodules develop inside the nasal passages, resulting in a thick, mucopurulent, sticky, yellowish discharge. This discharge can be copious, may be unilateral or bilateral, and can become bloody. The ulcers may coalesce over wide areas, and nasal perforation is possible. Healed ulcers become star-shaped scars, which may

be found concurrently with nodules and ulcers. The regional (submaxillary) lymph nodes become enlarged bilaterally or unilaterally. They are usually indurated in acute illness, and may occasionally suppurate and drain. Nasal infections can spread to involve the lower respiratory tract.

Pulmonary involvement occurs in most clinical cases, often in combination with other forms of glanders. Affected animals develop nodules and abscesses in the lungs, or bronchopneumonia in some cases. Some infections are inapparent; others are characterized by mild to severe respiratory signs (e.g., coughing, dyspnea), with fever or febrile episodes and progressive debilitation. If the upper respiratory tract was not involved initially, it may become infected via discharges from pulmonary abscesses.

In the cutaneous form (known as 'farcy') multiple nodules develop in the skin, along the course of lymphatic vessels. These nodules often rupture and ulcerate, discharging an oily, thick yellow exudate. Glanders ulcers heal very slowly, often continuing to discharge fluid, although dry ulcers may also be seen. The regional lymphatics and lymph nodes become chronically enlarged, and the lymphatics are filled with a purulent exudate. Some animals also have swelling of the joints, painful edema of the legs or glanderous orchitis (in intact males). While skin lesions may appear anywhere, they are reported to be most common on the inner thighs, limbs and abdomen. Animals with cutaneous glanders can remain in good condition for a time, but they eventually become debilitated and die.

Clinical cases are often a combination of forms, and may be acute (or subacute), chronic or latent, depending on the animal's resistance to disease. Donkeys and mules often develop acute glanders after exposure, although mules appear to be somewhat more resistant and the course of the illness may be slower. Acute glanders is characterized mainly by nasal and respiratory involvement, with clinical signs that commonly include a high fever, decreased appetite/ weight loss, depression, swelling of the nostrils, bouts of coughing and progressive dyspnea. An initial watery nasal discharge (often unilateral at first) can develop into the classic signs of the nasal form. There may also be a purulent ocular discharge. Neurological signs were reported in experimentally infected horses, possibly as the result of secondary bacterial (*Streptococcus zooepidemicus*) infection of the brain due to a compromised blood-brain barrier. Animals with the acute form of glanders usually die in a few days to a few weeks from septicemia and respiratory failure.

Horses usually develop chronic glanders. This form can also be seen in some mules. Chronic glanders develops insidiously and lasts for months to years, with periodic episodes of exacerbation, resulting in slowly progressive debilitation. Although the initial signs may be mild and easily overlooked (e.g., intermittent low fever and slightly labored breathing), progression of the lesions results in listlessness, generalized weakness and wasting, with an intermittent cough. Some animals become lame, with swelling of the joints in the hindquarters, or have hematuria, polyuria, diarrhea, epistaxis or orchitis. Signs of nasal glanders or skin involvement may be seen, and stressors can result in acute bronchopneumonia. Extension of lesions to the brain has been reported in at least one case. Chronic glanders is eventually fatal in most animals, although a few may recover clinically while remaining carriers. Animals that recover from glanders can relapse.

In latent cases, lesions may occur sporadically in the lungs and other internal organs. The clinical signs are usually minimal, and most often consist only of intermittent low fever, nasal discharge and/or occasional labored breathing. Latent glanders is most common in resistant species, such as horses.

Other species

The clinical signs in naturally infected dromedary camels were similar to those in equids, and included fever, lethargy, emaciation, and nodules and ulcers in the nasal passages, with severe mucopurulent discharge. In cats that ate infected meat, nodules and ulcers were found in the nasal passages and on the conjunctivae, as well as deeper in the respiratory tract. Affected cats also had a purulent yellowish nasal discharge that sometimes became bloody. Additional clinical signs included swelling of the lymph nodes and dyspnea, and affected cats usually died in 1 to 2 weeks. Similar respiratory, nasal and nonspecific signs (e.g., anorexia, depression) have been reported in large felids during outbreaks at zoos. Some of these animals also vomited, had skin ulcers or developed swelling of the face and head.

POST MORTEM LESIONS

Nodules, granulomas and/or ulcers may be detected in various tissues of equids with glanders. Glanders nodules are firm, round and usually about 1 cm. in diameter, with a caseous or calcified center. They are typically surrounded by areas of inflammation. The upper respiratory tract is often affected, with ulcers, nodules and/or stellate scars in the nasal passages, larynx and other tissues. Internally, nodules are most likely to be found in the lungs, particularly beneath the pleura. The lungs may also contain diffuse miliary granulomatous nodules, and in acute or exacerbated cases, there may be evidence of severe bronchopneumonia. In addition, nodules and other lesions may be detected in other visceral organs, particularly the liver and spleen. Some animals have had bone lesions, and abscesses were found in the muscles of infected racehorses. Swollen lymphatics, with chains of nodules and ulcerated nodules, may be noted in the skin, while the lymph nodes may be enlarged, congested and/or fibrotic, and can contain abscesses. Orchitis may be seen in males.

Similar lesions have been reported in other species.

DIAGNOSTIC TESTS

Glanders can be diagnosed by culturing B. mallei from lesions, lymph nodes, and nasal or other respiratory exudates. This organism is uncommonly detected in blood. Bacteriological diagnosis can be difficult when the animal is in the early stages of disease or subclinically infected. Detailed guidelines for isolating B. mallei, which grows best on media enriched with glycerol, have been published by the World Organization for Animal Health (OIE) and other sources. While this organism can also grow on ordinary culture media (though not well on MacConkey agar), its slow growth and the potential for overgrowth by other bacteria may make isolation difficult. If necessary, it can also be recovered by inoculation into guinea pigs. Once isolated, B. mallei is usually identified with biochemical tests. The absence of motility is important in distinguishing it from other members of the Pseudomonas group, including B. pseudomallei. It can be misidentified by automated bacterial identification systems. Due to the risks of human infection, isolates suspected to be B. mallei are typically sent to a reference laboratory for identification. Genetic techniques available in specialized laboratories (e.g., PCR-restriction fragment length polymorphism, pulse-field gel electrophoresis, 16S rRNA sequencing) can distinguish B. mallei from its close relative B. pseudomallei. Several PCR tests have been described, but many have not yet been thoroughly evaluated with clinical samples. A few are reported to differentiate B. mallei from B. pseudomallei. Antigen detection assays (e.g., latex agglutination, immunofluorescence) have been investigated.

B. mallei can sometimes be observed in smears from fresh lesions, where it is usually present in large numbers, although the staining may be weak or irregular. It can be difficult to find in older lesions or tissue sections. This organism can be stained with methylene blue, Wright or Gram stains, but some authors report that it stains best with Giemsa. It is a Gram negative, straight or slightly curved rod; organisms from clinical samples and young cultures appear as rods, while bacteria from older cultures can be pleomorphic. In tissue sections, it may have a beaded appearance.

A hypersensitivity reaction called the mallein test was used in glanders eradication programs, and is still used to detect infected equids in some countries. In the 3 versions of the mallein test, a protein fraction of B. mallei is either injected into the eyelid (intradermo-palpebral test), administered in eyedrops, or injected subcutaneously at a site other than the eye. The intradermo-palpebral test is considered to be the most reliable and sensitive version. Reactors in this test develop marked eyelid swelling after 1 to 2 days. There may also be a purulent ocular discharge and an elevated body temperature. Conjunctivitis occurs after administration in eyedrops, and a firm, painful swelling with raised edges is seen within 24 hours after subcutaneous (non-ocular) injection. Mallein testing can cause transient false positives in subsequent serological tests, and such reactivity could become permanent if the animal is tested repeatedly. It can give inconclusive results in acute glanders, or in the late stages of chronic disease. Cross-reactivity has also been reported.

A variety of serologic tests have also been used to diagnose glanders and/or detect infected horses in surveillance and import testing. Complement fixation and ELISAs are currently considered to be the most accurate and reliable assays in equids, although other tests may also meet this standard once they have been fully evaluated. Complement fixation has also been used to diagnose glanders in other animals, including camels and large zoo cats, and an ELISA test was positive in an infected camel. Immunoblotting appears promising in equids, and might be used in combination with other assays. A rose bengal plate agglutination test is sometimes employed in Russia. Cross-reactivity can be an issue in serological tests, and false negatives also occur, especially in chronically infected, debilitated, pregnant or old animals. Complement fixation is reported to detect chronically infected animals during episodes of exacerbation. Most serological tests cannot distinguish whether the animal has antibodies to *B. mallei* or *B. pseudomallei*.

TREATMENT

Some antibiotics may be effective against glanders, but treatment is often not allowed outside endemic areas. Treatment can be risky even in these regions, as infections can spread to humans and other animals, and treated animals may become asymptomatic carriers.

Designing effective treatments for glanders is complicated by differences in antibiotic susceptibility patterns between *B. mallei* isolates, and the inability of some drugs to penetrate into the host cells where this organism replicates. Treatment protocols that might be able to eliminate *B. mallei* have been published recently, but they have not yet been fully evaluated. Some require treatment for several months, using multiple drugs.

CONTROL

Disease reporting

A quick response is vital for containing outbreaks in glanders-free regions. Veterinarians who encounter or suspect this disease should follow their national and/or local guidelines for disease reporting. In the U.S., state or federal veterinary authorities should be informed immediately.

Prevention

During outbreaks in non-endemic regions, animals that test positive are usually euthanized, and the premises are quarantined, cleaned and disinfected. Carcasses, contaminated bedding and food should be safely destroyed (e.g., burned or buried), and equipment and other fomites should be disinfected. Import testing (e.g., by serology) is used to help exclude infected animals from regions where glanders has been eliminated.

In endemic areas, susceptible animals should be kept away from communal feeding and watering areas, since glanders is more common where animals congregate. Routine testing and euthanasia of infected animals can eradicate the disease or reduce its incidence. Meat from infected equids should not be fed to other animals (or used for human consumption). Vaccines are not available.

MORBIDITY AND MORTALITY

Glanders can spread widely when large numbers of animals are in close contact. This disease is also reported to be more common in animals that are undernourished or otherwise in poor condition. A high percentage of infections may be subclinical or latent. Although acute glanders is usually fatal within a short period, animals with the chronic form can sometimes survive for years. Mortality rates are thought to be high, but estimates are difficult to make because infected animals are usually euthanized to prevent them from spreading the disease.

Cases of glanders are reported infrequently in animals other than equids. Among carnivores, felids appear to be particularly susceptible: more than one outbreak has been reported in captive large felids, and cases have been seen in domesticated cats.

INFECTIONS IN HUMANS

INCUBATION PERIOD

The incubation period for acute glanders is reported to be 1 to 14 days, with most cases of localized disease becoming apparent within 5 days. Chronic cases can take months to appear.

CLINICAL SIGNS

Forms of glanders that have been described in humans include septicemia, pulmonary infection, acute localized infection and chronic disease. One form can progress to another, and combinations of syndromes occur. Some patients have had a biphasic illness, separated by remissions lasting a few days to several weeks.

Localized infections are characterized by nodules, abscesses and/or ulcers in the mucous membranes skin and/or subcutaneous tissues at the site of inoculation. In skin, the initial lesion may appear as a blister that gradually develops into an ulcer. Involvement of the lymphatics in the area results in lymphangitis with numerous foci of suppuration. When the mucous membranes are involved, a mucopurulent, sometimes blood-tinged, discharge may be seen. The nose and the face may swell if the nasal passages are affected, and local tissue destruction can occur. Localized lesions may be accompanied by systemic signs of illness, including fever (which may be low grade and fluctuating), sweats, malaise, headache and swelling of the regional lymph nodes, sometimes with abscesses.

Mucosal or skin infections may disseminate to other organs. The lungs, spleen and liver are often affected, but any tissue including the muscles can be involved. The clinical signs can be nonspecific in disseminated cases (e.g., nausea, dizziness, night sweats, myalgia, severe headache, weight loss). A papular or pustular rash may also be seen. Disseminated infections often progress to septicemia.

The pulmonary form can occur acutely after inhaling *B. mallei*, but organisms may also reach the lungs by localized or hematogenous spread from other forms. Pulmonary abscesses, pleural effusion and pneumonia are characteristic. The symptoms include fever and other nonspecific signs (e.g., chills, sweats, headache, myalgia), coughing and chest pain, progressing to dyspnea. Lymphangitis, nasal involvement and gastrointestinal signs may also be seen, and skin abscesses can develop up to several months after organisms are inhaled. Untreated pulmonary disease often develops into septicemia.

In the septicemic form, fever, chills, myalgia, headache and pleuritic chest pain may develop acutely. Other symptoms may include flushing, a pustular or papular rash, lymphadenopathy, cellulitis, cyanosis, jaundice, photophobia, diarrhea and granulomatous or necrotizing lesions, tachycardia and mild hepatomegaly or splenomegaly. Multi-organ failure is common, and death can occur rapidly.

Chronic glanders is characterized by multiple abscesses, nodules and ulcers in various tissues, with periodic recrudescence and milder symptoms than in acute cases. Weight loss, lymphadenopathy and lymphangitis are common. This form of the disease has been reported to last up to 25 years.

DIAGNOSTIC TESTS

Glanders can be diagnosed by culturing *B. mallei* from lesions, as in animals. This organism may also be found in sputum, blood or urine, although blood cultures are often negative. PCR assays or antigen detection tests could be useful, though they are not employed routinely. Serology can be employed in diagnosis, if tests are available; however, there can be unexplained high background titers in some normal sera, and seroconversion tends to occur late. Many serological tests cannot distinguish reactions to other species of *Burkholderia*, including *B. pseudomallei*. The mallein test is not used in humans.

Radiography is helpful in the pulmonary form, although it is not specific for glanders. The lesions can include bilateral bronchopneumonia, miliary nodules, segmental or lobar infiltrates, and cavitating lesions. Similar lesions may also be detected in other organs and tissues.

TREATMENT

Glanders is treated with antibiotics. The optimal treatment is still uncertain, but some treatment recommendations are available, and some cases have been treated successfully. Long-term treatment and/or multiple drugs may be necessary in some cases. Abscesses may need to be drained.

CONTROL

Strict precautions, including appropriate personal protective equipment (PPE), should be taken when handling infected animals and contaminated fomites. Biosafety level 3 practices are required for manipulating infected tissues and cultures. Postexposure prophylaxis with antibiotics might be used in some situations. No vaccine is available.

Although person-to-person transmission is rare, human glanders patients should be isolated. Infection control precautions should be taken, and PPE, including disposable surgical masks, face shields, and gowns, should be used as appropriate during nursing.

MORBIDITY AND MORTALITY

Glanders is a sporadic, and currently rare, disease that usually occurs in people who work with clinical samples or have frequent, close contact with infected horses and their tissues. Human epidemics have not been seen. Transmission from horses to humans may be inefficient; even when morbidity rates in horses are 5-30%, zoonotic disease is reported to be uncommon. However, some infections might be subclinical or mild; autopsy studies conducted in endemic areas found glanders-associated nodules in many people who had contact with horses. In laboratories, *B. mallei* is highly infectious, particularly when it is aerosolized. With aerosolized bacteria, morbidity rates up to 46% have been reported.

Mortality rates are reported to be high in untreated glanders, with a case fatality rate of 95% or greater in septicemia and 90-95% in the pulmonary form. With treatment, the case fatality rates for these forms are reported to be as high as 40-50%. The estimated mortality for localized disease is 20% when treated; untreated cases often progress to other forms. Chronic glanders is reported to be difficult to treat, with a case fatality rate as high as 50% in spite of treatment. It should be noted that these estimates were based on historical cases (and possibly extrapolated from melioidosis in some cases), and mortality could be lower with modern supportive care and effective antibiotics.

HEARTWATER

Cowdriosis, Malkopsiekte, Péricardite Exsudative Infectieuse, Hidrocarditis Infecciosa, Idropericardite dei Ruminanti

IMPORTANCE

Heartwater, a rickettsial disease of ruminants, is one of the most important diseases of livestock in Africa. This tick-borne illness can significantly decrease productivity in regions where it is endemic. It is particularly serious in non-indigenous livestock that are moved into heartwater areas; many of these animals may die. Wild ruminants can also be infected. Most wildlife species appear to carry the organism asymptomatically, but serious illness has been reported in lechwe moved into endemic areas, as well as in experimentally infected white-tailed deer.

Heartwater is readily introduced into new regions in infected animals or ticks. Known and potential host ticks are widely distributed, and can be found on a variety of animals including reptiles. On at least one occasion, leopard tortoises and African spurred tortoises imported into Florida were found to be carrying infected ticks. Once the tick vector becomes established, eradication of heartwater is difficult. One host tick, *Amblyomma variegatum*, was introduced into the Caribbean early in the 19th century. During the 1970s and early 1980s, this tick spread rapidly from island to island; in some cases, it may have been carried by cattle egrets. The presence of heartwater in the Caribbean increases the risk of introducing this disease into the Americas.

ETIOLOGY

Heartwater results from infection by *Ehrlichia* (formerly *Cowdria) ruminantium*, a small, Gram negative, pleomorphic coccus in the family Anaplasmataceae and order Rickettsiales. This organism is an obligate intracellular parasite. Strains of *E. ruminantium* are very diverse: while some strains are highly virulent, others appear to be non-pathogenic. Several different genotypes can co-exist in a geographic area, and may recombine to form new strains.

Closely related species of *Ehrlichia* (e.g., the Panola mountain *Ehrlichia*) exist in some areas. These organisms can complicate the diagnosis of heartwater, as cross-reactions occur in all serological tests, and false positives have been reported in some PCR assays, depending on the primers used. This has implications for various aspects of heartwater, including its geographic distribution and the species affected.

SPECIES AFFECTED

E. ruminantium affects cattle, sheep, goats and water buffalo. It can also infect some wild ungulates, with or without clinical signs. Wild species proven to be susceptible to natural and/or experimental infection include blesbok (*Damaliscus pygargus*), wildebeest (*Connochaetes gnou* and *C. taurinus*), African buffalo (*Syncerus caffer*), eland (*Taurotragus oryx*), giraffes (*Giraffa camelopardalis*), greater kudu (*Tragelaphus strepsiceros*), sable antelope (*Hippotragus niger*), lechwe (*Kobus leche kafuensis*), steenbok (*Raphicerus campestris*), springbok (*Antidorcas marsupialis*), sitatunga (*Tragelaphus spekii*), Timor deer (*Cervus timorensis*), chital (*Axis axis*) and white-tailed deer (*Odocoileus virginianus*). Some other ungulates, including various cervids, bison (*Bison* spp.), and wild relatives of sheep and goats are also thought to be susceptible, but confirmation is lacking. Reports of possible fatal heartwater in an African elephant (*Loxodonta africana*) and a dromedary camel are unproven, and could have occurred from other causes. The elephant was also infected with *Bacillus anthracis*, the agent of anthrax.

E. ruminantium nucleic acids were recently detected by PCR in a dog in Africa, but the susceptibility of this species remains to be confirmed. Experimental infections have been established in ferrets, laboratory mice, the four-striped grass mouse (*Rhabdomys pumilio*) and the southern multimammate mouse (*Mastomys coucha*). There is no evidence that any of these animals are important in the epidemiology of heartwater. Leopard tortoises (*Geochelone pardalis*) and helmeted guinea fowl (*Numida meleagris*) were reported to be susceptible in earlier studies, but this was not confirmed in a later report, and they are no longer considered to be hosts. The scrub hare (*Lepus saxatilis*) may be a host, but this has not been proven.

Zoonotic potential

Currently, the evidence that *E. ruminantium* may be zoonotic is limited to findings published in 2005, which reported positive PCR results for this organism in three fatal cases of human ehrlichiosis in Africa. Two cases occurred in children with encephalitis, vasculitis of the brain, and pulmonary edema. Clinical details were not available for the other case, an adult. *E. ruminantium* was not proven to be the cause of death in any of these three individuals, and it remains to be determined whether this organism can cause illnesses in humans. As of 2015, there appear to be no additional reports of possible zoonotic infections.

GEOGRAPHIC DISTRIBUTION

Heartwater is endemic in most of Africa south of the Sahara desert, as well as in surrounding islands such as Madagascar, and in some islands in the Caribbean (currently thought to be limited to Guadeloupe, Antigua and Marie Galante).

TRANSMISSION

Heartwater is transmitted by ticks in the genus *Amblyomma*. Transstadial transmission occurs in these ticks, which can remain infected for at least 15 months. Transovarial transmission is not thought to be epidemiologically significant in nature, although it has been demonstrated in the laboratory. *A. variegatum* (the tropical bont tick) is the major vector in Africa and the Caribbean. Other known vectors are *A. hebraeum* (the bont tick) in southern Africa, *A. lepidum* and *A. gemma* in East Africa, Somalia and the Sudan; and *A. astrion* and *A. pomposum*. Species demonstrated to be capable of transmitting *E. ruminantium* in the laboratory include *A. sparsum, A. cohaerans, A. marmoreum, A. tholloni,* and three North American ticks, *A. maculatum* (the Gulf Coast tick), *A. cajennense* and *A. dissimile. A. maculatum* is the most likely of the latter three species to act as a significant vector if *E. ruminantium* is introduced into North America. Based on PCR results, *E. ruminantium* might infect members of some other tick genera; however, these ticks are not thought to be capable of transmitting this organism to animals.

Ticks become infected with *E. ruminantium* by feeding on acutely ill or subclinically infected animals. Cattle, sheep, goats and some wild ungulates (e.g., blesbok, wildebeest, African buffalo, eland, giraffe, greater kudu, sable antelope) can continue to carry the organism at low levels for a time after recovery; reports of the carrier state after natural or experimental infections range from a month or two to almost a year. Vertical transmission is thought to occur, and *E. ruminantium* has been detected in colostrum. Iatrogenic transmission is possible (e.g., when unsterilized needles are reused between animals); however, significant transmission on fomites is otherwise considered unlikely in the field. *E. ruminantium* is very fragile and does not survive outside a host for more than a few hours at room temperature, although it has been reported to persist for as long as 72 hours at 4°C. Blood exposed to sunlight loses infectivity in less than 5 minutes.

DISINFECTION

There has been little or no research on the disinfectant susceptibility of *Ehrlichia* organisms.

INCUBATION PERIOD

The mean incubation period in natural infections is approximately 2-3 weeks (14 days in small ruminants and 18 days in cattle). Some infections can become apparent as late as 4-5 weeks after exposure.

CLINICAL SIGNS

Peracute cases of heartwater can be seen, although they are reported to be relatively rare, and are usually seen in non-native breeds of sheep, cattle and goats. This form of heartwater is characterized by sudden death, which may be accompanied by terminal convulsions, and preceded by a brief interval of fever, severe respiratory distress, hyperesthesia and lacrimation. Diarrhea has also been reported in some animals.

Acute disease is the most common form of heartwater in domesticated ruminants. The initial signs may include sudden fever, anorexia, listlessness, congested mucous membranes and respiratory signs (e.g., moist cough, bronchial rales, rapid breathing), which can progress to dyspnea. Some animals have diarrhea, which may be profuse and/or hemorrhagic. Neurological signs often develop in affected animals; commonly reported signs include chewing movements, protrusion of the tongue, twitching of the eyelids and circling, often with a high-stepping gait. Animals sometimes stand rigidly with muscle tremors. Some may become aggressive or anxious. As the disease progresses, the neurological signs become more severe, and the animal goes into convulsions. In the terminal stages, lateral recumbency with paddling or galloping movements, opisthotonos, hyperesthesia, nystagmus and frothing at the mouth are common. Animals with the acute form of heartwater usually die within a week. Heartwater can also present as a subacute disease with milder signs such as a prolonged fever, coughing and mild incoordination. CNS signs are inconsistent in this form. Subacute cases are reported to be infrequent (although some cases might not be recognized if diagnostic testing is not done). In this form, the animal either recovers or dies within 1 to 2 weeks.

Mild or subclinical infections may be seen in young calves, lambs or kids; partially immune livestock; some indigenous breeds; and some wild ruminants. Transient fever may be the only clinical sign in this form, which is known as "heartwater fever."

POST MORTEM LESIONS

Hydropericardium, with straw-colored to reddish pericardial fluid, gives heartwater its name; this lesion is more consistently found in sheep and goats than in cattle. Other common lesions include pulmonary and mediastinal edema, froth in the trachea (due to pulmonary edema and terminal dyspnea), hydrothorax, ascites, perirenal edema, and edema of the mediastinal and bronchial lymph nodes. There may also be congestion and/or edema in the gastrointestinal tract, especially in the abomasal mucosa of cattle. Subendocardial petechial hemorrhages are common, and submucosal and subserosal hemorrhages may also be seen in other organs. Splenomegaly may be noted, particularly in sheep and goats. Congestion and meningeal edema are sometimes found in the brain; however, gross lesions are usually subtle or absent in the CNS. Minimal or no lesions have also been reported in some cases.

Similar lesions have been reported in wild ruminants, with the most common lesions reported to be hydrothorax, hydropericardium, lung edema, ascites, splenomegaly and generalized congestion.

DIAGNOSTIC TESTS

Polymerase chain reaction (PCR) tests can identify *E. ruminantium* in tissues at necropsy, or in the blood of live animals from just before the onset of the fever to a few days after recovery. Nucleic acids may sometimes be detected in the blood or bone marrow of carrier animals, but this is inconsistent. Some PCR tests for *E. ruminantium* can react with some other *Ehrlichia*, including *E. chaffeensis*, *E. canis* and the Panola Mountain *Ehrlichia*, although there is usually lower reactivity to these organisms if the test is correctly calibrated. A PCR assay that can distinguish *E. ruminantium* and the Panola Mountain *Ehrlichia* was recently described. Loop-mediated isothermal amplification (LAMP) assays to detect *E. ruminantium* have also been published. Other DNA techniques may also be available, but are uncommonly used for clinical diagnosis.

Heartwater can also be diagnosed by observing *E. ruminantium* colonies in stained (Giemsa) smears from the brain or intima of blood vessels at necropsy. The best samples to collect from the brain are well-vascularized portions such as the cerebrum, cerebellum or hippocampus. *E. ruminantium* occurs as clumps of reddish-purple to blue, coccoid to pleomorphic organisms inside capillary endothelial cells. These organisms are often found close to the nucleus, and may be in a ring or horseshoe. *E. ruminantium* can also be detected in formalin-fixed brain sections using immunoperoxidase techniques, including combined immunostaining and counterstaining with hematoxylin. These techniques are more likely to detect small numbers of organisms than the use of tissue stains alone. Colonies can be difficult or impossible to find in some animals that have been treated with antibiotics. Only a few colonies may be found in peracute cases.

E. ruminantium can be isolated (e.g., from blood samples) in many primary ruminant endothelial cells or endothelial cell lines. The cultured organism is identified by microscopic examination or immunofluorescence/immuno-peroxidase staining. Heartwater may also be diagnosed by inoculating fresh blood from a suspected case into a susceptible sheep or goat. However, this technique is generally discouraged for animal welfare reasons.

Various serological tests for heartwater are available, including indirect immunofluorescence, enzyme-linked immunosorbent assays (ELISAs) and immunoblotting (Western blotting). Serology may be used to check the immune status of vaccinated animals, or as part of diagnosis on a herd basis; however, cross-reactions occur with various *Ehrlichia* species and other related organisms, such as some members of the genus *Anaplasma*. False negative results can also be seen, especially in cattle. Furthermore, infected animals typically seroconvert after recovery, and many animals die, making serology of limited use for clinical diagnosis in individual animals.

Heartwater carriers are difficult to detect. Rickettsial colonies are difficult to find in these animals, and animal inoculation may be unsuccessful except during the first few weeks after recovery. Carriers may sometimes be found by PCR, or by feeding ticks on the animal and testing the ticks by PCR. Some carriers can be seronegative.

TREATMENT

Tetracyclines are reported to be effective in the early stage of the disease. Prolonged treatment and/or larger doses may be needed if treatment is started later, and antibiotics are often ineffective once neurological signs appear. Sulfonamides also have activity against *E. ruminantium* but are less effective. Treated animals can remain carriers.

Supportive treatment (fluids, nutritional support) may also be needed. and additional drugs may be indicated to treat or mitigate conditions such as peripheral vascular collapse, increased capillary permeability, edema and convulsions. Animals should be kept quiet and undisturbed, in comfortable surroundings; stimuli may elicit fatal convulsions.

CONTROL

Disease reporting

A quick response is vital for containing outbreaks in regions free of heartwater, particularly where potential tick vectors exist. Veterinarians who encounter or suspect this disease should follow their national and/or local guidelines for disease reporting. In the U.S., state or federal veterinary authorities should be informed immediately.

Prevention

E. ruminantium cannot survive outside a living host for more than a few hours at room temperature. For this reason, heartwater is usually introduced in infected animals, including asymptomatic carriers, or in ticks. In heartwater-free countries, susceptible ruminants from endemic regions are tested before importation. Because serology is unreliable, the World Organization for Animal Health (OIE) currently recommends that the epidemiology of the importing herd be studied to determine that the animals and their resident ticks are free of *E. ruminantium*, and that the animals also be repeatedly tested by PCR. In addition, all animals that may carry *Amblyomma*, including species not susceptible to heartwater, must be inspected for ticks before entry. Wild animals such as birds may also be an issue. Cattle egrets (*Bubulcus ibis*) have been implicated in the dispersal of *Amblyomma* ticks in the Caribbean. Outbreaks occurring outside endemic regions are usually controlled with quarantines, euthanasia of infected animals and tick control. It is important to prevent ticks from feeding on infected animals, or the disease may be impossible to eradicate.

In endemic regions, clinical cases are prevented by prophylactic treatment of newly introduced animals with tetracyclines, strategic tick control and/or immunization. Tick control is usually employed at levels that prevent animals from being exposed to high doses of *E. ruminantium*, but allow continuous low level exposure. This helps establish immunity in young animals and maintains it in older members of the herd. Intensive tick control is no longer recommended in endemic regions, as it eliminates this immune boosting effect, and there can be serious losses if there is a break in tick control. Potential issues with tick control include the development of acaricide resistance, as well as seasonal increases in tick numbers and other problems that can make it difficult to control heartwater with this method alone.

Immunization currently consists of infecting animals with a commercial "vaccine" that contains a live, moderately virulent, *E. ruminantium* strain, then treating them with antibiotics when a fever develops. Alternatively, this vaccine may be given to young kids or lambs during their first week of life, or to calves during the first month. Such young animals are resistant to heartwater, and usually do not require treatment. (However, more valuable animals may still need to be monitored.) This vaccine does not protect animals from all field strains, and revaccination is risky due to the possibility of anaphylactic reactions. Other types of vaccines are in development, and some experimental vaccines have been tested in field trials.

It might be possible to eradicate heartwater from some regions by eliminating its vectors. However, *Amblyomma* ticks are difficult to eradicate due to their high rate of reproduction, the wide variety of hosts they infest, and the development of acaricide resistance. Regional *Amblyomma variegatum* eradication programs (the Caribbean *Amblyomma* Program and the POSEIDOM Vétérinaire Programme) were conducted in the Caribbean between 1994 and 2008. These programs succeeded in reducing the numbers of ticks on some islands and eradicating them from others, but complete eradication throughout the Caribbean was not achieved.

MORBIDITY AND MORTALITY

The mortality rate in susceptible livestock ranges from < 10% to 90%, depending on the animal's species, breed and previous exposures. Morbidity and mortality rates are normally higher in non-native than indigenous breeds, and sheep and goats are usually affected more severely than cattle. For example, up to 80% of merino sheep may die, but the mortality rate can be only 6% in Persian or Afrikander sheep. Angora and Saanen goats are also very susceptible to heartwater, while Creole goats in Guadeloupe are resistant. In cattle, reported mortality rates can be as high as 60-80%, and *Bos indicus* breeds tend to be less severely affected than *Bos taurus*. Genetic resistance has been demonstrated in some breeds. Young ruminants are resistant to heartwater. Sheep and goats are reported to be resistant during the first week of

life, while immunity can last up to 6-9 weeks in some calves. At least in calves, there appears to be a maternally-derived component in addition to innate immunity. Early resistance might be shortened in calves from heartwater-naïve dams.

Most infections in wild ruminants appear to be subclinical or mild, but high mortality rates have been reported in lechwe introduced into endemic areas, and in experimentally infected white-tailed deer. Occasional cases of heartwater have also been reported in other wild ruminants in Africa.

HENDRA VIRUS INFECTION

Equine Morbillivirus Pneumonia, Acute Equine Respiratory Syndrome

IMPORTANCE

Hendra virus infection is an emerging viral disease of horses and humans in Australia. Although this disease is uncommon, cases in horses have been reported with increasing frequency since it was first recognized in 1994. Hendra virus is maintained in asymptomatic flying foxes (pteropid fruit bats). Virus shedding from these bats appears to increase at unpredictable intervals, leading to spillover events that transmit Hendra virus to horses. Infected horses usually experience a brief, severe respiratory or neurological illness with a high case fatality rate, and are thought to be incidental hosts. Horse-to-horse transmission seems to be rare among animals kept on pastures, although infected horses brought into stables have spread the virus to a few animals in close contact. In some incidents, Hendra virus spread from horses to humans during close contact; human infections from other sources, including direct contact with flying foxes, have not been reported. Four of the seven clinical cases in humans were fatal. Other species may also be susceptible to Hendra virus. Infections without clinical signs have been reported rarely in dogs exposed to infected horses, and additional species, including cats, pigs, ferrets and pocket pets (hamsters, guinea pigs), can be infected experimentally. A vaccine was recently introduced for horses, but no vaccine or specific antiviral treatment has been found yet for humans. Uncertainty about the ability of Hendra virus to persist long-term has resulted in the euthanasia of infected horses and dogs in Australia even when the illness was not fatal.

ETIOLOGY

Hendra virus (HeV) is a member of the genus *Henipavirus* in the family Paramyxoviridae. This genus also includes Nipah virus, Cedar virus (an apparently nonpathogenic virus found in Australian bats) and additional uncharacterized henipaviruses in various locations. Multiple Hendra virus variants circulate in bats. Whether these viruses differ in virulence for other animals is unknown; however, several variants have been found in clinical cases in horses and humans.

SPECIES AFFECTED

Bats of the genus *Pteropus* (pteropid fruit bats/ flying foxes) appear to be the reservoir hosts. Hendra virus has been detected in all four species of Australian flying foxes: *Pteropus alecto, P. poliocephalus, P. scapulatus* and *Pteropus conspicillatus*. However, *P. alecto* and *P. conspicillatus* seem to be infected and/ or shed virus more often than *P. poliocephalus* or *P. scapulatus*.

Other mammals are thought to be incidental hosts. All clinical cases in animals, to date, have occurred in horses, but other species may also be susceptible. In an early experimental study, Hendra virus was pathogenic in cats and guinea pigs, but mice, rats, two dogs, rabbits and chickens did not develop clinical signs. Definitive seroconversion was only observed in the rabbits in this study, although one dog and three of four rats had equivocal neutralizing titers. However, naturally acquired subclinical infections were later detected in two dogs on properties with sick horses, and an unpublished study has confirmed that dogs can be experimentally infected without clinical signs. Aged (one-year-old) mice are now known to be susceptible to intranasal inoculation, and develop clinical signs. Other species that have been experimentally infected with Hendra virus include pigs, ferrets, guinea pigs, hamsters and African green monkeys (*Cercopithecus aethiops*). As of 2015, naturally acquired infections have not been reported in any species other than horses and dogs.

Zoonotic potential

Humans are susceptible to Hendra virus. To date, all clinical cases have been acquired during close contact with infected horses and/or their tissues. Necropsies are a particularly high-risk procedure, but any contact with blood, secretions or tissues also carries a risk. At least one case is thought to have resulted from contact with nasal fluids from an asymptomatic horse (while performing nasal cavity lavage for another condition) during the incubation period. No one has apparently been infected by direct or indirect exposure to infected flying foxes, and surveys have found no evidence of Hendra virus infections among people who care for these animals.

GEOGRAPHIC DISTRIBUTION

Hendra virus infections have been seen only in Australia, where this virus is endemic in flying foxes. Seropositive flying foxes have been found from Darwin in north central Australia to Melbourne in southeastern Australia. Cases in horses have only been reported from eastern Australia, in the states of Queensland and New South Wales. Antibodies detected in flying foxes in Papua New Guinea might be caused by Hendra virus or a related virus.

Currently there is no evidence that Hendra virus exists in other areas. However, henipaviruses or antibodies to these viruses have been detected in bats on several continents. Most of these viruses are poorly characterized.

TRANSMISSION

In flying foxes, infectious virus and/or viral nucleic acids have been found in urine, blood, throat swabs, saliva, feces, fetal tissues and uterine fluids. Urine is currently thought to be the most important source of this virus, with other secretions and excretions (e.g., feces, nasal and oral secretions) probably less significant in transmission. Virus prevalence appears to wax and wane in bat populations, with periodic pulses of high virus shedding in bat urine. One such pulse lasted for 2-3 months. Vertical transmission has been demonstrated, although a recent survey of archived flying fox tissues suggests that it might not be common. Whether Hendra virus persists in local populations of flying foxes (with periodic recrudescence), is transmitted between groups, or is maintained by some combination of these processes is uncertain.

Horses are thought to become infected by ingesting or inhaling Hendra virus from the environment, most likely when they feed in areas contaminated by flying fox urine and/or virus-contaminated fruits and spats (fibrous plant material that remains after chewing by bats). The index case is usually a horse kept outside, near flying fox activity. Hendra virus does not appear to be highly contagious among horses, and close contact seems to be necessary for it to spread. Infected horses on pastures have rarely transmitted the virus to their companions. In two outbreaks, however, infected animals in stables spread the virus to several contacts. In horses, there is evidence for Hendra virus shedding in nasal and oral secretions, urine, feces, blood and a wide variety of tissues, although the presence of infectious virus has not been confirmed in all secretions/excretions (some investigations only detected viral nucleic acids). Hendra virus appears to be widespread in the body by the time clinical signs appear, and it has been found in nasal secretions before the onset of clinical signs. Whether horses can remain persistently infected after recovery from clinical signs is currently uncertain.

There is limited information about Hendra virus infections in other animals, but several species are susceptible to experimental inoculation by the intranasal or oronasal routes. Cats could be infected intranasally, orally and by subcutaneous inoculation. How two dogs became infected under natural conditions is unclear, but both lived on properties with infected horses, and one dog had probably had been exposed to the blood of a sick horse. Viral nucleic acids were detected in the blood and tissues of one naturally infected pet dog, although this animal did not transmit the virus to people or to two other dogs on the property. Some experimentally infected dogs shed infectious virus for a short time in respiratory secretions. Experimentally infected cats were able to transmit Hendra virus to other cats or horses in close contact. In this experiment, the virus was detected in feline urine, but not in nasal secretions, oral secretions or feces. In experimentally infected pigs, Hendra virus was found primarily in the respiratory tract; pigs shed infectious virus in oral and nasal secretions and feces, and viral RNA was also detected in ocular secretions, but there was no evidence of virus excretion in the urine.

Humans have been infected during close contact with sick horses and during necropsies, probably via body fluids or aerosols. Person-to-person transmission has not been seen, but Hendra virus has been isolated from nasopharyngeal secretions and the kidneys, and detected by PCR in patients' urine. The virus may be shed for several weeks in acute cases. One person developed Hendra virus-associated neurological signs a year after infection, raising the possibility that this virus might persist in some body site(s) after recovery. A recent study found no evidence of long-term virus persistence in two survivors.

Transmission may be possible on fomites, particularly in closed environments such as stables. Under optimal laboratory conditions, Hendra virus survived for more than four days in flying fox urine at 22°C (72°F). This virus can also remain viable for a few hours to a few days (generally less than four days) in fruit juice or fruit. It does not survive well at higher temperatures, and it is inactivated in less then a day in either urine or fruit juice at 37°C (98.6°F). In one study, the half-life of this virus in cell culture medium was approximately 13 days at 4°C, 2 days at 22°C and 2 minutes at 56°C.

DISINFECTION

Like other paramyxoviruses, Hendra virus is expected to be susceptible to soaps, detergents and many common disinfectants including hypochlorite, iodophors, biguanidines (e.g. chlorhexidine), Virkon® and quaternary ammonium compounds. This virus is susceptible to desiccation or heat, but resists inactivation by acids or alkalis; it can survive a wide pH range from 4 to 11.

INFECTIONS IN ANIMALS

INCUBATION PERIOD

In horses, the incubation period ranged from 3 to 16 days, and was slightly longer in natural cases (5-16 days) than in experimentally infected animals. The incubation period in experimentally infected cats was 4 to 8 days.

CLINICAL SIGNS

Horses

Two syndromes, one characterized primarily by respiratory disease and the other mainly by neurological signs, have been reported in horses. Because Hendra virus causes vasculitis, other presentations might also be possible. Most known cases have been severe and acute, and progressed rapidly to death within days. A few infected horses were found dead, with no apparent signs of illness when they were last observed 12-24 earlier. Milder cases have also been seen, and a few horses recovered.

Nonspecific clinical signs, such as fever, anorexia and depression, were seen initially in experimentally infected horses. Fever and an elevated heart rate appeared to be the earliest signs in these animals. Apparent discomfort was also seen in some animals, which shifted their weight constantly from leg to leg, or alternated weight shifting with a rigid stance. Some experimentally infected horses had a slight nasal discharge early, became agitated or irritable, or developed respiratory signs before euthanasia, and one animal passed small amounts of blood and mucus in the feces. Nonspecific signs reported in naturally infected animals have included high fever, anorexia, depression, sweating and uneasiness.

In horses with respiratory signs, the respiration tends to be rapid, shallow and labored, and the mucus membranes may be congested. Jaundiced mucus membranes, ataxia, mild neurological signs or subcutaneous edema (e.g., facial edema or swelling of the lips) have also been seen. Just before death, animals may develop a copious nasal discharge, which becomes frothy and may be bloodstained. The clinical course is acute; death usually occurs one to three days after the initial signs. Some convalescent horses may develop neurological signs, but others seem to recover fully.

In other horses, neurological rather than respiratory signs have predominated. Some CNS signs reported in Hendra virus-infected horses have included an altered gait (e.g. high stepping), a "wobbly gait" that progresses to ataxia, altered consciousness or aimless walking, apparent blindness in one or both eyes, a head tilt, circling, muscle twitches or tremors, facial paralysis, a locked jaw, spasms of the jaw and involuntary chomping. Several horses have been found caught in fences, presumably as the result of neurological deficits, and were initially thought to have died as a result of accidents unrelated to Hendra virus infection.

Other reported clinical signs have included muscle tremors, colic and straining to defecate, foul odor to the breath, excessively warm hooves and delayed blood clotting times. Some horses have had difficulty urinating or dribbled urine in the terminal stages.

Other species

No clinical signs have been reported in naturally or experimentally infected dogs, with the possible exception of an episode of apparent discomfort in one animal. Despite the absence of clinical signs, this naturally infected dog had lesions at necropsy. The other naturally infected dog seroconverted with no evidence of virus replication. In experimentally infected cats, fever and increased respiratory rates were followed by severe illness and death within 24 hours. Experimentally infected pigs developed fever and depression. Some pigs also had respiratory signs (cough, respiratory distress), which were fatal in one severe case. One pig developed both respiratory signs and mild neurological signs, but recovered. Severe respiratory disease was seen in experimentally infected African green monkeys, while ferrets had a nonfatal illness with signs of fever, depression and generalized tremors. Some guinea pigs developed generalized, fatal vascular disease, with few clinical signs before death, while others had nonspecific signs (depression, anorexia) and recovered. Syrian golden hamsters (*Mesocricetus auratus*) had either fatal respiratory signs, or respiratory signs followed by neurological signs. Fatal illness with neurological signs (ataxia, muscle tremors) was also seen in one-year-old (aged) mice, while 2-month old mice were resistant.

Flying foxes (including pregnant animals) appear to remain asymptomatic, and all infected animals may not seroconvert.

POST MORTEM LESIONS

Necropsies have been linked to human cases, and should be performed only if they can be carried out safely, using recommended PPE and other precautions. Routine necropsy precautions may not be sufficient to protect people.

Horses

In horses with the respiratory syndrome, post-mortem lesions have been found mainly in the lower respiratory tract. Common lesions include marked pulmonary edema, dilation of the pulmonary lymphatics, and congestion and ventral consolidation of the lungs. Petechial hemorrhages have been seen on the pleural surfaces, and patchy hemorrhages may be found in the lung parenchyma. The airway often contains white or blood-tinged foam, and edema fluid oozes from cut tissues. Swollen and congested lymph nodes (especially lymph nodes associated with the respiratory tract), pleural and pericardial fluid, and visceral edema have also been reported. Scattered petechiae and ecchymoses may be found in the stomach, intestines and perirenal tissues. Yellowing of the subcutaneous tissue was reported to be common in some reports. Endometrial edema and purplish discoloration of the serosa of the uterus was reported in one experimentally infected mare. Vasculitis is the predominant lesion on histopathology.

Other animals

Post mortem lesions reported in a naturally infected, asymptomatic dog included respiratory lesions (diffuse reddening of the lungs, frothy fluid in the trachea and bronchi), enlargement and reddening of respiratory-associated lymph nodes, reddening of the tonsils, an enlarged liver and spleen, and prominent white streaks at the corticomedullary junction of the kidney. Severe pulmonary edema, hydrothorax and edematous bronchial lymph nodes were seen in experimentally infected cats. Some experimentally infected pigs had areas of consolidation in the lungs, with or without petechiae or larger, demarcated hemorrhagic areas. Petechial hemorrhages were also reported in other organs of some pigs, including the kidneys, bronchial and submandibular lymph nodes. Lesions found in experimentally infected ferrets included subcutaneous edema, petechial hemorrhages throughout the skin, the pulmonary parenchyma and the abdomen, and enlarged and hemorrhagic lymph nodes.

DIAGNOSTIC TESTS

Stringent precautions should be used when collecting and shipping any diagnostic samples from live or dead animals. Only those samples that can be collected safely should be taken. A description of the limited necropsy procedure used to collect diagnostic samples, as well as necropsy and sample collection recommendations, can be found on the Web sites maintained by some states in Australia.

Sampling a variety of sites increases the probability of detecting Hendra virus. A combination of blood and nasal, oral and rectal swabs for PCR and/or virus isolation, and serum for serology, can detect a high proportion of infections in live horses. Other samples that may be taken include urine (e.g., a urine soaked swab taken from the ground immediately after urination), conjunctival swabs and swabs of other orifices (vaginal, urethral). Similar swab samples have been recommended for dead horses, together with blood collected from the jugular vein, and sampling of the superficial submandibular lymph node. Additional tissue samples (e.g., lung, kidney, lymphoid tissues, brain) may be collected by people experienced in sampling for Hendra virus.

PCR on blood, secretions and excretions (swabs) or tissue samples is often used for rapid diagnosis. Virus isolation can also be attempted in live animals; however, Hendra virus is more likely to be recovered from the tissues after death. Because this virus is a biosafety level 4 (BSL4) pathogen, virus isolation can only be done in a limited number of laboratories. Vero cells are often employed, but a number of other cell lines or primary cultures can also be used. The isolated virus can be identified by methods such as immunostaining or virus neutralization. Electron or immunoelectron microscopy may also be helpful. Molecular methods (e.g., PCR), comparative immunostaining or differential neutralization assays can distinguish the closely related Hendra and Nipah viruses. Viral antigens can also be detected directly in tissues by immunoperoxidase or immunofluorescence assays.

Serology can be helpful, but horses may not have detectable titers until 10 to 14 days after infection. ELISAs and serum neutralization tests are used most often; the latter is considered to be the gold standard serological assay. False positives are common in ELISAs, which are often used as an initial screening test. Indirect immunofluorescence and immunoblotting have also been described. Cross-reactions can occur between Hendra and Nipah viruses in serological assays including virus neutralization; however, these reactions can be distinguished with comparative neutralization tests. Currently, there is no commercially validated test that can distinguish whether antibodies have resulted from infection or vaccination, but an experimental assay is reported to be available in Australia.

There is limited experience with diagnosis in animals other than horses. One naturally infected dog seroconverted without any virological evidence of infection. In another dog, PCR detected viral nucleic acids in blood and tissues, but not oral swabs, and virus isolation was unsuccessful. This animal was weakly seropositive at the time of euthanasia.

TREATMENT

Other than supportive therapy, there is no treatment for Hendra virus infections in animals. The current Australian policy is to euthanize surviving horses due to uncertainties about virus persistence. Infected dogs have also been euthanized for the same reason.

CONTROL

Disease reporting

A quick response helps reduce human and animal exposure to infected horses, and also decreases the risk of a wider outbreak. Veterinarians who encounter or suspect a Hendra virus infection should follow their national and/or local guidelines for disease reporting. In the U.S., state or federal veterinary authorities should be informed immediately. As of 2015, Australia also requires immediate notification of any infections in domesticated animals, although the virus is endemic in bats.

Prevention

A Hendra virus vaccine is now available for horses in Australia. Exposure to flying foxes, their tissues and secretions should also be minimized. Horse paddocks should not contain food trees favored by flying foxes, or trees planted in configurations that encourage roosting, and horses should be kept away from areas where flying foxes roost or are feeding. Whenever possible, feed bins and water troughs should be covered. Moving horses into stables or other enclosures designed to keep them away from flying foxes at night is expected to be helpful.

Horses that develop signs consistent with Hendra virus infection should be isolated; they should not be allowed to contact other domesticated animals, as well as other horses. Stringent infection control measures should be employed to avoid spreading the virus on fomites. Human exposure must also be minimized. In Australia, unvaccinated horses that may have been exposed are assessed and tested for the disease, and vaccination may be recommended. Authorities may also require that any companion animals (e.g., dogs and cats) exposed to an infected horse be isolated for a period. Quarantines and rigorous hygiene have been effective in containing past outbreaks. The low rate of horse-to-horse transmission also aids control.

Carcasses should also be isolated until Hendra virus infection can be ruled out. Necropsies should be avoided unless the operator can carry them out safely using recommended guidelines and PPE (see human Prevention section). Government authorities should be consulted for the most appropriate disposal method for carcasses; deep burial on the property is currently considered the option of choice, although other options such as burning may also be used.

MORBIDITY AND MORTALITY

The prevalence and shedding of Hendra virus seems to wax and wane in flying fox populations, but what causes these fluctuations is not known. Pregnancy, the birthing period and/or lactation were associated with Hendra virus infections in some studies, but not others, and their influence is currently uncertain. Other factors, such as nutritional stress, could also be involved, while environmental conditions such as the temperature might influence virus survival and transmission to horses. While Hendra virus can be shed year-round (though not constantly) in flying fox populations, infections appear to be seasonal in horses. Equine cases have occurred in the cooler months from May to October in subtropical areas, with a peak in July, although they have been seen year-round in the northern tropics.

Hendra virus infections seem to be uncommon in horses. As of July 2015, 94 cases had been reported in this species. The first cases were recognized during outbreaks in Hendra, Australia (Queensland) in 1994, but infections were rarely reported during the following decade; infected horses were found once in 1999, and on two occasions in 2004. The absence of any seropositive horses in two surveys, which tested approximately 4000 horses, also suggested that infections were rare. Hendra virus infections appeared more regularly between 2006 and 2009, with two incidents reported each year, and unexpectedly high numbers of cases were reported in 2011 (18 incidents with 23 cases) and 2012-2013 (12 incidents between January 2012 and July 2013). The reason for the recent increase in cases is unclear, although increased testing and recognition might play some role. The case fatality rate in recognized cases has been high and can approach 90%.

Other than in horses, the only naturally occurring infections that have been recognized (as of December 2015) were in two dogs on farms that had infected horses. In one of these incidents, only one of the three dogs on the farm became infected. In spite of their susceptibility to experimental infections, testing of cats on infected farms has revealed no natural infections in this species. A survey conducted in the Brisbane area, where the initial cases were reported in horses, also found no serological evidence of henipavirus infections in

500 cats. Likewise, an early survey reported that none of 100 swine herds tested in Queensland, Australia had antibodies to Hendra virus. Experimental infections in cats and guinea pigs have been fatal, but no clinical signs have yet been reported in naturally or experimentally infected dogs, and ferrets became ill but did not die.

INFECTIONS IN HUMANS

INCUBATION PERIOD

The initial symptoms occurred 5 to 16 days after exposure in six of the seven human cases. One person became ill after 21 days; however, he had been treated prophylactically with antiviral drugs, and developed encephalitis immediately afterward. It is possible that the treatment masked any initial influenza-like signs in this case. One person developed recurrent, fatal encephalitis a year after apparent recovery from the initial illness.

CLINICAL SIGNS

Hendra virus infections have been reported in seven people. The syndromes have included influenza-like illness, multiorgan failure and progressive encephalitis. The two initial cases were characterized by a serious influenza-like disease with fever, myalgia, respiratory signs and vertigo. One person died with pneumonitis, multiorgan failure and arterial thrombosis; the other recovered over the next six weeks. In the third case, a mild meningoencephalitic illness (drowsiness, headache, vomiting, neck stiffness) was followed by a long asymptomatic period before fatal encephalitis developed a year later. The fourth person reported a self-limited influenza-like illness with a dry cough, sore throat, cervical lymphadenopathy, fatigue, body aches and a fever that lasted for approximately one week.

Two cases in 2008-2009 were characterized by a biphasic illness that began with influenza-like signs (fever, myalgia and headache), followed by apparent recovery, then by recurrent fever and signs of encephalitis after 5-12 days. In one case, the neurological signs were limited to ataxia, mild confusion, bilateral ptosis and dysarthria, and the person survived, although with persistent neurological defects. The other person developed progressive, fatal neurological signs, beginning with ptosis, ataxia and mild confusion and progressing to seizures and coma. Another fatal case occurred in a person who had been treated prophylactically for 5 days with antiviral drugs after exposure. He developed encephalitis, with signs of ataxia, drowsiness and seizures, immediately after drug treatment, and died after 19 days.

DIAGNOSTIC TESTS

Hendra virus infections in humans have been diagnosed similarly to cases in horses, i.e., by tests such as PCR, virus isolation, antigen detection and immunohistochemistry.

TREATMENT

Treatment of Hendra virus infections, to date, has mainly been supportive. Antiviral drugs have been administered to some patients, as well as prophylactically in people at high risk of exposure; however, no antivirals have yet been shown to be effective against this disease. The efficacy of passively administered immunotherapy (monoclonal antibodies against Hendra virus) is under investigation.

CONTROL

Disease reporting

People who have been exposed to Hendra virus should seek medical advice. In Australia, the area health department should be contacted to report the case.

Prevention

Human infections have been reported after nursing or examining sick horses, or handling equine tissues at necropsy. Stringent precautions should be taken to prevent contact with blood, tissues, body fluids and excretions whenever Hendra virus is among the differential diagnoses. Personal protective equipment (PPE) recommendations are available from government sources in Australia (see Internet Resources). In general, the minimum recommendations during an investigation of a suspected case include impervious gloves, a particulate (P2 [N95] or higher) respirator, a face shield or safety eyewear to protect the eyes, splash-proof overalls (or cotton or disposable overalls with impervious or splash-proof apron) and impervious boots. [NB: splash-proof rather than impervious overalls are recommended in Australia, due to dangers from overheating in a hot climate] Excellent hygiene should be practiced at all times, and caution should be used to avoid generating aerosols or splashing material, both when examining the horse and during disinfection. Detailed recommendations for conducting investigations of suspected Hendra virus infections, as well as precautions to be used when the likelihood of Hendra virus is first revealed during an examination of the case, are available from authorities in Australia.

Because Hendra virus infections can look like other diseases and are often diagnosed retrospectively, good infection control precautions (standard precautions) should be used routinely with horses whenever there is a risk of contact with blood, body fluids, excretions, mucous membranes or breaks in the skin. Veterinarians in endemic areas should keep a dedicated Hendra virus field kit with appropriate PPE, disinfectants, waste disposal bags and other necessary items for use in unexpected cases. All human exposure should be minimized once the case is suspected, and any contamination should be washed off with soap and water. Investigations should be continued only if suitable precautions can be taken and PPE is available.

MORBIDITY AND MORTALITY

Hendra virus infections have been reported in seven people, all of whom had close contact with infected horses during their illness or at necropsy. Only a percentage of those exposed to infected horses have become ill. Two people, a stablehand and the trainer, were infected during an outbreak in 1994; the stablehand recovered but the trainer died. In a separate episode, a farmer who had close contact with two sick horses (both during their illness and at necropsy) became infected and died of the illness a year later. In 2004, a veterinarian who conducted the necropsy on an infected horse became ill but recovered. Two assistants at the necropsy remained seronegative. The same year, eighteen people were exposed to another infected horse or to its tissues at necropsy, but none seroconverted. No human infections were associated with the horses that died of this disease in 1999, 2006 or 2007, but illness was reported in a veterinarian and an animal nurse during one of the two clusters in 2008. A veterinarian was also infected during an outbreak in 2009. Two of the latter cases were fatal. Although there have been a number of people exposed to equine cases since that time (e.g., more than 60 people exposed to equine cases in 2011), no additional human cases were reported between 2010 and 2015. There has been no evidence of seroconversion in people who are often in close contact with flying foxes.

JAPANESE ENCEPHALITIS

IMPORTANCE

Japanese encephalitis virus (JEV) is a mosquito-borne agent that can cause encephalitis in equids and humans and reproductive disease in pigs. Rare clinical cases have also been reported in other species, such as cattle. Japanese encephalitis can be a very serious disease in people: although most infections are asymptomatic, clinical cases tend to manifest as severe encephalitis, and many survivors are left with neurological sequelae. All ages can be affected in a population without previous exposure; however, Japanese encephalitis tends to be a childhood disease in endemic areas, where most people develop immunity by the time they reach adulthood. Morbidity and mortality can be high in unvaccinated populations during epidemics. Approximately 4,000 people died during the 1924 epidemic in Japan, and nearly 2500 fatalities occurred in South Korea in 1949. Likewise, more than 3700 equids died during an epidemic in Japan in 1949.

Japanese encephalitis virus has gradually expanded its geographic range within Asia and spread to parts of the western Pacific region during the last 50 years. It could become endemic in additional regions, similarly to West Nile virus, which became established in the Americas in the 1990s.

Eradication is unlikely once JEV enters mosquito populations, as the virus is maintained and amplified in cycles between these vectors and various vertebrate hosts such as pigs and wild birds. Vaccination has reduced the number of clinical cases among horses in endemic areas, and is mandatory in certain animals (e.g., racehorses) in some countries. Childhood vaccination has, likewise, greatly decreased the number of human cases in some nations; however, vaccination rates vary, and this disease is still very common in some areas. Some regions have recently reported a relative increase in the percentage of cases seen in adults, leading to suggestions that vaccination campaigns also be conducted in this group.

ETIOLOGY

Japanese encephalitis virus (JEV) is an arbovirus (arthropod-transmitted virus) in the genus *Flavivirus* and family Flaviviridae. There is only one serotype of JEV, but at least five genotypes. Some genotypes are more common than others, and the dominant genotypes in an area can change over time. For example, genotype I has become common in some areas where genotype III used to be prevalent.

Japanese encephalitis virus is closely related to St. Louis encephalitis virus, Murray Valley encephalitis virus and West Nile virus; these viruses and a few others comprise the Japanese encephalitis serogroup of the flaviviruses.

SPECIES AFFECTED

Illnesses caused by JEV occur mainly in equids (e.g., horses, donkeys) and pigs; however, rare clinical cases have been reported in cows, and other species may be susceptible. Asymptomatic infections have been documented in many other domesticated and wild mammals (e.g., cattle, sheep, goats, rabbits, dogs, cats, wild boar, raccoons) and birds, as well as in reptiles and amphibians. Reports of infections in some species may be based on serology alone.

Ardeid birds (herons and egrets) and suids (domesticated and wild pigs) develop viremia sufficient to infect mosquitoes, and are considered to be important in maintaining and amplifying JEV. Other birds (e.g., young poultry, swallows) have also been suggested as possible reservoirs, and many avian species have never been examined for their ability to maintain or amplify this virus. There are also reports suggesting that bats might be significant in some cycles. An early study suggested that wild rodents are not important maintenance hosts.

Zoonotic potential

Humans are susceptible to Japanese encephalitis.

GEOGRAPHIC DISTRIBUTION

Japanese encephalitis is widespread in temperate and tropical regions of Asia, and also occurs in parts of the western Pacific. Its precise distribution in some areas is unclear, due to limited surveillance and/or cross-reactivity with other flaviviruses in serological tests. In Australia, the virus is endemic on the Torres Strait islands, and there have been reports of it on the northern mainland, but it may not be established in the latter location. There are also rare reports describing possible JEV in mosquitoes and birds in southern Europe. Specifically, a portion of the JEV genome was identified in dead birds in Italy in 2000, and JEV gene segments were detected by PCR in mosquitoes in Italy in 2010. However, the evidence to date is not definitive, and the presence of circulating live virus remains to be confirmed.

TRANSMISSION

Japanese encephalitis virus is usually transmitted by mosquitoes in the genus *Culex*. The specific mosquito vectors vary with the region; however, *Culex tritaeniorhynchus* is important in spreading this virus to humans and domesticated animals across a wide geographic range. *C. tritaeniorhynchus* breeds in rice paddies and connecting canals, and is active at twilight. Other culicine species can also be important locally and/or as minor vectors. For example, members of the *C. sitiens* subgroup, especially *C. annulirostris*, are the most important vectors in Australia. JEV has been reported in other genera of mosquitoes, and it was isolated from *Culicoides* midges in China, but the significance of these vectors is unclear.

JEV is usually transmitted in mosquito bites, although lizards and bats can also become infected by eating infected mosquitoes. Humans and most domesticated animals are incidental hosts, with low viremia, and are not considered to be important in virus transmission. For example, while horse-to-horse transmission via mosquitoes has been demonstrated in the laboratory, viremia is low and there are usually too few susceptible horses nearby to maintain the virus. Although both birds and suids can amplify JEV, domesticated pigs are considered to be particularly amplifying hosts, as large numbers of susceptible young swine are produced each year, sometimes in close proximity to people. Boars are reported to transmit the virus in semen.

In addition to mosquito bites, infections in people have been reported after exposure to JEV in the laboratory or during tissue sample collection. This virus can be transmitted through mucous membranes or broken skin, inhaled in aerosols, or acquired by needlestick injuries.

Japanese encephalitis virus does not survive well outside a living host. How the virus persists during the winter in temperate climates is uncertain, although various mechanisms have been suggested.

DISINFECTION

Agents reported to be effective for JEV disinfection include 70% ethanol, 2% glutaraldehyde, 3-8% formaldehyde, 1% sodium hypochlorite, iodine, phenol iodophors and organic solvents/detergents. This virus is also sensitive to heat, ultraviolet light and gamma irradiation.

INFECTIONS IN ANIMALS

INCUBATION PERIOD

The incubation period in experimentally infected horses is 4 to 14 days. Experimentally infected pigs can develop clinical signs after 3 days (with rising temperature detected in some animals as early as 24 hours after inoculation).

CLINICAL SIGNS

Most infections in horses are subclinical, and symptomatic cases vary in severity. Some horses have a mild illness with nonspecific signs such as a transient fever, anorexia, lethargy, and congested or jaundiced mucous membranes. This syndrome usually lasts for 2-3 days, and the horse recovers without complications. Other horses develop encephalitis. In the milder form, the animal is lethargic and anorexic, with a fluctuating fever and neurological signs that commonly include difficulty swallowing, incoordination, transient neck rigidity, radial paralysis or impaired vision. Signs of jaundice or petechial hemorrhages may be found on the mucous membranes. These horses often recover within a week. A more severe but uncommon form, called the "hyperexcitable form," is characterized by high fever, aimless wandering, violent and demented behavior, profuse sweating, muscle tremors and occasionally blindness. Although some horses with this form recover, many collapse and die in 1-2 days. Neurologic defects such as ataxia may persist in some animals after recovery.

Naïve pigs may have reproductive signs. The most common syndrome in this species is the birth of stillborn or mummified fetuses, usually at term. Infected piglets born alive often have tremors and convulsions, and die soon after birth. Pregnant sows may also abort. Nonpregnant pigs usually remain asymptomatic or experience a transient febrile illness, but signs of encephalitis are occasionally seen in pigs up to six months of age. A wasting syndrome was reported in one group of piglets with post-mortem evidence of nonsuppurative meningoencephalitis. In addition, disturbances of spermatogenesis can cause infertility in boars. Although this is usually temporary, it can be permanent in severely affected animals.

Other domesticated animals can be infected but typically remain asymptomatic. Rare cases of Japanese encephalitis in cattle were characterized by neurological signs, sometimes preceded by nonspecific signs (e.g., fever, depression, decreased appetite). Some of these cases were fatal; other animals were euthanized. Three experimentally infected dogs did not develop clinical signs, and the authors of this study reported that no clinical cases have been seen among dogs in Japan, even during epidemics in other species.

POST MORTEM LESIONS

Only nonspecific lesions are seen in horses, and there are no characteristic gross lesions in the brain. Diffuse nonsuppurative encephalomyelitis is the characteristic microscopic lesion. Nonsuppurative encephalitis was also reported in the few cattle reported to have Japanese encephalitis, but the macroscopic lesions varied. One animal had no gross lesions in the brain, spinal cord or other organs. In two other cases, hemorrhages and/or congestion were found in the brain. Additional lesions with uncertain relevance to Japanese encephalitis were reported in some cases, and included pulmonary emphysema in two cattle.

Mummified or stillborn fetuses can be found in litters from infected sows. Congenital neurological defects including hydrocephalus, cerebellar hypoplasia and spinal hypomyelinogenesis may be seen in some litters. Experimentally infected piglets with encephalitis had swelling and edema of the brain.

DIAGNOSTIC TESTS

A definitive diagnosis of Japanese encephalitis can be made by virus isolation. Isolating JEV from infected horses can be difficult, even from tissues collected at necropsy; however, it may be attempted from brain samples (e.g., corpus striatum, cortex or thalamus) and the spinal cord. Tissue samples should be very fresh, i.e., taken from animals that have been dead for less than 12 hours, or from animals killed during the acute stage of the disease. It may also be possible to isolate this virus from the blood, serum or CSF of living horses, but viremia is usually short-lived and this is rarely successful. In swine, JEV may be isolated from the brains of affected fetuses or piglets with encephalitis. The sow has usually cleared the virus by the time an affected litter is born. Various cell lines are suitable for virus isolation; some culture systems that have been used include chicken embryo, baby hamster kidney (BHK) cells, African green monkey kidney (Vero) cells, the MDBK cell line and mosquito cell lines (e.g. C3/36). Mouse inoculation is also used during virus isolation. JEV can be recognized as a flavivirus by hemagglutination inhibition or enzyme-linked immunosorbent assays (ELISAs), and its identity can be confirmed by virus neutralization, reverse transcription polymerase chain reaction (RT-PCR) assays, or immunofluorescence to detect viral antigens.

JEV can also be detected directly in tissues or blood by RT-PCR; however, there is little published information on the use of this technique with clinical samples. Immunohistochemistry has been used to identify viral antigens in the central nervous system (CNS). Histopathology is also helpful.

Serology is often used to diagnose Japanese encephalitis in endemic regions. Serological diagnosis can be complicated by pre-existing antibodies from vaccination or previous exposure to JEV, or cross-reactive antibodies to other viruses in the Japanese encephalitis serogroup. Tests that may be available include virus neutralization (e.g., the plaque neutralization test), hemagglutination inhibition, ELISAs to detect IgM (IgM capture ELISA) or IgG, and less commonly used assays such as complement fixation. Virus neutralization is the most specific assay, and has low cross-reactivity, but its availability may be limited. In endemic regions, a definitive serological diagnosis usually depends on a significant rise in titer with paired acute and convalescent samples. Sows usually seroconvert before the onset of reproductive signs, and rising titers may not be observed in these animals. A presumptive diagnosis may be made if a high titer is found in a single serum sample and supportive evidence suggests Japanese encephalitis. In horses, the detection of specific IgM and IgG in cerebrospinal fluid (CSF) is also good evidence of infection.

TREATMENT

There is no specific antiviral therapy for Japanese encephalitis. Affected animals are treated symptomatically. Infected animals may be euthanized in regions where this disease is not endemic.

CONTROL

Disease reporting

Veterinarians who encounter or suspect a Japanese virus infection should follow their national and/or local guidelines for disease reporting. In the U.S., state or federal authorities must be notified immediately.

Prevention

Japanese encephalitis vaccines can prevent disease in horses and pigs in endemic areas. Sows are widely vaccinated for Japanese encephalitis in some countries, but not in others. Maternal antibodies may interfere with vaccination during the short lifespan of young pigs. Although vaccines are cross-protective between genotypes, some reports suggest their relative efficacy might differ. Past vaccines generally contained genotype III viruses, but new genotype I vaccines are being developed in some areas where these viruses have become common, and may soon be commercially available. Various measures to reduce contact with mosquitoes, such as stabling animals in screened barns during peak mosquito biting activity, can be partially protective, particularly during outbreaks. Insecticide-treated mosquito nets have sometimes been used to help protect pigs. Environmental control of mosquitoes may temporarily help control these vectors during an outbreak, but large-scale use of insecticides is costly, difficult to implement well long-term, may have adverse effects on the environment, and is impractical in many areas.

Some control measures in swine are intended to help reduce the risk to other species. For example, pigs are sometimes relocated away from human population centers. Because JEV is also maintained in birds, some transmission can be expected to continue even if virus amplification in pigs can be controlled.

MORBIDITY AND MORTALITY

Japanese encephalitis may be a seasonal disease in endemic areas, depending on factors such as climate and rainfall patterns. In temperate regions, it may peak among horses in late summer and autumn when the virus spills over after being amplified in pigs and other animals. JEV circulates year-round in tropical areas, but there may be seasonal peaks of disease associated with irrigation, rainfall or other factors that affect the local abundance of mosquitoes and vertebrate amplifying hosts. In some areas, epidemics are associated with the rainy season.

In horses, cases usually occur sporadically or in small clusters, but epidemics may be seen when there are large numbers of susceptible animals. Inapparent infections are common in this species. Between 1948 and 1967, the morbidity rate in Asia was estimated to be approximately 0.045% (45 cases per 100,000 horses), but higher morbidity rates were reported during some outbreaks. During the 1948 epizootic in Japan, the morbidity rate in horses was 0.3% overall, and as high as 1.4% in some areas. The case fatality rate in horses is reported to be approximately 5% or less in some areas, and 5-15% in others. Case fatality rates as high as 30-40% have been reported in some outbreaks. For example, when one group of susceptible broodmares was introduced to an endemic area, a third of the mares died. Vaccination has reduced the incidence of clinical cases among horses in endemic regions.

Naïve pigs are reported to be highly susceptible to infection, with pregnant sows often aborting or giving birth to stillborn and mummified fetuses. During one epidemic in Japan, 50-70% of all pigs suffered reproductive losses. Affected piglets born alive often die; however, the mortality rate is close to zero in adult pigs. Japanese encephalitis may have much less impact on pigs in endemic regions, where they can develop immunity by the time they are bred. In one recent study, the only effects on reproductive performance occurred in young sows (i.e., animals < 1.5 years of age), and there was no impact when sows of all ages were analyzed. The number of swine in a region may affect the incidence of disease in other species, due to virus amplification in these animals. However, this varies with the type of husbandry practices, and modern pig farming does not necessarily increase the risk of infection. Where Japanese encephalitis is seasonal, serological surveillance in pigs can be used to help predict epidemics in humans. Some researchers have also suggested using serology in dogs, which are infected asymptomatically, to help predict human risk.

INFECTIONS IN HUMANS

INCUBATION PERIOD

The incubation period in humans is estimated to be 5 to 15 days.

CLINICAL SIGNS

The initial signs of Japanese encephalitis are usually nonspecific; they may include fever, chills, muscle aches and severe headache with vomiting. Children may appear to have a gastrointestinal illness, with nausea, vomiting and abdominal pain. Coryza and diarrhea are also mentioned by some authors. Some people recover after this stage, but others develop neurological signs. Signs suggestive of benign aseptic meningitis occur in a minority of the latter group, but most patients with neurological signs have encephalitis. Signs of encephalitis may develop gradually after the initial, nonspecific illness, or as a sudden onset of fever and convulsions. They may include a reduced level of consciousness, which can progress to coma; focal neurological signs; quadriplegia, hemiplegia or cerebellar disorders; and behavioral changes. Painful stiffness of the neck, and mild to severe convulsions, ranging from subtle focal signs to generalized seizures, are common. Movement disorders also occur frequently, and some people develop transient Parkinson's like signs (e.g., masking of the face, paucity of blinking, rigidity with or without tremor, akinesia). Various atypical presentations have been reported, and include isolated acute onset behavioral abnormalities that may be misdiagnosed as psychiatric illnesses. Occasionally patients can develop flaccid paralysis resembling polio; some of these patients may not have signs of encephalitis. Some case series also describe syndromes in other organs, such as pulmonary edema and upper gastrointestinal hemorrhage.

Convalescence can be prolonged, although some patients make a rapid, spontaneous recovery ("abortive encephalitis"). Up to 50% of the survivors have neurological sequelae such as epileptic seizures, a Parkinsonian syndrome with tremors and rigidity, or cognitive, behavioral or language impairment. Some survivors gradually improve, although this can take months or years. Miscarriages have been seen in pregnant women who were infected for the first time during pregnancy; however, this is reported to be uncommon in endemic areas.

DIAGNOSTIC TESTS

Serology is often used to diagnose Japanese encephalitis in endemic areas, typically by detecting IgM in acute phase serum and CSF with an ELISA. Some studies have reported that a few patients were seronegative in serum, CSF or both. Asymptomatic infections or vaccination usually result in the presence of IgM in the serum but not CSF. Cross-reactivity with other flaviviruses is an issue in some serological assays such as ELISAs and hemagglutination inhibition. Virus neutralization tests can also be used, and a fourfold rise in neutralizing antibody titer is diagnostic in retrospective cases.

Viremia in humans is usually transient and low level, and direct detection of viruses in the blood by virus isolation and/ or RT-PCR is reported to be difficult. RT-PCR may also detect viral RNA in the CSF; however, this method does not appear to be commonly employed.

Neuroimaging and electroencephalographic analysis can also be helpful, although they are not definitive.

TREATMENT

Treatment is supportive. There are currently no specific antiviral therapies for this disease.

CONTROL

Several vaccines are available for humans. Japanese encephalitis vaccines are cross-protective against all genotypes; however, there are reports that immunity against genotypes other than the vaccine strain may be weaker. Childhood vaccination is routine in some countries. With a relative increase in adult cases, some areas are also considering or conducting vaccination campaigns in adults. In non-endemic areas, vaccines are primarily given to laboratory workers at risk of infection and travelers to endemic region. Recommendations for the latter group vary, depending on factors such as the season, duration of travel, activities and lodging.

Other temporary preventive measures include the use of insect repellents, insecticide-impregnated bed nets, and long-sleeved shirts and pants to discourage mosquito bites. Environmental modifications to decrease mosquito populations (e.g., intermittent irrigation of rice fields, larvivorous fish, insecticide spraying) may be used in some areas or situations. Approaches to reduce amplification in pigs, as described above (Infections in Animals), have also been suggested or implemented.

MORBIDITY AND MORTALITY

Japanese encephalitis is an important cause of illness, death and disability in parts of Asia. Vaccination, changes in agricultural practices, improved standards of living and other factors have greatly reduced the incidence of this disease in some countries; however, it continues to be widespread in others. More than 27,000 cases were reported to the World Health Organization (WHO) between 2006 and 2009, and one recent analysis estimated the true worldwide incidence to be approximately 68,000 cases per year. As in animals, the patterns of disease in endemic regions vary with factors such as climate and rainfall. Human illnesses, like those in horses, may peak in late summer and autumn in some temperate regions, but can occur year-round in the tropics, with seasonal peaks caused by local factors such as rainfall.

The risk of developing encephalitis is affected by many factors including the person's age and immunity to flaviviruses. All ages can be affected in a population without previous exposure; however, clinical cases mainly occur in children (< 15 years) in endemic regions, where people usually develop immunity by the time they reach adulthood. An increasing proportion of cases have been reported in adults in some areas where children are vaccinated. The risk of infection also tends to be higher in rural areas than cities. Most human infections are asymptomatic: studies from endemic regions estimate that approximately one in every 100 to 1,000 infected people develops clinical signs. During some outbreaks (e.g., in people from nonendemic regions), this ratio can be as high as 1 in 25. The risk to all travelers visiting endemic regions has been estimated to be < 1 case per 1 million; however, the specific risk varies with the season, duration of travel, activities and lodgings. While most cases occur in people who visit an endemic area for a longer time, clinical cases have also occurred in short-term travelers.

In symptomatic cases, reported case fatality rates range from < 5% to 40% and occasionally higher. Some countries have reported that case fatality rates as well as morbidity rates have decreased significantly in recent years, possibly due to partial immunity from an incomplete vaccination series, better care and/or other factors. Up to 30-50% of survivors have mild to severe neurological sequelae. Some of these people gradually improve, although this can take months or years.

MAEDI-VISNA & CAPRINE ARTHRITIS AND ENCEPHALITIS

Ovine Progressive Pneumonia, Marsh's Progressive Pneumonia, Montana Progressive Pneumonia, Chronic Progressive Pneumonia, Zwoegersiekte, La Bouhite, Graff-Reinet Disease

IMPORTANCE

Maedi-visna and caprine arthritis and encephalitis are economically important viral diseases that affect sheep and goats. These diseases are caused by a group of lentiviruses called the small ruminant lentiviruses (SRLVs). SRLVs include maedi-visna virus (MVV), which mainly occurs in sheep, and caprine arthritis encephalitis virus (CAEV), mainly found in goats, as well as other SRLV variants and recombinant viruses. The causative viruses infect their hosts for life, most often subclinically; however, some animals develop one of several progressive, untreatable disease syndromes. The major syndromes in sheep are dyspnea (maedi) or neurological signs (visna), which are both eventually fatal. Adult goats generally develop chronic progressive arthritis, while encephalomyelitis is seen in kids. Other syndromes (e.g., outbreaks of arthritis in sheep) are also reported occasionally, and mastitis occurs in both species. Additional economic losses may occur due to marketing and export restrictions, premature culling and/or poor milk production. Economic losses can vary considerably between flocks.

ETIOLOGY

Small ruminant lentiviruses (SRLVs) belong to the genus *Lentivirus* in the family Retroviridae (subfamily Orthoretrovirinae). Two of these viruses have been known for many years: maedi-visna virus (MVV), which mainly causes the diseases maedi and visna in sheep, and caprine arthritis encephalitis virus (CAEV), which primarily causes arthritis and encephalitis in goats. (Note: In North America, maedi-visna and its causative virus have traditionally been called ovine progressive pneumonia and ovine progressive pneumonia virus.) A number of SRLV variants have been recognized in recent decades. As a result, this group of viruses is now classified into five genotypes, A to E. Genotype A is a heterogeneous group, divided into subtypes A1 to A13. It contains the 'classical' maedi-visna viruses and other SRLV variants, including some that infect both sheep and goats. Genotype B (subtypes B1 to B3) contains the classical CAEV strains. The other 3 genotypes, all found in Europe, are less common. Genotype C affects both sheep and goats, while genotypes D and E are divergent goat strains. Recombination can occur between different SRLVs, creating new variants.

SPECIES AFFECTED

SRLVs cause disease in sheep and goats. Classical strains of MVV mainly occur in sheep, but some other genotype A variants infect both species. Genotype C viruses also affect both sheep and goats, while classical CAEV isolates (genotype B), and genotypes D and E mainly occur in goats. The host specificity of SRLVs is not absolute: viruses transmitted from sheep to goats (or vice versa) sometimes adapt to and persist in the new species.

Wild relatives of small ruminants can be infected by SRLVs from domesticated animals. One virus, thought to be CAEV, caused disease in several captive Rocky Mountain goats (*Oreamnos americanus*) that had been fed goat milk as kids, and in another Rocky Mountain goat housed with this group. Mouflon *(Ovis gmelinii)* can be infected experimentally with SRLVs, and genotype B viruses have been detected in wild ibex (*Capra ibex*) in contact with goats. Serological evidence of SRLV infections has also been reported in some species including mouflon, ibex and chamois (*Rupicapra rupicapra*). Preliminary evidence suggests that some viruses in wild ruminants may be distinct from CAEV and MVV.

Other animals are not thought to be hosts for SRLVs. Newborn calves could be infected experimentally with CAEV; however, the infection was asymptomatic and the virus apparently disappeared after 4 months.

Zoonotic potential

There is no evidence that humans are susceptible to any SRLVs.

GEOGRAPHIC DISTRIBUTION

SRLV genotypes A and B, which contain the classical MVV and CAEV isolates, respectively, are widely distributed. MVV has been found in most sheep-raising countries other than Iceland, where it was introduced but eradicated, and Australia and New Zealand. CAEV has been detected in most industrialized countries. Genotypes C (Norway), D (Spain and Switzerland) and E (Italy) appear to be limited to small geographic areas in Europe, at present.

TRANSMISSION

MVV and CAEV can be transmitted to lambs, kids or other susceptible species in milk or colostrum. Lactogenic transmission was once thought to be the major route by which SRLVs spread, based on the ability to prevent most infections by removing lambs or kids from their dams at birth. However, this idea has been challenged by some recent studies, and the predominant route is currently unclear. It might differ with the host species, virus and/or management situation. In addition to milk, SRLVs have been found in respiratory secretions and feces, and infections have been demonstrated by intranasal or intraconjunctival inoculation, and via fecally-contaminated water. Most respiratory transmission is thought to occur during close contact; transmission of SRLVs beyond a few meters appears to be inefficient or absent. Coinfection with pulmonary adenomatosis (Jaagsiekte) virus increases contact transmission of MVV between sheep. Feed and water troughs, or the aerosolization of infectious milk in dairies might be additional sources of virus. Iatrogenic spread through the reuse of needles or other objects that contact blood and tissues (e.g., tail docking equipment) also seems possible. While SRLVs may be spread on fomites, they cannot survive for more than a few days in the environment, particularly under hot, dry conditions.

SRLVs can be found in semen and the female reproductive tract (e.g., uterus) of both sheep and goats, but they do not appear to directly infect oocytes or sperm. Shedding in semen can be intermittent. Sexual transmission is at least theoretically possible, but it does not seem to be common. Intrauterine infection of the fetus by SRLVs is also thought to be negligible or minor, although one study found evidence for MVV infections in 6% of lambs born by caesarean section. Despite the presence of virus in the reproductive tract, it is possible to harvest uninfected ova or early embryos from dams that are either infected or received contaminated semen, as well as to produce uninfected sheep or goat embryos from infected sires or dams by *in vitro* fertilization if certain precautions are taken.

Once an animal becomes infected, SRLVs are integrated into leukocyte DNA, and the animal carries the virus for life. Viral burdens vary between individual animals; however, both asymptomatic and symptomatic animals can transmit SRLVs.

DISINFECTION

Lentiviruses can be destroyed with most common disinfectants including lipid solvents, periodate, phenolic disinfectants, formaldehyde and low pH (pH < 4.2). Phenolic or quaternary ammonium compounds have been recommended for the disinfection of equipment shared between seropositive and seronegative herds.

INCUBATION PERIOD

The incubation period for SRLV-associated diseases is highly variable, and usually lasts for months to years. Sheep typically develop the clinical signs of maedi when they are at least 3-4 years of age. Visna seems to appear somewhat sooner, with clinical signs in some sheep as young as 2 years. Significant numbers of animals even younger than this were reported during recent outbreaks in Spain, where neurological signs mainly occurred in 1-2 year old sheep, and some cases were seen in lambs as young as 4-6 months.

CAEV-associated encephalitis usually occurs in kids 2 to 6 months of age, although it has also been reported in younger and older animals. Polyarthritis is generally seen in adult goats, although some cases have been reported in animals as young as 6 months.

CLINICAL SIGNS

Most SRLV infections in sheep and goats, including infections with classical MVV and CAEV, are asymptomatic. In animals with clinical signs, the disease can take several forms.

Maedi in sheep

Maedi is the most common form of disease in sheep infected with MVV, and usually occurs in adults. It is characterized by wasting and progressive dyspnea. Fever, bronchial exudates and depression are not usually seen. Maedi is eventually fatal; death results from anoxia or secondary bacterial pneumonia. Genotype C viruses can also cause lung lesions (chronic interstitial pneumonia) in sheep.

Visna in sheep

Visna also occurs in adult sheep. This syndrome was described during outbreaks among MVV-infected sheep in Iceland in the 1950s, but it has been reported only sporadically that time. However, it has been relatively common in a recent focus of infection among sheep and goats in northwestern Spain. Visna usually begins insidiously, with subtle neurological signs such as hindlimb weakness, trembling of the lips or a head tilt, accompanied by loss of condition. The clinical signs gradually progress to ataxia, incoordination, muscle tremors, paresis and paraplegia, usually more prominent in the hindlegs. Other neurological signs, including rare instance of blindness, may also be seen. The clinical course can be as long as a year. Unattended animals usually die of inanition.

Arthritis in sheep

MVV can occasionally cause slowly progressive arthritis with severe lameness in sheep, but this is uncommon. One genotype B virus (CAEV) caused an outbreak characterized by enlargement almost exclusively of the carpal joint. Pain and lameness occurred in a minority of the affected sheep. No respiratory signs were noted in this outbreak, although some animals had evidence of interstitial pneumonia at necropsy.

Encephalomyelitis in goats

Encephalomyelitis (progressive paresis) is sometimes seen in goats infected with CAEV. Most cases occur in 2-6 month-old kids, although this syndrome has occasionally been reported in younger or older animals. The initial clinical signs may include lameness, ataxia, hindlimb placement deficits, hypertonia and hyperreflexia. Initially, many kids are bright and alert, and continue to eat and drink normally. The signs gradually worsen to paraparesis, tetraparesis or paralysis. Some affected kids may also appear depressed or exhibit other neurological signs (e.g., head tilt, circling, blindness, torticollis, facial nerve deficits, dysphagia). Variable increases in body temperature have been reported. Affected kids are either euthanized for welfare/ economic reasons or eventually die of secondary causes such as pneumonia or exposure. Although it is rare, some goats have apparently recovered.

Neurological signs are uncommon in adult goats infected with CAEV. These cases are usually characterized initially by minor gait aberrations, lameness and knuckling, which progress to paralysis over weeks to months. The reflexes remain intact. Other signs (e.g., coarse tremors, nystagmus, trismus, salivation, blindness) are occasionally reported. Neurological signs may also be seen in goats infected with classical MVV.

Polyarthritis in goats

Chronic, painful polyarthritis, accompanied by synovitis and bursitis, is the main syndrome in adult goats infected with CAEV. This syndrome can occasionally occur in goats as young as 6 months. Early symptoms include distention of the joint capsule and a variable degree of lameness. The carpal joints are most often affected, but symptoms can also occur in other joints. Although the course of disease is slow, it is always progressive. In late stages, goats may walk with their front legs flexed or become recumbent. Affected animals also lose condition and tend to have coarse, dull coats.

Dyspnea in goats

Occasionally, goats with serological evidence of CAEV infection may develop chronic interstitial pneumonia and progressive dyspnea.

Mastitis in sheep and goats

SRLVs including MVV and CAEV can cause chronic indurative mastitis with a swollen, firm mammary gland and decreased production of normal-appearing milk. In severe cases, goats may produce no milk at parturition. The mammary gland may later soften and milk production may approach normal; milk yield remains low in other animals. There are some reports of decreased milk quality in sheep and goats due to reduced fat content. Sheep infected with genotype C viruses were also reported to have mastitis.

Other effects in sheep and goats

Some studies, but not others, have reported decreased fertility in SRLV-infected animals and lower birth weights in their offspring. Weight gain may be decreased in young animals, possibly due to lower milk yields from dams with indurative mastitis.

Infections in wild or captive wild species

Descriptions of clinical signs due to SRLVs are uncommon in wild species. Captive Rocky Mountain goats infected with CAEV developed signs of chronic pneumonia and wasting, with neurological signs and /or joint lesions in some animals.

POST MORTEM LESIONS

Maedi

In sheep with maedi, the lungs are enlarged, abnormally firm and heavy, and fail to collapse when the thoracic cavity is opened. They are typically emphysematous and mottled or uniformly discolored, with pale gray or pale brown areas of consolidation. Mottling may not be obvious in the earliest stages of the disease. Nodules may be found around the smaller airways and blood vessels, and the mediastinal and tracheobronchial lymph nodes are usually enlarged and edematous. Secondary bacterial pneumonia may mask the primary lesions.

Neurological forms

Apart from wasting of the carcass, the gross lesions of visna or the encephalitic form of caprine arthritis and encephalitis are usually limited to the brain and spinal cord. In severe cases, there may be focal, asymmetric, brownish pink areas in the white matter of the brain and spinal cord, as well as on the ventricular surfaces. The meninges may be cloudy and the spinal cord may be swollen. Only microscopic CNS lesions are apparent in some cases of neurological disease.

Arthritis

In goats with polyarthritis due to CAEV, the joint capsule is thickened, with proliferation of the synovial villi. The lesions mainly affect the carpal joints, and to a lesser extent the tarsal joints. The joint capsules, tendon sheaths and bursae may be calcified. In severe cases, there may be severe cartilage destruction, ruptured ligaments and tendons, and periarticular osteophyte formation. Goats with caprine arthritis and encephalitis may also have interstitial pneumonitis.

Similar but milder joint lesions, mainly limited to the carpal joints, were reported in an arthritis outbreak among sheep infected with one genotype B (CAEV) virus.

Mastitis

In animals with indurative mastitis, the udder is diffusely indurated and the associated lymph nodes may be enlarged.

DIAGNOSTIC TESTS

Diseases caused by SRLVs can be diagnosed by both virological and serological methods; however, all of the currently available tests have limitations. Some authors have suggested using at least 2 different tests for confirmation. Other sources suggest the combination of a diagnostic test (e.g., serology) and clinical signs, with histological examination of tissues when necessary.

Antibodies to SRLVs are usually diagnosed by various enzyme-linked immunosorbent assays (ELISAs) or agar gel immunodiffusion (AGID) tests, using either serum samples or milk. ELISAs have replaced AGID in many laboratories. A number of serological tests, based on different viruses, are available, and the test used should match the variants circulating in the region. Assays vary in their sensitivity and cross-reactivity for other genotypes, and can miss some viruses. Preliminary evidence from one study suggested that tests might also have different sensitivity in sheep and goats. Confirmatory tests may include immunoblotting (Western blotting) and radio-immunoprecipitation; however, these tests are not available in all laboratories. Animals generally seroconvert months after infection, at an unpredictable interval, and antibody titers can fluctuate and/or become intermittently negative in some animals. An additional complication is the existence of many subclinically infected animals, whose clinical signs may due to some other cause. Due to these limitations, serology may be of greater value in screening flocks than diagnosing clinical cases in individual animals.

Polymerase chain reaction (PCR) assays or virus isolation can also be used for diagnosis. These tests may be particularly useful before the animal seroconverts. SRLVs are usually cell-associated; free virus is rarely found in plasma or other fluids. In living animals, viruses can be detected in leukocytes in blood or milk, and possibly in joint fluid in animals with arthritis. Viral titers are variable and may fluctuate over time. At necropsy, SRLVs can be found in affected tissues, such as lung, mediastinal lymph node and spleen (maedi); brain and spinal cord (visna); choroid plexus, udder or synovial membrane. SRLVs can also be detected in alveolar macrophages collected by post-mortem bronchoalveolar lavage at necropsy. Limitations of diagnosis by PCR include the genetic variability between SRLVs (tests based on one set of primers may miss other viruses), and the low virus load. PCR can be confirmed by other

M

genetic techniques such as nucleic acid sequencing to rule out false positives from the host's own genome. Southern blotting or *in situ* hybridization may be performed in some cases, although these tests are not used routinely. SRLVs are isolated by co-culturing peripheral blood or milk leukocytes from live animals, or fresh tissues collected at necropsy, with sheep choroid plexus cells (MVV), sheep skin fibroblasts (MVV), goat synovial membrane cells (CAEV) or other appropriate cell lines. Virus isolation is not performed routinely and is not always successful.

Histology of affected tissues, using biopsy or necropsy samples, can help confirm the diagnosis in symptomatic animals.

TREATMENT

There is no specific treatment for diseases caused by SRLVs. Supportive therapy may be helpful in individual animals, but it cannot stop the progression of disease. Measures that may make animals with arthritis more comfortable include regular foot trimming, the provision of additional bedding material, and the administration of NSAIDs. Antibiotics may be used for secondary bacterial infections in cases of mastitis or pneumonitis. High-quality, readily digestible feed may delay wasting.

CONTROL

Disease reporting

Reporting requirements for SRLVs differ between countries, as well as between states, depending on the presence of official control programs for MVV and/or CAEV, and other factors. Veterinarians who encounter or suspect a reportable disease should follow their national and/or local guidelines for informing the proper authorities. In the U.S, state reporting guidelines should be consulted for caprine arthritis and encephalitis, or maedi-visna (ovine progressive pneumonia).

Prevention

MVV and CAEV are often introduced into a herd in live animals. Additions to uninfected herds should come from SRLV-negative herds. Other animals should be quarantined and tested before adding them to the herd (however, it is possible for tests to miss some viruses). Uninfected herds should also be kept from contact with untested or seropositive herds. Mixing sheep and goats, or feeding milk or colostrum from one species to another, can lead to the transfer of viruses between species. There are currently no vaccines for SRLVs.

If a herd has been infected, several methods can reduce the prevalence of infection or eliminate the virus from the herd. Once the prevalence of infection is low, clinical signs may not be seen. One approach is to completely depopulate the herd and replace it with uninfected animals. Another is to separate lambs or kids permanently from seropositive dams immediately at birth, and raise these animals on uninfected colostrum and pasteurized milk, milk replacer or milk from uninfected animals. The herd should be tested frequently for SRLVs, and seronegative and seropositive animals should be maintained separately. Any shared equipment should be disinfected before use with seronegative animals. Seropositive sheep and goats should eventually be culled. Other control methods (e.g., selective culling of seropositive animals, or early culling of seropositive animals with clinical signs) may also be helpful in reducing disease prevalence in an infected herd. In nationwide eradication programs, quarantines of infected herds aid the final stages of the program.

The discovery of genes associated with increased susceptibility to SRLVs may make it possible to produce disease-resistant flocks by selective breeding. Some authors caution that there may be difficulties due to the heterogeneity and high mutation rates of SRLVs, as well as the possibility that resistance is a polygenic trait. One newer approach to reduce or eradicate MVV from a herd is based on mating ewes to rams carrying genes for resistance, raising the lambs naturally until 7 months of age or older, and removing seronegative lambs to a separate flock at this time (see Leymaster et al, 2015 for details).

MORBIDITY AND MORTALITY

SRLVs are widely distributed among sheep and goats; however, the prevalence of infection in endemic regions can vary widely, ranging from < 5% to more than 60%. Infections tend to be more common in intensively raised herds or flocks, and in animals housed indoors. CAEV is common among dairy goats in most industrialized countries, and uncommon in meat- or fiber-producing goats. The reason for this disparity is unknown, but possible causes include genetic factors or management practices. CAEV is rarely found in the indigenous breeds of developing nations unless they have had contact with imported goats. Genotype C viruses are most common in goats, although they also regularly infect sheep. Control programs have significantly reduced the incidence of MVV and/or CAEV in some countries (e.g., from 60-80% to 1% among goats infected with CAEV genotype B in Switzerland).

Most MVV and CAEV infections are asymptomatic, and clinical signs are usually not seen in herds with a low prevalence of infection, When MVV is introduced into a new area (e.g., in Iceland in the 1950s), the morbidity and mortality rate may reach 20-30%. Morbidity and mortality have also been high in a recent focus of SRLV-associated neurological disease in sheep and goats in parts of Spain. The mortality rate is usually low in regions where classical MVV is endemic; annual losses rarely exceed 5% in a flock, even when nearly 100% of the flock is infected. Co-infection with Jaagsiekte virus, the retrovirus that that causes ovine pulmonary adenocarcinoma, results in more severe symptoms. Once clinical signs appear, diseases caused by SRLVs are progressive. While regression of MVV lesions has been documented under some experimental conditions, this is considered unusual. Dyspnea or neurological syndromes are usually fatal, and most animals with arthritis are eventually culled for welfare and/or economic reasons, or die from secondary causes. Milk production is estimated to decrease by 10% in herds of goats affected by CAEV.

Genetic factors, including breed, influence the outcome of infection in sheep; some breeds (e.g., Texel, Border Leicester, and Finnish Landrace) seem more likely to become ill, while others (e.g., Columbia, Rambouillet, and Suffolk) are more likely to remain subclinically infected. Genes associated with increased susceptibility to disease have also been identified in sheep. Some SRLV isolates also appear to be less virulent than others.

MALIGNANT CATARRHAL FEVER

Malignant Catarrh, Malignant Head Catarrh, Gangrenous Coryza, Catarrhal Fever, Snotsiekte

IMPORTANCE

Malignant catarrhal fever (MCF) is a serious, often fatal, disease that affects many species in the order Artiodactyla (even-toed ungulates) including cattle, bison, deer, moose, exotic ruminants and pigs. At least ten MCF viruses have been recognized, including two well-known viruses carried by sheep and wildebeest. Six of these viruses have been linked to disease, while the others have been found, to date, only in asymptomatic carriers. Each MCF virus is highly adapted to its usual host, and does not normally cause disease in that species, but can cause fatal infections if transmitted to susceptible animals.

Malignant catarrhal fever occurs in many countries worldwide. Sheep-associated MCF is the predominant form outside Africa. It is a particular problem in species such as farmed bison, deer and Bali cattle, although it occasionally affects relatively resistant hosts such as pigs and European breeds of cattle. Wildebeest associated MCF is an important disease among cattle in Africa, while zoos can be affected by either of these two forms, as well as by less common MCF viruses carried in various exotic ruminants. Malignant catarrhal fever is difficult to control, as the infections are widespread and asymptomatic in the reservoir species, and the incubation period can be long in susceptible animals. The only reliable methods of control are to separate susceptible species from carriers or breed virus-free reservoir hosts.

ETIOLOGY

Malignant catarrhal fever is caused by viruses in the genus *Macavirus* of the family Herpesviridae (subfamily Gammaherpesvirinae). There are two major groups of MCF viruses. The Alcelaphinae/Hippotraginae group contains alcelaphine herpesvirus 1 (AlHV-1), AlHV-2, hippotragine herpesvirus 1 (HiHV-1) and a virus carried in oryx (MCFV-oryx). The Caprinae group includes ovine herpesvirus 2 (OvHV-2), caprine herpesvirus 2 (CpHV-2), MCF virus-white tailed deer (MCFV-WTD), and the viruses carried by asymptomatic ibex (MCFV-ibex), muskox (MCFV-muskox) and aoudad (MCFV-aoudad). Most MCF viruses are named after their reservoir hosts; however, MCFV-WTD was found in sick white-tailed deer, and its carrier is unknown.

The two most important viruses are OvHV-2, which causes sheep-associated MCF, and AlHV-1, which causes the wildebeest-associated form of this disease. CpHV-2, MCFV-WTD, MCFV-ibex and AlHV-2 are also known to be pathogenic. No illness has been associated yet with MCFV-muskox, MCFV-oryx or MCFV-aoudad, which are carried in muskox (*Ovibos moschatus*), gemsbok/ South African oryx (*Oryx gazella*), and aoudads (*Ammotragus lervia*), respectively. Nevertheless, it is likely that these viruses can also cause MCF in some species of animals. HiHV-1, which was found in asymptomatic roan antelope (*Hippotragus equinus*), appears to be very similar or identical to MCFV-oryx.

SPECIES AFFECTED

MCF viruses are usually carried asymptomatically by their reservoir hosts, but can cause disease in other species. Wildebeest (*Connochaetes* spp.) are the carriers for AlHV-1. The blue wildebeest (*Connochaetes taurinus*) is the major reservoir host, but black wildebeest (*Connochaetes gnou*) are also carriers. All or most wildebeest appear to be infected by this virus. Domesticated sheep (*Ovis aries*) are the reservoir hosts for OvHV-2, and most individuals are infected. At least some species of wild sheep, such as Dall's sheep (*Ovis dalli*) and mouflon (*Ovis musimon*) are also carriers. Goats are the carriers for CpHV-2. Most goats are thought to be infected with this virus, based on high seroprevalence to MCF viruses; however, goats can also be infected asymptomatically with OvHV2, and serological tests cannot distinguish these two organisms. Alcelaphine herpesvirus-2 (AlHV-2) is carried subclinically in hartebeest (*Alcelaphus buselaphus*) and topi (*Damaliscus korrigum*). Nubian ibex (*Capra nubiana*) are known to be reservoir hosts for MCFV-ibex. The reservoir host for MCFV-WTD is uncertain, but goats may carry this virus.

MCF viruses cause illness in various members of the order Artiodactyla. Most susceptible animals belong to the subfamily Bovinae (e.g. cattle, bison, water buffalo, and exotic ruminants such as antelope, guar and banteng) and family Cervidae (e.g. deer, reindeer, moose), but other species such as giraffes (family Giraffidae) and pigs (family Suidae) are also affected.

M

A species can be susceptible to one MCF virus, but relatively resistant to others.

Most ruminants other than antelope of the subfamilies Alcelaphinae and Hippotraginae should be considered susceptible to AlHV-1. Significant numbers of cattle become ill if they are exposed to this virus.

European breeds of cattle (*Bos taurus* and *Bos indicus*) tend not to become sick when they are exposed to OvHV-2. When cases do occur, they often affect only a single animal. Water buffalo (*Bubalus bubalis*) and some species of deer are more susceptible to this virus than cattle, and American bison (*Bison bison*), Père David's deer (*Elaphurus davidianus*), white-tailed deer (*Odocoileus virginianus*), axis deer (*Axis axis*) and Bali cattle (*Bos javanicus*) are highly susceptible. OvHV-2 can also affect pigs, giraffes and exotic ruminants. OvHV-2 infections were recently reported in horses (order Perissodactyla) on a farm where these animals shared their feed with goats.

CpHV-2 associated disease has been seen in cervids including moose (*Alces alces)*, roe deer (*Capreolus capreolus*), sika deer (*Cervus nippon*), white-tailed deer and pronghorn antelope (*Antilocapra americana*), as well as in water buffalo.

Other MCF viruses have been linked only rarely to clinical cases. MCFV-WTD was found in sick white-tailed deer. The ibex-associated MCF virus has caused disease in several bongo antelope (*Tragelaphus euryceros*) and an anoa, and a virus resembling AlHV-2- was found in sick Barbary red deer (*Cervus elaphus barbarus*).

Although most cases of MCF have been reported in domesticated or captive animals, there are also reports of illness in wild animals such as moose and deer. A variety of ungulates, hamsters and rabbits can be infected experimentally with OvHV-2 and AlHV-1. In unusual cases, MCF viruses might be able to cause disease in their normal hosts. MCF-like disease was reported in domesticated sheep that were infected experimentally with high doses of OvHV-2. Rare clinical cases have been tentatively attributed to OvHV-2 in domesticated goats, and in Stone's sheep (*Ovis dalli stonei*) and Barbary sheep (*Ammotragus lervia*) at a zoo.

GEOGRAPHIC DISTRIBUTION

MCF viruses can be found worldwide, but illness occurs only where a carrier species can pass a virus to susceptible hosts. AlHV-1 associated disease is mainly seen in sub-Saharan Africa, in areas where wildebeest are present. This virus is reported to be the most important MCF virus in some parts of Africa, although OvHV-2 associated disease also occurs.

OvHV-2 is the major cause of MCF in domesticated animals outside Africa. Sheep-associated MCF is common among Bali cattle in Indonesia; however, cases in cattle are infrequent in countries where *Bos taurus* and *Bos indicus* are the predominant species. OvHV-2 is a serious concern in countries with bison and cervid farms, as these species

are very susceptible. Infections in pigs were, at one time, reported mainly from Norway, but sick pigs have now been found in other European countries and North America, and are likely to occur elsewhere.

OvHV-2 is reported to be the major cause of MCF among ruminants in zoos and wildlife parks. Several other MCF viruses, including AlHV-1, MCFV-ibex and other viruses carried in exotic species can also cause disease in these locations.

TRANSMISSION

MCF viruses, like other herpesviruses, establish lifelong, latent infections. In wildebeest, AlHV-1 occurs in both cell-free and cell-associated forms. These animals shed cell-free virus in nasal and ocular secretions for a short period after they become infected. After this time, the virus occurs mainly in the cell-associated form, which is transmitted only rarely to other animals. (However, cell-free virus can be isolated from the nasal secretions of some animals that are stressed or given corticosteroids.) AlHV-1 is spread mainly by wildebeest calves, which can become infected *in utero*, by direct contact with other wildebeest, or in aerosols during close contact. Virus shedding is most intense during the first 3-4 months of life, and most calves are thought to become infected from their cohorts. Contamination of pastures may also contribute to transmission. Neutralizing antibodies usually develop by approximately 3 months of age, and shedding declines after this time. After the age of six months, wildebeest shed little virus except when they are stressed or during parturition,

Most cases of wildebeest-associated MCF are seen when susceptible animals are exposed to parturient wildebeest or young calves. This usually occurs after close contact, but transmission has been reported when the animals were separated by at least 100 meters. Inhalation is thought to be the primary means of transmission for all MCF viruses, although ingestion might also be possible. Cell-associated AlHV-1 is very fragile, and infectivity disappears after 72 hours in the environment. Cell-free virus has been reported to survive for more than 13 days in humid environments. MCF viruses are inactivated quickly by sunlight.

Like AlHV-1, OvHV-2 seems to be excreted mainly in nasal and ocular secretions. The virus is shed intermittently for short periods, typically lasting less than 24 hours. While sheep of all ages may transmit OvHV-2, one study found that the highest virus levels and most frequent shedding occurred in 6-9 month old lambs. Most lambs in naturally infected flocks do not seem to become infected until they are at least two months of age. Circumstantial evidence (antibodies to MCF viruses in a survey of some gnotobiotic and specific pathogen- free sheep), and the identification of virus-infected cells in colostrum and milk, suggest that vertical transmission of OvHV-2 is possible. However, transmission by these routes seems to be uncommon. Viral DNA has also been reported in the semen of rams.

Cases of sheep-associated-MCF increase during the spring lambing season. Because there are no reports that sheep shed more virus during parturition, and shedding does not seem to be common in very young lambs, some authors suggest that this phenomenon might be caused by improved virus survival at cool temperatures, or seasonal variations in stock densities. Other sources suggest that the dynamics of infection might vary between flocks. As OvHV-2 has never been cultured, its survival in the environment is unknown. In general, enveloped viruses such as herpesviruses survive better under moist conditions.

Susceptible animals usually become infected with OvHV-2 when they are in close contact with sheep, but cases have been reported when sheep and cattle were separated by 70 meters. One outbreak in bison occurred in herds up to 5 km from a lamb feedlot.

CpHV-2 transmission in goats seems to resemble OvHV-2 transmission in sheep. In one infected goat herd, 94% of the goats became infected by the age of 10 months. In this herd, CpHV-2 DNA was first detected in goat kids at 3 months of age, approximately 50% had seroconverted by 7 months of age, and more than 80% by 9 months. There was no evidence of infection at birth, and no goats became infected if they were removed from the infected herd at one week of age. Adult goats also became infected readily when they were exposed to a CpHV-2 infected herd.

Ruminants that develop malignant catarrhal fever are usually dead end hosts. A few instances of animal-to-animal transmission have been suspected in cattle, pigs and OvHV-2 infected deer, although there is no definitive evidence that this is possible. In pigs, large amounts of OvHV-2 DNA have been found in the semen of asymptomatic boars and in the nasal mucosa and skin of sick animals. Case reports have also suggested that some non-reservoir hosts might be able to transmit MCF viruses to their offspring. One recent study suggested that horizontal transmission does not occur between bison.

Subclinical infections with OvHV-2 have been reported in some incidental hosts including cattle, bison, cervids and pigs. Recrudescence might be possible in these animals, although it seems to be uncommon even in animals that are stressed.

DISINFECTION

Many common disinfectants can inactivate MCF viruses. If heavy organic debris is present, the World Organization for Animal Health (OIE) recommends 3% sodium hypochlorite.

INCUBATION PERIOD

The incubation period varies with the virus, host and other factors, and is incompletely understood. Cattle became sick 11-34 days after inoculation with AlVH-1, and 11-73 days after the administration of blood from OvHV-2 infected, sick cattle. In bison exposed to sheep, the incubation period is often a month or more, with peak losses reported to occur 40-70 days after exposure. The incubation period was 2-6 weeks in pregnant bongos affected by ibex-associated MCF in a zoo, and 21 to 40 days in one-week-old piglets inoculated intranasally with OvHV-2.

Latent infections and recrudescence might also be possible. Epidemiological evidence suggests that some cattle may be infected subclinically for more than 20 months before developing disease. In one outbreak in subclinically infected bison, clinical cases tended to occur 3-14 days after the animals were stressed by handling.

CLINICAL SIGNS

Malignant catarrhal fever can present with a variety of clinical sign in different species, depending on their susceptibility to the virus. Subclinical infections are usual in the reservoir hosts. Asymptomatic infections have also been reported in some incidental hosts such as cattle, bison, deer and pigs.

Almost any organ can be affected in clinical cases, although the gastrointestinal tract, eye and central nervous systems are often involved in domesticated ruminants. Peracute disease, which tends to occur in highly susceptible species, progresses very rapidly, with few clinical signs before death. In some animals, death may be preceded by 12-24 hours of depression, weakness, diarrhea or dysentery. Clinical signs are more apparent in animals that survive longer, such as cattle, which may be ill for a week or more before dying. In addition to high fever and inappetence, cattle often have bilateral corneal opacity, beginning at the corneoscleral junction and progressing inward. Serous oculonasal discharge is common early; later, this discharge becomes mucopurulent. The muzzle and nares are usually encrusted, and dyspnea, open-mouthed breathing and salivation may be seen. The oral mucosa is often hyperemic, and may contain multifocal or diffuse areas of necrosis. Erosions may be found at the tips of the buccal papillae. The superficial lymph nodes are often markedly enlarged in cattle. The skin is sometimes erythematous or ulcerated, and hardened scabs may develop, particularly on the perineum, udder and teats. In some animals, the horn and hoof coverings may be loosened or sloughed. The joints may be swollen, and milk production often drops. Diarrhea, hemorrhagic gastroenteritis or hematuria may also be seen, although these signs are less common than in bison and deer. Occasionally, animals develop neurological signs, especially in the terminal stages. Although many or most animals die, chronic infection or recovery is possible. Persistent eye lesions may be seen in surviving cattle. Skin lesions have been reported in cattle without other clinical signs, and may resolve spontaneously.

The clinical signs are similar in other species, but often vary in some aspects. For example, corneal opacity is reported to be inconsistent in water buffalo with MCF, although mild to moderate conjunctivitis seems to be common. Bison often die rapidly, without developing purulent rhinitis or keratoconjunctivitis. Anorexia, depression, corneal opacity, lacrimation, mild serous nasal and ocular discharge, coughing, salivation, diarrhea and neurological signs may be seen in some cases, but in many bison herds, the symptoms are subtle. Hematuria and hemorrhagic enteritis are more common than in cattle, but lymphadenomegaly is usually minimal. In the last stage of the disease, bison often develop an edematous band at the corneoscleral junction; this lesion is difficult to recognize in live animals. Bison attempt to mask the clinical signs until they are near death. Inhalation pneumonia is common in the last stage of the disease, and some sick bison may be attacked by herdmates, resulting in trauma. Recumbent animals generally die within a few hours.

In deer, malignant catarrhal fever is often peracute, with death within a few days, and the characteristic signs may not be seen. In other outbreaks or in more resistant species, more typical MCF symptoms including depression, loss of condition, a rough hair coat, nasal discharge, corneal opacity, transient loose stools, hemorrhagic diarrhea and bloody urine have been reported, with some animals surviving for up to three weeks after the onset of disease. Unusually, skin lesions were the primary complaint in some deer infected with CpHV-2. In white-tailed deer infected with this virus, the major lesions were widespread alopecia; thickening, crusting, hyperkeratosis, and focal ulceration of the skin; weight loss; and impaired vision. The hoof walls were shed in some animals. Similarly, sika deer infected with CpHV-2 developed skin lesions including extensive alopecia, as well as weight loss and diarrhea. One sika deer had seizures but no other clinical signs before it was euthanized. Neurological signs including abnormal behavior, apathy and incoordination have been reported in wild moose and roe deer.

Most OvHV-2 infections reported in pigs have been acute or peracute, with high fever and dyspnea the most consistent signs. Subclinical infections and chronic cases lasting for several weeks have also been reported. In some but not all outbreaks, pigs developed crusting rhinitis or foul-smelling nasal discharge, erosions on the nasal and oral mucosa, corneal edema or uveitis. Other reported signs were hematuria, reproductive losses (abortions, stillbirths and smaller-than-normal litters) reddened foci on the skin and neurological signs. In some outbreaks, only pregnant animals were affected. One-week old, experimentally infected piglets developed fever, apathy, anorexia, adipsia, skin rashes and seizures, but there was no evidence of nasal or ocular discharge, corneal opacity or diarrhea. However, these piglets may have been euthanized before some clinical signs developed. Although OvHV-2 infections in pigs are often fatal, some pigs have recovered.

Sporadic cases have been documented in other species. Possible MCF was reported in an OvHV-2 infected alpaca with apathy, dehydration, anorexia and emaciation. In a zoo, 3 periparturient bongo antelope with MCF became acutely

inappetent and developed respiratory distress, dying within 24-72 hours. Illnesses attributed to possible MCF in Stone's sheep (Ovis dalli stonei) in a zoo were sudden death in one animal, and neurological signs including hind limb weakness, unusual aggression to humans and seizures in another. Three goats infected with OvHV-2-developed a fever and neurological signs, and one animal had diarrhea and bilateral corneal opacity. Unusually, PCR evidence of OvHV-2 infections was reported in a sick, 6-month-old foal and asymptomatic adult horses on a farm in Brazil. The foal had neurological signs and severe dyspnea, which progressed rapidly to death.

POST MORTEM LESIONS

Malignant catarrhal fever is characterized by inflammation and epithelial necrosis, with lymphoproliferation, infiltration of nonlymphoid tissues by lymphoid cells, and vasculitis.

The extent of the lesions varies with the severity and course of the disease. In cattle that die suddenly, there may be few abnormalities other than hemorrhagic enterocolitis. In less acute cases, the carcass may be dehydrated, emaciated or normal. Diffuse or focal bilateral corneal opacity is common, and corneal ulcers are sometimes present. The muzzle is often raw and encrusted with a serous, mucopurulent or purulent nasal discharge. Hyperemia, edema and small focal erosions or ulcers may be found on the nasal mucosa. Dermatitis and skin ulcers may be found in some animals. The lymph nodes are usually markedly enlarged in cattle, although the degree of involvement varies. On cut surface, they may be firm and white, hemorrhagic or necrotic. Petechiae or ecchymoses may be present on various serosal surfaces. Prominent raised white foci, 1-5 mm in diameter, may be seen in some tissues, particularly the kidney. These nodules are sometimes surrounded by a thin hemorrhagic zone. The gastrointestinal tract can contain erosions and hemorrhages; in severe cases, the intestinal contents may be hemorrhagic. However, lesions in the gastrointestinal tract may be difficult to identify, especially when the carcass is autolyzed. The upper respiratory tract often has catarrhal exudates and erosions, and a diphtheritic membrane may be present. Ecchymotic hemorrhages, hyperemia and edema are common in the mucosa of the urinary bladder. In more chronic cases, the small arteries in multiple organs can be very prominent and tortuous, with thickened walls.

Similar lesions have been reported in other species, but some species-specific differences have been noted. In bison, vasculitis tends to be milder than in cattle and the lymph nodes are less likely to be markedly swollen, but hemorrhagic cystitis and hemorrhagic colitis are more common. Bison that die with few clinical signs may have advanced lesions on necropsy. Unique features of MCF in 3 periparturient bongos included necrotizing cholangio-hepatitis and neutrophilic, necrotizing myocarditis, together with more characteristic lesions. Severe perirenal hemorrhage and multiple renal infarcts were seen in Stone's sheep thought to have MCF, together with petechial hemorrhages in multiple tissues, and serosanguineous to fibrinous effusion in some body cavities.

DIAGNOSTIC TESTS

Sick animals

Malignant catarrhal fever is often suspected based on microscopic lesions in tissues collected at necropsy. Because some MCF viruses cannot be isolated from infected animals, polymerase chain reaction (PCR) assays are often the method of choice for confirmation. Lymphoid tissues such as spleen and lymph node are optimal for this test, but other tissues can also be used. Most PCR tests detect AlHV-1 and/or OvHV-2, but some can also detect other MCF viruses. Epidemiological information (e.g., contact with sheep but not wildebeest) should guide the choice of PCR assay.

Infections with viruses in the Alcelaphinae/ Hippotraginae group, such as AlHV-1, can also be diagnosed by isolating this virus from the blood of live animals, or from the lymph nodes, spleen and other affected tissues at necropsy. AlHV-1 is inactivated quickly in dead animals, and samples should be taken as soon as possible. The most useful samples are collected immediately after euthanasia of a dying animal. The viability of the host cells must be maintained after sample collection, as the virus cannot be recovered from dead cells. AlHV-1 can be isolated in bovine thyroid cells or other susceptible cell lines, and can be identified by immunofluorescence or immunocytochemistry. OvHV-2 and CpHV-2 cannot be isolated in cell culture.

Serological tests for MCF viruses include virus neutralization (VN), immunoblotting, enzyme-linked immunosorbent assays (ELISAs) and immunofluorescence or immunoperoxidase tests. All of these assays are based on antigens from alcelaphine herpesviruses (mainly AlHV-1), which can be propagated in cell culture. While they also detect antibodies to other MCF viruses (e.g., OvHV-2 and CpHV-2), such tests cannot distinguish reactions to different viruses. Most of the serological tests can be used in sick animals; however, the VN test cannot be employed, as these animals do not usually develop neutralizing antibodies. Cross-reactions with other herpesviruses (e.g., bovine herpesvirus-4) are possible, especially in tests that use polyclonal antibodies. Most, but not all, sick cattle and bison are seropositive. Because healthy animals can also have antibodies to MCF viruses, serology should be used in conjunction with histopathology and clinical findings.

It is difficult to substantiate a diagnosis of MCF in the reservoir host for a virus. Critical components include histopathology and the elimination of other possible causes of the illness.

Reservoir hosts

PCR can be used to document the absence of infection in some reservoir hosts (for example, when producing OvHV-2 free sheep). Highly sensitive PCR assays should be employed. The peripheral blood leukocytes of most infected sheep contain sufficient OvHV-2 DNA to be detected by PCR, but this is not the case in infected oryx or black wildebeest. PCR was reported to be positive in 85% of goats with antibodies to CpHV-2.

Serology can also be used to identify infected reservoir hosts. Seroconversion may take more than 4 weeks in animals that received a low dose of virus. Maternal antibodies can be a problem in lambs under 4 months of age. All of the serological tests, including VN, can be used in wildebeest. VN is not useful in sheep and goats infected with OvHV-2, CpHV-1 or related viruses, as they have low or no titers of neutralizing antibodies to AlHV-1.

In wildebeest calves, cell-free virus can be found in nasal secretions for a short period after infection. The virus can also be isolated from peripheral blood leukocytes at this time. It is less likely to be successful in older wildebeest, except when they are immunosuppressed (e.g., by stress or drug treatment). Cell-associated AlHV-1 can be isolated by establishing cultures of tissues from wildebeest. Subclinically infected, susceptible species

The levels of OvHV-2 DNA are very low in subclinically infected bison and cattle, and may not be detected readily by PCR. However, such infections are not expected to be clinically significant, as these animals are expected to be dead end hosts for the virus. In surveillance, such animals can be detected more readily by serology than PCR.

TREATMENT

No specific antiviral therapy is available. Antibiotics to control secondary infections and supportive therapy may occasionally help, but many affected animals die.

CONTROL

Disease reporting

Veterinarians who encounter or suspect malignant catarrhal fever should follow their national and/or local guidelines for disease reporting. In the U.S., malignant catarrhal fever is a reportable disease in many states. State authorities should be consulted for more specific information

Prevention

Malignant catarrhal fever can be prevented by separating susceptible animals from sheep, goats, wildebeest or other suspected reservoir hosts. Wildebeest seem to transmit AlHV-1 readily, and should always be separated from cattle. Susceptible animals should not be allowed on pastures where these animals have recently grazed, particularly near the time wildebeest calve. To prevent sheep-associated MCF, it is important to separate sheep from bison, some deer and other highly susceptible species. Although this form of MCF can also occur in European breeds of cattle, cases are uncommon, and separation of cattle and sheep is not always necessary. Some flocks of sheep have been associated with recurring transmission to cattle, lasting for years, and separation or culling of such flocks should be considered.

In zoos and wild animal parks, control is complicated by the number of potentially susceptible animal species and MCF virus carriers, which are often poorly characterized. In addition to OvHV-2 and AlHV-1, there have been at least two incidents involving transmission from Nubian ibex to bongo. Increased susceptibility (e.g., during pregnancy) or increased virus shedding (e.g., recently acquired animals stressed by a new environment) might be factors in some outbreaks.

The minimum distance needed for separation is unknown. Although most infections occur when the carrier host and susceptible animals are in close contact, transmission of AlHV-1 has been reported when animals were separated by a distance of at least 100 meters. OvHV-2 was reported in cattle separated from lambs by 70 meters. This disease was also reported in bison herds up to 5 km from a lamb feedlot. Separation by longer distances is likely to be more important when the host is highly susceptible and the concentration of virus is high. Transmission on fomites must also be avoided, particularly when the species is highly susceptible. In some cases, the production of virus-free hosts may also be considered. OvHV-2 free domesticated sheep and mouflon have been produced by early weaning, isolation and testing for virus. CpHV-2-free goats were produced by separating them from the infected herd at 7-10 days of age. One outbreak at a zoo was successfully controlled by the removal of infected sheep species, followed by the reintroduction of virus-free mouflon sheep derived from the infected flock. Commercial vaccines are not currently available for any species.

During outbreaks, susceptible animals should be separated immediately from the suspected source of the virus to prevent further cases. Although there is some uncertainty about the possibility of horizontal transmission in some species, most incidental hosts are thought to be dead end hosts. The current consensus is that sick animals they do not need to be culled or separated from other susceptible animals. Because the incubation period can be very long, cases can continue to occur for months, even after the animals have been separated from the source of virus. Stress reduction can help prevent disease in subclinically or mildly affected animals.

MORBIDITY AND MORTALITY

AlHV-1, OvHV-2 and CpHV-2 seem to be carried in many, most or all individuals of the reservoir species, and the virus spreads readily within infected herds. In wild wildebeest, an intense epizootic occurs during the perinatal period,

and all calves are thought to become infected with AlHV-1 before they reach 6 months of age. Uninfected wildebeest are thought to be rare in zoos, if they exist. Similarly, most sheep are infected with OvHV-2, although infection usually seems to occur later than in wildebeest, and OvHV-2 free herds have been created by early weaning. Most goats in CpHV-2 infected herds are thought to carry this virus by the age of 10 months. The prevalence of MCF viruses in wild sheep and goats is poorly understood, and may vary with the species or population. For example, antibodies to MCFV were found in 95% of a group of wild Dall's sheep in Alaska. but one population of bighorn sheep (*Ovis canadensis*) had no evidence of infection. Illness in reservoir hosts is thought to be possible, but very rare.

In MCF-susceptible species, AlHV-1 infections are often associated with exposure to wildebeest herds around the time of calving. Wildebeest-associated MCF is uncommon when all wildebeest in the herd are older than 6 months. Outbreaks of sheep-associated MCF (OvHV-2) have been seen most often during lambing season, although the reason is still unclear. Certain sheep flocks may continue to infect other animals for years. However, cases of MCF can be unpredictable; and sometimes develop in animals that were exposed to carriers without incident for years. The conditions leading to such outbreaks are often speculative. Stress might increase virus shedding, and environmental conditions such as high humidity might increase virus survival. In one outbreak, concentration of the virus by a barn fan was suggested as a possible contributing factor. Pregnancy might increase animals' susceptibility. In some pig herds, most or all of the affected animals were pregnant. Similarly, MCF occurred in 3 periparturient bongo antelope exposed to a healthy adult male Nubian ibex, but neither a bongo calf exposed to this ibex, nor male bongo exposed to other Nubian ibexes became ill.

In Africa, morbidity from AlHV-1 is approximately 6-7% in most cattle herds, although it can be as high as 50%. In European breeds of cattle, sheep-associated MCF usually occurs sporadically in only one to a few animals in the herd. The morbidity rate from this form is usually less than 1%. A few outbreaks affecting 16-50% of the herd have been reported, but this is unusual. In highly susceptible species such as farmed cervids and bison, both the number of affected animals and the case fatality rate are higher. Morbidity rates as high as 50-100% have been reported in bison, in outbreaks where there is close contact with sheep. The case fatality rate from MCF viruses is 80-90% in symptomatic cattle, and approaches 100% in symptomatic bison, deer and water buffalo. Residual corneal opacity is often seen in recovered cattle, but complete recovery is also possible.

Healthy animals, including those from MCF-susceptible species, may have antibodies to MCF viruses. Subclinical infections have been reported in bison, deer, cattle, pigs, wild cervids and other species. In one study, 24% of healthy bison had antibodies to MCF viruses, and OvHV-2 DNA was found in the blood of 11% of the seropositive bison. Genetic susceptibility to illness has been identified in bison. On Norwegian farms where outbreaks had occurred previously in cattle and/or swine, antibodies to OvHV-2 were found in 25% of the cattle and 43% of the pigs. Up to 35% of some wild cervid populations are also reported to have antibodies to MCF viruses.

PUBLIC HEALTH

There is no evidence that any of the MCF viruses can infect humans.

MELIOIDOSIS

Pseudoglanders, Whitmore Disease

IMPORTANCE

Melioidosis is a bacterial disease that affects humans and many species of animals. While some infections are subclinical, others result in localized acute or chronic disease, or fatal septicemia. Because it can affect almost any organ, melioidosis can mimic many other diseases; it is sometimes called "the great imitator." Infections can also remain asymptomatic for months or years, and emerge to cause disease at a later time. A misdiagnosis may be fatal; the causative organism, *Burkholderia pseudomallei,* is susceptible to a limited number of antibiotics.

In endemic areas, melioidosis is an important cause of illness and death in humans and animals. Outside these regions, it can be a concern in travelers, immigrants and imported animals. In 1975, a panda is thought to have introduced melioidosis to the Paris Zoo, where it caused a severe outbreak. The epidemic spread to other zoos in Paris and Mulhouse, and to equestrian clubs throughout France. It decimated some zoo populations and caused at least two human deaths. More recently, melioidosis was reported in three pet iguanas in the U.S. and the Czech Republic, all of which had resided in a non-endemic region for more than a year. The importance of considering melioidosis among the diagnostic possibilities is highlighted by such reports, even outside areas of known endemicity. An additional concern about *B. pseudomallei* is that has been identified as a potential biological weapon.

ETIOLOGY

Melioidosis results from infection by *Burkholderia pseudomallei,* a Gram negative bacillus in the family Burkholderiaceae. This organism was formerly known as *Pseudomonas pseudomallei.* The genus *Burkholderia* contains numerous soil organisms, some of which are closely related to *B. pseudomallei*. It includes *B. oklahomensis* sp. nov., which has been cultured from the soil in North America, and caused two human cases originally identified as melioidosis in the U.S. *B. pseudomallei* is also a close relative of *B. mallei,* the agent of glanders.

SPECIES AFFECTED

Many terrestrial and aquatic mammals, as well as marsupials, birds, reptiles and fish, can be affected by melioidosis. Goats, sheep and pigs are the most commonly infected species in Australia; sheep and goats seem to be particularly susceptible to clinical signs. Cases of melioidosis have also been reported in other species including dogs, cats, cattle, buffalo, camels, alpacas, horses, mules, bison (*Bison bison*), zebra (*Equus burchelli*), deer, kangaroos, wallabies, koalas, hog badger (*Arctonyx collaris*), large felids (e.g., cheetah, *Acinonyx jubatus*, and flat-headed cat, *Prionailurus planiceps*), various nonhuman primates, captive marine mammals, crocodiles, snakes, iguanas and tropical fish. This disease has been documented in some species of birds including psittacine birds, penguins, ratites and chickens. Some reports suggest that, among birds, species not native to endemic regions may be more likely to develop melioidosis. Rodents and rabbits can be infected experimentally.

Zoonotic potential

Humans are susceptible to *B. pseudomallei*. This organism is usually acquired from environmental sources, but a few zoonotic cases have been described.

GEOGRAPHIC DISTRIBUTION

The exact distribution of *B. pseudomallei* is uncertain, due to factors such as limited laboratory support and/or low clinical suspicion in some areas. Melioidosis is mainly reported in parts of Asia (e.g., Southeast Asia, South Asia, China, Singapore, Taiwan) and northern Australia. However, indigenous cases in animals or humans, or organisms in the environment, have been documented in many other regions including the Middle East, South and Central America, Africa and various islands, such as the Philippines, Puerto Rico, the Caribbean, New Caledonia, Madagascar and Mauritius. Rare cases of melioidosis have been reported from the U.S. and Mexico, in people who had not traveled outside this region. To date, environmental sampling has not detected *B. pseudomallei* in North America, and it is possible that these individuals were exposed to an unknown, imported source of the organism. Cases in three iguanas in the U.S. and the Czech Republic were attributed to chronic infections in animals most likely imported from Latin America. Soil sampling in France detected *B. pseudomallei* in several locations after an outbreak in the 1970s, but whether it still exists there seems to be unclear.

M

TRANSMISSION

Animals and humans usually acquire melioidosis from organisms in the environment. *B. pseudomallei* is a saprophyte that occurs in soil and water in endemic areas. Its environmental niches are still incompletely understood. Although this organism is particularly common in moist soils, it can also survive for prolonged periods in intermittently irrigated soils. It is reported to be common in garden soil in some areas. There are occasional reports of its isolation from an arid location after flooding, although there was no evidence for its presence before that event.

B. pseudomallei can enter the body by ingestion, via inhalation, or through wounds and abrasions. Both animals and humans can become chronically infected, with or without clinical signs. Infected animals can shed this organism in various sources such as wound exudates, nasal secretions, milk, feces and urine. Transplacental transmission has been documented in several species (goats, a pig and a spider monkey). Nosocomial transmission was reported in four cats at a veterinary hospital, possibly via contamination of a multidose injectable solution. Insects are not thought to play any significant role in transmission, although *B. pseudomallei* could be transmitted by mosquitoes (*Aedes aegypti*) and rat fleas (*Xenopsylla cheopsis*) in laboratory experiments.

There have been a few reports of zoonotic transmission, often after skin lesions were exposed to infected animals, tissues (including meat) or milk. However, most people become infected directly from the environment. This occurs through skin wounds in many cases, but humans can also acquire *B. pseudomallei* via ingestion (from sources such as contaminated, unchlorinated water supplies) or inhalation. Inhalation may be particularly important during periods of heavy rainfall and strong winds, or during exposure to soil organisms from artificial turbulence (e.g., winds generated by helicopter blades). Person-to-person transmission has rarely been described, and generally occurred to family members who had been in close contact through activities such as nursing the patient. Possible sexual transmission was suggested in rare cases. Some infants seem to have been infected from human milk, and transmission may also occur *in utero*, although vertical transmission has rarely been proven in people.

B. pseudomallei can survive for months or years in contaminated soil and water. In one report, this organism remained viable in triple distilled water at 25°C for 16 years. Other groups have reported that, under laboratory conditions, it can survive in room temperature water for as long as 8 weeks, in muddy water for up to 7 months, in soil for up to 30 months, and in soil with a water content of less than 10% for up to 70 days. *B. pseudomallei* is acid tolerant, and has been recovered from water sources ranging in pH from 2 to 9 (with good survival in the laboratory at pH ≥ 4). It was also reported to remain viable for up to a month in water containing salt concentrations as high as 0.4%, with little loss in cultivable cell numbers, and to persist for at least 4 weeks in a 4% salt solution, although the number of viable organisms decreased significantly at this concentration. How long *B. pseudomallei* can persist at low temperatures is unclear. In two experiments, some strains survived for as long as 42 days at 0-2°C.

B. pseudomallei is capable of existing in a viable but non-cultivable state in the environment. While these organisms cannot be cultured, they can still cause disease. This phenomenon occurs in acid pH, as well as under other conditions. The morphology of the viable but non-cultivable organisms can change. In acid pH, for instance, they can appear as Gram-positive, coccoid organisms, which revert to conventional Gram-negative-bacilli in neutral pH. *B. pseudomallei* can also enter the cells of some protozoa or the mycorrhizal fungus *Gigaspora decipiens*, a characteristic that might help it survive environmental stresses.

DISINFECTION

B. pseudomallei is stated to be susceptible to numerous disinfectants including 1% sodium hypochlorite, 70% ethanol, glutaraldehyde and formaldehyde. However, unpublished experiments suggest that it can remain viable for some time in 0.3% chlorhexidine, and one outbreak was associated with a contaminated container of commercial hand-washing detergent. Recent experiments documented its susceptibility to a commercial peracetic acid disinfectant and Virkon®. Disinfectants may not completely eliminate this organism from drinking water, particularly when it is protected within protozoa or found in biofilms. Chlorination reduces the number of *B. pseudomallei* in water, but small numbers of bacteria have been isolated from water containing up to 1000 ppm. free chlorine. Strains can differ in their sensitivity to this agent.

B. pseudomallei is also reported to be susceptible to inactivation by sunlight. It can be killed by moist heat of 121°C (249°F) for at least 15 min or dry heat of 160-170°C (320-338°F) for at least one hour.

INFECTIONS IN ANIMALS

INCUBATION PERIOD

The incubation period ranges from days to months or years.

CLINICAL SIGNS

Subclinical infections are common in animals, and asymptomatic abscesses may be found at slaughter. Symptomatic melioidosis may be acute, subacute or chronic, and mild or severe. The lungs, spleen, liver and associated lymph nodes are often involved in animals, but any organ can be affected. The effects vary with the site. Acute melioidosis, which is most often seen in young animals, often occurs as septicemia. Localized respiratory signs, gastrointestinal signs, septic arthritis, osteomyelitis, mastitis, orchitis, neurological signs, mycotic aneurysms and other syndromes may be also seen. Septicemia or extensive involvement of the vital organs can be fatal.

Forms of melioidosis reported in mammals and birds

Pulmonary melioidosis is common in sheep, with clinical signs that can include fever, severe coughing, respiratory distress and profuse mucopurulent yellow nasal and ocular discharge. Some sheep become arthritic and lame. In others, the only signs may be fever and generalized weakness. Neurological signs have also been reported. Orchitis with testicular nodules can occur in rams. In goats, respiratory disease is reported to be less severe than in sheep, and coughing may not be a prominent sign. Progressive emaciation, lameness or hindleg paresis, aortic aneurysms and abortions have also been documented in this species. Mastitis appears to be a common syndrome in goats.

Pigs may be relatively resistant to melioidosis when husbandry and nutrition are good. Adult pigs tend to develop chronic infections with few clinical signs; however, enlarged lymph nodes (particularly the submandibular nodes) may be palpable. Progressive emaciation, neurological signs, incoordination, multiple skin ulcers and diarrhea have also been reported. Young pigs can develop acute septicemia with fever, anorexia, coughing and nasal and ocular discharge. Occasional abortions or stillbirths have been seen in sows, and orchitis can occur in boars. In endemic regions, asymptomatic splenic abscesses are often found in pigs at slaughter.

Various forms of melioidosis have been reported in horses. Generally, the disease lasts approximately a few weeks to a few months, with clinical signs that may include weakness, emaciation, edema and lymphangitis of the limbs, mild colic, diarrhea, and signs of pneumonia including coughing and nasal discharge. Skin infections can initially resemble fungal eczema, but later become papular. Hyperacute septicemia with high fever, limb edema, diarrhea and rapid death has also been seen. Acute meningoencephalitis has been reported in rare cases.

Melioidosis has rarely been described in cattle. Most cases in adult cattle have been chronic. Fever, dyspnea, continuous profuse salivation and neurologic signs were reported in one animal. In two other cases, abscessation or acute, localized arthritis occurred after wound contamination. Acute melioidosis was reported in a calf.

Camels may develop chronic respiratory disease with a hacking cough, purulent nasal discharge and dyspnea. Other animals had hindleg ataxia and a wasting disease with severe emaciation. Acute septicemia has been seen in both camels and alpacas.

Acute, subacute or chronic melioidosis can occur in dogs. Acute cases in this species are often characterized by septicemia. Signs may include fever, severe diarrhea and fulminant pneumonia. Subacute disease can begin as a skin lesion with lymphangitis and lymphadenitis; untreated cases may progress to septicemia over a week to several months. Respiratory disease can also be the initial syndrome. In addition, chronic disease can occur in any organ; it may be accompanied by anorexia, myalgia, edema of the limbs and skin abscesses.

Abscesses have also been reported in various organs in cats. In two published cases, the clinical signs were not strongly suggestive of an infectious disease. One cat presented with jaundice and anemia, and died soon after it was seen. Fatal neurological disease was reported in the second cat, possibly after dissemination from an infected foot wound.

Nonspecific signs of illness, fever, generalized lymphadenopathy and respiratory signs were common in affected zoo mammals and marsupials in Thailand. Most cases in captive marine mammals have been characterized by acute septicemia with fever, inappetence, anorexia and listlessness followed by death. Unlike other species, respiratory distress was not reported. Enteric disease with diarrhea and liver abscesses has been seen in some dolphins. Three cases in iguanas were characterized by masses in internal organs and/ or external abscesses. Some animals had recurrent or repeated abscess formation.

Although birds may be relatively resistant to melioidosis, fatal cases with lethargy, anorexia and diarrhea have been reported in various avian species in Australia. Experimentally infected chickens remained asymptomatic; however, facial abscesses were reported in a naturally infected chicken.

POST MORTEM LESIONS

At necropsy, the major findings are multiple abscesses containing thick, caseous greenish-yellow or off-white material. These abscesses are generally not calcified. The regional lymph nodes, lungs, spleen, liver and subcutaneous tissues are most often involved, but abscesses can occur in most organs. Splenic abscesses are reported to be common in asymptomatic pigs at slaughter. In animals with respiratory disease, exudative bronchopneumonia, consolidation and/or abscesses may be found in the lungs. Suppurative lesions including nodules and ulcers may also be detected on the nasal mucosa and septum, as well as on the turbinate bones. These nodules may coalesce to form irregular plaques. Meningoencephalitis, severe enteritis, suppurative polyarthritis, mycotic aneurisms, mastitis and other syndromes have also been documented in animals. Diffuse pinpoint nodules in the liver and spleen are reported to be common lesions in birds.

DIAGNOSTIC TESTS

Culturing B. pseudomallei is currently considered to be the gold standard test for melioidosis in both animals and people. This organism may be found in various sites including abscesses and wound exudates, milk, feces, throat swabs, blood, urine, and tissues collected at necropsy. It will grow on most media including blood agar. Selective media such

M

as Ashdown's medium are often used in endemic regions. Ashdown's medium selects for gentamicin resistance, a characteristic of most *B. pseudomallei*; however, gentamicin-susceptible strains were recently reported to be common in some areas. Colonies of *B. pseudomallei* can be identified by biochemistry combined with microscopic and culture appearance. On microscopic examination, the organisms are classically described as motile, short Gram negative bacilli, with bipolar or irregular staining. However, their form can differ from this description, for instance in older cultures or clinical samples. PCR and antigen detection tests (e.g., latex agglutination, immunofluorescence) are also used for identification. There have been multiple reports of the misidentification of *B. pseudomallei* by automated identification systems, although some sources indicate that these systems can identify most isolates. It is also possible to mistake this organism for *Pseudomonas* or a contaminant during manual culture and identification. Misidentification is a particular concern in non-endemic areas, where the isolation of *B. pseudomallei* is unexpected. *B. pseudomallei* is a biosafety level 3 organism, and not all laboratories are equipped to safely culture and identify this organism.

Other tests that can be used to identify *B. pseudomallei* in clinical samples include antigen detection assays such as direct immunofluorescence, latex agglutination or ELISAs, and PCR tests to detect nucleic acids. The specific tests available can differ between regions, and PCR does not appear to be widely used at present. Genetic techniques that may be used for epidemiological purposes include PCR–restriction fragment length polymorphism, pulse-field gel electrophoresis, 16S rRNA sequencing, variable number tandem repeat polymorphism and multilocus sequence typing (MLST). These tests may be available mainly in research laboratories.

Serology is sometimes used to diagnose melioidosis in animals, but it is not considered to be definitive. Animals in endemic areas often have pre-existing titers to this organism, and there may be cross-reactions with closely related species such as *B. mallei* or *B. cepecia*. False positives have also been reported from other Gram negative bacteria including *Legionella* spp. Some of the available serological tests include indirect hemagglutination, immunofluorescence and complement fixation.

Environmental samples are sometimes taken from soil and/or water during outbreaks or case investigations. Recommended methods and sampling protocols for surveillance have been published.

TREATMENT

B. pseudomallei is susceptible to some antibiotics; however, this organism is intrinsically resistant to many drugs, including some that are commonly used to treat bacterial infections. Because relapses can occur when treatment is stopped, animals given antibiotics may need to be monitored afterward.

Treatment regimens similar to those currently used in humans, with intravenous therapy followed by an eradication stage, may be effective in animals; however, there are no published reports evaluating their use.

Because treatment can be expensive and protracted, and it may not eliminate the organism, some animals are euthanized instead. Treatment of infected animals may not be allowed in some areas.

CONTROL

Disease reporting

Veterinarians who suspect melioidosis should follow their national and/or local guidelines for disease reporting. In the U.S., this disease is reportable in animals in some states. State or federal authorities should be consulted for specific regulations and information.

Prevention

Melioidosis is usually acquired from the environment, particularly after contact with soil or water. To minimize contact with dirt, animals can be raised on wooden slats, concrete or paved floors. Providing safe drinking water (e.g., by filtration and chlorination) is also important in endemic areas. Carnivores and omnivores should not be allowed to eat contaminated carcasses. Licensed vaccines are not available.

Euthanasia of infected animals is often recommended even in endemic areas, because melioidosis is difficult to treat and can be zoonotic. After culling infected animals, the premises should be disinfected. Disinfecting some environments may be difficult. The soil in one exhibit at a Thai zoo was decontaminated by mixing in quicklime (calcium oxide) and left for approximately one year, after which time repeat cultures found no evidence of *B. pseudomallei*. If infected animals are not euthanized, precautions should be taken to protect people and other animals. Strict hygiene is necessary to prevent transmission from infected horses in stables. The feces should be removed several times a day, and the premises, and the hooves and lower legs of the animals should be disinfected regularly. Food and water should be provided as aseptically as possible. Standing water should be allowed only in limited quantities or disinfected immediately.

MORBIDITY AND MORTALITY

Susceptibility to melioidosis may differ between species and individual animals. Immunosuppression may predispose cats and dogs to this disease. Pigs generally seem to be more resistant to clinical signs than sheep and goats, and infections in cattle are very rarely reported. One report indicated that, among zoo animals, orangutans (*Pongo pygmaeus*) appeared to be unusually susceptible, with cases usually developing into septicemia and ending in death within a week. Although melioidosis does not appear to be a problem in marine mammals in the wild, an outbreak occurred in marine mammals at a Hong Kong oceanarium after heavy summer rains washed soil into the animals' water.

The mortality rate varies with the site of the lesions, but can be high in sheep. Extensive abscesses and involvement of the vital organs can be fatal. Septicemia has a high case fatality rate, but it seems to be less common in animals than humans. Most cases of septicemia are seen in young animals.

INFECTIONS IN HUMANS

INCUBATION PERIOD

The incubation period in humans varies from less than a day (after very high exposure) to several months or years. In one study, most acute cases became apparent within 21 days after exposure, with a mean of 9 days. A few cases have remained subclinical for up to 29 years, and one infection apparently became symptomatic after 62 years.

CLINICAL SIGNS

B. pseudomallei can cause a wide spectrum of clinical signs in people. While many infections seem to be inapparent, some result in acute pulmonary disease, septicemia, or localized acute or chronic suppurative infections. The frequency of the various syndromes can differ between regions. For example, parotid abscesses are common among children in Thailand, but rare in Australia. One syndrome can develop into another if the organisms spread to other sites.

Acute localized infections sometimes occur at the site of inoculation. In Australia, localized skin disease was reported to be a common form of melioidosis in children. Lesions in the skin typically appear as gray or white, firm nodules and ulcers, which are often but not always single. The nodules may caseate, and are often surrounded by inflammation. They may be accompanied by regional lymphadenopathy and lymphangitis. Other forms of acute localized disease include suppurative parotitis/parotid abscesses, destructive corneal ulcers seen after corneal trauma, and cellulitis or infections that resemble necrotizing fasciitis. Genitourinary infections often manifest as prostatic abscesses. Localized infections can disseminate, but systemic infections are not always preceded by localized signs. Skin and subcutaneous infections can also result from the hematogenous spread of organisms from other sites.

Pulmonary disease is a common syndrome in people. It can occur as either the primary syndrome or a component of septicemia, and may develop either suddenly or gradually after a nonspecific prodromal illness. Pulmonary melioidosis ranges in severity from mild acute or subacute pneumonia to respiratory distress with overwhelming septic shock. Common symptoms include fever, coughing, pleuritic chest pain and, in some cases, hemoptysis. However, patients with pneumonia as a component of septicemia often have little coughing or pleuritic pain, although they are febrile and severely ill. Chronic pulmonary melioidosis can wax and wane and resembles tuberculosis, with weight loss, fevers, night sweats, and a productive cough, sometimes with blood-tinged sputum. Ulcerative lesions and nodules are sometimes found in the nose, and the septum may perforate. Complications may include pneumothorax, empyema and pericarditis. Untreated cases can progress to septicemia.

Septicemia is the most serious form of melioidosis. It is most common in people with pre-existing diseases such as diabetes, cancer and kidney failure. The onset is usually acute, with fever, rigors and other typical signs of sepsis. However, it may develop more gradually in some patients, with a fluctuating fever often associated with severe weight loss. Common symptoms of septicemic melioidosis include fever, severe headache, disorientation, pharyngitis, upper abdominal pain, diarrhea, jaundice and notable muscle tenderness. Pulmonary signs including dyspnea are common, and arthritis or meningitis may be seen. Some patients have a disseminated pustular rash with regional lymphadenopathy, cellulitis or lymphangitis. Septic shock is common and life-threatening..

In chronic cases, abscesses and suppurative lesions can occur in a variety of organs. Although the liver, spleen, skeletal muscle and prostate gland are often affected, lesions may be found in a variety of other organs including the skin, lung, kidney, myocardium, bone, joints, lymph nodes and testes. Mycotic aneurysms are also seen. Uncommonly, melioidosis can result in brain abscesses, encephalomyelitis (with various syndromes including flaccid paralysis) or meningitis. There may be severe residual defects in cases of encephalitis.

DIAGNOSTIC TESTS

Isolation of *B. pseudomallei* in culture is considered to be the gold standard test for melioidosis in people, as it is in animals, and the techniques are the same. In human clinical cases, *B. pseudomallei* can be recovered from sources such as blood, sputum, throat or rectal swabs, urine, skin lesions or ulcer swabs, tissues and wound exudates. Sampling multiple sites, rather than limiting samples to the apparent focus of the infection, is more likely to detect the organism. *B. pseudomallei* can sometimes be found in samples such as urine even if there are no signs associated with the urinary tract. Culture is not successful in all cases of melioidosis.

B. pseudomallei antigens may be identified directly in tissues, wound exudates or body fluids by assays such as direct immunofluorescence or latex agglutination, particularly if the number of bacteria is high. Lateral flow immunoassays have also been developed. PCR is reported to be no more sensitive than culture for detecting melioidosis in humans, and does not seem to be widely used at present. Matrix-assisted laser desorption ionization time-of-flight mass spectrometry (MALDI-TOF MS) methods are being investigated. As

M

in animals, specialized genetic techniques can be used in epidemiological studies.

Serological tests may be helpful in some circumstances, particularly when paired sera are available. In some cases, a high single titer in the presence of clinical signs may be suggestive. However, most of the population is seropositive in some (but not all) endemic areas, limiting the value of these assays. A number of serological tests have been described in humans, including agglutination, indirect hemagglutination, immunofluorescence, ELISAs, and immunochromatographic tests (ICT). Test availability differs between regions, but indirect hemagglutination is a commonly used test. People with symptomatic melioidosis are occasionally seronegative, and cross-reactivity with other organisms is possible.

TREATMENT

Although a few cases with only localized skin lesions were reported to heal spontaneously, melioidosis is treated even when it is localized or mild, due to the risk that the organism may persist and/or disseminate.

B. pseudomallei is not susceptible to some drugs that are often used empirically to treat infections. Combinations of drugs were generally used for treatment in the past, but some newer single antibiotics are equally effective. At present, the recommended protocol is a two-stage therapy. Initially, patients receive intravenous antibiotics for a minimum of 10-14 days (longer in some conditions). This is followed by prolonged antibiotic treatment, usually with oral drugs, for several months or longer. The purpose of the second stage is to eliminate the organisms from the body. Prolonged oral treatment alone was reported to be effective in some milder conditions in healthy people. Some patients also require adjunct treatments, such as supportive therapy for septic shock. Pulmonary resection or drainage of abscesses is occasionally necessary.

At one time, up to 30% of patients relapsed after being treated for melioidosis. However relapses are much less common with newer treatment regimens, and tend to occur mainly in cases where the course of antibiotics is not completed.

CONTROL

B. pseudomallei is widely distributed in soil and standing water in endemic regions. Skin wounds (including abrasions or burns) should be protected from potential contamination, and promptly and thoroughly cleansed if they become exposed. Gloves and rubber boots are recommended for anyone doing agricultural work. Because *B. pseudomallei* can be found in milk from infected ruminants, only pasteurized dairy products should be consumed. Chlorination of the water supply decreases the risk of infection from this source, and carcasses with signs of melioidosis are condemned and not used for human food. People who process meat should wear gloves and disinfect their knives regularly. Veterinarians

should also take precautions to avoid exposure, including the use of gloves and protective clothing, when working with infected animals or collecting diagnostic samples. People with diabetes or other predisposing conditions should be especially vigilant in avoiding exposure, including potential inhalation during severe weather events. Screening for melioidosis has been recommended for patients who will be starting immunosuppressive therapy in an endemic area.

Laboratory workers may be exposed in clinical samples from patients, even where melioidosis is not endemic. Practices such as sniffing opened culture plates should be discouraged. Postexposure prophylaxis may sometimes be given after laboratory exposure, but its effectiveness is currently uncertain. In hospitals, ordinary precautions to prevent transmission in blood and body fluids should be taken. No vaccine is currently available for humans.

MORBIDITY AND MORTALITY

Melioidosis can occur as sporadic cases or outbreaks in endemic regions. The number of cases typically increases after heavy rainfall or flooding. While this disease is most common in tropical and subtropical areas, it has been reported in arid regions after floods. Some outbreaks have been linked to contaminated drinking water supplies, and occasionally to unusual sources, such as a container of contaminated hand washing detergent. Occasional cases occur outside endemic areas in immigrants and travelers. Most human illnesses seem to appear soon after exposure; however, *B. pseudomallei* can persist asymptomatically in the body and cause disease at a later time, typically when another condition causes the person to become debilitated or immunosuppressed. One study in Australia suggested than < 4% of recognized cases potentially result from the reactivation of latent lesions.

The incidence of melioidosis is reported to peak between the ages of 40 and 60 among adults in Thailand. This disease is particularly common in people with diabetes. Other chronic conditions including thalassemia, kidney disease, chronic lung disease, cancer and alcoholism, as well as the use of immunosuppressive drugs (e.g., steroids), also increase the risk of illness. However, some cases occur in previously healthy people. Children account for 5-15% of melioidosis cases in Australia, and do not have any risk factors in most cases. Seroprevalence rates vary widely in endemic regions: while > 50% of the population may be seropositive in parts of Thailand, one study reported that antibodies to *B. pseudomallei* occurred in < 10% of people at high risk of exposure in Australia. It is currently unclear how many seropositive people without clinical signs might be carrying this organism. Colonization without disease is currently considered unlikely, although there are reports suggesting that it might occur.

The severity of melioidosis is influenced by factors such as the host's immunity, the form of the disease, and the dose and possibly the strain of the organism. For example, acute suppurative parotiditis or localized skin disease in children usually has a good prognosis. Conversely, septic shock is rapidly fatal without treatment, and has a high risk of death even with good care. Case fatality rates for melioidosis have decreased in recent years in some areas, most likely due to improved recognition and treatment. Recent estimates of the overall mortality rate for all patients range from approximately 10% in Australia to 40% in Thailand, and can be higher in other areas where only limited medical care is available. Australia reports that deaths are currently uncommon in patients without known risk factors for melioidosis, provided there is prompt recognition of the condition, treatment with appropriate antibiotics, and state-of-the-art management of sepsis. In one large prospective study from Australia, the case fatality rate ranged from 4% in patients without septic shock to 50% in patients with septic shock. Cases in infants can also be severe. One review reported a case fatality rate of 73% in published cases of neonatal melioidosis.

MONKEYPOX

IMPORTANCE

Monkeypox is a zoonotic viral disease that can infect nonhuman primates, rodents and some other mammals. This disease is endemic in western and central Africa, where it circulates in unknown animal hosts and emerges periodically as a zoonosis in humans. Outbreaks have also been seen occasionally among captive nonhuman primates in other parts of the world. The only outbreak of human monkeypox to be reported outside Africa occurred in the United States in 2003. The virus entered North America in exotic African rodents imported as pets, and spread to pet prairie dogs, which were highly susceptible to infection. The monkeypox virus subsequently infected approximately 70 people who had been in contact with these animals. No outbreaks have been reported in the U.S. since that time, and there is no evidence that the virus has become endemic in North America. Prompt diagnosis of monkeypox is essential, both to prevent this disease from becoming established outside Africa, and because it resembles smallpox, a potential bioterrorist weapon.

ETIOLOGY

Monkeypox results from infection by the monkeypox virus, a member of the genus *Orthopoxvirus* in the family Poxviridae (subfamily Chordopoxvirinae). Two clades of monkeypox viruses, the West African and Congo Basin viruses, have been identified. The Congo Basin viruses are more virulent. Monkeypox virus is closely related to some other orthopoxviruses such as variola (smallpox) virus, and it cannot be distinguished from these viruses in some laboratory tests.

Monkeypox should not be confused with benign epidermal monkeypox (BEMP), a poxviral disease of primates caused by tanapox virus, an antigenically unrelated virus in the genus *Yatapoxvirus* of the family Poxviridae.

SPECIES AFFECTED

The monkeypox virus's full host range is unknown. Species known to be susceptible include Old and New World monkeys and apes, a variety of rodents and other small mammals. Among captive primates, infections have been reported in rhesus macaques (*Macaca mulatta*), cynomolgus monkeys (*Macaca fascicularis*), langurs, baboons (*Papio* spp.), chimpanzees (*Pan* spp.), orangutans (*Pongo* spp.), marmosets, gorillas (*Gorilla* spp.), gibbons (family Hylobatidae), owl–faced monkeys (*Cercopithecus hamlyn*), squirrel monkeys (*Saimiri* spp.) and others.

In 2003, a West African strain of monkeypox virus was introduced into the U.S. in a shipment of imported exotic mammals from Africa. Infected animals in this shipment included Gambian giant pouched rats (*Cricetomys* spp.), rope squirrels (*Funisciurus* sp.) and dormice (*Graphiurus* sp.). Whether a species originally harbored the virus or became infected during shipment is unknown. Two cusimanse (*Crossarchus obscurus*), a genet (*Genetta genetta*) and 27 sun squirrels (*Heliosciurus gambianus*) from this shipment had no evidence of infection. North American black-tailed prairie dogs (*Cynomys ludovicianus*) were readily infected by this virus. Infections were also documented in a groundhog/woodchuck (*Marmota monax*), an African hedgehog (*Atelerix* sp.), a jerboa (*Jaculus* sp.) and two opossums (*Didelphis marsupialis*, a species native to South America, and the gray short-tailed opossum, *Monodelphis domestica*). Species that developed antibodies after exposure, but had no evidence of viral DNA or infectious virus, included chinchillas (*Chinchilla lanigera*) and coatimundis (*Nasua nasua*). Many other species were exposed but did not become seropositive. Experimental infections have been established in prairie dogs, dormice, ground squirrels (*Spermophilus tridecemlineatus*), the cotton rat (*Sigmodon hispidus*) and the multimammate mouse (*Mastomys natalensis*). Anteaters were thought to have been involved in an outbreak among primates at the Rotterdam Zoo, the Netherlands in 1964.

The natural reservoir hosts for the monkeypox virus remain to be determined. In Africa, antibodies to this virus have been found in various species of rodents and shrews, as well as nonhuman primates. Two genera of African squirrels, *Funisciurus* spp. (rope squirrels) and *Heliosciurus* spp. (sun squirrels), have high seroprevalence rates, and have been suggested as possible maintenance hosts or vectors. Rope squirrels were among the infected species during the outbreak in the U.S. Sun squirrels in the same shipment had no evidence of infection; however, it is possible that they are reservoir hosts only for the Congo Basin clade and not the

M

West African clade. It is also possible that all of these species are incidental hosts. A recent study in Ghana examined rodents in the area where the animals involved in the U.S. outbreak were collected. This study found serological and/or molecular evidence of intermittent orthopoxvirus exposure in rodents of the genera *Cricetomys*, *Graphiurus* and *Funisciurus*, as well as in African ground squirrels (*Xerus* spp.). This study did not implicate any single species as the reservoir host.

Zoonotic potential

Humans are susceptible to monkeypox, and most cases occur after exposure to infected animals.

GEOGRAPHIC DISTRIBUTION

Monkeypox is endemic in central Africa (the Congo Basin) and West Africa. An outbreak of human monkeypox occurred in the U.S. in 2003. In the U.S., cases were seen in pet prairie dogs, other small mammals in captivity, and people who had been exposed to infected prairie dogs. There have been no reports of infections among humans or domesticated animals in North America since 2003, and limited surveys suggest that the virus probably did not enter wild animal populations.

TRANSMISSION

In prairie dogs, monkeypox virus or its nucleic acids have been found in skin lesions, urine, feces, and oral, nasal and conjunctival exudates. For epidemiological purposes, infected animals are assumed to be contagious one day before and up to 21 days after the initial signs, or until all skin lesions have formed scabs and no other clinical signs are present. In two experiments, shedding of West African clade viruses began 6-12 days after intranasal inoculation. West African or Congo Basin monkeypox viruses could be shed until 21 days after inoculation. In terminal cases, the virus appears to be widespread in the tissues. Prairie dogs are susceptible to infection by intranasal inoculation or contact with fomites (bedding from an animal with lesions).One study suggested that aerosol transmission could also occur between these animals; however, this is still not entirely certain, as the experimental design did not rule out the possibility of nose-to-nose contact between cages.

There is little published information on transmission in other small animal pets, but monkeypox virus has been found in most tissues of dormice. Limited evidence suggests that some small animals, such as dormice and Gambian giant pouched rats, might carry this virus for a few weeks or months.

Humans usually become infected by contact with animals. This virus is thought to be transmitted to people in bites from animals, in aerosols during close contact, or by direct contact with lesions, blood or body fluids. In Africa, human outbreaks have often been linked to handling, preparing and eating wild animals. In the U.S., most cases occurred among people who had close direct contact with prairie dogs; some

infections were apparently acquired in scratches and bites, or through open wounds. Human-to-human transmission can also occur. Potential routes of transmission between people include contact with skin lesions or infectious body fluids, or aerosol transmission during prolonged face-to-face contact. Transmission between humans appears to relatively inefficient, and sustained person-to-person spread has not been reported. Until 2005, the longest documented chain was four serial transmissions. More efficient person-to-person spread, with six serial transmissions, was recently reported from an outbreak in the Republic of Congo.

DISINFECTION

The U.S. Centers for Disease Control and Prevention (CDC) recommends disinfection of contaminated surfaces with 0.5% sodium hypochlorite or other EPA-approved high-level disinfectants. Incineration or autoclaving is appropriate for some contaminated materials. Burial without decontamination is not recommended.

INFECTIONS IN ANIMALS

INCUBATION PERIOD

Reported incubation periods are 4 to 13 days in experimentally infected black-tailed prairie dogs, 11 to 18 days in 3 prairie dogs infected by exposure to fomites, and 4 to 5 days in experimentally infected ground squirrels. In two studies, experimentally infected cynomolgus monkeys developed clinical signs 3 to 7 days after aerosol exposure.

CLINICAL SIGNS

Nonhuman primates

In nonhuman primates, the predominant syndrome is a self–limiting rash. The initial clinical signs are a fever and 1-4 mm cutaneous papules, which develop into pustules, then crust over. A typical monkeypox lesion has a red, necrotic, depressed center, surrounded by epidermal hyperplasia. These "pocks" can be seen over the entire body, but may be more common on the face, limbs, palms, soles and tail. The number of lesions varies from a few individual pocks to extensive, coalescing lesions. The crusts over the pustules eventually drop off, leaving small scars. Some animals have only skin lesions. In more severe cases, coughing, nasal discharge, dyspnea, anorexia, decreased body weight, facial edema, oral ulcers or lymphadenopathy may also be seen. Disseminated disease with visceral lesions is uncommon in natural infections among nonhuman primates. Pneumonia is common only in monkeys infected experimentally via aerosols.

Most naturally infected animals recover; however, fatalities are sometimes seen, particularly in infant monkeys. Asymptomatic infections also occur.

Prairie dogs

In prairie dogs, the clinical signs may include fever, depression, anorexia, weight loss, nasal discharge, sneezing and/or coughing, respiratory distress, diarrhea, a nodular skin rash and oral ulcers. During the outbreak in the U.S., blepharoconjunctivitis was often the first sign. Lymphadenopathy has been reported in naturally infected prairie dogs, but did not occur in all experimentally infected animals. Elevated serum levels of liver enzymes have also been seen. In experimentally infected prairie dogs, skin lesions appeared first on the head or extremities, followed by the trunk (a centrifugal pattern), similarly to humans. On the trunk and limbs, characteristic monkeypox lesions developed from macules through vesicles and pustules before forming scabs. Macules and vesicles also occurred on the face in this experiment, but pustules were not seen.

Infected prairie dogs may either recover or become fatally ill. Some experimentally infected prairie dogs died 1-2 weeks after infection without developing lesions on the skin or mucous membranes.

Other rodents

Experimental infections have been reported in several species of rodents. In dormice inoculated intranasally, the clinical signs were limited to lethargy, an unkempt hair coat, a hunched posture, conjunctivitis and dehydration. Many infections were fatal. Experimentally infected cotton rats developed an acute illness with rhinitis, conjunctivitis, dyspnea, coughing and progressive emaciation, often ending in death. In ground squirrels, the first signs were anorexia and lethargy. Nasal hemorrhages and dyspnea were common in ground squirrels inoculated with a Congo Basin isolate. In contrast, most ground squirrels inoculated with a West African strain did not develop nasal hemorrhages, and respiratory distress occurred only terminally. Both stains were uniformly fatal at the dose used.

Fatal infections were reported among rope squirrels and one Gambian giant pouched rat in the shipment of exotic African rodents to the U.S. Mild symptoms, with no respiratory signs and limited skin lesions, were seen in another Gambian giant pouched rat in the shipment. Other pouched rats that appeared healthy were also seropositive.

POST MORTEM LESIONS

Due to the risk of infection, the Centers for Disease Control and Prevention (CDC) recommends that practicing veterinarians avoid performing necropsies or biopsies on suspected cases. Pending necropsy, whole carcasses should be double-bagged and frozen. Animals should be necropsied only by individuals who have a current smallpox vaccination, and the biological safety guidelines recommended by the CDC (http://www.cdc.gov/poxvirus/monkeypox/) should be followed.

At necropsy, the skin may contain papules, umbilicated pustules ("pocks") with central necrosis, or crusts over healing lesions. The skin lesions may vary from barely detectable, single small papules to extensive lesions. In some animals, visceral lesions including (but not limited to) multifocal necrotizing pneumonitis, orchitis and peripheral lymphadenopathy may be seen.

In cynomolgus monkeys infected with monkeypox by aerosols, necropsy lesions commonly included both skin lesions and fibrinonecrotic bronchopneumonia. The lungs were heavy, congested and failed to collapse, and a dark red, lobular, mottled pattern of edema, atelectasis and necrosis was seen throughout all lobes. In some cases, fibrinous pleuritis or a clear pericardial effusion was also present. Peripheral lymphadenopathy; facial exanthema; ulcerative cheilitis; gingivitis; papulovesicular pharyngitis; necrotic lesions on the mucosa of the trachea, larynx or esophagus; and ulcerative stomatitis occurred in some animals. The oral lesions, which were most common on the hard palate and the dorsal surface of the tongue, were described as depressed, reddened foci of necrosis, erosion or ulceration surrounded by pale tan to white, slightly raised margins. Some animals had gastritis or 2-3 mm raised lesions with umbilicated necrotic centers on the mucosa of the distal colon or rectum. In some cases, necrotizing lesions were also reported in the lymph nodes, spleen and other lymphoid organs; in the gonads; and infrequently in other organs including the prostate gland, uterus, skeletal muscle and urinary bladder.

Blepharoconjunctivitis is a common finding in prairie dogs. As well as skin lesions, ulcers may be found on the tongue and hard palate. Bronchoalveolar pneumonia with patchy red-brown consolidation, and enlargement of the cervical and thoracic lymph nodes, have been reported in some animals. The visceral pleura may contain 1-3 mm white plaques, and small (2-3 mm) white, firm, deeply embedded foci with umbilicated necrotic centers have been reported in the intestines and glandular portion of the stomach.

In intranasally inoculated dormice, the gross lesions at necropsy included hepatomegaly, lymphadenopathy and hemorrhages in the upper gastrointestinal tract, nasal cavity, gall bladder and brain. Pulmonary edema and hemorrhages were reported in experimentally infected ground squirrels. In multimammate mice, hemorrhagic pleuritis or peritonitis and inflammatory hyperemia were described in many organs after intraperitoneal inoculation.

DIAGNOSTIC TESTS

In the U.S., diagnostic samples for monkeypox are submitted through the state health department, which should be contacted before collecting or shipping any samples. Tissues and other specimens must be packaged and shipped under secure conditions to prevent infections in humans

M

and animals. Shipment must comply with all local, state and federal regulations.

Monkeypox can be tentatively diagnosed if the characteristic skin lesions are present, or if other clinical signs consistent with the disease are seen during an outbreak. Histopathology provides supportive evidence. The diagnosis can be confirmed by virus isolation or PCR. Monkeypox virus can be recovered in mammalian cell cultures, and may be identified using PCR followed by RFLP analysis or sequencing. Monkeypox-specific PCR assays are available in some laboratories. PCR can also be performed directly on clinical samples. If the animal has not been exposed to other orthopoxviruses, monkeypox can be tentatively diagnosed by detecting orthopoxvirus virions with electron microscopy or orthopoxvirus antigens by immunohistochemistry.

Serum, samples of skin lesions and conjunctival swabs may be collected from live animals. Monkeypox virus has also been detected in blood, and sometimes in oral and nasal secretions (e.g., oropharyngeal swabs), urine and feces. At necropsy, tissues should be collected from all organs that have lesions. One set of tissues should be collected into 10% formalin for histopathology. A second set should be collected aseptically for virus isolation. Transport medium should not be used with the latter set of tissues. In prairie dogs, monkeypox viruses, viral DNA or antigens have been detected in skin lesions, eyelid and tongue samples, and in many internal organs including the lung, liver, spleen and lymph nodes. In dormice, monkeypox viruses have been found in most organs and tissues. One study suggested that the liver contained particularly large amounts of virus in this species. In experimentally infected ground squirrels, monkeypox antigens could be detected by immunohistochemistry in the lung, liver, lymphoid organs, esophagus and intestines.

TREATMENT

During the 2003 outbreak in the U.S., the CDC recommended that all animals with suspected monkeypox be euthanized to prevent zoonotic infections and reduce disease transmission to other animals. Nonhuman primates are not necessarily euthanized during outbreaks in facilities. Treatment is supportive. Some animals recover spontaneously.

CONTROL

Disease reporting

Veterinarians who encounter or suspect monkeypox should follow their national and/or local guidelines for disease reporting. In the U.S., state or federal authorities must be notified immediately.

Prevention

Six types of African rodents—sun squirrels (*Heliosciurus* sp.), rope squirrels (*Funisciurus* sp.), dormice, Gambian giant pouched rats, brush-tailed porcupines (*Atherurus* sp.), and striped mice (*Hybomys* sp.)—can no longer be imported into the U.S. except for scientific purposes, education or exhibition under a permit from the government. This ban applies to these animals whether they were born in Africa or on another continent. In addition, prairie dogs cannot be captured from the wild for use as pets. Restrictions also prevent the sale, exchange, transport and release of all seven species, with the exception of animals taken to a veterinarian or animal control officer for veterinary care, quarantine or euthanasia. Exceptions to the restrictions are allowed, by permit, for organizations such as zoos.

Good infection control measures, including the isolation of new animals, help prevent outbreaks in primate facilities. Care should be taken to avoid spreading the virus on fomites. Vaccination with vaccinia virus is protective. Because infections have been reported in Asian monkeys mixed with primates from Africa, these species should not be housed in the same area. Anyone who has been exposed to monkeypox should avoid contact with animals, particularly rodents and nonhuman primates, to avoid transmitting the virus to them.

During an outbreak, monkeypox may be controlled by quarantines of infected animals and tracing of their contacts. In the U.S., the CDC has recommended that animals exposed to monkeypox be quarantined for six weeks after exposure. Areas where these animals have been kept should be cleaned and disinfected; specific instructions are available from the state or local health department, or the CDC Web site. Animals that have been in contact with a monkeypox-infected animal may be placed under quarantine for 6 weeks from the date of the last exposure.

During outbreaks, veterinarians should remain aware of current recommendations from their state and local health departments. During the 2003 outbreak in the U.S., some states recommended that animals with suspected monkeypox not be taken to veterinary hospitals, to prevent human exposure. Animals that may have this disease should never be brought to a veterinary clinic without first contacting the clinic so that precautions may be taken. To avoid exposing other people and animals, the animal should enter the facility through a separate area. When it is transported, it should be kept in a cage (or box with air holes) and handled using heavy rubber gloves and a long-sleeved shirt to prevent scratches and exposure to body fluids. If the animal is likely to bite, heavier gloves would be appropriate. In the clinic, monkeypox suspects should be kept isolated, and handled using PPE. If the animal has died, the carcass should be double-bagged and frozen pending necropsy. For additional preventative measures, see "Infections in Humans."

MORBIDITY AND MORTALITY

The prevalence of infection in wild primates is unknown. In one study, 8% of nonhuman primates in Africa were seropositive. Few outbreaks have been reported among captive primates. The morbidity rate is usually high and the mortality rate low; most adult animals recover. More severe illness may be seen in infants, which may die, as well as in cynomolgus monkeys, orangutans, and primates of all ages infected experimentally via aerosols. Cynomolgus monkeys developed more severe clinical signs after inoculation with a Congo Basin virus than a West African strain.

Prairie dogs appear to be very susceptible to monkeypox. In black-tailed prairie dogs, the mortality rate was 50% in animals inoculated subcutaneously with a Congo Basin strain, and 25% in animals inoculated intranasally. Prairie dogs infected with a West African strain by either route did not die in this experiment. Other experiments have, however, demonstrated fatal disease in prairie dogs infected with West African strains. In one study, intranasal inoculation of a West African strain resulted in 60% mortality, and intraperitoneal inoculation was uniformly fatal. In the U.S. outbreak, which was caused by a West African strain, some prairie dogs died rapidly, but others recovered.

In Africa, monkeypox infections may be particularly common among squirrels; antibodies have been found in 24-50% of rope squirrels (*Funisciurus* spp.) and 15-50% of *Heliosciurus* spp. squirrels. Fatal infections have been reported in rope squirrels, but the mortality rate in this species is unknown. Infections have also been documented among Gambian giant pouched rats and dormice. In one study, 16% of giant pouched rats in Africa were seropositive. During the outbreak in the U.S., monkeypox virus was found in one giant pouched rat that died soon after arrival. Another member of this species had a very mild illness, and orthopoxvirus antibodies were found in 12 of 18 healthy animals after the outbreak. In dormice inoculated intranasally with 2-200 PFU of virus per animal, the mortality rate was dose-dependent and varied from 38% to 100%. A lower dose (0.2 PFU/dormouse) did not result in any deaths.

Experimental infections have been reported in other species of rodents. Cotton rats inoculated by the intranasal route developed acute disease with a mortality rate of 50% after intranasal inoculation and 100% after intravenous inoculation. Ground squirrels had more severe clinical signs after inoculation with a Congo Basin strain than a West African strain, but both strains resulted in 100% mortality.

INFECTIONS IN HUMANS

INCUBATION PERIOD

The incubation period is reported to be 7 to 17 days, with a mean of 12 days, in Africa. In the U.S. outbreak, the incubation period was 4 to 24 days, with a mean of 14.5 days.

CLINICAL SIGNS

In humans, monkeypox resembles smallpox; however, the symptoms are generally milder, and unlike smallpox, the lymph nodes are usually enlarged. The initial symptoms are flu-like and may include malaise, fever, chills, headache, sore throat, myalgia, backache, fatigue, lymphadenopathy (most often affecting the submandibular, postauricular, cervical and/or inguinal lymph nodes) and a nonproductive cough. Nausea, vomiting and conjunctivitis were also reported from some cases in the U.S. A rash, initially characterized by macules and papules, develops one to several days after the prodromal signs; these lesions develop into vesicles and pustules ("pocks"), which umbilicate, form scabs and are eventually shed. The number of skin lesions varies from less than 25 to more than a hundred. They are usually concentrated on the extremities (a centrifugal pattern) but can also be seen on the head and torso. Lesions may develop on the mucous membranes, as well as on the palms, soles and genitalia. Confluent rashes and recurrent febrile periods can occur in severe cases. Corneal ulceration, coagulation disorders, respiratory complications including dyspnea, encephalitis (rarely) and multiorgan failure have also been reported. Although most patients survive, some cases end in death. In patients who recover, the illness generally lasts for 2 to 4 weeks, and the skin lesions usually resolve within 14 to 21 days. Residual varioliform scarring, with hypopigmented and/or hyperpigmented skin lesions may be a sequela. Severe scarring, as seen in smallpox, is rare. Subclinical and very mild cases have also been reported.

The 2003 monkeypox outbreak in the U.S., which was caused by a West African strain of the virus, differed in some respects from the classical description of the disease in Africa. Most people in the U.S. had a relatively mild form of the disease, with less marked lymphadenopathy than reported in Africa, relatively few lesions and a self-limiting course. In many patients, the skin lesions were localized and confined to the extremities; generalized rash was rare. Some pustules had prominent erythematous flares; such flares have not been noted in African cases, possibly because most affected people have darker skin. In the U.S., skin lesions sometimes occurred at a bite or scratch, the apparent inoculation site, before systemic signs developed. The skin lesions usually healed without dyspigmented scars in this outbreak. Two severe cases were reported, both in children. One child developed encephalitis, a complication that had been reported only once before. The other child had generalized lesions including lesions in the oropharynx, and severe cervical and tonsillar lymphadenopathy, which caused difficulty in breathing and swallowing. An adult developed complications of keratitis and corneal ulceration, and received a corneal transplant. Patients with other symptoms of monkeypox and immunological evidence of exposure, but no skin lesions, were described in this outbreak. All patients recovered.

DIAGNOSTIC TESTS

Monkeypox can be tentatively diagnosed if the characteristic skin lesions are present and there is a history of exposure. Electron microscopy identifying orthopoxviruses in skin lesions and immunohistochemistry for orthopoxvirus antigens are suggestive, but the specific virus cannot be identified with these techniques. A definitive diagnosis can be made by isolating the monkeypox virus from skin lesions (e.g., in scabs or material from vesicles) or throat and nasopharyngeal swabs. This virus can be recovered in mammalian cell cultures, and may be identified using PCR followed by restriction fragment-length polymorphism (RFLP) analysis or sequencing. Monkeypox-specific PCR assays are available in some laboratories, and a DNA oligonucleotide microarray can identify this virus rapidly and specifically. PCR can also be performed directly on clinical samples.

Serology may also be helpful. Convalescent-phase serum can be tested for orthopoxvirus-specific IgM with an enzyme-linked immunosorbent assay (ELISA) if the lesions have resolved. Cross-reactions between orthopoxviruses, including smallpox and monkeypox viruses, can occur in serological tests. Cross-adsorbed virus neutralization, immunofluorescence or hemagglutination inhibition assays, as well as immunoblotting (Western blotting), can be used to distinguish reactions between monkeypox virus and smallpox virus. However, cross-adsorption assays are not always easy to interpret. The possibility of exposure to undiscovered orthopoxviruses also complicates the interpretation of serology in endemic areas. A specific ELISA that may detect monkeypox antibodies in people vaccinated for smallpox has been reported in the literature.

TREATMENT

Treatment of monkeypox is mainly supportive. The antiretroviral drug cidofovir has been promising *in vitro* and in animal studies, but its efficacy against monkeypox in humans is unknown. The toxic effects of this drug must also be considered. The efficacy of vaccinia immune globulin (which was used to treat smallpox) in cases of monkeypox is unknown.

CONTROL

As a routine preventive measure, care should be taken to treat and cover breaks in the skin when working with nonhuman primates or other animals that may be hosts. Smallpox vaccination, particularly when recent, appears to provide some protection from monkeypox. Post-exposure vaccination also seems to be helpful. The CDC currently recommends this vaccine only for people who have been or are likely to be exposed to monkeypox. The general population is not currently vaccinated in endemic areas of Africa. Any consideration of routine vaccination in healthy people must evaluate the risks and expense of the vaccine, as well as the benefits, in that population. Some people, including those with severe T cell immunodeficiencies, may not be able to receive the smallpox vaccine.

Isolation of infected patients, good infection control measures and ring vaccination are helpful in preventing person-to-person transmission. Because the full host range of monkeypox virus is uncertain, infected individuals should also limit their contact with any pet, particularly species known to be susceptible.

Infection control procedures such as good hygiene, frequent hand washing, and disinfection of surfaces and equipment are important during contact with animals suspected to have monkeypox. As few people as possible should be exposed. Veterinarians and staff should use personal protective equipment (PPE) including gloves and a gown when examining or treating these animals. Eye protection such as tightly fitted goggles or a face shield is advisable if body fluids might be sprayed. Aerosol transmission can be prevented with a N-95 filtering or comparable disposable respirator. If no respirator is available in the clinic, a surgical mask gives some protection from transmission by contact or large droplets. Veterinarians who do not wish to examine or treat any animal with monkeypox may refer clients to the local or state health department for guidance. Anyone who has been in contact with a monkeypox suspect should contact a health care provider immediately. The local or state health department must also be informed.

Necropsies should be done in Biosafety Level 2 laboratories, using a certified Class II Biological Safety Cabinet. The person performing the necropsy should have a recent smallpox vaccination and wear PPE. The CDC recommends that veterinarians in private practice avoid performing necropsies or biopsies due to the zoonotic risk. PPE should be used when collecting other types of clinical samples.

MORBIDITY AND MORTALITY

Case fatality rates of 0% to 33% have been reported during outbreaks of monkeypox in Africa. Congo Basin (Central African) strains of the virus, such as those found in the Democratic Republic of Congo (DRC), seem to cause more severe disease than the West African clade. In recent surveillance from the DRC, the case fatality rate was approximately 10-17%. The highest risk of death is in young children. Monkeypox seems to be less severe in people who have been vaccinated for smallpox, although the protection might decrease with time.

In Africa, monkeypox is usually seen in rural populations, particularly in children. Most cases occur among people who live in or near heavily forested areas, where the virus is thought to be endemic in animals. Infections tend to occur after contact with wild small mammals, which are caught for food and other purposes. In the past, monkeypox was thought to be a rare disease; however, recent data from the Congo Basin may challenge that assumption. Active surveillance conducted in the DRC between 1981 and 1986 indicated an incidence of < 1 case per 10,000 population. In contrast, the average annual incidence in the central DRC was 5.5 cases per 10,000 population (760 cases) during active surveillance from 2005 to 2007. Passive surveillance programs reported 215 possible monkeypox cases to the DRC Ministry of Health between 1998 and 2002, and 88 were subsequently confirmed by laboratory testing. Sporadic cases and outbreaks have also been documented in neighboring countries. Because most of these cases occurred in young people born after smallpox vaccination ended, some authors suggest that waning immunity may be contributing to an increase in the prevalence rate. Other societal factors (e.g., changes resulting from poverty or war) that increase exposure to the reservoir hosts are also plausible.

Current information on monkeypox in residents of West Africa is limited. No outbreaks have been reported recently in endemic areas; however, these viruses are thought to cause milder illness than the Congo Basin clade, and cases might be underreported. In a recent survey from Ghana, antibodies to orthopoxviruses were found in 36% of young people who had not been vaccinated against smallpox and lived near a forest where monkeypox is endemic. These individuals frequently entered these forests, but reported no previous illness suggestive of this disease. Because it is difficult to distinguish antibodies to the various orthopoxviruses, the study could not exclude reactivity to other, unknown orthopoxviruses circulating in the area. Another study reported serological evidence of recent exposure to orthopoxvirus(es) among young, unvaccinated individuals in Sierra Leone.

Most monkeypox outbreaks in Africa have been short-lived and self-limiting, with only limited person-to-person spread. Through the mid-1980s, estimates of the human-to-human transmission rates ranged from 3.3% to 30%. In 1996-1997, an outbreak in the DRC continued for more than a year, with a person-to-person transmission rate estimated at 78%. However, epidemiological evidence suggests that many of the cases in this outbreak may have been chickenpox (varicella), resulting in an inflated estimate of the transmission rate for monkeypox. Person-to-person transmission with six serial transmissions was reported during an outbreak in the Republic of Congo (RCG) in 2003; before this time, the maximum number of serial transmissions was four. Sustained transmission of monkeypox virus in human populations has not been reported.

The monkeypox outbreak in the U.S. was caused by a West African strain of the virus. In this outbreak, people became infected after direct contact with pet prairie dogs. One case was originally thought to have been acquired from a rabbit, but testing (unpublished) by the CDC determined that the rabbit was not infected. African rodents were not implicated in direct transmission to humans in this outbreak, although some of these animals had high viral titers. The types of behavioral interactions with humans may have contributed to this phenomenon. Seventy-two human infections were reported in this outbreak, with 37 of these laboratory confirmed. Most clinical cases were relatively mild. Severe disease occurred in two children, as the result of encephalitis or generalized monkeypox, but no deaths were reported. The availability of advanced health care facilities and good supportive care, as well as the absence of poor nutrition and concurrent diseases, may have contributed to the survival rate. The route of inoculation might also contribute to differences in clinical signs or severity; some people in Africa may be infected by ingestion during food preparation.

NEWCASTLE DISEASE

Avian Paramyxovirus-1 Infection, Goose Paramyxovirus Infection, Ranikhet Disease

IMPORTANCE

Newcastle disease is a viral disease of birds caused by avian paramyxovirus 1 (APMV-1). For official control purposes, this disease is currently defined as the most severe form of the illness, which is caused only by certain viral strains. Many less virulent strains of APMV-1 also circulate among domesticated and wild birds. These viruses usually cause much milder clinical signs or infect birds asymptomatically. However, they can sometimes evolve to become the highly virulent strains that cause Newcastle disease.

Newcastle disease is considered to be one of the most important poultry diseases in the world. Chickens are particularly susceptible, and may experience morbidity and mortality rates up to 100%. Outbreaks can have a tremendous impact on backyard chickens in developing countries, where these birds are a significant source of protein and this disease is endemic. In developed countries, where highly virulent APMV-1 strains have usually been eradicated from poultry, trade embargoes and restrictions cause significant economic losses during outbreaks. Newcastle disease can also affect other commercial poultry, game birds, ratites, and various pet, hobby and zoo birds. Some of these birds become ill, while others carry and shed virulent viruses asymptomatically. Subclinically infected birds, particularly illegally imported psittacines, can introduce Newcastle disease into countries where it does not usually exist.

A number of recent studies have examined the epidemiology of APMV-1 in wild birds. Although these birds are mainly infected with low pathogenicity strains of APMV-1, highly virulent strains circulate in some cormorant populations in North America. Outbreaks occur periodically in cormorants, with severe illness and deaths in young birds. Viruses from cormorants can also infect nearby gulls, and could spread to other wild or domesticated birds. Strains of APMV-1 maintained in wild (and domesticated) Columbiformes may also be a concern, although these particular viruses generally tend to cause serious disease only in pigeons and doves. Recently, several papers described sporadic infections with virulent APMV-1 viruses in various wild birds throughout the world. The significance of this finding is still uncertain.

ETIOLOGY

Avian paramyxoviruses belong to the genus *Avulavirus* in the family Paramyxoviridae. Twelve serotypes of these viruses (APMV-1 through APMV-12) have been identified in birds. The viruses that cause Newcastle disease belong to avian paramyxovirus type 1 (APMV-1), and are also called Newcastle disease viruses (NDV). APMV-1 strains maintained in Columbiformes (pigeons and doves) have some antigenic differences from other isolates, and are often called pigeon paramyxovirus type 1 (PPMV-1).

APMV-1 viruses have been classified into three or more pathotypes based on their virulence in chickens. Lentogenic strains are the least virulent, mesogenic strains are moderately virulent, and velogenic strains are the most virulent. Most strains cluster toward the two extremes of virulence, and are either lentogenic or velogenic. Some authors also identify an "asymptomatic enteric" group, while others consider these to be lentogenic viruses. Velogenic viruses can be subdivided into two groups: strains that cause a neurotropic form, typically associated with respiratory and neurologic signs, and strains that cause a viscerotropic form with hemorrhagic intestinal lesions. However, these clinical forms are not necessarily clear-cut and can overlap

The World Organization for Animal Health (OIE) has defined Newcastle disease as an infection caused by highly virulent APMV-1 viruses – isolates that have either an intracerebral pathogenicity index (ICPI) of at least 0.7 in day-old chicks, or amino acid sequences in the viral fusion (F) protein that resemble those seen in previously isolated, highly virulent viruses. Such viruses must be reported to the OIE and have severe repercussions for international trade. This definition has been widely adopted by many countries, although other definitions were sometimes used in the past. For example, the term "Newcastle disease" has also been used for the illness caused by any APMV-1 strain (including

lentogenic viruses), and the U.S. formerly defined "exotic Newcastle disease" as the disease caused only by velogenic viscerotropic strains.

Two different classification systems have been used to divide APMV-1 into genotypes for epidemiological purposes, although a unified system was recently proposed. For this reason, an APMV-1 isolate can have more than one designation. One system, as well as the unified system, separates APMV-1 isolates into two clades, called class I and class II. Each of these classes is further divided into genotypes. The vast majority of APMV-1 strains belong to class II, which contains both highly virulent and nonpathogenic strains. Class I isolates have been found mainly in wild waterfowl and some live bird markets, and are usually of low pathogenicity. Some virulent APMV-1 genotypes are particularly significant, as they have spread widely and have been identified as possible panzootic viruses.

SPECIES AFFECTED

APMV-1 viruses are known to infect more than 250 species of birds in 27 orders; other avian species are also likely to be susceptible.

Wild birds

The epidemiology of APMV-1 is incompletely understood; however, the vast majority of the viruses found in wild birds have been lentogenic. Some species, particularly aquatic birds such as waterfowl, may be reservoir hosts for these viruses. Lentogenic viruses appear to be capable of developing into the velogenic viruses that cause Newcastle disease. The circulation of lentogenic APMV-1 viruses around the world is still under investigation; however, there is evidence that some viruses can spread between continents or hemispheres in wild birds, as well as in poultry. Strains of viruses that seem to originate from live vaccines (i.e., low virulence isolates) have also been found in wild birds in some locations.

In North America, virulent APMV-1 viruses have become established in some cormorant (*Phalacrocorax* sp.) populations. These viruses can also infect gulls, and there is a risk that they could spread to poultry. Other velogenic APMV-1 strains have been found sporadically in wild birds in other parts of the world. Reports have described infections in diverse avian species, including shorebirds, waterfowl, passerines and wild pheasants. Some of these birds seem to have been infected by contact with poultry during local outbreaks. In other cases, authors have speculated that wild birds might transmit virulent viruses during migration, or even act as reservoirs for some genotypes. In the past, velogenic APMV-1 viruses were thought to be endemic in wild psittacine populations; however, it now appears that their high prevalence in imported psittacines is the result of infections spreading subclinically among these birds after capture.

Domesticated birds

Lentogenic, mesogenic and velogenic APMV-1 viruses can have been reported to infect domesticated birds and a number of captive wild species. Poultry and some other birds are important in maintaining these viruses. However, some species are more likely to develop Newcastle disease than others. Chickens are highly susceptible to velogenic strains and usually become severely ill if they are infected. Turkeys develop less severe signs than chickens, and the susceptibility of other gallinaceous game birds (pheasants, partridges, peacocks, quail and guinea fowl) is variable. Infections are usually inapparent in ducks and geese; however, some isolates have caused outbreaks among geese in China since the 1990s. Outbreaks have also been reported recently among ducks in China, although the pathogenicity of these viruses remains to be completely investigated. One isolate caused severe signs in intramuscularly inoculated ducks, but the signs were much milder when the virus was administered by a more natural (oronasal) route. Newcastle disease has also been reported in ratites and various species of zoo, pet and hobby birds, such as owls, raptors, penguins and corvids. It is reported to be an important cause of illness among captive falcons in the Middle East. Among psittacine birds, cockatiels (*Nymphicus hollandicus*) are reported to be highly susceptible, but illnesses have also been reported in conures (*Aratinga* spp.), some parrots and experimentally infected budgerigars (*Melopsittacus undulates*).

Pigeon Paramyxovirus 1

PPMV-1 circulates in domesticated pigeons and some populations of wild pigeons and doves. While these viruses mainly affect Columbiformes, occasional outbreaks or clinical cases have been documented in other species including captive game birds (pheasants, partridges), chickens and turkeys. PPMV-1 viruses may cause only mild signs initially in poultry, but can become more virulent as they continue to circulate. PPMV-1 viruses have also been isolated from other birds, including passerine birds, waterfowl and raptors.

Mammals

Naturally occurring APMV-1 infections were once thought to be rare or nonexistent in mammals. However, one virus was isolated from a calf in the 1950s, and more recently, lentogenic viruses were detected in two healthy sheep, and isolated multiple times from pigs in China. Several isolates from pigs shared high homology with vaccine strains used in poultry. These viruses may have spread to pigs from nearby poultry, or from piglets treated for diarrhea with Newcastle disease vaccines, a practice employed in some parts of China. The significance of APMV-1 infections in mammals, if any, is uncertain, but additional isolations seem likely as more surveillance is conducted.

Experimental infections with APMV-1 viruses have been reported in cattle, nonhuman primates, rabbits, ferrets and small mammals (guinea pigs, hamsters).

Zoonotic potential

Newcastle disease viruses can infect humans, although this seems to occur only after exposure to particularly high concentrations of virus.

GEOGRAPHIC DISTRIBUTION

Velogenic APMV-1 viruses are endemic among poultry in much of Asia, Africa and the Middle East, and some countries in Central and South America. Virulent strains are maintained in wild cormorants in the U.S. and Canada, but commercial poultry are free of velogenic isolates. Lentogenic isolates occur in poultry and wild birds throughout the world.

TRANSMISSION

APMV-1 can be transmitted by inhalation or ingestion, and birds shed these viruses in both feces and respiratory secretions. Gallinaceous birds are thought to excrete APMV-1 for 1-2 weeks, but psittacine birds often shed these viruses for several months, and sometimes for more than a year. Prolonged shedding has also been reported in some members of other orders, including owls (more than four months) and cormorants (one month). Shedding can be sporadic. While aerosol transmission can occur between nearby birds, its importance in long distance transmission is controversial. In one study, APMV-1 was detected 64 meters but not 165 meters downwind of an infected farm. The survival of aerosolized virus is probably dependent on humidity and other environmental factors, as well as on the concentration of infected poultry.

APMV-1 is present in all parts of the carcass, and can persist for some time at cold temperatures. When the temperature is just above freezing (1-2°C [34-35°F]), this virus was reported to survive on chicken skin for up to 160 days and in bone marrow for nearly 200 days. Some Newcastle disease outbreaks in raptors have been linked to eating infected birds, and in 1984, a PPMV-1 outbreak among chickens in the U.K. was caused by chicken feed contaminated by infected pigeons. Some APMV-1 isolates can also be transmitted through the egg to hatching chicks. Egg-associated transmission of highly virulent isolates is possible but uncommon, as the embryo usually dies unless the viral titer in the egg is low. Other sources of virus for newly hatched chicks are feces-contaminated eggshells and cracked or broken eggs. Flies may be able to transmit APMV-1 mechanically.

APMV-1 is readily transmitted on fomites. Survival is prolonged on eggshells and especially in feces, compared to an inorganic surface (filter paper). Published information on the persistence of these viruses is highly variable, probably because it can be affected by many factors such as humidity, temperature, the suspending agent and exposure to light, as well as the technique used to detect the viruses. One study reported that APMV-1 survived in contaminated, uncleaned poultry houses for up to 7 days in summer, as long as 14 days in the spring, and 30 days during the winter. Another group reported virus isolation up to 16 days after depopulation of an unvaccinated flock. However, one study found that APMV-1 remained viable for up to 255 days in a henhouse, at ambient temperatures of –11°C (12°F) to 36°C (97°F). At 23-29°C (73-84°F), APMV-1 is reported to survive in contaminated litter for 10 to 14 days, and at 20°C (68°F) in soil for 22 days. Virus has also been recovered from earthworms for 4 to 18 days, and from experimentally contaminated lake water for 11 to 19 days.

DISINFECTION

Effective disinfectants for APMV-1 include sodium hypochlorite, phenolic disinfectants, glutaraldehyde, chlorhexidine and oxidizing agents (e.g. Virkon®). Quaternary ammonium compounds may be effective if used in the presence of sodium carbonate. APMV-1 can also be inactivated by heat of 56°C (133°F) for 3 hours, or 60°C (140°F) for 30 minutes, and is susceptible to acid (pH 3), ether and formalin. The effectiveness of formalin varies with the temperature.

INCUBATION PERIOD

The incubation period for APMV-1 infections in poultry ranges from 2 to 15 days, and is commonly 2-6 days in chickens infected with velogenic isolates. Incubation periods up to 25 days have been reported in some other avian species. In pigeons, PPMV-1 causes clinical signs after 4 to 14 days, with some authors reporting incubation periods as long as 3-4 weeks.

CLINICAL SIGNS

APMV-1 viruses can cause varying clinical signs, depending on the pathogenicity of the isolate and the species of bird. Lentogenic strains usually infect chickens subclinically or cause mild respiratory disease, with signs such as coughing, gasping, sneezing and rales. Illnesses caused by mesogenic strains can be more severe in this species. There may be respiratory signs, decreased egg production, and in some cases, neurological signs, but the mortality rate is usually low. With both lentogenic and mesogenic viruses, the illness can be more severe if the flock is co-infected with other pathogens.

Velogenic strains cause severe, often fatal, illnesses in chickens, but the clinical signs can be highly variable. Early signs may include lethargic, inappetence, ruffled feathers, and conjunctival reddening and edema. Some birds develop watery, greenish or white diarrhea, respiratory signs (including cyanosis) or swelling of the tissues of the head and neck. Egg laying often declines dramatically, and eggs may be misshapen, abnormally colored, and rough or thin-shelled, with watery albumen. Sudden death, with few or no preceding clinical signs, is also seen frequently. Neurological signs (e.g., tremors, clonic spasms, paresis or paralysis of the wings and/or legs, torticollis, circling) are common in some outbreaks. CNS signs can occur concurrently with other signs of illness, but

are generally seen later in the course of the disease, and the birds may be bright and alert. Surviving chickens may have permanent neurological damage and/or a permanent decrease in egg production. Clinical signs caused by velogenic APMV-1 viruses are sometimes reported in vaccinated flocks, but these signs may be less severe.

Similar clinical signs occur in other birds; either neurological signs or respiratory signs may be more prominent in some species. Newcastle disease is generally milder in turkeys than chickens, but some strains can cause significant disease. Game birds sometimes become severely ill. Neurological signs, diarrhea and/or respiratory signs, as well as nonspecific signs of illness, have been reported in pheasants. Guinea fowl may develop clinical signs, but they can also carry velogenic isolates subclinically. Respiratory signs tend to predominate in ostriches and emus, and these birds are usually less severely affected than chickens. Geese and ducks are usually infected subclinically, even with velogenic strains of APMV-1, although there are reports of clinical cases or outbreaks. Reported clinical signs in waterfowl include nonspecific signs such as anorexia, neurological signs, diarrhea, ocular and nasal discharges, decreased egg production, and sudden death.

In psittacine birds, Newcastle disease may be acute, subacute, chronic or inapparent, with highly variable signs that can include respiratory signs (including dyspnea), neurological signs, diarrhea and sudden death. Neurological signs, including talon convulsions, the inability to coordinate flight and numerous other CNS signs, are prominent in raptors. Additional signs reported in captive falcons are inappetence, regurgitation and the excretion of metallic green urates. Some falcons have only nonspecific signs, sometimes accompanied by mucoid-hemorrhagic diarrhea, before they die, and some raptors die suddenly with few or no preceding signs.

In cormorant colonies, Newcastle disease is usually characterized by neurological signs, and illness is almost always limited to juveniles. Affected birds may be weak, with paresis or paralysis of one or both legs and/or wings, incoordination, tremors, torticollis and/or drooping of the head. Sick or dead birds can be found in the same nest as apparently normal nestmates. Older fledged cormorants may be seen trying to walk, fly, swim or dive. Neurological signs and deaths were also reported in gulls infected with this virus during some outbreaks. Sick juvenile white pelicans with neurological signs have been seen near affected cormorant colonies; however, it has not been proven that these symptoms were caused by APMV-1.

PPMV-1 and other viruses in pigeons and doves

Outbreaks caused by PPMV-1 in pigeons vary in severity. Neurological signs with a high mortality rate are often seen, but some strains can cause kidney disease with initial signs of polyuria, and sporadic cases of neurological disease in the flock. These signs may be preceded by severe drops in egg production. Bloody diarrhea can occur in some birds, and feather development may be abnormal if the infection occurs during molting. Strains of APMV-1 from chickens, including velogenic strains, often cause little or no disease in pigeons, although there have been reports of neurological signs.

Mammals

No clinical signs have been linked to APMV-1 infections in naturally infected mammals, as of 2015, although some of the infected pigs in China were reported to come from sick herds. Most experimentally infected mammals had few or no clinical signs. Mice showed nonspecific signs of illness and significant weight loss, without mortality.

POST MORTEM LESIONS

Necropsy lesions caused by velogenic APMV-1 viruses have mainly been characterized in poultry, especially chickens. The head or periorbital region may be swollen, and the interstitial tissue of the neck can be edematous, especially near the thoracic inlet. Congestion or hemorrhages are sometimes found in the caudal pharynx and tracheal mucosa, and diphtheritic membranes may occur in the oropharynx, trachea and esophagus. Petechiae and small ecchymoses may be seen in the mucosa of the proventriculus. Hemorrhages, ulcers, edema and/or necrosis often occur in the cecal tonsils and lymphoid tissues of the intestinal wall (including Peyer's patches); this lesion is particularly suggestive of Newcastle disease. Thymic and bursal hemorrhages may also be present, but can be difficult to see in older birds. The spleen may be enlarged, friable and dark red or mottled. Some birds also have pancreatic necrosis and pulmonary edema. The ovaries are often edematous or degenerated, and may contain hemorrhages. Some birds, particularly those that die suddenly or mainly have neurological signs, have few or no gross lesions.

Similar lesions have been reported in geese, turkeys, pheasants and other birds infected with velogenic strains. In some experimentally infected guinea fowl, the only significant lesions were hemorrhages at the tip of the glands of the proventriculus and in the cecal tonsil.

DIAGNOSTIC TESTS

Newcastle disease can be diagnosed by isolating APMV-1 from live or recently dead birds. Tracheal and cloacal swabs are usually taken from live birds, although fresh feces may replace cloacal swabs if collecting the latter might harm the bird. Commonly collected tissues at necropsy include spleen, lung, intestines (particularly the cecal tonsil), intestinal contents, liver, kidneys, heart and brain. The OIE also recommends collecting oronasal swabs from the carcass. APMV-1 viruses are usually isolated in embryonated chicken eggs, although cell cultures can also be used for some viruses. In particular, some PPMV-1 strains can be isolated in cell cultures but not embryonated eggs, and both culture systems should be used

when this virus is suspected. The presence of hemagglutinating activity in chorioallantoic fluid from the eggs may indicate that APMV-1 viruses are present, and these eggs can be tested with a hemagglutination inhibition (HI) assay for APMV-1. Some isolates (e.g., cormorant isolates in North America, and some velogenic viruses collected from zoo birds in Iran) do not agglutinate red blood cells. APMV-1 can cross-react with some other avian paramyxoviruses, particularly APMV-3 and APMV-7, in the HI test. A panel of monoclonal antibodies against these viruses can help resolve this issue. Reverse-transcription polymerase chain reaction (RT-PCR) assays are increasingly used to identify APMV-1 in cultures, but these tests do not necessarily detect all strains, including some that are highly virulent. Other molecular tests, such as gene sequencing and restriction enzyme analysis, may also be employed during the identification process.

The pathogenicity of an APMV-1 isolate can be quantified with several different assays. Most velogenic strains have a particular sequence, 112R/K-R-Q/K/R-K/R-R116 (multiple basic amino acids) at the C-terminus of the viral F2 protein and phenylalanine at residue 117 of the F1 protein. The presence of this genetic sequence is enough to classify an isolate as highly virulent for the purposes of international trade. If this pattern is not present, the pathogenicity of the virus must be determined in live birds. The intracerebral pathogenicity index (ICPI), which evaluates illness and death in 1-day old chicks, is currently the international standard test. This test generates values from 0 to 2.0; the most virulent viruses approach 2.0, while lentogenic strains usually have a value close to 0.0. The intravenous pathogenicity index (IVPI), which evaluates virulence in 6-week old chickens, and produces values from zero (lentogenic) to 3.0, was also in the past. However, some viruses that cause severe disease in chicken flocks have IVPI values of zero, and this test has generally fallen out of favor. Another test used more often in the past is the mean death time (MDT) in chicken embryos. In this assay, velogenic isolates have an MDT of less than 60 hours, mesogenic strains have an MDT of 60-89 hours, and lentogenic viruses have an MDT greater than 90 hours. Estimates of virulence for viruses isolated from birds other than chickens (e.g., PPMV-1 from pigeons) may not be accurate when assessed with these assays, including ICPI. There are no standardized tests to evaluate virulence for species other than chickens, but the OIE suggests experimental inoculation with a standard dose of virus, administered by a natural route such as oronasal inoculation.

RT-PCR tests can be used to identify APMV-1 directly in clinical specimens. Tracheal or oropharyngeal swabs are generally the preferred samples, as false negative results are less likely, but tissues and feces can also be employed. In the U.S., a separate RT-PCR test must be used to detect cormorant isolates, as the standard assay for other velogenic APMV-1 does not recognize these viruses. Similar results have been reported for some other isolates of APMV-1. Other types of molecular tests, such as RT loop-mediated isothermal amplification assays (RT-LAMP), have been described in the literature.

Serological assays may be useful in some circumstances. Hemagglutination inhibition is used most often, but other tests such as virus neutralization, hemagglutination or enzyme-linked immunosorbent assays (ELISA) may be employed. Vaccination or previous exposure to other APMV-1 viruses (e.g., lentogenic strains) can interfere with serological testing.

Additional tests not performed routinely for diagnosis in chickens, such as immunohistochemistry and *in situ* hybridization, may occasionally be employed.

CONTROL

Disease reporting

Veterinarians who encounter or suspect an APMV-1 infection should follow their national and/or local guidelines for disease reporting. In the U.S., state or federal authorities must be notified immediately of any suspected cases of highly virulent (velogenic) Newcastle disease.

Prevention

Good biosecurity can help protect poultry flocks from Newcastle disease. Flocks should not be allowed to contact domesticated poultry of unknown health status, any pet birds (particularly psittacines), and wild or feral birds (particularly cormorants, gulls and pigeons). Whenever possible, workers should avoid contact with birds outside the farm. Biosecurity measures include bird-proofing houses, feed and water supplies, minimizing travel on and off the facility, and disinfecting vehicles and equipment that enter the farm. Pests such as insects and mice should also be controlled. If possible, employees should shower and change into dedicated clothing for work. All in/ all out breeding (one age group per farm), with disinfection between groups, is also advisable. More detailed biosecurity guidelines are available from sources in the online factsheet.

Similar biosecurity measures can help protect birds kept in zoos or aviaries, or as pets (see Internet Resources). Pet birds should be bought only from suppliers who can certify that the birds have been imported legally or bred in the country, and are healthy. In the U.S., legally imported pet birds have been quarantined and tested for velogenic strains of APMV-1. Domestically raised birds are usually closed-banded. Vendors who are selling large numbers of young birds that belong to difficult-to-raise species (particularly when they are bargain-priced) without adequate documentation should be viewed with caution. Newly acquired birds should be isolated or quarantined for at least 30 days, and they should be monitored closely for signs of illness. Illegally imported psittacines should be reported, because many of them may be carrying velogenic APMV-1. Avian carcasses (of any species) that could be infected with velogenic Newcastle disease should never be fed to raptors, chickens or other birds.

Vaccines are commonly used to protect chickens, pheasants, some exotic birds (e.g., in aviaries or zoos) and other species from Newcastle disease. Vaccines are widely used in regions where velogenic viruses circulate among poultry. Some Newcastle disease-free countries allow vaccination to protect birds from lentogenic strains. Vaccination can protect birds from clinical signs, and may decrease virus shedding and transmission; however, some viruses can spread and/or be maintained in some vaccinated flocks. Although other factors are sometimes involved in poor vaccine efficacy in the field, there have been some concerns about whether the currently available vaccines protect birds adequately against distantly related APMV-1 genotypes. Sentinel chickens are sometimes used to monitor vaccinated flocks.

Outbreaks of Newcastle are eradicated with quarantines and movement controls, depopulation of all infected and exposed birds, thorough cleaning and disinfection of the premises, and other measures (e.g., fly control) as needed. Farms must generally remain empty for a few weeks before restocking; the specific time may vary with the climate, season and other factors. During some eradication programs, government agencies may collect and test birds that die suddenly in any facility. This measure can be helpful in recognizing new cases.

MORBIDITY AND MORTALITY

Morbidity and mortality rates vary greatly depending on the virulence of the strain and susceptibility of the host. Lentogenic and mesogenic viruses usually kill few birds; in healthy poultry, the mortality rate is approximately 10% for mesogenic strains and negligible with lentogenic strains. However, concurrent illnesses may increase the severity of illness and result in a higher death rate. In contrast, velogenic isolates have morbidity and mortality rates as high as 100% in unvaccinated, fully susceptible chickens. The onset of disease is usually rapid, and the virus often spreads quickly, particularly in group-housed flocks. Outbreaks are sometimes reported in vaccinated birds, with reduced morbidity and mortality rates. In one epidemic mainly affecting vaccinated chickens, flock mortality rates ranged from 30% to 90%.

Other species of birds tend to be less severely affected. Velogenic isolates can kill up to 100% of experimentally infected pheasants, but some individual birds may be resistant to disease, and the mortality rate reported during outbreaks is highly variable. Affected pheasant flocks lost 22% to 77% of the birds during one epizootic in Denmark, but in another outbreak in the U.K., the mortality rate was less than 3% even in the most severely affected pen. Variable mortality rates have also been reported in other species, including ostriches and guinea fowl. Newcastle disease is rarely severe in waterfowl; however, some velogenic strains circulating in China have an average morbidity rate of 17.5% and an average mortality rate of 9% in geese. One virus isolated from an outbreak in ducks in China caused very little mortality in experimentally infected ducks challenged by oronasal inoculation, although severe signs occurred after intramuscular inoculation.

APMV-1 (PPMV-1) is endemic in pigeons and doves in many countries. In these birds, morbidity rates may approach 70% or higher, and mortality rates may be as high as 40% to 100%, depending on the virus, composition of the flock and coinfections with other pathogens. Young birds are more severely affected, and some authors estimate that morbidity is approximately 10% in adult pigeons, with minimal mortality in the absence of coinfections. However, more virulent strains may exist. One strain was reported to cause > 70% mortality in healthy, experimentally infected pigeons.

The prevalence of all APMV-1 viruses in wild birds, including lentogenic strains, is often ≤ 5%, although it is reported to be higher in some surveys. To date, highly pathogenic strains have been uncommon or absent in most surveys, with the exception of North American cormorants. Outbreaks in this species are reported to only affect young cormorants; adult birds do not appear to develop clinical signs or die. The estimated mortality in juvenile cormorants during several outbreaks ranged from less than 1% to 92%. Up to 90% of juvenile white pelicans near these colonies died in some outbreaks; however, it has not been proven that the disease in pelicans was caused by APMV-1. One study that tested dead birds near outbreaks in cormorants found no evidence that APMV-1 was responsible for deaths in other species, with the exception of some gulls.

PUBLIC HEALTH

Velogenic strains of APMV-1 can cause conjunctivitis in humans, usually when the person has been exposed to large quantities of virus. Laboratory workers and vaccination crews are affected most often. Poultry workers are rarely infected, and handling or consuming poultry products does not appear to be a risk. The conjunctivitis usually resolves rapidly without treatment, but APMV-1 is shed in the ocular discharges for 4 to 7 days. All direct or indirect contact with birds should be avoided during this time.

Mild, self-limiting influenza-like disease with fever, headache and malaise has also been reported in humans; in some cases, it is uncertain whether the illness was caused by APMV-1 or misdiagnosed by cross-reactions in serologic tests. One report, confirmed by virus isolation, suggested that APMV-1 could cause serious opportunistic infections in people who are severely immunosuppressed. A patient developed fatal pneumonia 18 days after receiving a peripheral blood stem cell transplant. There was no history of contact with poultry, and the isolate was most closely related to APMV-1 viruses from pigeons.

NIPAH VIRUS INFECTION

Nipah Virus Encephalitis, Porcine Respiratory and Encephalitis Syndrome, Porcine Respiratory and Neurologic Syndrome, Barking Pig Syndrome

IMPORTANCE

Nipah virus infection is an emerging disease endemic in Southeast Asia. This virus is carried subclinically in fruit bats of the genus *Pteropus*, a host to which it seems well adapted. Illnesses caused by Nipah virus were first described in 1998-1999, during widespread outbreaks among pigs and people in Malaysia. The virus had apparently been transmitted from bats to pigs around 1996, and was thereafter maintained in swine populations. It was not detected immediately, as the mortality rate was low and the illness resembled other pig diseases. Nipah virus subsequently spread to pig farmers and abattoir workers in Malaysia and Singapore, causing severe, often fatal, encephalitis in more than 250 people. Some other species, including cats, dogs and goats, were also affected. The Malaysian outbreaks were controlled in both domesticated animals and humans by culling more than one million pigs. In addition, pig farming was permanently banned in some high-risk areas.

While Nipah virus encephalitis has not been documented in Malaysia since that time, human cases have been reported regularly in Bangladesh and a neighboring region of northern India since 2001. Many of these cases seem to be acquired directly from bats by drinking raw date palm sap, a widely consumed local delicacy. The sap is thought to become contaminated when bats visit and drink from unprotected sap collection sites at night. Person-to-person transmission also occurs after close, unprotected contact. How widely Nipah virus circulates in bats is still uncertain; however, viral RNA and seropositive bats have also been identified in areas where no clinical cases have ever been reported. A recent outbreak of neurological disease in horses and humans in the Philippines appears to have been caused by this virus.

ETIOLOGY

Nipah virus is a member of the genus *Henipavirus* in the family Paramyxoviridae. This genus also includes Hendra virus, Cedar virus (an apparently nonpathogenic virus found in Australian bats) and additional uncharacterized henipaviruses in various locations.

There seem to be multiple strains of Nipah virus. At least two major strains were isolated from pigs in Malaysia, and the strains that cause human cases in Bangladesh and India differ from outbreak strains isolated in Malaysia. A henipavirus that recently caused an outbreak in the Philippines is also thought to be Nipah virus, based on RT-PCR results. It appears to be most similar to the viruses from Malaysia.

N

SPECIES AFFECTED

Fruit bats of the genus *Pteropus* (flying foxes) are the main reservoir hosts for Nipah virus. *P. vampyrus*, the Malayan flying fox, and *P. hypomelanus*, the island flying fox, are known to carry this virus in Malaysia. *P. giganteus* is thought to be an important host in Bangladesh and India and possibly other locations. Although live virus has not yet been isolated from this species, Nipah virus RNA has been detected and many bats are seropositive. Nipah virus also occurs in *P. lylei* in Thailand and Cambodia, and *P. poliocephalus* has been infected experimentally. Viral RNA and/or antibodies have been found in a few other species of fruit or insectivorous bats, although their significance is unclear

Many domesticated mammals seem to be susceptible to Nipah virus. This virus can be maintained in pig populations, but other domesticated animals appear to be incidental (spillover) hosts. Sick goats, dogs, cats and horses were observed in the outbreak area in Malaysia, and infections in dogs, a cat, a horse and goats were confirmed by immunohistochemistry. Sheep might also have been affected, but there are no confirmatory data, and no evidence of infections could be found in rats. Nipah virus seems to have affected horses in the Philippines in 2014, based on clinical signs in the horses and epidemiological links to human patients; however, no tissues were available from the horses for confirmation. Several cats and a dog that had eaten tissues from sick horses in the Philippines also died, and seropositive dogs were reported in the outbreak area. Another study reported seropositive cattle, pigs and goats in Bangladesh; however, these antibodies did not neutralize Nipah virus, and could have been caused by related henipaviruses.

Experimental infections with Nipah virus have established in pigs, cats, ferrets, nonhuman primates, guinea pigs, golden hamsters (*Mesocricetus auratus*) and mice.

Zoonotic potential

Nipah virus can cause serious illnesses in people. A number of cases have been linked to drinking raw date palm sap, which had probably been contaminated by bats. Drinking fermented date palm sap (alcohol content approximately 4%) appeared to be a risk factor in a few cases. Zoonotic cases were acquired from pigs in Malaysia (bat to human transmission appears to be uncommon or absent in this area), while people who became infected in the Philippines had either eaten undercooked meat from sick horses or participated in their slaughter. A few cases in Bangladesh and Malaysia might have been acquired from sick animals of other species (a dog, various livestock), but the evidence in these cases was speculative and/or circumstantial.

GEOGRAPHIC DISTRIBUTION

Nipah virus might be endemic across much of Southeast Asia; however, confirmed cases in humans and/or domesticated animals have only been reported in Malaysia, Bangladesh and nearby areas of northern India. The virus that caused an outbreak in the Philippines has not been completely characterized yet, but it also appears to be Nipah virus. Abattoir workers in Singapore became ill after contact with infected pigs imported from Malaysia; however, there is no evidence that this virus is endemic among pigs in Singapore. Nipah virus has been isolated from bats in Cambodia, and viral RNA has been detected in bats in Thailand and East Timor. Antibodies to Nipah virus or other henipaviruses have been found in bats in additional Asian countries (e.g., China, Vietnam) and on other continents; however, viral and serological evidence suggests that at least some of these viruses might be distinct viral species.

TRANSMISSION

In *Pteropus* bats, Nipah virus has been found repeatedly in urine, and viral RNA has been detected rarely in oropharyngeal swabs and rectal swabs from naturally or experimentally infected bats. It has also been found in fruit that had been partially eaten by bats. Despite high seroprevalence rates, only a few bats in a colony may shed the virus at any given time, and excretion from the colony may be sporadic.

How bats transmit this virus to domesticated animals is uncertain, but ingestion of contaminated fruit, water, or aborted bat fetuses or birth products (e.g., by pigs) is suspected. Nipah virus is highly contagious in swine, which can act as amplifying hosts and shed this virus in respiratory secretions and saliva. Experimental infections suggest that shedding may start as early as 2 days after infection and persist for up to 3 weeks. During the Malaysian outbreak, Nipah virus appeared to be transmitted within a farm by aerosols and direct contact between pigs; virus spread between farms was usually associated with pig movements. Although this virus has not been reported, to date, in the urine of pigs, it can occur in the kidneys, and exposure to pig urine is a risk factor for human infections. Anecdotal evidence suggests that vertical transmission may occur across the placenta. Transmission in semen may be possible, and re-used vaccination needles may have contributed to the spread of the virus between pigs in Malaysia.

Cats can be infected experimentally by intranasal and oral inoculation, and they can shed Nipah virus in respiratory secretions and urine. Cats and a dog that died in the Philippines had recently eaten meat from infected horses. *In utero* transmission has been demonstrated in cats, with the detection of virus in the placenta and embryonic fluids. Although experimental studies have not been published in dogs, serological surveys in Malaysia suggest that Nipah virus did not spread horizontally in dogs during this outbreak.

Humans can be infected by direct contact with infected swine, probably through the mucous membranes, but possibly also through skin abrasions. During a recent Nipah-like outbreak in the Philippines, most patients had been involved in slaughtering sick horses or had eaten undercooked horsemeat from sick horses. In Bangladesh, human cases have been linked to drinking unpasteurized date palm sap (juice). Oral transmission, using artificial palm sap spiked with Nipah virus, and respiratory transmission were both demonstrated in a hamster model. Person-to-person transmission can occur after close direct contact, and has been common during some outbreaks in Bangladesh and India. Humans can shed Nipah virus in respiratory secretions, saliva, and urine, and contact with respiratory secretions is thought to be the main route of spread. Some people also became ill after unprotected contact with deceased patients, such as during preparation of the corpse for burial. Nosocomial transmission has been documented in hospitals where infection control measures are inadequate; however, the risk to healthcare workers appeared to be low in Malaysian hospitals.

How long Nipah virus can remain viable in the general environment is uncertain; however, it can survive for up to 3 days in some fruit juices or mango fruit, and for at least 7 days in artificial date palm sap (13% sucrose and 0.21% BSA in water, pH 7.0) held at 22°C. This virus is reported to have a half-life of 18 hours in the urine of fruit bats.

DISINFECTION

Like other paramyxoviruses, Nipah virus is readily inactivated by soaps, detergents and many disinfectants. Routine cleaning and disinfection with sodium hypochlorite or commercially available disinfectants is expected to be effective. Sodium hypochlorite was recommended for the disinfection of pig farms in Malaysia.

The effect of heat may depend on the substrate. Nipah virus concentrations decreased but the virus was not completely eliminated in artificial palm sap held at 70°C for 1 hour. However, it was completely inactivated by heating at 100°C for more than 15 minutes.

INFECTIONS IN ANIMALS

INCUBATION PERIOD

The incubation period in pigs is estimated to be 7 to 14 days, but it may be as short as four days. Experimentally infected cats developed clinical signs after 6-8 days and experimentally infected ferrets after 6-10 days.

CLINICAL SIGNS

Pigs

Subclinical infections appear to be common in pigs. Symptomatic infections are usually acute febrile illnesses, but fulminating infections and sudden death have also been seen. In general, mortality is low except in young piglets.

A respiratory syndrome appears to be the most common presentation in 1-6 month old pigs, with clinical signs that may include fever, nasal discharge, open mouthed breathing, rapid and labored respiration and a loud barking cough. Hemoptysis can occur in severe cases. Pigs in this age group occasionally develop neurological signs such as trembling, twitching, muscle spasms, myoclonus, weakness in the hind legs, spastic paresis, lameness, an uncoordinated gait when they are driven or hurried, and generalized pain that is particularly evident in the hind quarters. One experiment suggested that bacterial meningitis might be a contributing factor in some animals, especially when the neurological signs develop later in the course of the disease.

Similar clinical signs can occur in sows and boars, although neurological signs appear to be more common in sows than younger animals. Reported signs in these pigs include agitation, head pressing, nystagmus, chomping of the mouth, tetanus-like spasms, seizures and apparent pharyngeal muscle paralysis. Some sows aborted during Nipah virus outbreaks, generally during the first trimester. Sudden death may also be seen.

In piglets, common signs include open-mouthed breathing, leg weakness with muscle tremors, and twitching. Deaths may also occur due to starvation if the dam is ill.

Other species

Horses thought to be infected with Nipah virus in the Philippines either developed acute, fatal neurological signs or died suddenly with no apparent preceding illness. Although significant numbers of dogs and cats may have been infected on farms in Malaysia, clinical cases have been published for only two dogs. One of these animals had died of the illness, and the clinical signs were not described. In the other dog, the disease resembled canine distemper; the clinical signs included fever, respiratory distress, conjunctivitis, and mucopurulent nasal and conjunctival discharges. Experimental inoculation of cats with Nipah virus resulted in severe respiratory signs with fever, depression, an increased respiratory rate and dyspnea. Three cats thought to have been infected during an outbreak in the Philippines were found dead, while a fourth was moribund with terminal bleeding from the nose and mouth. Experimentally infected ferrets developed severe depression, serous nasal discharge, coughing, dyspnea, tremors and hind limb paresis. Neurological and/or respiratory signs, which can be severe, have also been reported in some experimentally infected hamsters.

An unproductive cough, poor growth, severe respiratory signs and deaths were documented in naturally infected goats in Malaysia. Two goats associated with a Nipah case in Bangladesh had a febrile neurological syndrome, but whether their illness was caused by Nipah virus or another disease is unknown.

Infections in fruit bats appear to be asymptomatic.

POST MORTEM LESIONS

In pigs, lesions may be found in the lungs, brain or both organs. Lung lesions range from mild to severe, and

N

can include varying degrees of consolidation, petechial or ecchymotic hemorrhages, and emphysema. On cut surface, the interlobular septa may be distended. The bronchi and trachea may contain frothy, sometimes bloodstained, fluid. In the brain, there may be congestion of the cerebral blood vessels and meningeal edema. Mottled, enlarged and congested lymph nodes were also reported in some experimentally infected pigs. The kidneys may be congested with petechiae in the renal capsule and cortex, but are often normal.

In dogs, necropsy lesions have been reported only for two animals. In one dog, diffuse red-pink mottling and consolidation were seen in the lungs, with exudates in the bronchi and trachea. The visceral pleura were yellowish-cream and opaque. Irregular reddening was noted in the renal capsules and cortices. In addition, nonsuppurative meningitis, signs of cerebral and hepatic vascular degeneration, and necrosis and inflammation of the adrenal gland were seen. Similar lesions were reported in the other dog, although there was severe autolysis.

Lesions in experimentally infected cats included hydrothorax, consolidation and edema in the lungs, edema of the pulmonary lymph nodes and froth in the bronchi. Meningitis was reported in some cats after histopathological examination. More subtle lesions were seen in earlier stages of the disease; they included numerous small hemorrhagic nodules in the lungs, scattered hemorrhagic nodules on the visceral pleura, and, in one cat, edema of the bladder serosa with dilation of the serosal lymphatic vessels. Generalized vasculitis was seen in one naturally infected cat in Malaysia, particularly in the brain, kidney, liver and, to a lesser extent, the lung.

Nonsuppurative meningitis was reported in an infected horse in Malaysia.

DIAGNOSTIC TESTS

Nipah virus infections can be diagnosed by virus isolation, the detection of antigens or nucleic acids, and serology. Histopathology also aids diagnosis. In swine, Nipah virus has been detected in respiratory secretions, blood and various tissues including the bronchial and submandibular lymph nodes, lung, spleen, kidney and brain. In experimentally infected cats, this virus has been found in the lung and spleen, and less often, in the kidney, lymph nodes and other organs. It can also be detected in feline blood, urine and respiratory secretions. In dogs, viral antigens or RNA have been found in the brain, lung, spleen, kidney, adrenal gland and liver. Stringent precautions should be used to protect people when collecting samples from animals. Standardized sampling procedures, including limited sampling techniques to help safeguard personnel (e.g., 'keyhole' sampling of target tissues such as lung and lymph nodes), have been published for the closely related Hendra virus, but do not appear to be available for Nipah virus.

Reverse transcription-polymerase chain reaction (RT-PCR) assays on blood, secretions, excretions or tissue samples can be used for a rapid diagnosis. Virus isolation is available in a limited number of laboratories, as Nipah virus is a BSL4 pathogen and must be cultured under high-security conditions. This virus is often isolated in Vero cells, but many other cell lines (e.g., RK-13, BHK and porcine spleen cells) can also be used. Nipah virus can be cultured in embryonated chicken eggs; however, this system is not generally employed due to the ease of culture in cells. Isolated viruses can be identified by methods such as RT-PCR, immunostaining or virus neutralization. Electron or immunoelectron microscopy may also be helpful. Molecular methods (e.g., RT-PCR), comparative immunostaining or differential neutralization assays can distinguish Hendra and Nipah viruses. Viral antigens can be detected directly in tissues with immunoperoxidase or immunofluorescence assays.

Serology can be helpful, especially in pigs, which are often infected subclinically. Both virus neutralization and ELISAs have been used in animals. Nipah virus can cross-react with Hendra virus and other henipaviruses in these assays. These reactions can be distinguished with comparative neutralization tests.

TREATMENT

No specific antiviral treatment is available for Nipah virus. Infected animals have generally been killed to prevent the virus from being transmitted to human caretakers.

CONTROL

Disease reporting

Veterinarians who encounter or suspect a Nipah virus infection should follow their national and/or local guidelines for disease reporting. In the U.S., state or federal veterinary authorities should be informed immediately.

Prevention

Good biosecurity is important in preventing infections on pig farms; strategies should target routes of contact with other pigs as well as fruit bats. Fruit tree plantations should be removed from areas where pigs are kept. Wire screens can help prevent contact with bats when pigs are raised in open-sided pig sheds. Run-off from the roof should be prevented from entering pig pens. Fruits that may have been contaminated by bats should not be fed to pigs or other livestock. Feeding spoiled or contaminated date palm sap to livestock, as is sometimes done in endemic areas, also appears to be a dangerous practice.

Early recognition of infected pigs can help protect other animals and humans. Due to the highly contagious nature of the virus in swine populations, mass culling of seropositive animals may be necessary. Quarantines are also important in containing an outbreak; in Malaysia, Nipah virus mainly seemed to spread between farms in infected pigs. Fomites and equipment should be cleaned and disinfected. Other animals, including dogs and cats, should be prevented from contacting infected pigs or roaming between farms. No vaccines are currently available for any species.

MORBIDITY AND MORTALITY

There are few studies on the epidemiology of Nipah virus infections in flying foxes. Studies from Malaysia reported that 9-17% of *Pteropus vampyrus* and 21-27% of *P. hypomelanus* had antibodies to this virus; however, the frequency and timing of virus shedding in bats is unknown. Some studies have suggested that it may be uncommon and/or intermittent.

Nipah virus was widespread in pigs during the 1998-1999 outbreak in Malaysia. Before this virus was eradicated from domesticated swine, seropositive animals were found on approximately 5.6% of all pig farms. On one farm, more than 95% of all sows and 90% of the piglets had antibodies to this virus. The morbidity rate is estimated to approach 70-100%, but the mortality rate is low (e.g., 1-5% in 1-6 month old pigs) except in piglets. Mortality in the latter age group was approximately 40% in Malaysia, although neglect of the piglets by sick sows may have also played a role.

The frequency of Nipah virus infections in other species is unknown, although other domesticated animals were infected from pigs during outbreaks in Malaysia. While clinical cases were only confirmed in two dogs, a number of dogs are said to have died on infected farms. Farmers also reported illnesses in cats and goats. Serological surveys found seroprevalence rates of 15%-55% in dogs, 4%-6% in cats, and 1.5% in goats in the outbreak area. Infections in horses seemed to be rare during this outbreak: only five horses out of more than 3200 were positive by serology, and viral antigens were found in a single horse that died with signs of meningitis. Direct bat to animal transmission might be uncommon. In 2004, no feral cats living near an infected bat colony on Tioman Island, Malaysia had antibodies to Nipah virus.

There have apparently been no significant outbreaks among domesticated animals during human outbreaks in Bangladesh and India, and there are no published reports of proven cases in animals from this region. Whether this is due to little or no virus transmission to these animals, or limited surveillance and diagnostics is unclear. A recent human outbreak in the Philippines was linked to contact with sick horses, although it could not be confirmed that the horses were infected (no tissues were available). Four cats and one dog died soon after eating tissues from sick horses during this outbreak. Antibodies to Nipah virus were detected in dogs but not cats in the area.

INFECTIONS IN HUMANS

INCUBATION PERIOD

Clinical cases in humans usually become apparent several days to 14 days after exposure; however, incubation periods as short as 2 days or as long as a month or more have been reported. Some people with mild or subclinical infections can develop late-onset encephalitis months or years later. One such case occurred after 11 years.

CLINICAL SIGNS

Although some Nipah virus infections can be asymptomatic or mild, most recognized clinical cases have been characterized by respiratory disease and/or acute neurological signs. The initial symptoms are flu-like, with fever, headache, sore throat and myalgia. Nausea, vomiting and a nonproductive cough may also be seen. This prodromal syndrome may be followed by encephalitis, with symptoms such as drowsiness, disorientation, signs of brainstem dysfunction, convulsions, coma and other signs. Segmental myoclonus was common in patients with encephalitis in Malaysia, and cases of meningitis, as well as encephalitis, were documented in the Philippines. Nipah virus infections in some patients appear as respiratory disease, including atypical pneumonia or acute respiratory distress syndrome. These patients may or may not develop neurological signs. Septicemia, bleeding from the gastrointestinal tract, renal impairment and other complications are possible in severely ill patients. Survivors of encephalitis may have mild to severe residual neurological deficits, or remain in a vegetative state.

Some people infected with Nipah virus develop relapsed encephalitis or late-onset encephalitis, months or years later. The latter syndrome occurs in a person who was initially asymptomatic or had a non-neurological illness. The clinical signs usually develop acutely, with symptoms that may include fever, headache, seizures and focal neurological signs. Some cases are fatal.

DIAGNOSTIC TESTS

Nipah virus infections in people can be diagnosed by virus isolation, serology and RT-PCR, as in animals. In humans, this virus has been isolated from blood, throat or nasal swabs, cerebrospinal fluid (CSF) and urine samples, as well as from a variety of postmortem tissues. It is most likely to be recovered from clinical samples early in the illness, and virus isolation from the CSF is a poor prognostic sign. In patients who have died, immunohistochemistry can also be used to detect viral antigens in tissues. Nipah virus antigens are most likely to be found in the central nervous system (CNS), followed by the lung or kidney.

Serological tests used in humans include ELISAs to detect henipavirus-specific IgM or IgG, and serum neutralization.

N

Antibodies to Nipah virus occur in serum and/or CSF. IgM can be found in a significant number of patients during the illness. A rising titer, using acute and convalescent sera, is also diagnostic.

TREATMENT

Treatment is supportive, with some patients requiring measures such as mechanical ventilation. Ribavirin appeared to be promising in some outbreaks, but had little or no effect on the outcome in animal models, and its efficacy is currently considered to be uncertain. Other potential treatments, such as the administration of antibodies to Nipah virus, are being investigated in preclinical studies.

CONTROL

Pigs seem to be important amplifying hosts for Nipah virus, and preventing infections in this species can decrease the risk of infection for humans. Sick animals should not be used for food, even if the meat is to be cooked, as the slaughter process can increase human exposure to viruses in the tissues. Close contact with fruit bats and their secretions and excretions should also be avoided. Bats have been observed visiting date palm sap collection sites at night, and can contaminate collection pots with urine and saliva. While the general recommendation is to avoid drinking any unpasteurized juices in endemic regions, keeping bats away from sap collection sites with protective coverings (e.g., bamboo sap skirts) may be helpful in areas where people are unlikely to stop drinking raw date palm sap. Smearing lime on the collection area to discourage bats appeared to have little inhibitory effect in one study. Fruit should be washed thoroughly, peeled or cooked before eating. Good personal hygiene, including hand washing, is likely to reduce the risk of infection from the environment.

Nipah virus has been classified as a Hazard Group 4/ BSL4 pathogen; infected animals, body fluids and tissue samples must be handled with appropriate biosecurity precautions. People who come in close contact with potentially infected animals should wear protective clothing, impermeable gloves, masks, goggles and boots. Because Nipah virus can be transmitted from person to person, barrier nursing should be used when caring for infected patients. Patients should be isolated, and personal protective equipment such as protective clothing, gloves and masks should be used. Good hygiene and sanitation are important; in one study, hand washing helped prevent disease transmission. Vaccines are currently not available for humans.

MORBIDITY AND MORTALITY

Nipah virus has emerged repeatedly into humans in Southeast Asia, with more than 500 cases identified as of 2016. The first known cases occurred in Malaysia (and abattoir workers in Singapore) in 1998-1999, although retrospective diagnosis shows that human infections also occurred in 1997. Approximately 283 cases of encephalitis (including late onset cases) were reported in Malaysia during these outbreaks, with 109 deaths. Most people were infected by contact with pigs, and human cases were not seen after seropositive animals had been culled. However, sporadic cases and clusters have been reported most years from Bangladesh, and occasionally from India, since 2001. These infections tend to be clustered in certain regions, although isolated cases have been reported from other areas. Outbreaks in Bangladesh are seasonal and occur mainly between December and May, which is also the period when date palm sap is harvested. Drinking raw date palm sap is thought to be responsible for a number of cases, but person-to-person transmission is also significant, and nosocomial outbreaks have occurred in hospitals where barrier nursing precautions were inadequate. Additional routes of exposure, such as contact with bat excretions when climbing trees, have been suspected in some cases.

Serological studies suggest that some human infections may be asymptomatic or mild, although the prevalence of such cases is currently unclear. In the Malaysian outbreak, the subclinical infection rate was estimated to be 8%-15%. In clinical cases, the fatality rate has ranged from 38% to approximately 70-75% in various outbreaks, with higher rates reported from some small case series. The case fatality rate is reported to be much higher in Bangladesh and India than Malaysia, but whether this is due to strain variability or to differences in healthcare is uncertain. One study reported a higher mortality rate in people with diabetes. Among surviving patients, an estimated 19-32% have residual neurological deficits, and higher rates have been reported in patients with more severe neurological signs. In Malaysia, late onset or relapsed encephalitis occurred in < 5% and < 10% of patients, respectively, with an overall case fatality rate of 18%.

PESTE DES PETITS RUMINANTS

Ovine Rinderpest, Pseudorinderpest, Goat Plague, Pest of Small Ruminants, Pest of Sheep and Goats, Kata, Stomatitis-Pneumoenteritis Syndrome, Pneumoenteritis Complex

IMPORTANCE

Peste des petits ruminants (PPR) is a highly contagious viral disease that mainly affects sheep and goats. Heavy losses can be seen, especially in goats, with morbidity and mortality rates sometimes approaching 80-100%. At one time, peste des petits ruminants was thought to be restricted to the Middle East and limited areas of Africa and Asia. Recently, its range has expanded in both Africa and Asia. In addition, infections and clinical cases have been recognized in other ungulates, particularly antelope and wild relatives of sheep and goats, but also camels and water buffalo. Some clinical cases and outbreaks in these animals have been severe, and there is a risk that PPR could threaten the conservation of certain wildlife.

ETIOLOGY

Peste des petits ruminants virus (PPRV) is a member of the genus *Morbillivirus* in the family Paramyxoviridae. Four genetic lineages (lineages 1-4) and a number of viral strains have been identified. Lineage 4 viruses have become especially prevalent in recent years. PPRV is closely related to rinderpest virus, which has been eradicated.

SPECIES AFFECTED

Among domesticated animals, peste des petits ruminants is primarily a disease of goats and sheep. PPRV has also been implicated, either alone or with other pathogens, in a few outbreaks in camels and water buffalo. Cattle can be infected but they do not seem to develop clinical signs, and are not known to transmit PPRV to other animals. No clinical signs were reported in experimentally infected pigs, which also appear to be dead-end hosts.

Many species of antelope (e.g., gazelle, impala, bushbuck, springbuck) and wild relatives of domesticated small ruminants are susceptible to PPRV. Clinical cases have been reported in gazelles (e.g., Dorcas gazelle, *Gazella dorcas*; Thomson's gazelle, *Gazella thomsoni;* Rheem gazelle, *Gazella subgutturosa marica*; Arabian gazelle, *Gazella gazella*), bushbuck (*Tragelaphus scriptus*), impala (*Aepyceros melampus*), springbuck (*Antidorcas marsupialis*), gemsbok (*Oryx gazella*), bharal (*Pseudois nayaur*), Sindh ibex (*Capra aegagus blythi*), wild goats/ bezoar ibex (*Capra aegagrus*), Nubian ibex (*Capra nubiana*), Afghan Markhor goat (*Capra falconeri*), Barbary sheep (*Ammotragus lervia*) and Laristan sheep (*Ovis gmelini laristanica*). PPRV is thought to have been responsible for an outbreak that affected both gazelle and deer in Saudi Arabia in the 1980s, and white-tailed deer (*Odocoileus virginianus)* can be infected experimentally. Subclinical infections were reported in captive nilgai (Tragelophinae). Evidence of infection (antibodies and/or virological evidence of infection) has been demonstrated in additional species, such as goitered gazelle (*Gazella subgutturosa subgutturosa*), African grey duiker (*Sylvicapra grimmia*), Bubal hartebeest (*Alcelaphus buselaphus*), waterbuck (*Kobus ellipsiprymnus*), kob (*Kobus kob*) and African buffalo (*Syncerus caffer*). Whether wild ruminants are important in the epidemiology of this disease is unknown. Currently, there is no evidence that the virus circulates in wild ruminants independently of its presence in domesticated sheep and goats.

PPRV (lineage IV) nucleic acids were recently detected in the tissues of an Asiatic lion (*Panthera leo persica*) that died of trypanosomiasis.

Zoonotic potential

There is no evidence that humans are susceptible to PPRV.

GEOGRAPHIC DISTRIBUTION

Peste des petits ruminants occurs in parts of Africa and Asia, and most of the Middle East. At present, lineages 1 through 4 have been reported in parts of Africa, and lineages 3 and 4 occur in the Middle East. In Africa, PPRV was once restricted to areas south of the Sahara desert and north of the equator, and most cases were reported in West Africa. However, viruses have now spread north, south and east of these boundaries (including into North Africa). Likewise, PPRV has historically existed on the Indian subcontinent in Asia, but recently caused outbreaks in additional countries including Nepal, Vietnam and China. Only lineage 4 is currently known to exist in Asia. Lineage 3 was detected in southern India in 1992, but it has not been reported since that time.

TRANSMISSION

Transmission of PPRV mainly occurs during close contact. Inhalation is thought to be an important route of spread. This virus can be shed during the incubation period, and has been found in nasal and ocular secretions, saliva, urine and feces. It probably occurs in milk. While long-term carriage is not thought to occur, some recent studies have detected viral antigens and/or nucleic acids in the feces of clinically recovered goats for as long as 1 to 3 months. Whether live virus is also present, and if so, for how long, has not been determined. Little is known about virus shedding and transmission in other species, such as camels and antelope. PPRV is relatively fragile in the environment, and long distance aerosol transmission is unlikely; in cool temperatures and in the dark, this virus has been shown to spread for approximately 10 meters.

Fomites such as water, feed troughs and bedding can probably transmit PPRV for a short time, but do not remain infectious for long periods. There is very little information on the survival of PPRV in the environment; however, this virus is very similar to rinderpest virus, which is inactivated by ultraviolet light and desiccation within 3-4 days or less (depending on the specific environment), and normally survives for very short periods in carcasses. Temperatures above 70°C, as well as pH less than 5.6 or greater than 9.6, are also expected to inactivate PPRV. Rinderpest virus has been reported to survive for a time in refrigerated meat, and for several months in salted or frozen meat, and the survival of PPRV in meat might be similar.

DISINFECTION

PPRV can be inactivated by many disinfectants including alkalis (sodium carbonate, sodium hydroxide), halogens (sodium hypochlorite), phenolic compounds, citric acid, alcohols and iodophores.

INCUBATION PERIOD

The incubation period can range from 2 to 10 days; in most cases, clinical signs appear in 3-6 days.

CLINICAL SIGNS

The severity of the clinical signs can vary with the animal's species, breed and immunity to PPRV. Immunosuppression caused by this virus can exacerbate concurrent infections, contributing to the clinical signs.

Sheep and goats

Peracute cases can be seen when PPRV first infects naïve populations of sheep or goats. In this form, the clinical signs are generally limited to high fever, severe depression and death. More often, the illness is subacute or acute. In acute cases, the initial signs include a sudden high fever, inappetence, marked depression and somnolence. Serous nasal and ocular discharges appear soon after the onset of clinical signs; these discharges generally become mucopurulent from secondary bacterial infections. Matting is common around the eyes, and the nose may become obstructed. Within a few days, the gums become hyperemic, and small, gray, necrotic foci, covering shallow erosions, begin to appear in the mouth. (If these lesions are difficult to find, rubbing a finger across the gums and palate may recover foul-smelling exudates and shreds of tissue.) The oral lesions are painful, and animals may resist opening their mouths. Salivation is usually increased. In some cases, the mouth lesions resolve rapidly. In others, they enlarge, spread and coalesce. While lesions are most common on the lips and gums, they can also be found on the dental pad, palate, cheeks and their papillae, and tongue. In severe cases, the mouth may be completely covered in thick, cheesy material. The lips are often swollen, cracked and crusted, and the breath of animals with severe stomatitis is fetid. Necrotic lesions may also be detected on other mucous membranes, including those of the nasal cavity, vulva and vagina.

Many animals also develop profuse diarrhea, which may be watery, fetid and/or blood-stained, and sometimes contains shreds of tissue. Severely affected animals can become dehydrated and emaciated. Rapid respiration is also common, and dyspnea, coughing and other signs of pneumonia may be seen. Pasteurellosis is a frequent complication. In addition, some animals may abort. In the late stages of the disease, small nodules resembling contagious ecthyma or sheep/goat pox can appear in the skin around the muzzle. The cause of these lesions is unknown. Deaths are usually the result of dehydration and/or pneumonia. Animals that do not die often have a prolonged convalescence.

Some animals have subacute or mild cases of PPR, which can last up to 2 weeks. The clinical signs are variable, but often include respiratory signs. Asymptomatic infections are also seen.

Camels

Respiratory disease was the predominant syndrome in PPRV-infected camels during one outbreak in Ethiopia. This outbreak may have been complicated by *Streptococcus equi*. Concurrent infections with PPRV and other respiratory pathogens were found in the lungs of apparently healthy camels sampled from abattoirs in Sudan.

An outbreak among camels in Sudan was characterized by sudden death in some animals, and a more prolonged course in others. The most prominent clinical signs in the latter cases were yellowish diarrhea, which later became bloody, and abortions. Other reported signs included subcutaneous edema, submandibular swelling, "chest pain," infrequent coughing, decreased milk production, weight loss and increased water consumption. Although all ages were affected, fatal cases were most common in animals that were pregnant or had recently given birth.

Water buffalo, cattle and pigs

A highly fatal outbreak in water buffalo was characterized by depression, profuse salivation and conjunctival congestion; however, the animals were not reported to be febrile. Experimentally infected 3-5-month-old water buffalo calves developed a fever but no other clinical signs, and died in 30- 35 days. Gastrointestinal lesions were found in these calves at necropsy.

Cattle are usually asymptomatic; however, clinical signs have been reported in experimentally infected calves, and it is possible that some cattle in poor condition might become symptomatic. If they did, the syndrome would probably resemble rinderpest.

Experimentally infected pigs remained asymptomatic.

Wild ungulates

Clinical signs have been described in a few exotic species. Deer can have signs similar to sheep and goats, but subclinical infections have also been reported. Captive gazelles became severely ill during one outbreak. The initial signs were anorexia and depression, followed by fever, lacrimation, congested mucous membranes, nasal discharges, small erosions on the tongue, salivation and diarrhea. All affected animals died. Similar signs were reported in Sindh ibex. Elevated respiratory rates, lacrimation, congested mucous membranes, ocular and nasal discharges, sneezing and ocular lesions (ulcerative keratitis and conjunctivitis) were documented in wild goats. Clinical descriptions of live animals were not available from one outbreak in the United Arab Emirates; however, necropsy findings indicated involvement of the lower gastrointestinal tract (e.g., catarrhal to hemorrhagic colitis) and lungs (congestion, subacute bronchointerstitial pneumonia with occasional suppurative or fibrinopurulent pneumonia). However, no lesions were found in the upper digestive and respiratory tracts, including the oral mucous membranes, during this outbreak. Lameness has been reported in some wild ruminants, but not definitively linked to PPR.

POST MORTEM LESIONS

The postmortem lesions are characterized by inflammatory and necrotic lesions in the oral cavity and throughout the gastrointestinal tract. The respiratory tract is also affected in many cases.

The carcass is often emaciated and/or dehydrated, and there may be evidence of diarrhea, serous or mucopurulent oculonasal discharges, crusted scabs on the lips, and necrotic stomatitis. Erosions, which are shallow and sharply demarcated from normal epithelium, may be found in the mouth, and sometimes in the pharynx and upper esophagus. Similar lesions may be detected on the vulva and vaginal mucous membranes of some animals. Erosions are common in the abomasum, but the rumen, reticulum and omasum are not significantly involved (although erosions are occasionally found on the pillars of the rumen). Hemorrhagic streaks and erosions may also occur in the duodenum and the terminal ileum, but other segments of the small intestine are generally spared. The Peyer's patches often have extensive necrosis, which can lead to ulceration. The most severe lesions are seen in the large intestine, particularly around the ileocecal valve, at the cecocolic junction and in the rectum. "Zebra stripes" or "tiger stripes" of congestion, hemorrhage or darkened tissue are sometimes found in the posterior part of the colon on the mucosal folds. (These stripes can also be seen in animals with diarrhea and tenesmus from other causes). Respiratory lesions are also common, and may include congestion of the lungs; small erosions and petechiae in the nasal mucosa, turbinates, larynx and trachea; and bronchopneumonia. Blood-tinged, frothy exudates have been reported in the tracheas of some experimentally infected goats. The lymph nodes, particularly those associated with the respiratory and gastrointestinal tracts, are generally congested, enlarged and edematous, and the liver and spleen may have necrotic lesions. In peracute cases, the lesions may be limited to congestion of the ileocecal valve and bronchopneumonia.

The most prominent lesions in an outbreak among camels in Sudan included congestion and consolidation of the lungs (primarily the apical lobes), and inflammation and hemorrhages of the small intestine and stomach, together with enlarged lymph nodes and a pale, fragile liver. Oral lesions (swelling of the lips and hemorrhagic ulcers on the tongue) were reported in one animal.

The gross lesions in wild small ruminants and water buffalo are generally reported to be similar to those in sheep and goats. However, hemorrhagic and edematous gastroenteritis was found to involve the abomasum and all segments of the intestines in infected water buffalo. The presence of oral lesions might also be inconsistent in some wild species. Small erosions were found on the tongue of gazelles in one outbreak, and the esophagus contained thick mucoid deposits along the walls.

However, oral lesions and erosive mucosal lesions were absent from the upper intestinal and respiratory tracts of affected ungulates during another outbreak. In addition, congestion has been reported in visceral organs such as the liver, kidney, pancreas, spleen and brain of wild ruminants.

DIAGNOSTIC TESTS

PPRV, its nucleic acids or antigens can be detected in whole blood, swabs of ocular and nasal discharges and/or swabs of buccal and rectal mucosa. In one study, nucleic acids were detected in the buffy coat, but serum was much less likely to be diagnostic. Samples for virus isolation should be collected during the acute stage of the disease, preferably from animals with a high fever that have not yet developed diarrhea. At necropsy, samples can be collected from lymph nodes (particularly the mesenteric and bronchial nodes), lungs, spleen, tonsils and affected sections of the intestinal tract (e.g. ileum and large intestine).

In endemic regions, PPR is often diagnosed by detecting viral nucleic acids with RT-PCR assays. This disease can also be confirmed by virus isolation, but recovery of the virus is not always successful. At present, PPRV is usually isolated in African green monkey kidney (Vero) cells, although other cell lines have also been employed. The identity of the virus can be confirmed by virus neutralization or other methods.

PPRV antigens can be detected by immunocapture ELISA (ICE), counter immunoelectrophoresis (CIEP) or agar gel immunodiffusion (AGID). CEIP and ICE can distinguish PPRV from rinderpest virus, but the AGID test cannot differentiate these two viruses. AGID is also relatively insensitive, and may not be able to detect small quantities of viral antigens in milder forms of PPR. Immunofluorescence and immunochemistry can be used on conjunctival smears and tissue samples collected at necropsy.

Serological tests include virus neutralization and competitive ELISA assays. Both tests can distinguish peste des petits ruminants from rinderpest; this is not always possibly with older serological tests such as complement fixation. Whenever possible, paired sera should be taken rather than single samples. However, in countries that are PPRV-free, a single serum sample (taken at least a week after the onset of clinical signs) may be diagnostic.

TREATMENT

There is no specific treatment for PPR; however, supportive care and treatment of bacterial and parasitic coinfections may decrease mortality.

CONTROL

Disease reporting

A quick response is vital for containing outbreaks in PPRV-free regions. Veterinarians who encounter or suspect

P

this disease should follow their national and/or local guidelines for disease reporting. In the U.S., state or federal veterinary authorities should be informed immediately.

Prevention

PPRV is a short-lived virus in the environment, and it is usually spread by direct contact, and introduced by infected animals. Import controls, movement restrictions, testing and quarantine are used to exclude the virus from nonendemic areas.

In regions where peste des petits ruminants is not endemic, it can be eradicated with a combination of quarantines, movement controls, euthanasia of infected and exposed animals, and cleaning and disinfection of infected premises. Ring vaccination and/or vaccination of high-risk populations may also be helpful. The rapid inactivation of PPRV in the environment aids eradication; this virus is thought to remain viable for less than four days outside the animal. Carcasses are generally buried or burned. Care should be taken to prevent the virus from spreading to susceptible or potentially susceptible wild populations such as deer, gazelles, wild sheep or feral goats.

Peste des petits ruminants is controlled in endemic areas by vaccination. Animals that recover develop good immunity, which persists for at least four years and possibly lifelong. Some vaccines are also reported to be highly effective and provide long-term immunity. Animals may shed some vaccine strains.

To help protect susceptible wildlife and captive wild animals in endemic regions, they should not be allowed to have contact with sheep and goats. It might also be possible to vaccinate exotic species, but there is currently little information on the safety and efficacy of sheep/goat PPR vaccines in other animals. One outbreak among Sindh ibex at a wild animal part seemed to be controlled by vaccinating domesticated small ruminants and disinfecting common water sources in nearby villages.

MORBIDITY AND MORTALITY

Exposure to PPRV can be common among small ruminants in endemic regions, with seroprevalence rates ranging from < 2% to greater than 50%. These rates are often higher in sheep than goats. Several studies reported that up to 20% of camels and cattle also had antibodies to PPRV, and one study from Pakistan found that 42% of cattle and 67% of water buffalo (most born after rinderpest had been eradicated) were seropositive.

Peste des petits ruminants is highly contagious when it first occurs in a naïve population. Periodic outbreaks may also be seen in endemic regions, particularly when animals are mixed or new animals are introduced into a herd. Some epizootics are associated with changes in weather, such as the beginning of the rainy season or a cold, dry period. How this virus is maintained between outbreaks is uncertain. Some sources suggest that it might circulate subclinically in small ruminant

populations, emerging when immunity wanes or naïve animals are introduced.

The severity of the disease varies with the host's species, immunity, breed, age and concurrent illnesses or infections. Some isolates can cause serious illness in one breed of goats, but mild disease in another. At least two comparative experimental studies, as well as some outbreaks in the field, have suggested that clinical cases are more severe in goats than sheep; however, there have also been reports of outbreaks among sheep where signs in goats were mild. In endemic regions, animals between three months and two years of age are most severely affected; young animals that are still nursing and older animals tend to be spared.

The morbidity and case fatality rates in small ruminants can reach levels of 80-90% or greater, particularly in naïve herds and young animals; however, these rates tend to be lower in endemic areas, and morbidity and mortality rates in some individual flocks are reported to be as low as 10-20%. Few cases have been reported in other domesticated ruminants. In an outbreak among water buffalo in India, the case fatality rate was 96%. Fifty of 385 water buffalos were affected; most (38) of these cases occurred in animals that had been recently introduced into the herd and were not yet vaccinated against rinderpest. During a countrywide outbreak among camels in Ethiopia, the morbidity rate was greater than 90%, and the mortality rate ranged from 5% to 70%. In another outbreak affecting camels in Sudan, mortality rates were 0% to 50%, and fatalities were most common in animals that were pregnant or had recently given birth.

High case fatality rates have been reported in some exotic ungulates. During one outbreak in captive gazelles, the morbidity rate was 51% and the case fatality rate was 100%. High case fatality (100%) was also reported among wild ungulates, including various antelope species. in an outbreak in the United Arab Emirates. An outbreak among wild Sindh ibex in Pakistan was likewise severe.

PLAGUE

Peste, Black Death, Bubonic Plague, Pneumonic Plague, Septicemic Plague, Pestis Minor

IMPORTANCE

Plague is an important zoonotic bacterial disease, and a cause of significant mortality in wild rodents and rabbits. In some animals such as prairie dogs, outbreaks may kill nearly all of the animals in a colony. Sporadic cases also occur in other wild and domesticated mammals, particularly felids. Infections in animals can be transmitted to humans, resulting in life-threatening disease. Pneumonic plague, which is a particularly deadly form of the disease, is usually fatal if antibiotics are not started very soon after the symptoms appear. Bubonic plague, the most common form, is less fulminant, but also has a high mortality rate if left untreated.

At least three major plague pandemics have been seen in human populations. The Justinian plague occurred in the Mediterranean region in the 6th century AD and caused an estimated 100 million deaths, and the Black Death killed a third of the European population beginning in the 14th century. The most recent pandemic, which began in China in the late 1800s, spread worldwide and caused an estimated 12 million fatalities by 1930. The organisms that caused these three pandemics still exist in wild animal reservoirs in parts of the world, and occasionally spill over from these reservoirs to affect people or other animals. More than a thousand human cases and 100 to 200 deaths are reported annually to the World Health Organization (WHO), and many additional cases are probably not diagnosed. Most outbreaks occur in Asia and Africa, but sporadic cases and outbreaks can be seen in any endemic region. Plague may reoccur after a long period when the disease seems to disappear; recent outbreaks in India, Indonesia and Zambia followed quiescent periods of 30 to 50 years. An additional concern is that the agent of plague has been identified as a potential biological weapon.

ETIOLOGY

Plague results from infection by *Yersinia pestis*, a Gram negative bacillus in the family Enterobacteriaceae. Only one serotype is recognized. *Y. pestis* can be divided into three biovars: Antiqua, Medievalis, and Orientalis. The Antiqua strains are more variable than isolates in the other two biovars. Other classification schemes have also been proposed, and some recent analyses classify isolates using genetic markers.

There are three principal forms of plague, defined mainly by the syndrome in humans. Bubonic plague is the most common form, and usually results from the inoculation of *Y. pestis* into the skin. Patients with bubonic plague typically develop a swollen and very painful draining lymph node, called a bubo, in addition to other clinical signs. Pneumonic plague occurs after the inhalation of bacteria (primary pneumonic plague) or after blood–borne spread to the lungs (secondary pneumonic plague). The third form, septicemic plague, may occur without obvious involvement of the lymph nodes (primary septicemic plague) or as the result of dissemination of the other two forms.

Recent evidence suggests that attenuated strains of *Y. pestis* used in research might be virulent in some circumstances. One of these strains (*Y. pestis* KIM) caused fatal septicemic plague in a researcher who was an insulin-dependent diabetic and also had evidence of hereditary hemochromatosis. There is some evidence that hemochromatosis might have been a predisposing factor, possibly by providing iron deposits this organism was able to exploit. Immunosuppression from the diabetes might also have played a role.

SPECIES AFFECTED

Rodents and lagomorphs are the most important host species for plague. These animals are infested with fleas that can transmit *Y. pestis*, and develop bacteremia high enough to infect those fleas. Infections have been documented in more than 200 species and subspecies of rodents. Significant rodent hosts include prairie dogs (*Cynomys* spp.), ground squirrels/susliks (*Spermophilus* spp.), antelope ground squirrels (*Ammospermophilus* spp.), chipmunks (*Tamias* spp.), rats (*Rattus* spp.), wood rats (*Neotoma* spp.). mice (*Peromyscus* spp.), Siberian marmots (*Marmota sibirica*), voles (*Microtus* spp.), jerboas, and some gerbils (*Rhombomys opimus* and *Meriones* spp.). The principal rodent hosts vary with the geographic region. Pikas (*Ochotona* spp.), which are lagomorphs, are also important hosts in Asia.

Many other species of mammals also become infected, but the majority are incidental hosts. Some species are more likely to develop clinical signs than others. Felids seem to be particularly susceptible to plague; fatal disease has been reported in housecats and wild cats including bobcats (*Lynx rufus*) and mountain lions (*Puma concolor*). Black-footed ferrets (*Mustela nigripes*) are also very susceptible. Infrequent cases of plague have been described in ungulates including camels (*Camelus bactrianus* and *Camelus dromedarius*), various species of deer, pronghorn antelope (*Antilocapra americana*), at least one llama, and goats. *Y. pestis* infections have also been reported in dogs, coyotes (*Canis latrans*), foxes, badgers, skunks and nonhuman primates.

Zoonotic potential

Humans are susceptible to infection with *Y. pestis* as incidental hosts, and are not involved in the natural cycle of this organism outside epidemics.

GEOGRAPHIC DISTRIBUTION

Y. pestis can be found in parts of Africa, the Middle East, Asia, and North and South America, as well as Madagascar.

P

The distribution of this organism is patchy. In North America, *Y. pestis* occurs in the western third of the continent, from British Columbia and Alberta, Canada to Mexico, and as far east as Dallas and the western borders of Kansas, Nebraska, Oklahoma and South Dakota. In South America, active foci have been identified mainly in Brazil and the Andes mountain region of Bolivia, Peru and Ecuador. In Asia, plague has been reported from areas in the former U.S.S.R. east through China, and south to Southwest and Southeast Asia. In Africa, this disease occurs primarily in the eastern and southern regions, but foci are also found in the west and north. Plague is not endemic in Europe or Oceania.

The distribution of each biovar varies. The Antiqua biovar occurs in Africa and Central Asia, and the Medievalis biovar seems to be found mainly in Central Asia (however, one isolate was reported in northern Africa). The Orientalis biovar can be found in most regions where plague occurs

TRANSMISSION

Plague is usually transmitted by the bites of infected fleas. More than 30 species of fleas are capable of transmitting *Y. pestis*, but they vary in their efficiency as vectors. The oriental rat flea, *Xenopsylla cheopis*, is a particularly effective biological vector. Other species of rodent fleas are also important in transmission. Dog and cat fleas (*Ctenocephalides* spp) can be infected, but are poor vectors compared to species such as *X. cheopis*. Human fleas (*Pulex irritans*) can also carry *Y. pestis*. Fleas are usually short-lived; however, some may survive for several months, or even a year or more, in rodent burrows after their host have died. During epizootics, there is a high risk that fleas leaving dead animals will bite species they do not usually infest, such as humans. Other arthropods have also been proposed as potential vectors. *Y. pestis* has been detected in human lice during outbreaks in people, and lice were able to transmit the infection between rabbits in the laboratory. Ticks have been suggested as possible mechanical vectors in some countries.

Direct transmission can also occur between animals or people, but the importance of this route varies with the form of the disease. *Y. pestis* is present in tissues, draining lesions and some body fluids, and these bacteria may enter the body through mucous membranes and broken skin. Person-to-person spread of bubonic plague seems to be rare or nonexistent, though theoretically possible. In contrast, people or animals with the pneumonic form may transmit *Y. pestis* in respiratory droplets. In humans, this occurs most readily in crowded, poorly ventilated conditions. Pnuemonic plague is most contagious during its final stages, when the number of bacteria in the sputum increases. In the earlier stages, transmission does not seem to occur as readily.

Animals, including cats, can transmit bacteria in bites. Carnivores and omnivores, including humans, may also be infected by eating tissues from infected animals. In camels and other herbivores, this might occur when dead rodents or their excretions contaminate the animal's feed. At present, there is little information about the survival and growth of *Y. pestis* in food products. In one study, an attenuated *Y. pestis* strain (*Y. pestis* KIM5) was able to persist without growth in raw meat (ground pork) for at least 2 months at 4°C, and to grow in this product at 10-30°C.

Y. pestis can be transmitted on fomites at least for short periods; however, its long-term survival in the environment, particularly in soil, is still poorly understood. This organism is not resistant to desiccation or heat, and on surfaces such as glass and steel, it usually persists for less than 72 hours. However, it is reported to survive for long periods of time in organic material; it may remain viable for up to 100 days in blood and for as long as 9 months in human bodies. Viable *Y. pestis* was recently found after 24 days in soil that had been contaminated by the blood of a dead mountain lion. In the laboratory, this organism can survive for many months, and possibly years, in autoclaved soil, and for long periods in water. Rodents have been infected experimentally by burrowing in or running over recently contaminated soil, but whether this is an important maintenance mechanism for plague remains to be determined.

Epidemiology

In the wild, *Y. pestis* seems to be maintained in cycles between wild rodents or lagomorphs (e.g., pikas) and fleas. Periodically, these animals experience epizootics, increasing the risk of transmission to other species. What triggers these epizootics, and how *Y. pestis* persists during interepizootic periods, is poorly understood. Whether this organism circulates in its epizootic hosts between outbreaks, or in a different 'maintenance' host, is controversial.

Sporadic cases of plague occur in people who are exposed to tissues from wild animals, or to their fleas. Domesticated animals can act as 'bridges' that carry *Y. pestis* closer to humans. These animals may become infected themselves, or they can simply act as temporary hosts for infected fleas. Infection of rodents in urban areas, particularly rats, can result in epidemic plague in humans. The importance of different transmission routes during human epidemics (e.g., aerosols, or transmission via ectoparasites) is still incompletely understood.

Human infections

Most human cases are associated with wild rodents or lagomorphs, but other species have also been involved. Among domesticated animals, cats seem to be most likely to transmit plague to humans. Unusually, a recent case of primary pneumonic plague in China, which then spread to 11 human contacts, was attributed to close contact with a severely ill, *Y. pestis* (Antiqua biovar) infected dog. One study suggested that extended contact with dogs may increase the risk of plague, possibly by bringing infected rodent fleas into the household. Small outbreaks have also been reported in people who ate uncooked tissues from infected hosts (e.g., uncooked camel liver or guinea pig flesh). A few human cases have been attributed to contact with wild animals including bobcats, coyotes, mountain lions, foxes and badgers. In these cases, it may sometimes be difficult to determine whether the organism was acquired directly from an animal or from infected fleas.

DISINFECTION

Y. pestis is susceptible to a number of disinfectants including 1% sodium hypochlorite, 70% ethanol, 2% glutaraldehyde, formaldehyde, and iodine–based and phenolic disinfectants. It can also be inactivated by moist heat (121° C [250° F] for at least 15 minutes) or dry heat (160-170° C [320-338°F] for at least 1 hour).

INFECTIONS IN ANIMALS

INCUBATION PERIOD

Clinical signs usually develop within 1 to 4 days in cats. Few cases have been reported in other species.

CLINICAL SIGNS

The three principal forms of plague - bubonic plague, septicemic plague and pneumonic plague - seem to occur in animals as well as humans; however, plague should be a consideration in any animal with a systemic infection and a history of potential exposure in an endemic area.

Most cats infected with *Y. pestis* develop the bubonic form. This form is usually characterized by fever, anorexia and lethargy, with an enlarged lymph node (bubo) near the site of inoculation. Many cats are probably infected by ingestion, and the submandibular lymph nodes are most often involved. The affected lymph node may develop abscesses, ulcerate and drain. Some cats also have cellulitis, abscesses at sites other than lymph nodes, mouth lesions including ulcers, or necrotic tonsillitis. Vomiting, diarrhea, ocular discharges, dehydration and weight loss have been reported. Bubonic plague can progress to septicemic plague, with typical signs of sepsis. Disseminated intravascular coagulation (DIC) and/ or respiratory distress may be seen. Primary septicemic plague, without a bubo, has also been reported in cats. Pneumonic plague can develop in cats with bubonic or septicemic plague, and is characterized by respiratory signs including dyspnea and hemoptysis. Neurological signs such as incoordination have been reported in some infected cats. Studies in experimentally infected cats and serological surveys suggest that some animals might have mild or asymptomatic infections after exposure.

Dogs seem less likely to become ill than cats, and subclinical infections may be more common. Only rare descriptions of plague in naturally infected dogs have been published: the clinical signs included fever, lethargy, submandibular lymphadenitis, lesions in the mouth and coughing. Two recent, linked cases in China were characterized by prostration, anorexia, and severe coughing and vomiting with blood in the nose and mouth, and death within a few days. Experimentally infected dogs inoculated by the subcutaneous or oral routes developed a fever and other signs of illness, but recovered spontaneously during the next week. However, two dogs exposed via aerosols died.

In rodents, the outcome varies from subclinical infection or mild illness to severe, rapidly fatal disease. Epizootics with high mortality rates are reported among some rodents and lagomorphs. Infections in other wild animals are poorly understood. Infected mountain lions, bobcats, coyotes, foxes and other animals have occasionally been found dead. Fever and lethargy, without bacteremia, were reported in experimentally infected raccoons in one study. In another experiment, neither fever nor deaths were seen in this species, or in coyotes and striped skunks infected by the oral route. Whether individual susceptibility or other factors (e.g., dose or route of exposure, or underlying illness) affect the outcome in these species is not known.

Occasional cases of plague have been reported in domesticated or wild ungulates. Ocular plague, characterized by keratoconjunctivitis, endophthalmitis and panophthalmitis, has been documented in mule deer (*Odocoileus hemionus*) and black-tailed deer (*Odocoileus hemionus columbianus*). Septicemia and pneumonia have also been seen in mule deer, either with or without ocular signs. Overall, plague is not reported to be an important cause of morbidity and mortality in this species. Goats and camels can become ill and die, and a death was reported in a llama in New Mexico. Clinical cases have not been reported in the literature in cattle, horses or pigs.

POST MORTEM LESIONS

In cats, necrotic foci may be found in the liver, spleen, lungs and other internal organs. The liver may be pale and the spleen enlarged. Affected lymph nodes can be markedly swollen, with necrosuppurative inflammation, edema and hemorrhages. Diffuse interstitial pneumonia, focal congestion, abscesses and hemorrhages may be found in the lungs.

In wild animals, reported lesions have included hemorrhagic buboes and splenomegaly in some acute cases, or caseous buboes and necrotic lesions in the spleen, liver and lungs when the disease progresses more slowly. Keratoconjunctivitis, endophthalmitis and panophthalmitis, as well as septicemic lesions, pneumonia and lymphadenitis have been reported in deer.

DIAGNOSTIC TESTS

A presumptive diagnosis can be made by identifying the characteristic organisms in clinical samples such as lymph node (bubo) aspirates or swabs of draining lesions. Some types of samples, such as lymph nodes, may contain a relatively homogenous population of bacteria. *Y. pestis*

P

is a Gram negative, facultative intracellular coccobacillus or bacillus with bipolar staining. Bipolar staining is particularly evident when Wright-Giemsa or Wayson stains are used. Bacteria in clinical samples can be identified by immunofluorescence. Rapid immunoassays can also be used to detect *Y. pestis* antigens in clinical samples, and PCR may be used to identify nucleic acids. *Y. pestis* can sometimes be detected by PCR or other techniques in fleas collected from the animal.

Plague can also be diagnosed by isolating *Y. pestis* from blood, nasal/oral swabs, lymph node aspirates, swabs of draining lesions, transtracheal aspirates and/or tissue samples including the liver, spleen, lungs and affected lymph nodes. Specimens for culture should be collected before antibiotics are started. *Y. pestis* will grow on ordinary media including blood agar, MacConkey agar, nutrient agar or brain-heart infusion broth. *Yersinia*-specific CIN agar can also be used; this medium is particularly helpful with contaminated samples. *Y. pestis* can be identified with routine biochemical tests and other methods. It should be kept in mind that automated systems may misidentify this bacterium, as it grows slowly and biochemical reactions may be delayed. A specific bacteriophage that lyses only *Y. pestis* and not *Y. pseudotuberculosis* is used as a rapid diagnostic test in reference laboratories. Although animal assays are generally discouraged if there are other alternatives, *Y. pestis* may also be recovered in laboratory animals such as mice, particularly when the sample is contaminated with other organisms.

Serology using paired serum samples can be helpful. A single sample, together with consistent clinical signs, may also be supportive. Various serological tests including latex hemagglutination and passive hemagglutination may be available.

TREATMENT

Early treatment with antibiotics can be successful. Some antibiotics that have been used to treat plague in animals include streptomycin, gentamicin, doxycycline, tetracycline and chloramphenicol. Drug availability may vary with the country.

CONTROL

Disease reporting

Veterinarians who encounter or suspect a case of plague should follow their national and/or local guidelines for disease reporting. In endemic areas, prompt reporting helps prevent exposure of other animals and humans. In addition to any other state reporting requirements, all suspected cases of animal or human plague in the U.S. should be reported to the local or state public health department. The state public health laboratory or U.S. Centers for Disease Control (CDC) laboratory should be contacted before collecting or shipping samples.

Prevention

A good flea control program should be established for dogs and cats, and they should be kept from eating tissues from animals that may be infected. Allowing animals to hunt or roam increases the risk of infection in endemic areas. Animals that become ill should be examined by a veterinarian. Barrier precautions are necessary during examination and treatment, and suspected cases are isolated. The most stringent measures are needed before antibiotics are begun and during the initial stages of treatment. PPE may include gloves, surgical masks to prevent droplet infection, protective clothing, and eye protection if splashes or sprays are expected. Excellent hygiene should be practiced.

Vaccination has been used to protect endangered black-footed ferrets, which are highly susceptible to plague, during epizootics. Vaccines (in food bait) were also given to prairie dogs, which are the food source for these ferrets, and prairie dog burrows were dusted with an insecticide. Vaccines have been tested in other wildlife species susceptible to plague, and they might be promising for controlling *Y. pestis* in rodents near human environments. Vaccines are not currently available for domesticated animals.

MORBIDITY AND MORTALITY

In endemic areas, epizootics occur periodically in susceptible rodents and lagomorphs. Resistance to plague differs between rodent species, and the percentage of individuals that survive *Y. pestis* infection can vary. The mortality rate in some species can approach 100%. Between epizootics, plague persists in wild animals without causing high mortality. Populations that live in endemic areas may be more resistant than those outside these regions.

Among domesticated animals, cats seem to be particularly susceptible to plague. One study reported that the mortality rate was 14% in housecats with bubonic plague, 70% in cats with septicemic plague (or cases that were not classified into a form), and 83% in the pneumonic form. In experimentally infected cats with bubonic plague, the case fatality rate can be as high as 60% if the disease is left untreated. Subclinical infections also seem to occur. Surveillance has reported antibodies in healthy cats, and some cats have survived experimental infections. In one study, 20 of 25 cats inoculated by ingestion or subcutaneous inoculation became ill, but three cats seroconverted without clinical signs. Dogs do not seem to be as susceptible to plague as cats. Ten experimentally infected dogs that were inoculated by subcutaneous or oral inoculation experienced only a brief illness and recovered on their own. However, severe illness is possible. Two dogs infected by aerosols died, and fatal cases of plague have been reported rarely in naturally infected dogs.

Serological evidence suggests that wild carnivores are frequently exposed to *Y. pestis*, probably through hunting. Fatal cases of plague have been reported in large cats including bobcats and mountain lions. A recent survey from the western U.S. found that 2% of apparently healthy bobcats and mountain lions in California, and 21% to 46% of these animals in different regions of Colorado, had antibodies to *Y. pestis*. Seroprevalence rates of 13-14% in raccoons and coyotes, and 55% in badgers, have also been reported. Endangered black-footed ferrets (*M. nigripes*) are very susceptible to plague, and have a high mortality rate. In contrast, experimentally infected domesticated ferrets (*Mustela putorius furo*) and Siberian polecats (*M. eversmanni*) did not become ill.

INFECTIONS IN HUMANS

INCUBATION PERIOD

Pneumonic plague develops rapidly, within 1 to 4 days. The incubation period for bubonic plague is 1 to 10 days, but in most cases, the symptoms usually appear in 2 to 5 days.

CLINICAL SIGNS

Bubonic plague is the most common form of plague in humans. It begins with the sudden onset of high fever, chills, headache, malaise and myalgia. Dizziness, nausea and vomiting may also be seen, in addition to an infected, swollen and very painful draining lymph node (the bubo). Although it can occur anywhere, the bubo is often one of the femoral or inguinal lymph nodes. In some cases, a pustule, vesicle, eschar or papule may be found at the site of the flea bite; however, this is often absent or missed. People who become infected by ingestion can develop severe pharyngitis and tonsillitis, with swelling of a submandibular lymph node and the neck. Vomiting, diarrhea and abdominal pain may also be seen. In a recent outbreak linked to eating undercooked camel meat, gastrointestinal signs without prominent pharyngeal signs were the primary syndrome. If it is not treated, bubonic plague often progresses to septicemia and/or secondary pneumonia.

Approximately 10-25% of human plague cases are characterized by primary septicemia. In addition to high fever and other signs in common with bubonic plague, this form has signs of sepsis, but there may be no obvious involvement of the lymph nodes. Epistaxis, hematuria petechiae, DIC and neurological signs may also be seen, and the course of the disease can be rapid, with multiorgan failure. Secondary septicemia is similar, but results from disseminated bubonic plague. Meningitis is a relatively rare form of plague; it occurs in approximately 6% of people with the septicemic or pneumonic forms.

Pneumonic plague occurs after the inhalation of bacteria or after blood–borne spread to the lungs. The symptoms of pneumonic plague develop acutely and include high fever, chills, headache (often severe), myalgia, malaise and an increased respiratory rate. Within 24 hours, a cough develops; it is initially dry but becomes productive, then bloodstained and/or purulent.

The sputum contains only specks of blood at first but eventually becomes foamy and pink or red from blood. Pneumonic plague is rapidly fatal, with dyspnea, stridor and cyanosis ending in respiratory failure and circulatory collapse.

Pestis minor is a benign form of bubonic plague, usually seen only among people in regions where plague is common. Pestis minor is characterized by fever, lymphadenitis, headache and prostration, which resolve spontaneously within a week.

DIAGNOSTIC TESTS

A presumptive diagnosis can be made, as for animals, by identifying the characteristic organisms in sputum, bronchial/tracheal washings, blood, lymph node (bubo) aspirates, cerebrospinal fluid (CSF) or postmortem tissue samples. Rapid immunoassays employed with human samples include an F1 antigen test used in Africa.

Plague can also be diagnosed by isolating *Y. pestis*. Organisms may be recovered from respiratory secretions, blood and/or aspirates of affected lymph nodes, depending on the form of the disease, as well as from lungs and other tissues postmortem. Organisms are usually present in blood only during septicemia; however, bacteria are sometimes released intermittently from lymph nodes into the blood, and a series of blood samples collected 10-30 minutes apart may be diagnostic. Specimens for culture should be collected before antibiotics are started.

Serology is occasionally helpful. Serological tests include ELISAs, passive hemagglutination, hemagglutination-inhibition, latex agglutination and complement fixation. A fourfold rise in titer is diagnostic.

TREATMENT

Antibiotics are effective for the treatment of plague; however, their efficacy in the pneumonic form is often limited if the symptoms have been present for more than 20 hours. Buboes are occasionally drained but usually resolve with antibiotic treatment. Although antibiotic resistant strains of *Y. pestis* have been detected, they seem to be rare. In a recent study, no resistant *Y. pestis* was found among approximately 400 isolates from the Americas, Asia and Africa, including nearly 300 organisms isolated between 1995 and 2009.

CONTROL

In endemic areas, rodents should be controlled around human homes, workplaces and recreational areas. Buildings should be rodent-proofed, and access to food sources should be prevented. Brush, rock piles, junk and cluttered firewood should not be allowed to accumulate, as they may provide nesting places for rodents. Campers and hikers should not approach rodents or their carcasses, and should avoid sleeping beside rodent burrows. Prevention methods for pets (see Animal section) can help keep them from becoming infected or carrying infected fleas into the home. Game meat, as well as tissues

P

from domesticated animals that might be infected, should be cooked thoroughly if they are eaten (however, eating tissues from sick animals is not recommended). Die-offs of rodents or lagomorphs should be reported.

Personal protective equipment (PPE) should be worn when handling animals if there is any risk that they might be infected. More stringent precautions are necessary when pneumonic plague is suspected or higher risk procedures such as necropsies are performed. Good hygiene, including frequent hand washing, should be practiced. Insect repellents can also be applied to clothing and skin if exposure to rodent fleas is expected. Specific recommendations for protective measures are available from the CDC and other groups.

In endemic regions, rodents that host *Y. pestis* may be monitored and/or controlled. Concurrent insecticidal treatment is often necessary when hosts die or are killed, as fleas leave the carcasses to seek new hosts. People who have been exposed to *Y. pestis* are treated prophylactically with antibiotics. Good infection control procedures, including the use of disposable surgical masks, are used to prevent transmission from patients with pneumonic plague.

Human vaccines may be used in some countries or high risk groups, but there are concerns about their safety and efficacy, and their availability is limited. Efforts to create safe and effective human vaccines, as well as vaccine baits to reduce environmental load, are areas of current research.

MORBIDITY AND MORTALITY

Y. pestis is endemic in populations of wild rodents and lagomorphs, and occasionally spills over to affect people or other animals. Worldwide, approximately 1,000 to 2,000 human cases of plague and 100 to 200 deaths are currently reported annually to the World Health Organization (decreased from a high of 5,000 cases in 1997). The exact number of plague cases is, however, uncertain. Some reported cases are not laboratory confirmed, and conversely, many cases are probably not diagnosed. Most outbreaks occur in Asia and Africa, but sporadic cases and outbreaks can be seen in any endemic region. On average, fewer than 20 cases of plague are reported annually in the U.S., but up to 40 cases have been reported in some years. Plague may reoccur after a long period when the disease seems to disappear; recent outbreaks in India, Indonesia and Zambia followed quiescent periods of 30 to 50 years.

Bubonic plague accounts for 80-95% of the cases seen worldwide. Without treatment, the case fatality rate for this form is estimated to be 40-70%; some sources suggest it may be as high as 90%. The availability of treatment lowers the case fatality rate in bubonic or septicemic plague to approximately 5-15%. Untreated pneumonic or septicemic plague is almost always fatal, often within a few days. If appropriate treatment is given very soon after the onset of symptoms, most people survive; however, the narrow window for treatment means that the case fatality rate for the pneumonic form remains greater than 50%.

RABIES AND RABIES-RELATED LYSSAVIRUSES

Hydrophobia, Lyssa

IMPORTANCE

Rabies is a viral disease that affects the central nervous system (CNS) of mammals and has an extremely high case fatality rate. Once clinical signs develop, there are very few survivors. Vaccines can protect pets, as well as people exposed to these animals, but the maintenance of rabies viruses in wildlife complicates control. In humans, illness can be prevented by administering anti-rabies antibodies and a series of vaccinations, provided exposure is recognized before the symptoms appear. However, people in impoverished countries do not always have access to effective post-exposure prophylaxis. Due to this and other factors, such as inadequate levels of vaccination in dogs and cats, the annual incidence of human rabies is estimated to be 40,000 or more cases, worldwide. A few cases occur even in nations with good medical care, typically in people who did not realize they were exposed.

Closely related lyssaviruses circulate among bats in the Eastern Hemisphere, and can cause an illness identical to rabies in people and domesticated animals. Rabies vaccines and post-exposure prophylaxis are thought to provide some protection against some of these viruses, but not others. Rabies-related lyssaviruses can be found even in countries classified as rabies-free.

ETIOLOGY

Rabies is caused by the rabies virus, a neurotropic virus in the genus *Lyssavirus*, family Rhabdoviridae. There are many variants (or strains) of this virus, each maintained in a particular reservoir host. The reservoir host may be reflected in the case description. For example, if a virus maintained in skunks caused rabies in a dog, it would be described as skunk rabies in a dog, rather than canine rabies.

Closely related lyssaviruses, which are known as rabies-related lyssaviruses or nonrabies lyssaviruses, can cause a neurological disease identical to rabies. Lagos bat virus, Duvenhage virus, European bat lyssavirus (EBLV) 1, EBLV 2, Australian bat lyssavirus (ABLV), Mokola virus and Irkut virus have caused clinical cases in humans or domesticated animals, and Ikoma virus was detected in the brain of an African civet (*Civettictis civetta*) with neurological signs. Shimoni bat virus, Aravan virus, Khujand virus, Bokeloh virus and West Caucasian bat virus have been found, to date, only in bats, but might be pathogenic in other species. Additional rabies-related lyssaviruses are likely to exist.

Rabies virus and the rabies-related lyssaviruses have been classified into two or more phylogroups, based on their genetic relatedness. Viruses that are more closely related to rabies virus can be neutralized, at least to some extent, by antibodies to rabies virus. Phylogroup I contains rabies virus, Duvenhage virus, EBLV 1, EBLV 2, Australian bat lyssavirus, Irkut virus, Aravan virus and Khujand virus. Bokeloh virus also appears to belong to this group. Phylogroup II consists of Lagos bat virus, Mokola virus and probably also Shimoni bat virus. West Caucasian bat virus has been provisionally placed in a new group, phylogroup III. Ikoma virus seems to be related to West Caucasian bat virus, although a full analysis is not yet available.

SPECIES AFFECTED

All mammals are susceptible to rabies, but only a limited number of species also act as reservoir hosts. They include members of the families Canidae (dogs, jackals, coyotes, wolves, foxes and raccoon dogs), Mustelidae (e.g., skunks), Viverridae (e.g., mongooses), and Procyonidae (raccoons), and the order Chiroptera (bats). Although cats can be affected by rabies, cat-adapted variants have not been seen. Each rabies variant is maintained in a particular host, and usually dies out during serial passage in species to which it is not adapted. However, any variant can cause rabies in other species. Occasionally, a virus adapted to one species becomes established in another.

Rabies is maintained in two epidemiological cycles, one urban and one sylvatic. In the urban rabies cycle, dogs are the main reservoir host. This cycle predominates in areas where the proportion of unvaccinated and semi-owned or stray dogs is high, such as some parts of Africa, Asia, the Middle East and Latin America. The urban rabies cycle has been virtually eliminated in the U.S., Canada and Europe; although sporadic cases occur in dogs infected by wild animals, the urban cycle is not perpetuated in canine populations. However, the canine rabies variant is apparently established in some wildlife populations (e.g., foxes and skunks in North America) and it could be re-established in dogs from these reservoirs.

The sylvatic (or wildlife) cycle is the predominant cycle in Europe and North America. It is also present simultaneously with the urban cycle in some parts of the world. The epidemiology of this cycle is complex; factors affecting it include the virus strain, the behavior of the host species, ecology and environmental factors. In any ecosystem, often one and occasionally up to 3 wildlife species are responsible for perpetuating a particular rabies variant. The disease pattern in wildlife can either be relatively stable, or occur as a slow moving epidemic. Some wildlife maintenance hosts include skunks and bats in the Americas, raccoons (*Procyon lotor*) in North America, raccoon dogs (*Nyctereutes procyonoides*) in Europe and Asia, and wolves in northern Europe. Various foxes are reservoir hosts in Europe, North America, the Middle East and Asia, and mongooses maintain rabies viruses in Asia

and the Caribbean. Coyotes are reported to be reservoir hosts in Latin America, and jackals in the Middle East and Asia. Several species including jackals, foxes, mongooses and genets might maintain viruses in Africa.

Rabies-related Lyssaviruses

With the possible exception of Mokola virus, rabies-related lyssaviruses seem to be maintained in insectivorous bats and fruit bats. They also cause illness in these animals. Mokola virus has been detected in shrews and wild rodents, but not bats, and its reservoir host is still uncertain. The reservoir host for Ikoma virus is also unknown.

The susceptibility of other mammalian species to rabies-related lyssaviruses is incompletely understood. Like rabies virus, they might be able to infect all mammals. As of 2012, fatal neurological disease has been reported in cats, dogs and a water mongoose (*Atilax paludinosis*) infected with Lagos bat virus; cats and dogs infected with Mokola virus; cats, sheep and a stone marten infected with EBLV 1; and an African civet infected with Ikoma virus. Experimental infections with EBLV-1 were established in mice, sheep, foxes, ferrets, dogs and cats. It is likely that domesticated animals can also be affected by other lyssaviruses, such as Duvenhage virus, which has caused fatal illness in people.

Zoonotic potential

All rabies variants are thought to be zoonotic. Clinical cases have also been caused by Duvenhage virus, EBLV 1, EBLV 2, Australian bat lyssavirus, Mokola virus and Irkut virus. Humans are likely to be susceptible to other rabies-related lyssaviruses.

GEOGRAPHIC DISTRIBUTION

With some exceptions (particularly islands), rabies virus is found worldwide. Some countries such as the United Kingdom, Ireland, Sweden, Norway, Iceland, Japan, Australia, New Zealand, Singapore, most of Malaysia, Papua New Guinea, the Pacific Islands and some Indonesian islands have been free of this virus for many years. According to the World Health Organization (WHO), a country is considered to be free of rabies if there have been no indigenously acquired cases in humans or animals during the previous 2 years, in the presence of adequate surveillance and import regulations. Using this definition, several additional countries are considered to be rabies-free. In some cases, these nations have conducted rabies vaccination programs in wildlife, but are susceptible to the reintroduction of the virus from neighboring countries. Official lists should be consulted for the current list of rabies-free countries and areas, as it may change.

Rabies related lyssaviruses have been found only in the Eastern Hemisphere. There is limited information on the distribution of individual viruses within this area. EBLV 1, EBLV 2 and Bokeloh virus occur in Europe, Irkut virus and

West Caucasian bat virus were detected in Russia, and Aravan virus and Khujand virus have been found in Asia. Antibodies to West Caucasian bat virus were also found in Africa, suggesting that it or a related virus might circulate there. Viruses that have been reported only from Africa include Duvenhage virus, Lagos bat virus, Mokola virus, Shimoni bat virus and Ikoma virus. Australian bat lyssavirus seems to be limited to Australia, but neutralizing antibodies to this or a related virus were found among bats in the Philippines. Rabies-related lyssaviruses have not been detected in the Americas, where the classical rabies virus is common among bats. The presence of a rabies-related lyssavirus does not prevent a nation from being listed as rabies-free.

TRANSMISSION

Rabies virus has an unusual dissemination pattern in the body, which influences its transmission, diagnosis and prevention. Immediately after infection, the virus enters an eclipse phase during which it replicates in non-nervous tissue (e.g., muscle), and is not easily detected. It does not usually stimulate an immune response at this time, but it is susceptible to neutralization if antibodies are present. After several days or months, the virus enters the peripheral nerves and is transported to the CNS. After dissemination within the CNS, where clinical signs develop as the neurons are infected, the virus is distributed to highly innervated tissues via the peripheral nerves. The virus is concentrated in nervous tissue, salivary glands, saliva and cerebrospinal fluid (CSF), which should all be handled with extreme caution. Limited amounts of virus have been detected in a number of other tissues and organs. Because the virus is contained within neurons, handling most body fluids or intact organs is thought to be low risk. However, a few cases of rabies have been reported in organ transplant recipients. Corneas were often involved, but various internal organs have also transmitted rabies. Needles or other sharp objects might transmit the virus if they pass through tissues, because there is a possibility they may have pierced nervous tissue. Feces, blood, urine and other body fluids are not thought to contain infectious virus.

Rabies virus is usually spread between animals in the saliva, during a bite from an infected animal. Less often, an animal or person is infected by contact with infectious saliva or neurological tissues, through mucous membranes or breaks in the skin. This virus is not transmitted through intact skin. The efficiency of transmission varies with the behavior of the infected animal. Animals with the furious form are more likely to spread rabies than animals with the paralytic form. Carnivores are also more efficient vectors, in general, than herbivores.

Not all rabid animals will transmit the virus to animals they bite. Virus shedding is estimated to occur in 50-90% of infected animals, and the amount of virus in the saliva varies from a trace to high titers. It can be influenced by the species of animal and the viral strain. Shedding can begin before the onset of clinical signs. Cats have been reported to excrete virus for 1-5 days before the signs appear, cattle for 1 to 2 days, skunks for up to 14 days and bats for 2 weeks. Virus shedding in dogs is usually said to be limited to 1-5 days before the onset of clinical signs; however, in some experimental studies (using viruses of Mexican or Ethiopian origin), the virus was present in the saliva for up to 13 days before the dogs became ill. In very rare cases, it has been suggested that bats or dogs animals might be able to carry lyssaviruses asymptomatically, but this is controversial, and has not been unequivocally demonstrated.

Human saliva contains rabies virus, and transmission between people is theoretically possible, but unproven. Activities that could pose a risk for exposure include bites, kisses or other direct contact between saliva and mucous membranes or broken skin, sexual activity, and sharing eating or drinking utensils or cigarettes. It is not known how long humans can shed the virus before becoming symptomatic; the U.S. Centers for Disease Control and Prevention (CDC) recommends post-exposure prophylaxis for anyone who had at-risk contact with a person during the 14 days before the onset of clinical signs.

There are rare reports of transmission by other routes. Aerosol transmission has been documented under special circumstances, such as in laboratories and a bat cave with an unusually high density of aerosolized, viable virus particles. Rabies viruses have been transmitted by ingestion in experimentally infected animals, and there is anecdotal evidence of transmission in milk to a lamb and a human infant from their mothers. (More conventional routes could not be ruled out in the latter case.) Some authors have speculated that ingestion might play a role in rabies transmission among wild animals. In one epizootic among kudu (*Tragelaphus strepsiceros*), the virus may have spread between animals when they fed on thorn trees. There is no evidence that people have ever been infected by eating rabies virus (with the possible exception of the case described in the infant).

Rabies-related Lyssaviruses

There is little information on the transmission of rabies-related lyssaviruses, although it is probably similar to rabies. Infections with these viruses have been reported after bites, scratches or close contact with bats. Bats inoculated with Eurasian bat lyssaviruses shed virus in saliva shortly before clinical signs developed. In one experiment, there was no evidence for transmission to uninoculated bats kept in the same cage.

DISINFECTION

Rabies virus can be inactivated by sodium hypochlorite, 45-75% ethanol, iodine preparations, quaternary ammonium compounds, formaldehyde, phenol, ether, trypsin, β-propiolactone, and some other detergents. It is also inactivated by a very low pH (below 3) or very high pH (greater than 11). This virus is susceptible to ultraviolet radiation. It is rapidly inactivated by sunlight and drying, and (in dried blood and secretions) it does not survive for long periods in the environment.

INFECTIONS IN ANIMALS

INCUBATION PERIOD

The incubation period varies with the amount of virus transmitted, virus strain, site of inoculation (bites closer to the head have a shorter incubation period), pre-existing host immunity and nature of the wound. In dogs, cats and ferrets, the incubation period is usually less than 6 months; most cases in dogs and cats become apparent between 2 weeks and 3 months. In cattle, the vampire bat variant is reported to have an incubation period of 25 days to more than 5 months. The incubation period is also usually less than 6 months in bats, although some individuals can remain asymptomatic for much longer.

CLINICAL SIGNS

The initial clinical signs are often nonspecific and may include fearfulness, restlessness, anorexia or an increased appetite, vomiting, diarrhea, a slight fever, dilation of the pupils, hyperreactivity to stimuli and excessive salivation. The first sign of post-vaccinal rabies is usually lameness in the vaccinated leg. Animals often have behavioral and temperament changes, and may become either unusually aggressive or uncharacteristically affectionate. Pigs frequently have a very violent excitation phase at the onset of disease. After 2 to 5 days, these signs may be followed by a stage during which either the paralytic or the furious form of rabies predominates. Survival is extremely rare in either form of the illness.

The paralytic ("dumb") form of rabies is characterized by progressive paralysis. In this form, the throat and masseter muscles become paralyzed; the animal may be unable to swallow, and it can salivate profusely. Laryngeal paralysis can cause a change in vocalization, including an abnormal bellow in cattle or a hoarse howling in dogs. There may also be facial paralysis or the lower jaw may drop. Ruminants may separate from the herd and can become somnolent or depressed. Rumination may stop. Ataxia, incoordination and ascending spinal paresis or paralysis are also seen. The paralytic form of rabies may be preceded by a brief excitatory phase, or none at all. Biting is uncommon. Death usually occurs within 2 to 6 days, as the result of respiratory failure.

The furious form of rabies is associated with infection of the limbic system, and is the more common form in cats. Large animals with this form, such as horses, are extremely dangerous due to their size. Furious rabies is characterized

by restlessness, wandering, howling, polypnea, drooling and attacks on other animals, people or inanimate objects. Affected animals often swallow foreign objects such as sticks and stones. Wild animals frequently lose their fear of humans, and may attack humans or animal species they would normally avoid (e.g., porcupines). Nocturnal animals may be visible during the day. In cattle, unusual alertness can also be a sign of this form. Some animals have convulsions, especially during the terminal stages, and death sometimes occurs during a seizure. In most cases, however, the illness eventually progresses to incoordination and ascending paralysis. Animals with furious rabies usually die 4 to 8 days after the onset of clinical signs.

The signs of rabies can be highly variable, and many cases do not fit neatly into either the classic furious or paralytic presentation. The most reliable diagnostic signs are behavioral changes and unexplained paralysis, but rabies should be a consideration in all cases of unexplained neurological disease. For example, there have been cases in cats where no behavioral changes were noticed, and the illness appeared only as ataxia or posterior weakness, followed by ascending paralysis. Horses and mules are often in distress and extremely agitated, which may be interpreted as colic. Diagnosis can be particularly difficult in rabbits and rodents unless there is a history of exposure to a potentially rabid animal, such as a raccoon. Some infected rabbits developed obvious neurological signs, often of the paralytic form, but others had signs that were not initially suggestive of rabies, or experienced only nonspecific illness before death. In one report, sudden death was the only sign in many infected squirrels.

Rabies-related Lyssaviruses

Information about rabies-related lyssaviruses is currently limited to a handful of case reports and a few reports of experimental inoculation. In the case reports, these viruses caused fatal neurological disease in various wild and domesticated animals. Various inoculation routes, including intracerebral, intravenous and intramuscular injection, were used in several species of experimentally infected animals. Some animals developed severe neurological signs and died, while others were asymptomatic or had milder clinical signs and survived. Some mild cases might have resulted from using less virulent viruses (e.g., less pathogenic strains, or attenuated viruses propagated in the laboratory). For example, early studies suggested that phylogroup II viruses were less virulent than phylogroup I viruses; however, this is no longer thought to be true. Pre-existing immunity might also have contributed to survival in wild-caught bats.

The occurrence of healthy carriers among bats is controversial. There is one report that apparently healthy bats shed EBLV-1.

POST MORTEM LESIONS

There are no characteristic gross lesions. The stomach may contain unusual objects that were ingested. The typical histological signs, found in the CNS, are multifocal, mild, polioencephalomyelitis and craniospinal ganglionitis with mononuclear perivascular infiltrates, diffuse glial proliferation, regressive changes in neuronal cells, and glial nodules. Aggregates of viral material in neurons (Negri bodies) can be seen in some but not all cases.

DIAGNOSTIC TESTS

In animals, rabies virus is usually identified by detecting viral antigens in a brain sample taken at necropsy. The virus might also be found in other tissues such as the salivary gland, skin (tactile facial hair follicles) and corneal impression smears, but detection is less efficient. Immunofluorescence is the most commonly used assay, and is most effective on fresh samples. It can identify 98-100% of cases caused by all genotypes of the rabies and rabies-related lyssaviruses, using brain tissues. The usual immunofluorescence assay cannot, however, distinguish these viruses. Immunohistochemistry and enzyme-linked immunosorbent assays (ELISAs) can also be used to detect antigens. RT-PCR can be useful, particularly when the sample is small (e.g., saliva) or when large numbers of samples must be tested in an outbreak or epidemiological survey. Histology to detect Negri bodies is nonspecific, and it is not recommended if more specific techniques are available.

A single negative test does not rule out infection; therefore, virus isolation in cell culture (e.g., mouse neuroblastoma cells) is often done concurrently. Mouse inoculation may also be used in some circumstances, but cell culture is preferred. Identification of rabies virus variants or other species of lyssaviruses is done in specialized laboratories using monoclonal antibodies, specific nucleic acid probes, or RT-PCR followed by DNA sequencing.

Serology is occasionally used to test seroconversion in domesticated animals before international travel, as well as during wildlife vaccination campaigns or in research. It is rarely useful for diagnosing clinical cases, as the host usually dies before developing antibodies. Serological tests include virus neutralization tests and ELISAs. Rabies virus and rabies-related lyssaviruses cross-react, but the assays do not detect antibodies to most other rhabdoviruses. Some cross-reactive epitopes have been reported in members of the *Ephemerovirus* genus (bovine ephemeral fever virus and closely related viruses).

TREATMENT

There is no treatment once the clinical signs appear. Post-exposure prophylaxis of animals, as described below for humans, is usually considered inadvisable because it may increase human exposure. Post-exposure prophylactic procedures for animals have not been validated and are either prohibited or not recommended in the U.S. and many European countries. This is not the case in all parts of the world, and commercial vaccines are licensed for this purpose in some countries.

CONTROL

Disease reporting

A quick response is important for minimizing exposure to a rabies case, even in endemic regions. Veterinarians who encounter or suspect rabies should follow their national and/or local guidelines for disease reporting. In the U.S., state authorities must be notified immediately.

Prevention

In animals, rabies prevention is based on vaccination and the avoidance of contact with infected animals (e.g., preventing pets from roaming, housing pet rabbits and rodents indoors). Rabbits kept outside should be in an elevated, double-walled hutch that does not have exposed wire mesh floors. Bats caught by cats should be submitted for rabies testing. Six-month quarantines have been recommended for all wild-caught mammals added to collections. This is expected to identify most infected animals, though rare cases may become apparent after this time.

Vaccination is recommended for dogs, cats and ferrets, to reduce human exposure as well as to protect the animal. Both inactivated and modified live vaccines are effective in dogs and cats, but rare cases of post-vaccinal rabies have been reported with modified live vaccines. Rabies vaccines are also available for livestock. Vaccines have not been validated in rabbits or rodents, although they might be used extralabel in petting zoos or other facilities where animals are in contact with the public. Vaccination programs in wildlife, using oral vaccines, protect domesticated animals as well as people. In countries with large stray dog populations, similar oral vaccines may be useful.

Rabies vaccines are all based on rabies virus, and seem to provide little or no protection from rabies-related lyssaviruses in phylogroup II or those provisionally classified in phylogroup III. Limited vaccination and challenge studies suggest that they may provide some cross-protection against rabies-related lyssaviruses in phylogroup I. Within phylogroup I, the amount of protection may vary with the specific virus.

The specific regulations for domesticated animals exposed to a rabid animal vary with the country, species of animal and vaccination status. If an unvaccinated animal is exposed to rabies virus in the U.S., authorities recommend that it be euthanized and tested. This prevents unnecessary prophylaxis in people who may have been exposed, and also reduces the risk that it will infect other people or animals. If the owner is unwilling to allow euthanasia, the animal may be placed in strict isolation for 6 months. If a vaccinated animal is exposed to rabies in the U.S., it is revaccinated and confined under observation for 45 days. Animals with expired vaccinations are evaluated on a case-by-case basis.

Most countries have regulations to prevent the importation of rabies in animals. These regulations vary with the country and animal species, and may include quarantine or testing for vaccine-induced seroconversion.

MORBIDITY AND MORTALITY

The incidence of rabies in domesticated animals varies with the region. Canine rabies was once very common worldwide, but it has been controlled, or even eradicated, in some countries. In some countries (e.g., the U.S.), cats are now more likely to develop rabies than dogs, probably due to the lower vaccination rates in this species, combined with greater exposure to wildlife. Rabies is reported infrequently in ferrets, and rarely documented in rabbits and rodents. Sylvatic and urban rabies cycles occur concurrently in some regions, while the sylvatic cycle predominates in others. For example, wild animals accounted for more than 90% of the animal rabies cases reported in the U.S. and Canada in 2010. Rabies can be a serious concern in some rare or endangered species. In Africa, the Ethiopian wolf (*Canis simensis*) and African wild dogs (*Lycaon pictus*) are threatened by this virus. Although cases of rabies tend to be sporadic, epizootics are possible. Outbreaks occur among cattle bitten by vampire bats (*Desmodus rotundus*) in South America. Epizootics have also been reported occasionally among wildlife, such as kudu in Africa.

All animals exposed to rabies virus do not become ill. Factors that may affect the outcome of exposure include the virus variant, presence in saliva at the time of the bite, dose of virus, route and location of exposure, and host factors such as the species of animal, age and existing immunity to lyssaviruses. Experiments in bats and dogs suggest that some animals can survive and become resistant to reinfection. Antibodies have also been found in a few cats with no history of vaccination. Reports of animals surviving after the development of clinical signs are very rare, but do exist. In one well-documented case, an experimentally infected ferret (skunk origin virus) developed neurological signs and had evidence of infection in the CSF, but recovered with persistent hindlimb paralysis. There was no evidence of any residual virus at the time of euthanasia.

Rabies-related Lyssaviruses

Although some rabies-related lyssaviruses are common in bats, only a few clinical cases have been reported in domesticated animals. All of these cases were fatal.

INFECTIONS IN HUMANS

INCUBATION PERIOD

In humans, the incubation period can be a few days to several years. Most cases become apparent after 1-3 months.

CLINICAL SIGNS

Nonspecific prodromal signs may be seen during the early stage of rabies. They can include malaise, fever or headache, as well as discomfort, pain, pruritus or other sensory alterations at the site of virus entry. After several days, anxiety, confusion and agitation may appear, and progress to insomnia, abnormal behavior, hypersensitivity to light and sound, delirium, hallucinations, slight or partial paralysis, hypersalivation, difficulty swallowing, pharyngeal spasms upon exposure to liquids, convulsions and other neurological signs. Either an encephalitic (furious) form with hyperexcitability, autonomic dysfunction and hydrophobia, or a paralytic (dumb) form characterized by generalized paralysis, may predominate. Death usually occurs within 2 to 10 days.

Survival is extremely rare in clinical cases, and survivors are often left with severe neurological deficits. However, there are a few documented cases where patients with relatively mild neurological signs recovered well.

Rabies-related Lyssaviruses

Only a few infections with rabies-related lyssaviruses have been reported. These patients developed neurological signs, similar to rabies, and nearly all cases were fatal.

DIAGNOSTIC TESTS

Antemortem diagnosis is sometimes possible in people with rabies symptoms. RT-PCR or immunofluorescence may detect viral nucleic acids or antigens in saliva, or in skin biopsies taken from the nape of the neck. In skin, the virus occurs in the cutaneous nerves at the base of the hair follicles. Rabies virus is sometimes found in corneal impressions or eye wash fluid, and RT-PCR may occasionally detect nucleic acids in CSF or urine. Virus isolation is sometimes possible from the saliva, conjunctival secretions/tears, corneal impressions, skin biopsies or (less often) CSF in living patients. More than one test is usually necessary for an antemortem diagnosis, as the virus is not invariably present in any tissue other than the CNS. Detecting antibodies to rabies virus in CSF is definitive, and indicates that the virus is replicating in the CNS. Neutralizing antibodies do not usually appear in the blood until late, and infected people may still be seronegative when they die. Rabies is usually undetectable during the incubation period.

After death, rabies virus can be detected in the brain, as in animals.

Rabies-related Lyssaviruses

Infections with rabies-related lyssaviruses are easily misdiagnosed as rabies. The immunofluorescence test used for postmortem rabies diagnosis can detect these viruses, but does not recognize them as different from rabies virus. The specific virus can, however, be identified with tests based on monoclonal antibodies, or by PCR.

TREATMENT

Post-exposure prophylaxis consists of immediate wound cleansing, followed by the administration of human rabies immunoglobulin and several doses of human rabies vaccine. Fewer vaccine doses and no rabies immunoglobulin are given if the person was previously vaccinated. In unvaccinated patients, the recommended number of vaccine doses can vary with the availability of high quality biologicals, the performance of initial wound care, and whether the patient is immunocompetent or immuno-suppressed. Post-exposure prophylaxis is highly effective if it is begun soon after exposure.

There is no single, recommended treatment once rabies symptoms develop. The ideal treatment is unknown, and both aggressive treatment and supportive therapy have a very high risk of failure. A number of experimental therapies (e.g., vaccines, antiviral agents, antibodies to rabies virus, ketamine and/or the induction of a therapeutic coma) have been tried in the past, but were usually ineffective. Some treatments, such as therapeutic coma, are controversial. One young patient who recovered well was treated with ribavirin, amantadine and supportive care including therapeutic coma (the "Milwaukee protocol"); however, the same treatment protocol has been unsuccessful in a number of other patients. Two young patients recently recovered with only supportive therapy. Currently, the CDC does not advocate either supportive therapy or aggressive treatment, and instead states that either may be offered. If treatment is successful in sustaining life, the patient may be left with permanent, and possibly severe, neurological deficits.

CONTROL

Controlling rabies in domesticated and wild animals, mainly through vaccination, reduces the risk of exposure in humans. Wild animals should not be handled or fed; wildlife behaving abnormally should especially be avoided. Bats should be kept out of houses and public buildings. Although pasteurized milk and cooked meat are not expected to contain infectious rabies virus, which is inactivated by heat, ingesting any product from a rabid animal is not recommended.

Veterinarians and animal control officers should handle potentially rabid animals with extreme caution. In addition to the risk of contracting rabies, these animals can be very unpredictable and can attack without warning. Protective clothing such as thick rubber gloves, eye goggles and a plastic or rubber apron should be worn when doing autopsies, or in other circumstances when exposure to infectious tissues could occur. Sick animals, including rabbits and rodents, should not be sent home if they have been exposed to potentially rabid wildlife, even if the clinical signs do not immediately suggest rabies.

Bites, needlestick injuries, and other exposures should be reported immediately so that they may be evaluated, and any necessary post-exposure prophylaxis can begin promptly. Non-bite exposures, defined as the contamination of mucous membranes or broken skin with saliva, nervous tissue, or other potentially infectious material, are evaluated for prophylaxis on a case-by-case basis.

To protect people from animals that may be in the early stage of rabies, asymptomatic dogs, cats or ferrets that have bitten humans are confined under observation for a short period (e.g., for 10 days in the U.S.). If the animal develops signs of rabies during this time, it is euthanized and tested. It is not known whether the rabies status of lagomorphs and rodents can be determined by observation during a 10-day confinement. Until research establishes the viral shedding period in these species, human bites and scratches are evaluated individually for post-exposure prophylaxis. Factors that are considered include the animal's species, the circumstances of the bite and the epidemiology of rabies in the area, as well as the biting animal's history, current health status and potential for exposure to rabies. Similar considerations also apply when the companion animal belongs to other species in which the disease is incompletely understood.

Inactivated human vaccines are available for at risk veterinary staff, other animal handlers, wildlife officers, laboratory workers and others at high risk of exposure. International travelers may be vaccinated, depending on their destination and other risk factors. People in high risk occupations should have their antibody titers monitored periodically, with revaccination as needed. The recommended monitoring interval varies with the type and frequency of exposure. Vaccination does not eliminate the need for post-exposure prophylaxis, but fewer treatments are needed. It may also provide some protection if the person is unaware of the exposure or post-exposure prophylaxis is delayed.

Rabies-related Lyssaviruses

All currently licensed vaccines are based on rabies virus, and do not contain antigens from other lyssaviruses. Nevertheless, limited, preliminary studies in animals suggest that these vaccines may provide some protection against other phylogroup I viruses. In Europe, vaccination is recommended for people who regularly handle bats and may be exposed to lyssaviruses. Precautions should also be taken to avoid bites and scratches. If an injury occurs, the wound should be cleansed and brought to the attention of a physician. Some sources recommend rabies booster vaccination/ post-exposure prophylaxis if the bat is not available for testing.

MORBIDITY AND MORTALITY

The risk of developing rabies varies with factors such as a person's occupation, recreational activities and geographic location. Rabies is a very common disease in some parts of the developing world. Worldwide, 10 million people are estimated to receive post-exposure prophylaxis each year, and 40,000 or more to die of this illness. Most of these cases occur in Africa and Asia, and over 90% are caused by rabid dogs. In contrast, human rabies is rare in countries where canine rabies has been controlled or eliminated, and effective post-exposure prophylaxis (with high quality reagents) is available. In the U.S., only 0-3 cases of rabies are usually reported in people, each year. In developed countries, rabies typically occurs in people who did not realize they were exposed, or for some other reason, did not seek medical treatment.

Without post-exposure prophylaxis, an estimated 20% of humans bitten by rabid dogs develop rabies. Once the symptoms appear, rabies is almost always fatal, regardless of treatment. There are currently less than a dozen well-documented cases of survival, and only a few of these patients made a good recovery. Until recently, all rabies survivors were people who received vaccine before the onset of symptoms (it is also possible that some of these patients had post-vaccinal encephalomyelitis rather than rabies). Most were left with severe neurological complications. Since 2004, there have been at least 3 reports of young patients who survived with few or no residual neurological signs. All three had neutralizing antibodies to rabies virus at diagnosis, although none had been vaccinated. They also had relatively mild neurological signs when they were seen by a physician. One patient was treated aggressively with antiviral drugs and the induction of a therapeutic coma, but the other two received only supportive therapy. One of these patients appeared to have been infected 2 years earlier. The reasons for their good outcomes are uncertain, but potential factors include the patients' young age and good health, the mild neurological signs at presentation, or the type/origin of the virus (e.g., a less virulent strain). Based on limited serological evidence, especially in one South American population, it appears that subclinical infections might also be possible in humans. However, this remains to be proven.

Rabies-related Lyssaviruses

Infections with rabies-related lyssaviruses seem to be rare, but might be underdiagnosed, as they can easily be mistaken for rabies. Some of these viruses also occur in areas where diagnostic capabilities and surveillance are limited. Almost all symptomatic cases have been fatal. One child thought to have been infected with Mokola virus recovered; however, there is some question whether this child was actually infected with the virus. Recently, another child did not become ill after receiving a bite from an Ikoma virus-infected civet with neurological signs. The child received wound care and post-exposure rabies vaccination, but its efficacy against this virus is not known. It is uncertain whether the civet was shedding virus at the time of the bite.

RIFT VALLEY FEVER

Infectious Enzootic Hepatitis of Sheep and Cattle

IMPORTANCE

Rift Valley fever (RVF) is a zoonotic viral disease that can affect a variety of species, including ruminants and camels, causing high mortality in young animals and/or abortions in adults. The RVF virus is endemic mainly in subSaharan Africa, but it has also been seen in North Africa, and may have become established in Egypt. There are concerns that this virus might be spreading, after outbreaks were reported in Saudi Arabia and Yemen in 2000. Rift Valley fever tends to occur in periodic epidemics, which typically occur after heavy rainfalls and may be devastating to domesticated livestock. These outbreaks are thought to begin when dormant, infected mosquito eggs hatch in flooded areas. However, the epidemiology of Rift Valley fever is incompletely understood, and low levels of infection have now been identified during interepidemic periods.

Rift Valley fever outbreaks in domesticated animals are often accompanied by human disease. Many human cases are caused by occupational exposure to blood and tissues from infected animals, but mosquito-borne transmission can also occur. The most common form of the disease is a self-limiting, flu-like illness. Complications in a minority of cases include ocular disease, neurological signs, kidney dysfunction and a life-threatening hemorrhagic syndrome with hepatic dysfunction. Although overall case fatality rates are thought to be low ($\leq 2\%$), there may be very large number of cases during some epidemics, resulting in hundreds of serious cases and significant numbers of deaths.

ETIOLOGY

Rift Valley fever results from infection by the Rift Valley fever virus, an RNA virus in the genus *Phlebovirus* in the family Bunyaviridae. There are several genetic lineages of this virus, some of which may co-circulate, in endemic regions. Some viral isolates differ in virulence in laboratory rodents and possibly other species.

SPECIES AFFECTED

Rift Valley fever can affect many species of animals including sheep, cattle, goats, African buffalo (*Syncerus caffer*), water buffalo (*Bubalus bubalis*), camels, some species of monkeys, and a number of rodents (various wild African rodents), rats (*Rattus rattus*), nonnative gray squirrels (*Sciurus carolinensis*) and laboratory rodents including hamsters, gerbils, rats and mice, but not guinea pigs. Severe disease can be seen in newborn puppies and kittens, although adult dogs and cats seem to be unaffected. Some experimentally infected ferrets developed febrile reactions. Limited information suggests that some wild ruminants other than African buffalo are also susceptible to disease.

Sheep, goats and cattle are thought to be the primary amplifying hosts among domesticated animals, although other species such as camels could also be involved. The role of wildlife is still being investigated, but some animals might amplify the virus, or help maintain it during interepidemic periods. In addition to African buffalo, serological evidence of infection has been reported in other wild ruminants (e.g., Thomson's gazelle [*Gazella thomsonii*], lesser kudu [*Tragelaphus strepsiceros*], impala [*Aepyceros melampus*] and waterbuck [*Kobus ellipsiprymnus*]), as well as in black rhinocerus (*Diceros bicornis*), African elephant (*Loxodonta africana*) and warthog (*Phacochoerus aethiopicus*). Some wild species, such as giraffe, seem to become infected mainly during outbreaks in domesticated animals, and may be unlikely to maintain the virus. Wild rodents have been proposed as possible hosts for RVF virus, but their role (if any) is currently uncertain. There is also evidence for infection in other species including bats. Birds do not become infected in laboratory experiments, and surveillance has not detected any evidence of infection in nature.

Zoonotic potential

Humans are susceptible to infection with Rift Valley fever virus, and can develop clinical signs. The viremia may be sufficient to infect mosquitoes.

GEOGRAPHIC DISTRIBUTION

The Rift Valley fever virus is endemic in Africa south of the Sahara desert. Although outbreaks are most common in southern and eastern Africa, they also occur in other regions. Outbreaks or infections have been reported sporadically in Egypt and various islands off the coast of Africa (e.g., Madagascar, Mayotte), and a major outbreak occurred on the Arabian peninsula (Saudi Arabia and Yemen) in 2000-2001. Rift Valley fever might have become endemic in some of these regions, including Egypt; however, this can be difficult to determine, both because the virus is not necessarily found during interepidemic periods, and because some reported infections may result from illegal animal importation.

TRANSMISSION

Rift Valley fever is transmitted by mosquitoes, which act as biological vectors. This virus has been detected in many genera of mosquitoes in endemic regions; however, laboratory experiments suggest that some of these species are not competent vectors for transmission. At present, the major hosts appear to be members of the genera *Aedes, Culex* and *Anopheles*. Other biting insects might also be able to transmit this virus from viremic animals, although their role (if any) in nature is still uncertain. Potential mechanical and/or biological

vectors include stable flies (*Stomoxys* spp.), tsetse flies (*Glossina morsitans*), sandflies (*Lutzomyia longipalpis*), biting midges (*Culicoides variipennis),* blackflies and ticks. RVF virus was not detected in approximately 1000 ticks collected from livestock during one recent outbreak.

The mechanisms that maintain RVF virus in nature and cause it to emerge in epidemic form are incompletely understood, and might differ between areas. Transmission cycles are best understood in savannah regions, where the virus is thought to survive between outbreaks in the dried eggs of *Aedes* mosquitoes found in shallow depressions in the soil (dambos). Infected mosquitoes are thought to hatch when the dambos fill after heavy rainfall, and initiate transmission cycles involving additional mosquito species, and animals that act as amplifying hosts. The vertebrate amplifying hosts are thought to be critical in propagating epidemics. Virus transmission has also been demonstrated at low levels in livestock, wildlife and humans during interepidemic periods. Infection cycles in some other climates, such as forested regions, are poorly understood and might differ from this pattern.

RVF virus can be transmitted *in utero* to the fetus of ruminants, camels and other species. This virus may also infect other animals exposed to abortion or birth products, which contain large amounts of virus; however, the importance of this route is controversial. Although RVF virus can enter the body through mucous membranes, and might occur in milk, one attempt to inoculate puppies, kittens and lambs with virus-spiked milk was unsuccessful. Virus shedding in secretions and excretions from infected ruminants is poorly understood, although it is not thought to be important in spreading Rift Valley fever. Some studies have, nevertheless, detected small amounts of virus in oral fluids and nasal discharge, as well as in semen, and sentinel sheep were infected by unknown route(s) during 2 laboratory experiments. There was evidence for horizontal transmission during experiments in cats and dogs, and virus was detected in the saliva of puppies. RVF virus has not been reported in the urine or feces of any species except when these excretions are contaminated by blood.

Humans can acquire RVF virus by direct contact with infected tissues, contact with aerosolized viruses generated in laboratories or during slaughter, or from mosquitoes. The relative importance of mosquito-borne exposure and exposure to infected animal tissues continues to be debated. Drinking raw (unpasteurized) milk is a significant risk factor for human infection, although definitive proof for this route is lacking. Vertical transmission to human infants has been demonstrated in at least 2 cases. Person-to-person (horizontal) transmission does not seem to occur, but the blood and tissues of patients might be sources of exposure for medical personnel.

In vitro experiments suggest that RVF virus can persist for a few days in some protein-rich environments such as tissues. In a neutral or alkaline pH, mixed with serum or other proteins, the virus may survive for as long as four months at 4°C (40°F) and eight years below 0°C (32°F). It is quickly destroyed by pH changes in decomposing carcasses. Under optimal conditions, RVF virus remained viable in aerosols for more than an hour at 25°C (77°F).

DISINFECTION

The Rift Valley fever virus is susceptible to low pH (≤ 6.2), lipid solvents and detergents, and solutions of sodium or calcium hypochlorite with residual chlorine content greater than 5000 ppm.

INFECTIONS IN ANIMALS

INCUBATION PERIOD

The incubation period in sheep, goats and cattle is thought to be approximately 1-3 days, based on laboratory experiments. Young ruminants and puppies can develop clinical signs as early as 12 hours after inoculation.

CLINICAL SIGNS

In endemic regions, epidemics of Rift Valley fever are characterized by high mortality rates in newborn animals and abortions in adults. Between epidemics, this virus can circulate without apparent clinical signs in susceptible species, or there may be sporadic abortions that could be confused with other diseases.

Rift Valley fever is usually most severe in young animals. Nonspecific signs of fever, anorexia, weakness and lymphadenopathy are common in lambs. Hemorrhagic or fetid diarrhea, melena, regurgitation, signs of abdominal pain, a serosanguineous or bloodstained mucopurulent nasal discharge and elevated respiratory rate may also be seen. Very young lambs and kids with clinical signs rarely survive longer than a few days, and often die with 24 hours. Older animals may die acutely or peracutely, recover from the illness, or become infected with few or no clinical signs. Similar signs have been reported in young calves, although some sources have reported that icterus is more likely, and survival rates appear to be higher.

Abortions, apparently unrelated to the gestation period, are the most characteristic sign in adult sheep, goats and cattle. There are also reports of abortions in wild ruminants including African buffalo, a waterbuck (*Kobus ellipsiprymnus*), a springbuck (most likely *Antidorcas marsupialis*) and a blesbuck (probably *Damaliscus dorcas*). Some pregnant animals have few or no clinical signs other than abortion, while others become ill or die.

Experimental infections in nonpregnant older lambs and adult sheep suggest that some animals may have may minimal clinical signs (e.g., fever in some animals, slight lethargy), while others may have a more severe illness with fever, depression, diarrhea, nasal discharge, and neurological signs in some cases. Ocular signs (corneal opacity/ edema and erosions, and anterior uveitis) occurred 8-9 days after inoculation in some minimally affected animals. Hemorrhagic diarrhea has been seen in both naturally and experimentally infected sheep, and may be more severe in some breeds. A hemorrhagic syndrome reported in 7-11-month-old, experimentally infected Yansaka sheep (an indigenous Nigerian breed) was characterized by petechiae and ecchymoses on mucous membranes and unhaired skin, severe respiratory distress with epistaxis, severe bloody diarrhea and conjunctival hemorrhage. Infections are often subclinical in adult cattle, but some animals can have a few days of fever, anorexia, weakness, excessive salivation, lacrimation, nasal discharge, bloody or fetid diarrhea, and decreased milk production.

In the past, camels were thought to abort but not become ill; however, clinical signs reported during a recent outbreak included sudden death or an acute syndrome characterized by fever, neurological signs (e.g., ataxia), expiratory wheeze, ventral positional dyspnea, edema at the base of the neck, icterus, blood-tinged nasal discharge, hemorrhages on the oral mucosa and abortions. Camels that developed hemorrhagic signs usually died within a few days. Severe conjunctivitis and blindness occurred in some animals. Foot lesions were also documented in the outbreak report, but whether they were caused by Rift Valley fever seems uncertain.

Descriptions of illnesses in other species are based mainly on laboratory infections. Some wild or laboratory rodents, including rats, mice and hamsters, have nonspecific signs (e.g., weight loss, fever) of varying severity, with neurological signs and deaths in some cases. Kittens 3 weeks of age and younger developed neurological signs of ataxia and paddling, and many died soon afterward. Some very young puppies (≤ 1 week of age) also had neurological signs, while other pups of this age died rapidly with few or no clinical signs. Adult cats, puppies 2 weeks of age and older, and adult dogs appear to be unaffected (with the possible exception of reduced fertility in female dogs), while a fever was reported in experimentally infected ferrets. RVF virus can cause nonspecific signs of illness (fever, anorexia, depression), neurological signs, or hemorrhagic signs (petechiae, ecchymoses and bleeding from the nose, gums or venipuncture sites) in some species of nonhuman primates, while some other species seem to be unaffected or minimally affected.

POST MORTEM LESIONS

The most consistent lesion in all species is hepatic necrosis, which tends to be more extensive and severe in younger animals. In aborted fetuses and newborn lambs, the liver may be very large, yellowish-brown to dark reddish-brown, soft and friable, with irregular patches of congestion. Multiple gray to white necrotic foci are usually present, but may not be grossly visible. The liver lesions are often less severe and more localized in calves and adult animals, and may consist of numerous pinpoint reddish to grayish-white necrotic foci. The walls of the gallbladder may be edematous, and can contain visible hemorrhages. Hepatic necrosis is also the most prominent and consistent microscopic lesion, and eosinophilic oval or rod-shaped intranuclear inclusion bodies may be found in the liver in up to 50% of cases.

Additional gross lesions may include jaundice, widespread subcutaneous hemorrhages, petechial and/or ecchymotic hemorrhages on the surface of other internal organs (including the serosa of the heart in experimentally infected puppies and kittens), and fluid in the body cavities. The peripheral lymph nodes and spleen are typically enlarged, congested and/or edematous to some degree, and may contain petechiae. A variable degree of inflammation or hemorrhagic enteritis can sometimes be found in the intestines of ruminants and experimentally infected puppies and kittens. Ruminants may have hemorrhages and edema in the abomasal folds, sometimes with blood in lumen of the intestine. The hemorrhagic syndrome reported in 7-11-month-old, experimentally infected Yansaka sheep included unusual lesions of pulmonary edema/hemorrhage, and thrombosis in the heart, kidneys and brain. Aborted fetuses are often autolyzed.

DIAGNOSTIC TESTS

Rift Valley fever can be diagnosed by detecting the virus in the blood of febrile animals, or the tissues of dead animals and aborted fetuses. Some recommended tissues for sampling include the liver (the major site of replication), spleen and brain, with some sources also recommending kidney and lymph nodes; however, the virus may also be found at other sites.

Several RT-PCR tests including loop-mediated isothermal amplification (LAMP) techniques can detect Rift Valley fever viral RNA. Virus isolation is also possible, although this virus is a hazard to laboratory personnel, and biosecure facilities are required. Rift Valley fever virus can be grown in numerous cell lines including baby hamster kidney cells, monkey kidney (Vero) cells, chicken embryo-related (CER) cells and AP61 mosquito cell lines, as well as in primary kidney or testis cultures from calves or lambs. Although animal inoculation is avoided whenever possible, hamsters, adult or suckling mice, embryonated chicken eggs or two-day-old lambs can also be used. Viral antigens can be detected by immunostaining or with enzyme immunoassays (ELISAs, lateral flow assays). Some ELISAs are commercially available. In addition, the high viral titers in some samples (e.g., tissues from aborted fetuses or blood) may allow a rapid diagnosis to be made with serological tests such as virus neutralization, using organ suspensions as the antigen. The latter test should be supplemented with other, more definitive, assays.

ELISAs and virus neutralization can detect antibodies to RVF virus. Virus neutralization tests that require live virus are generally not recommended outside endemic regions or in laboratories not capable of biocontainment, but alternative neutralization tests that do not require highly virulent viruses are in development. Indirect immunofluorescence is used less frequently, while other serological assays employed in the past (hemagglutination inhibition, complement fixation, agar gel immunodiffusion) are generally no longer used. Cross-reactions with other phleboviruses can occur in serologic tests other than virus neutralization; however, the latter test has few or no issues with cross-reactivity.

TREATMENT

No specific treatment, other than supportive care, is available.

CONTROL

Disease reporting

Animals that may be infected with Rift Valley fever virus must be reported immediately, to protect humans who may be exposed and aid in controlling the outbreak. In endemic areas, animal cases also act as a warning that human outbreaks may be imminent, and public health messages and prevention advice should be issued.

Prevention

Vaccines are generally used to protect animals from Rift Valley fever in endemic regions. Vaccination of susceptible animals may protect people as well as animals by reducing amplification of the virus. Attenuated and inactivated Rift Valley fever vaccines are both available. An advantage to inactivated vaccines is their safety; however, they are less immunogenic than attenuated vaccines, and if quality control fails, an incompletely inactivated vaccine could introduce the virus to livestock. Attenuated RVF vaccines produce better immunity, but vaccine viruses might reassort with wild type RVF viruses, contributing to viral diversity. Attenuated RVF vaccines can also cause abortions and birth defects in pregnant animals. A newer inactivated vaccine, called Clone 13, did not cause abortions or fetal deformities in pregnant ewes vaccinated at 15 days of gestation. Vaccination campaigns conducted in resource-poor areas face additional challenges such as mechanical transmission from already infected animals when needles are reused. For this reason, some sources including the World Health Organization do not recommend that vaccination campaigns be initiated once an epidemic has begun.

Because epidemics typically follow heavy rainfall, weather prediction models may give some advance warning when conditions are favorable for outbreaks. Sentinel herds have also been used as part of early warning systems in some areas. Movement bans or restrictions, and the closure of livestock markets during outbreaks, may help prevent virus transmission to unaffected regions. Larvicides are the most effective form of vector control, if mosquito breeding sites can be identified and are limited in size. However, breeding sites are usually extensive, making vector control impractical.

MORBIDITY AND MORTALITY

Epidemics of Rift Valley fever tend to occur at intervals, when heavy rainfalls cause infected mosquito eggs to hatch and a susceptible animal population is present. In Africa, outbreaks typically occur in savannah regions every 3 to 15 years, and less frequently in some other areas. Low levels of infection can also be seen in livestock and wildlife during interepidemic periods. Some regions may mainly experience low-level virus activity during each rainy season, without explosive epidemics.

The morbidity rate varies between outbreaks, and is influenced by factors such as pre-existing immunity, pregnancy status, and the age of the animals. In some cases, illnesses are widespread in herds throughout the country, and most of the animals in infected herds are affected. Among domesticated animals, infections seem to be most severe in sheep and goats. Abortion rates in sheep range from 5% to nearly 100%, but they are generally lower in cattle (e.g., < 10%). Widespread abortions have also been reported sometimes in camels; 10% of camels aborted in one outbreak.

The case fatality rate can be very high in young animals, with fatalities decreasing in older age groups. The mortality rate may reach 70% to 100% in newborn lambs and kids, while estimated mortality in calves, and older lambs and kids, varies from 10% to 70%. Overall, the mortality rate is estimated to be 10-30% in adult sheep and < 10% in adult cattle, but higher rates have been reported in some outbreaks or herds. Deaths are most common in pregnant ewes that abort. Some experiments suggest that there may be breed-specific differences in the severity of clinical signs; however, naïve sheep of breeds not indigenous to Africa (e.g., European breeds) do not necessarily become severely ill. Mortality rates were 81% in experimentally infected young kittens (≤ 2 weeks of age), and 50-100% in young puppies (≤ 1 week of age), but no adult cats or dogs 2 weeks of age or older died.

INFECTIONS IN HUMANS

INCUBATION PERIOD

In humans, the incubation period is estimated to be 3 to 6 days. This is based on a limited number of cases, almost all acquired in the laboratory or by contact with the tissues of infected animals, rather than after exposure to mosquitoes.

CLINICAL SIGNS

Most people are infected subclinically with RVF virus or develop a mild to moderate, non-fatal, febrile flu-like illness with liver abnormalities The symptoms of uncomplicated infections are usually nonspecific and may include fever, headache, generalized weakness, dizziness, weight loss, myalgia and back pain. Some patients also have stiffness of the neck, photophobia and vomiting or diarrhea. Most people recover spontaneously within a week. A clinical syndrome that appears to be characteristic of severe Rift Valley fever was described

in several patients during the 2006-2007 epidemic in Kenya, and included nonspecific signs of fever, malaise and headaches, together with arthralgia in the large joints (elbows, knees and shoulders), gastrointestinal signs (nausea, vomiting, mid-epigastric pain), progressing to tender hepatomegaly, jaundice and delirium. Lymphadenopathy and diarrhea appeared to be absent in these patients.

Complications including renal dysfunction, meningoencephalitis, ocular disease, or a hemorrhagic syndrome with liver involvement occur in a small percentage of patients. The hemorrhagic syndrome is the most serious form, and may be seen in up to 1% of patients, with symptoms usually developing 2-4 days after the initial signs. Jaundice may be the first indication of this syndrome, followed by signs such as hematemesis, melena, menorrhagia, a macular or purpuric rash, petechiae and bleeding from the gums. These patients often progress to frank hemorrhages, shock and death within 3-6 days. Acute kidney dysfunction is a new complication reported in severe cases during recent outbreaks, and can also lead to death. Whether the kidney dysfunction is caused directly by the virus or a consequence of complications such as shock is still unclear. Survivors of this syndrome did not develop chronic kidney disease.

Ocular disease and meningoencephalitis can be late complications of Rift Valley fever. The ocular form is estimated to occur in up to 2% of patients, typically begins 1-3 weeks after the initial symptoms, and is characterized by retinal lesions and blurred vision. While ocular lesions disappear after 10-12 weeks in some patients, others experience some degree of permanent visual impairment, which may include blindness. Encephalitic signs are seen in less than 1%, and usually begin 1-4 weeks (but occasionally later) after the initial signs. The symptoms can include intense headache, memory loss, vertigo, hallucinations, confusion, disorientation, coma or seizures. Some patients have permanent neurological damage, which may be severe, but deaths are uncommon.

Some authors indicate that increased mortality or abortions in pregnant women have not been seen during outbreaks. However there are at least two reports of maternal transmission to the fetus. One infant, whose mother was also ill with malaria, was born with a rash and jaundice. The infant in the other case died soon after birth.

DIAGNOSTIC TESTS

Rift Valley fever virus can be detected in the blood, brain, liver or other tissues, but viremia usually occurs only during the first three days of fever. There are also reports of virus detection in other samples, such as throat swabs, cerebrospinal fluid, pericardial and peritoneal fluid. Tests to detect RVF virus in humans are similar to those used in animals, and can include PCR assays, virus isolation and various antigen detection assays. During some outbreaks, RT-PCR was able to identify people with high levels of viremia in the blood, who were more likely to progress to severe illness. ELISAs and other serological tests can detect specific IgM or rising titers.

TREATMENT

No specific treatment, other than supportive care, is available. Some animal studies have suggested that antiviral drugs or other therapies such as passive antibodies might be effective; however, these treatments have not been tested in humans. Most cases of Rift Valley fever are thought to be relatively mild, brief illnesses and resolve on their own.

CONTROL

Public education about transmission methods can help reduce infections during outbreaks. Milk should be pasteurized or boiled, and all other animal tissues including blood and meat should be cooked, and not consumed raw. Home slaughter of livestock is not recommended during outbreaks.

Barrier precautions should be used whenever contact may occur with infectious tissues or blood from animals; recommended measures include gloves and other barriers to prevent direct contact with tissues and/or aerosols. The precautions can depend on the form of exposure, with necropsies considered high risk procedures. Diagnostic tissue samples should be processed by trained staff in appropriately equipped laboratories. An inactivated vaccine has been used in some at-risk individuals (e.g., laboratory workers), but has had limited availability, and is no longer manufactured by one former supplier. Although person-to-person transmission has not been reported, there is a risk of transmission by contact with viruses in human blood and tissues. Standard (universal) precautions (e.g., barriers to prevent direct contact with blood and other potential sources of virus) have been recommended for healthcare workers who care for patients with confirmed or suspected Rift Valley fever.

Mosquito repellents, long shirts and trousers, bednets, and other arthropod control measures should be used to prevent transmission by mosquitoes and other potential insect vectors. Outdoor activities should be avoided, if possible, during periods of peak mosquito activity.

MORBIDITY AND MORTALITY

Humans are highly susceptible to Rift Valley fever. Specific risk factors include assisting in animal births, having contact with tissues (e.g., slaughtering or skinning an animal, preparing meat for cooking, handling abortion products, conducting necropsies), drinking raw (unpasteurized) milk, and sheltering animals within the home. Clinical cases are often seen in veterinarians, abattoir workers and others who work closely with blood and tissue samples from animals. Laboratory workers are also at risk. Human infections tend to occur mainly during Rift Valley fever epidemics in livestock, and are typically preceded by cases in animals; however,

illnesses were first diagnosed in people during some outbreaks. Sporadic cases may also be seen during interepidemic periods.

The vast majority of human infections appear to be asymptomatic or mild. However, the number of infections in some epidemics can be very large (e.g., possibly more than 180,000 infections in Kenya in 2006-2007), resulting in hundreds of serious cases and significant numbers of deaths. The overall case fatality rate for all patients with Rift Valley fever is estimated to be between 0.5% and 2%, but case fatality rates in hospitalized patients with more severe symptoms may be much higher (e.g., 31% of 747 hospitalized patients in Sudan in 2006-2007). Case fatality rates up to 50% have been reported in the hemorrhagic syndrome, and the case fatality rate in people with acute renal dysfunction was 40% during an outbreak in Sudan.

RINDERPEST

Cattle Plague

Note: *The World Organization for Animal Health (OIE) declared rinderpest eradicated worldwide, as of May 2011. However, samples of rinderpest virus are still believed to be present in laboratories.*

IMPORTANCE

Rinderpest is an acute, highly contagious, viral disease of cattle, domesticated buffalo and some species of wildlife. The classical form of rinderpest is one of the most lethal diseases of cattle, and can have a catastrophic effect on naïve herds. At one time, epidemics of rinderpest occurred regularly in Eurasia. In 1889, cattle shipped from India carried the rinderpest virus to Africa, causing an epidemic that established the virus on the continent. Initially, approximately 90% of the cattle in sub-Saharan Africa and many sheep and goats died. Wild buffalo, giraffe and wildebeest populations were decimated. The loss of plow animals, herds and hunting resulted in mass starvation, killing a third of the human population in Ethiopia and two-thirds of the Maasai people of Tanzania. The reduction in the number of grazing animals also allowed thickets to form in grasslands. These thickets provided breeding grounds for tsetse flies, resulting in an outbreak of sleeping sickness in humans. Some consider this epidemic to have been the most catastrophic natural disaster ever to affect Africa.

Although the rinderpest virus was eradicated from Europe early in the 20th century, epidemics continued to occur in sub-Saharan Africa and many parts of Asia. In areas where it persisted, rinderpest became the main constraint to livestock production. Several eradication campaigns have been conducted since World War II. One international project, started in the 1960s, eradicated or controlled the virus in much of Africa; however, in the 1970s, the termination of vaccination campaigns and surveillance efforts allowed the disease to emerge from two remaining pockets of infection and recolonize large areas. A similar event happened in Asia in the 1980s. In 1992, the Food and Agriculture Organization (FAO) of the United Nations began the Global Rinderpest Eradication Programme, with the goal of complete eradication by the year 2010. As of 2011, rinderpest was declared eradicated. Rinderpest is the first worldwide eradication of an animal pathogen; only one other virus, human smallpox, has ever been completely eliminated from nature.

ETIOLOGY

Rinderpest results from infection by rinderpest virus, a member of the genus *Morbillivirus* of the family Paramyxoviridae. There is just one serotype of this virus, but three genetically distinct lineages – lineage 1, lineage 2, and lineage 3 – have been identified. In the past, these lineages were found in different geographic areas.

SPECIES AFFECTED

Most cloven-hooved animals (order Artiodactyla) are susceptible to rinderpest virus to some degree. Cattle, water buffalo, yaks, African buffalo, giraffes, warthogs and Tragelaphinae (spiral-horned antelope) are particularly susceptible to disease. Wildebeest and East African zebus are moderately susceptible, and gazelles, sheep and goats are mildly susceptible. Asian breeds of pigs appear to be more susceptible than African or European breeds. Rinderpest is rare in camelids.

Cattle are the most important maintenance hosts for rinderpest virus. Sheep and goats are relatively unimportant in the epidemiology of this disease. Among wildlife, African buffalo seem to be the most important hosts. Although there is some disagreement on the length of time the virus can persist in this population, some studies suggest that it disappears after approximately three years. In at least one environment where African buffalo were infected, the virus did not spread to other susceptible species in the area, including wildebeest. Currently, it is believed that wildlife populations cannot maintain the rinderpest virus indefinitely.

Zoonotic potential

Rinderpest has not been reported to infect humans.

GEOGRAPHIC DISTRIBUTION

Rinderpest was eradicated from Europe early in the 20th century. Lineage 1 has been reported only in Africa and the Middle East, and was last seen in 2001. Lineage 3 (the "Asian lineage") was found in Russia, Turkey, and parts of Asia and the Middle East. This lineage has not been seen since 2000.

Lineage 2 was once reported from many parts of Africa and has now been eradicated from the region.

TRANSMISSION

Transmission of rinderpest virus usually occurs through direct or close indirect contact with infected animals. Small amounts of virus can be found in nasal and ocular secretions, saliva, milk, urine and feces beginning 1-2 days before the onset of fever. Blood and all tissues are also infectious before the clinical signs appear. Large amounts of rinderpest virus can be found in the animal's secretions and excretions (including nasal and ocular discharges, saliva, feces, milk, semen, vaginal discharges and urine), as well as expired air, during the first week of clinical signs, but virus shedding decreases as specific antibodies develop and the animal recovers. Pigs can be infected if they ingest contaminated meat, and infected pigs can transmit the virus to cattle. Rinderpest virus can remain viable for at least a week in meat kept at 4°C. Aerosol transmission is insignificant in the epidemiology of the disease, and is typically only seen over short distances in confined spaces. However, some sources suggest that rinderpest virus may occasionally be transmitted up to 100m or more at night, when the humidity is very high. Infected animals do not become carriers; the virus maintains itself by passing from animal to animal in a large, susceptible population. Vertical transmission does not occur.

Although fomites can spread rinderpest virus, this virus is readily inactivated by sunlight and drying, and fomite-mediated transmission is relatively unimportant. Rinderpest virus can remain viable on unshaded pastures for six hours or shaded pastured for 18-48 hours. Bare enclosures usually lose their infectivity within 48 hours and contaminated buildings within 96 hours. In Africa, transmission was thought to be facilitated by the nomadic husbandry system and the use of common watering areas. Because rinderpest virus is inactivated quickly by autolysis and putrefaction, this virus is destroyed within 24 hours in carcasses; however, freezing or chilling of the carcass in some climates could slow these processes and allow the virus to survive longer.

DISINFECTION

Rinderpest virus can be killed by most common disinfectants including phenol, cresol, sodium hydroxide (2% for 24 hours) and lipid solvents. The FAO recommends that premises, equipment and clothing be cleaned, then decontaminated with oxidizing agents such as sodium or calcium hypochlorite, or alkalis such as sodium hydroxide or sodium carbonate. Feces and effluents should be treated with sodium carbonate, before they are burned or buried. Pasteurization or heat treatment can inactivate the virus in milk.

INCUBATION PERIOD

The incubation period for rinderpest ranges from 3 to 15 days; 4 to 5 days is typical. The virulence and dose of virus and the route of exposure affect the incubation period. Mild forms of the disease can have an incubation period between one and two weeks. The World Organization for Animal Health (OIE) has established a maximum incubation period of 21 days for zoosanitary measures.

CLINICAL SIGNS

Rinderpest infections can vary in severity depending on the virulence of the strain and resistance of the infected animal. A peracute form, characterized primarily by high fever and sudden death, is mainly seen in young and newborn animals. In the acute (classical) form in cattle, a prodromal period of fever, depression, decreased appetite, decreased milk yield, congestion of mucous membranes, and serous ocular and nasal discharges is followed in approximately 2-5 days by the development of necrotic oral lesions. Necrotic epithelium can be found on the lips, tongue, gums, buccal mucosa, soft and hard palates. These lesions begin as pinpoints but enlarge rapidly to form gray plaques or a thick, yellow pseudomembrane. They slough to form shallow, nonhemorrhagic erosions. The muzzle eventually dries and develops cracks, and the animal becomes anorexic and develops mucopurulent ocular and nasal discharges. The breath is fetid. Necrotic lesions may also be found on the nares, vulva, vagina and preputial sheath. Diarrhea usually starts a few days after the onset of oral necrosis; it is typically profuse and watery at the onset, but may contain mucus, blood and shreds of epithelium in the later stages. Severe abdominal pain, thirst and tenesmus often accompany the diarrhea, and animals may die from dehydration. Dyspnea may be seen, and a maculopapular rash has been described on sparsely haired areas such as the groin and axillae. Mortality varies with the strain. Convalescence can be prolonged and may be accompanied by secondary infections. Pregnant cows often abort during this period.

In endemic areas, cattle may also develop mild subacute disease or atypical forms of rinderpest. Lineage 2 viruses can appear in cattle as mild, short-lived fever with slight congestion of the mucous membranes. Small, focal areas of raised, pale epithelial necrosis may be seen on the lower gum, and a few eroded cheek papillae can occur in some animals; these lesions are transient. A slight, serous ocular or nasal discharge may also be seen; this discharge does not usually become mucopurulent. Most animals are not noticeably depressed, and can continue to graze and behave normally. Lineage 2 infections can be difficult to recognize in cattle; however, these viruses can cause severe disease if they spread to susceptible wildlife such as Asian buffalo, giraffe, eland, and lesser kudu.

Rinderpest is usually milder in sheep and goats than cattle, and some infections are subclinical. The clinical signs may include fever and anorexia, with diarrhea in some animals. Severe cases with necrotic stomatitis, oculonasal discharge, conjunctivitis, pneumonia and diarrhea (similar to classical disease in cattle) may also be seen.

Peracute disease, with fever and sudden death, can be seen in Asiatic breeds of pigs. These animals can also have acute disease characterized by the sudden onset of fever, depression, inappetence, shivering, vomiting and epistaxis. Mucosal necrosis and erosions can develop, and diarrhea with rapid dehydration and emaciation may be seen. Some pigs may die. Subclinical infections have been reported in European pigs.

In susceptible wildlife, the clinical signs can include fever, nasal discharge, erosive stomatitis, gastroenteritis, and death; however, the symptoms can vary with the species. In buffalo, rinderpest generally resembles the disease in cattle, but lymphadenopathy, plaque-like keratinized skin lesions and keratoconjunctivitis might also be seen. Similar signs can be seen in lesser kudus, and severe keratoconjunctivitis often causes blindness, but diarrhea is uncommon in this species.

POST MORTEM LESIONS

In the classical form of rinderpest, the carcass is often dehydrated and emaciated, and shows evidence of diarrhea and mucopurulent nasal discharges. The eyes may be sunken. Depending on the stage of the disease and strain of the virus, congestion, pinhead or larger gray necrotic foci, or extensive necrosis and erosions may be seen in the oral cavity. Necrotic areas are sharply demarcated from healthy mucosa. In some cases, the necrotic lesions extend to the soft palate, pharynx and upper esophagus. Necrotic plaques are occasionally found on the pillars of the rumen, but other areas of the rumen and reticulum are usually unaffected. Occasionally, erosions and hemorrhages may be seen in the omasum. Severe congestion, petechiation and edema may be found in the abomasum, particularly in the pyloric region. White necrotic foci may be seen in Peyer's patches; necrosis, erosions and sloughing can be seen in the adjacent areas. The small intestine is otherwise unaffected. In the large intestine, blood and blood clots may be found in the lumen, and edema, erosions and congestion may be seen in the walls, particularly in the upper colon. The ileocecal valve, cecal tonsil and crests of the longitudinal folds of the cecal, colonic and rectal mucosae can be greatly congested in animals that die acutely, and may be darkened in more chronic cases, a lesion known as 'tiger striping' or 'zebra striping'. (Tiger striping can also occur in other diarrheas, and is probably caused by tenesmus.) The lymph nodes are usually enlarged and edematous, and the spleen may be slightly larger than normal. Petechiae and ecchymoses may be found in the gall bladder, and emphysema, congestion and secondary bronchopneumonia are sometimes present in the lungs.

MORBIDITY AND MORTALITY

Rinderpest is highly contagious in species such as cattle; the classical form of the disease can affect all exposed animals within a short time. In endemic areas where animals have developed immunity from exposure or vaccination, rinderpest is often a disease of young animals. Maternal antibodies to rinderpest can persist for 6-11 months, and young animals may become ill after maternal immunity wanes but before they are vaccinated. During epidemics in naïve populations, the virus usually infects most susceptible animals. Rinderpest epidemics can affect different species at different rates. In some outbreaks, only a single species may be affected; in others, multiple concurrent epidemics can occur in different species at different rates. Outbreaks of rinderpest are self-limiting unless the virus can be passed from animal to animal in a large susceptible population. Animals that survive are immune for life.

Morbidity and mortality vary with the strain of the virus, and the susceptibility and immunity of the animal. In endemic areas, the morbidity rate is low and the clinical signs are frequently mild. However, in naïve animals, some strains can cause morbidity and mortality rates up to 100%. During the early stage of the outbreak, the mortality rate is often 10-20%, but it rises are more animals are exposed. Repeated epidemics that occurred in Eurasia before the virus was eradicated typically killed 30% of an affected herd. Lineage 2 strains can be mild and cause no mortality or significant morbidity in cattle, but these strains can cause severe disease with high morbidity and mortality rates in susceptible wildlife. For this reason, severe outbreaks in wildlife can be a sign that rinderpest viruses are being maintained in cattle populations.

DIAGNOSTIC TESTS

Laboratory tests

Rinderpest can be diagnosed by a variety of tests; however, the Global Rinderpest eradication campaign required that the virus be isolated and identified during any outbreak. Rinderpest virus can be isolated in B95a, a marmoset lymphoblastoid cell line, or other cell lines.

Rinderpest can also be confirmed by demonstrating viral antigens or RNA in clinical samples. Rinderpest antigens can be detected with agar gel immunodiffusion (AGID) tests, counterimmunoelectrophoresis or the immunocapture enzyme-linked immunosorbent assay (ELISA). The AGID test can be useful under field conditions, but it does not differentiate between rinderpest and peste des petits ruminants. The immunocapture ELISA can be used for definitive diagnosis and the differentiation of rinderpest from peste des petits ruminants. A monoclonal antibody-based, latex particle agglutination test for field use has also been described. Antigens can be identified in tissues by immuno-peroxidase or immunofluorescence staining. Reverse-transcription polymerase chain reaction (RT-PCR) assays can be used to identify the virus, distinguish the three viral lineages, or differentiate rinderpest virus from peste des petits ruminants virus. A real-time RT-PCR assay has also been described.

Serological tests include the competitive ELISA and virus neutralization. These tests can be used for surveillance, but cannot distinguish infected from vaccinated animals. An indirect ELISA method has also been developed, and could be useful for rinderpest surveillance, particularly where lineage 2 viruses might be found.

Samples to collect

Viremia can be seen a day or two before the fever begins, and can continue for 1-2 days after the fever begins to wane. Samples for virus isolation and antigen or RNA detection should ideally be collected when a high fever and oral lesions are present, but before the onset of diarrhea – the period when viral titers are highest. Blood (in heparin or EDTA) is the preferred sample for virus isolation in live animals. Whenever possible, samples should be submitted from more than one animal. Serum, swabs of lacrimal fluid, necrotic tissues from oral lesions, and aspiration biopsies of superficial lymph nodes should also be collected. At necropsy, samples should be taken from the spleen, lymph nodes (prescapular or mesenteric) and tonsil. The ideal post-mortem lesions come from an animal that has been euthanized during the febrile stage. A second choice would be a moribund animal that has been euthanized. Samples for RT-PCR can be taken from the lymph nodes, tonsils or blood (peripheral blood lymphocytes). The spleen is less desirable due to its high blood content. An additional set of tissue samples should be collected for histopathology and immuno-histochemistry. In addition to other tissues, it should include the base of the tongue, retropharyngeal lymph node and third eyelid. Samples for virus isolation should be kept cold on ice during transport, but should not be frozen.

CONTROL

Disease reporting

2016: Rinderpest was declared eradicated from the world, as of May 2011. If any rinderpest infections are identified, it is of the utmost importance to report them to national authorities immediately.

Prevention

Rinderpest was controlled in the past by annual vaccination of all cattle and domesticated buffalo more than a year of age. Maternal antibodies to rinderpest can persist for 6-11 months. Unvaccinated animals can serve as sentinels if outbreaks occur.

Rinderpest is usually introduced into an area by infected animals. Outbreaks can be controlled with quarantines and movement controls, euthanasia of infected and exposed animals, decontamination of infected premises, and intensive focal vaccination. Although it is not a desirable option, quarantine and ring vaccination without slaughter can also eradicate the disease. Vaccination for one strain is protective against all strains of the virus. Vaccinated animals should be marked.

Rinderpest virus is inactivated rapidly in the environment, and decontamination is not difficult. This virus can remain viable on unshaded pastures for six hours or shaded pastured for 18-48 hours. Bare enclosures usually lose their infectivity within 48 hours and contaminated buildings within 96 hours. The FAO recommends that the premises, equipment and clothing be cleaned, then decontaminated with oxidizing agents such as sodium or calcium hypochlorite, or alkalis such as sodium hydroxide or sodium carbonate. Feces and effluents should be treated with sodium carbonate, before they are burned or buried. Pasteurization or heat treatment can inactivate the virus in milk. During an outbreak, carcasses from infected or exposed animals should be burned or buried. However, because rinderpest virus is inactivated quickly by autolysis and putrefaction, this virus is usually destroyed within 24 hours in carcasses. Restocking should be delayed for at least 30 days after cleaning and disinfection.

SCREWWORM MYIASIS

IMPORTANCE

Screwworms are fly larvae (maggots) that feed on living flesh. These parasites infest all mammals and, rarely, birds. Two different species of flies cause screwworm myiasis: New World screwworms (*Cochliomyia hominivorax*) occur in the Western Hemisphere, and Old World screwworms (*Chrysomya bezziana)* are found in the Eastern Hemisphere. However, the climatic requirements for these two species are similar, and they could become established in either hemisphere. New World and Old World screwworms have adapted to fill the same niche, and their life cycles are nearly identical. Female flies lay their eggs at the edges of wounds or on mucous membranes. When they hatch, the larvae enter the body, grow and feed, progressively enlarging the wound. Eventually, they drop to the ground to pupate and develop into adults. Screwworms can enter wounds as small as a tick bite. Left untreated, infestations can be fatal. Screwworms have been eradicated from some parts of the world, including the southern United States, Mexico and most of Central America, but infested animals are occasionally imported into screwworm-free countries. These infestations must be recognized and treated promptly; if the larvae are allowed to leave the wound, they can introduce these parasites into the area.

ETIOLOGY

New World screwworm myiasis is caused by the larvae of *Cochliomyia hominivorax* (Coquerel). Old World screwworm myiasis is caused by the larvae of *Chrysomya bezziana* (Villeneuve). Both species are members of the subfamily Chrysomyinae in the family Calliphoridae (blowflies).

SPECIES AFFECTED

All warm-blooded animals can be infested by screwworms; however, these parasites are common in mammals and rare in birds.

Zoonotic potential

Humans can be hosts for screwworm larvae.

GEOGRAPHIC DISTRIBUTION

Screwworms are very susceptible to freezing temperatures or long periods of near-freezing temperatures. These organisms are seasonal in some areas, and can spread into colder climates during the summer. The ideal environmental conditions for survival and activity are temperatures of 25-30°C and relative humidity of 30-70%.

New World screwworms are found only in the Western Hemisphere, primarily in the tropical and semitropical regions of South America and the Caribbean. They are rare above 7,000 feet. Eradication programs have eliminated these parasites from the North and Central America, Puerto Rico, the Virgin Islands, and Curacao. A sterile fly release program (see Prevention) is maintained at the Darien Gap, between Panama and Colombia, to prevent screwworms from spreading north from South America. However, screwworms occasionally pass this barrier and are detected in Panama. An eradication program is ongoing in Jamaica. New World screwworms were detected in Libya in 1988, but have since been eradicated.

C. bezziana, the Old World screwworm, can be found in parts of Asia, much of tropical and sub–Saharan Africa and some countries in the Middle East. Old World screwworms have never become permanently established in Europe, Australia, New Zealand or the Western Hemisphere.

Occasional cases or outbreaks are reported in screwworm-free countries.

TRANSMISSION

Although they are members of different genera, New World and Old World screwworms fill the same parasitic niche and have nearly identical life cycles. Screwworm larvae are obligate parasites of live animals. Infestations are transmitted when a female fly lays her eggs on a superficial wound or mucous membrane. Occasionally, Old World screwworms also lay their eggs on unbroken soft skin, particularly if it has blood or mucous on its surface. The larvae hatch and burrow into the flesh, where they feed on living tissues and fluids Wounds infested by screwworms often attract other female screwworms, and multiple infestations are common. After feeding through two molts (5- 7 days), the larvae leave the wound and fall to the ground, then burrow into the soil to pupate. The adults that emerge feed on wound fluids and mate after three to five days. Female flies mate usually only once, but can lay more than one batch of eggs at intervals of a few days. New World screwworms usually deposit 2 masses of eggs, but are capable of laying 6-8 batches or more. The length of the life cycle varies with the temperature. At the high temperatures that occur in the tropics, it may be completed in less than three weeks; at low temperatures, maturation can take up to 2-3 months. Freezing or a soil temperature consistently below 8°C (46°F) will destroy the pupae. The lifespan of a male fly is up to 14 days; 10 days is common for a female, but some female flies may live up to 30 days or more.

Female screwworms are attracted to all warm-blooded animals. A fly may travel up to 10-20 km in tropical environments with a high density of animals (though 3 km is more usual). In arid environments, flies can travel 20-25 km in search of a new host, and journeys up to nearly 300 km have been documented. Flies tend to travel along river valleys and other bodies of water in dry regions.

INCUBATION PERIOD

Screwworm larvae emerge from the eggs in 12 to 24 hours, but they are difficult to detect in wounds for the first day or two.

CLINICAL SIGNS

Screwworms can infest a wide variety of wounds, from tick bites to cuts and dehorning or branding wounds. Infestations are very common in the navels of newborns, and the vulval and perineal regions of their dams. If a screwworm deposits its eggs on mucous membranes, the larvae may enter any orifice including the nostrils, sinuses, mouth, orbits of the eye, ears or genitalia.

In the first day or two, screwworm infestations are difficult to detect. Often, all that can be seen is slight motion inside the wound. As the larvae feed, the wound gradually enlarges and deepens. Infested wounds often have a serosanguineous discharge and sometimes a distinctive odor. By the third day, the larvae may be easily found; as many as 200 vertically oriented parasites can be packed deep inside the wound. Screwworm larvae do not generally crawl on the surface, and tend to burrow deeper when disturbed. Sometimes, there may be large pockets of larvae with only small openings in the skin. Screwworms may be particularly difficult to find inside the nasal, anal, preputial and vaginal openings. In dogs, the larvae often tunnel under the skin. Larvae from other species of flies, which feed on dead and decaying tissues, may also infest the wound. These larvae are often found more superficially than screwworm larvae. Secondary bacterial contamination is also common.

Infested animals usually separate from the herd and lie down in shady areas. Fawns with screwworms in their navels may stand in water up to their abdomen. Discomfort, decreased appetite, and lower milk production are common. Untreated animals may die in 7 to 14 days from toxicity or secondary

infections. Because repeated infestations can occur, up to 3,000 larvae have been found in a single wound.

POST MORTEM LESIONS

Screwworms may be found post-mortem in any wound.

DIAGNOSTIC TESTS

Laboratory diagnosis is by identification of the parasites under the microscope. Any eggs on the edge of the wound should be carefully removed with a scalpel. The samples of eggs, larvae, or flies should be placed in 70% alcohol (not formalin) and transported to the laboratory. New World screwworm eggs are creamy and white, and are deposited in a shingle-like array on or near the edges of superficial wounds. The egg masses of Old World screwworms are similar but larger. The eggs from other species of flies are usually not well organized.

Larvae should be collected from the deepest parts of the wound; more superficial larvae may be other parasites and not screwworms. The second and third instar larvae of screwworms resemble a wood screw. They are cylindrical, with one pointed end and one blunt end, and have complete rings of dark brown spines around the body. Younger larvae are creamy white, while fully mature third-stage larvae may have a reddish-pink tinge. In third-stage *C. hominivorax* larvae, dark tracheal tubes can be found on the dorsum of the posterior end. Field diagnosis of screwworm larvae, even with a microscope or magnifying glass, is difficult.

Female screwworm flies are larger than a housefly. The thorax of a New World screwworm is metallic dark blue to blue-green and the head is reddish-orange. On the back of the thorax, there are three longitudinal dark stripes. The Old World screwworm is metallic blue, bluish-purple or blue-green, with two transverse stripes on the thorax. Adult screwworms are uncommonly seen. They are also difficult to distinguish from other flies.

Other techniques used mainly in research laboratories include cuticular hydrocarbon analysis, analysis of mitochondrial DNA, and random amplified polymorphic DNA polymerase chain reaction (RAPD-PCR) assays. Serology is not used.

TREATMENT

Screwworm infestations are treated in both endemic and non-endemic regions; the animal is not euthanized. Although some wounds may be surgically excised, most are treated with a suitable larvicide and allowed to heal without closure. Treatment is usually repeated at intervals until the wound has healed. Removal of necrotic tissue may be necessary, and antibiotics may be given when secondary bacterial contamination is present. In non-endemic regions, the animal is quarantined until treatment is complete and the wound has healed. Treatment of the environment may also be necessary. Larvae that are removed from the wound must be placed in alcohol preservative or destroyed. If any larvae leave an infested wound and mature into adults, screwworm can become established in an area.

CONTROL

Disease reporting

Veterinarians who encounter or suspect screwworms should follow their national and/or local guidelines for disease reporting. In the U.S., screwworm infestations should be reported to state or federal authorities immediately upon diagnosis or suspicion of the disease.

Prevention

Screwworms can enter non-endemic areas in infested animals or as adult flies. Vehicles that may contain adults or immature screwworms should be sprayed with insecticides. Imported animals (including pets) must be inspected for infestations, and treated if necessary, before they are allowed to enter. As a precaution, wounds that do not appear to be infested may be treated with an insecticide. Animals may also be sprayed or dipped. Any infestations that become apparent after an animal enters the country must be treated promptly.

In endemic areas, animals must be inspected for screwworms every few days. Livestock can also be protected by regular spraying or dipping with insecticides, or by subcutaneous injections of ivermectin and related compounds. Insect growth regulators have also shown good results. Organophosphate insecticides are effective against newly hatched larvae, immature forms and adult flies. Other insecticides, such as carbamates and pyrethroids have also been used; however, there are concerns about the development of insecticide resistance. In areas where screwworms are seasonal, breeding can be scheduled to avoid births when these flies are numerous. Whenever possible, procedures that leave wounds should not be performed during screwworm season, and sharp objects should be removed from livestock pens. No vaccine is available.

Screwworms can be eradicated from a region by repeatedly releasing sterile male flies that mate with wild female screwworms to produce unfertilized eggs. (Because it is usually impractical to separate irradiated male and female flies, both males and females are usually released.) This technique leads to a reduction in screwworm numbers and eventually results in eradication. In addition, infested animals are treated and their movements are controlled.

MORBIDITY AND MORTALITY

The morbidity from screwworms varies, but it can be very high when the ecological conditions are favorable. In some areas, screwworms may infest the navel of nearly every newborn animal. A single deposition of eggs, or a treated infestation, is not usually fatal; however, deaths may occur in smaller animals or from secondary infections. Untreated wounds usually develop multiple infestations and may be fatal within 7 to 10 days. Deaths seem to be more common with New World than Old World screwworms. In the 1950s, when screwworm was still endemic in south Texas, the annual mortality rate in fawns on one ranch varied from 20% to 80%.

PUBLIC HEALTH

Humans can be affected similarly to animals. The disease can quickly become debilitating if it affects the eyes, mouth, nasal or frontal sinuses or the ears.

SURRA

Murrina, Mal de Caderas, Derrengadera, Trypanosomosis, El Debab, El Gafar, Tabourit

IMPORTANCE

Surra, caused by *Trypanosoma evansi*, is one of the most important diseases of animals in tropical and semitropical regions. While surra is particularly serious in equids and camels, infections and clinical cases have been reported in most domesticated mammals and some wild species. *T. evansi* is transmitted mechanically by various tabanids and other flies, and it can readily become endemic when introduced into a new area. The morbidity and mortality rates in a population with no immunity can be high. In the early 1900s, an outbreak in Mauritius killed almost all of the Equidae on the island. More recently, severe outbreaks have been reported in the Philippines, Indonesia and Vietnam. In addition to illness and deaths, surra causes economic losses from decreased productivity in working animals, reduced weight gain, decreased milk yield, reproductive losses and the cost of treatment.

ETIOLOGY

Surra is caused by the protozoal parasite *Trypanosoma evansi*. This organism belongs to the subgenus *Trypanozoon* and the Salivarian section of the genus *Trypanosoma*. Two genetic types of *T. evansi*, type A and type B, have been recognized. Most isolates worldwide belong to type A. Type B, which is not recognized by some diagnostic tests, has only been detected in parts of Africa as of 2015. Whether *T. evansi* should be considered a distinct species, separate from *T. brucei*, is controversial.

SPECIES AFFECTED

The principal hosts and reservoirs for *T. evansi* are reported to differ between regions; however, camels, equids, water buffalo and cattle are generally considered to be the major hosts among domesticated animals. Equids, Bactrian camels (*Camelus bactrianus*) and dromedaries (*Camelus dromedarius*) are highly susceptible to disease. Infections are usually mild or asymptomatic in cattle, water buffalo and related species in the Bovinae (the genera *Bos, Bubalus, Syncerus*, and *Poephagus*) in Africa or Latin America, but cattle and water buffalo regularly become ill in Asia. Many other mammals and marsupials are also susceptible to varying degrees; clinical cases have been reported in South American camelids, deer, sheep, goats, pigs, dogs, cats, tigers (*Panthera onca*), jaguars (*Panthera onca*), elephants, Sumatran rhinoceroses (*Dicerorhinus sumatrensis sumatrensis*), Himalayan black bears (*Selenarctos thibetanus*), coati (*Nasua nasua*), and experimentally infected wallabies (e.g., *Macropus agilis* and *Thylogale brunii*) and bandicoot rats (*Bandicota bengalensis*).

Infections have been documented in many wild mammals (e.g., various cervids, other large ungulates, wild pigs, lagomorphs, felids, canids, primates, small mammals) and marsupials, with or without disease, and some of these animals may help maintain *T. evansi*. In particular, vampire bats (*Desmodus rotundus*) are considered to be reservoirs as well as vectors in South America. Various small mammals, including capybara (*Hydrochaeris hydrochaeris*), have also been proposed as possible maintenance hosts. Some birds (e.g., young pigeons, chicks) can be infected experimentally, but their susceptibility in nature is uncertain.

Zoonotic potential

While *T. evansi* is not currently considered to be zoonotic, a few cases have been reported in humans (see Public Health section for details). It is uncertain whether all of these infections occurred in people who are unusually susceptible or the disease is underdiagnosed.

GEOGRAPHIC DISTRIBUTION

Surra is enzootic in Africa, the Middle East, many parts of Asia, and Central and South America. It also occurs in the Canary Islands of Spain, although control programs appear to have limited the organism to one small region.

TRANSMISSION

T. evansi does not require a biological vector. This organism, which can be found in blood and tissues, is transmitted mechanically by biting insects. Members of the deerfly and horsefly family, Tabanidae (e.g., the genera *Tabanus, Atylotus, Chrysops, Lyperosia, and Haematopota*) and flies in the genus *Stomoxys* spp. are thought to be the most important vectors. Transmission by other biting insects (e.g., *Hippobosca* spp., mosquitoes in the family Culicidae, and midges in the family Ceratopogonidae) has been reported experimentally or suspected in the field, and might contribute to local spread. Sucking flies, such as *Musca sp.,* may spread *T. evansi* when they visit contaminated wounds. Other organisms proposed as potential vectors include ticks and leeches, such as buffalo leeches in Asia.

Additional means of transmission include iatrogenic spread on contaminated needles or surgical instruments, and the ingestion of infected tissues by carnivores. Vampire bats can both maintain *T. evansi* and act as mechanical vectors in South and Central America. Transplacental transmission has been demonstrated in ruminants and donkeys, and transmission in milk and colostrum was reported in experimentally infected sheep. Trypanosomes cannot survive for long periods outside the host, and disappear relatively quickly from the carcass after death. In one recent study, organisms were detected as long as 13-15 hours in the heart blood of mice, although their viability had decreased to ≤ 5% by this time.

DISINFECTION

There is limited need for disinfectants, due to the fragility of trypanosomes in the environment, and no studies appear to have examined disinfectant susceptibility specifically for *T. evansi*. The closely related organism *T. brucei* can be inactivated by various agents including 0.05% sodium hypochlorite, 70% ethanol, 2% TriGene™, 0.1% hand soap, 2% formaldehyde and 0.05% glutaraldehyde. The temperature reported to kill 100% of trypomastigotes is 50°C.

INCUBATION PERIOD

In the Equidae, the incubation period ranges from approximately one week to 2 months, with most cases appearing in 1-4 weeks.

CLINICAL SIGNS

Surra can be an acute, subacute or chronic disease, with the severity of the clinical signs differing between individual animals, as well as between species. Some animals die rapidly, especially among highly susceptible species such as horses and camels; in other cases, clinical signs may persist for months or years. Such chronic illnesses can occur in less susceptible species, but they may also be prevalent among equids and camels in endemic regions. Animals can also carry *T. evansi* subclinically.

Common clinical signs include fever (which can be intermittent in chronic cases), weight loss or wasting, lethargy, signs of anemia and enlargement of the lymph nodes. There may also be dependent edema, jaundice, petechial hemorrhages of the mucous membranes and abortions or stillbirths. Neurological signs have been documented in a number of species, especially in the late stages, and ataxia, with gradually progressive paresis of the hindquarters accompanied by muscle atrophy, is reported to be a common sign among horses in South America. Horses may have episodes of urticaria, and this sign was also reported in an outbreak among pigs. Testicular lesions in camels and experimentally infected goats suggest that, in some species, male fertility might also be impaired.

Additional signs documented in individual species include facial and laryngeal edema and ocular signs (e.g., conjunctivitis, keratitis, corneal opacity, anterior uveitis and/or hemorrhages) in dogs; diarrhea and conjunctivitis in some water buffalo; decreased milk production in dairy cattle; facial edema in Asian elephants; nasal hemorrhages in rhinoceroses; respiratory signs (dyspnea, coughing), diarrhea, ocular signs or arthritis in some experimentally infected goats; and diarrhea, vomiting, ocular signs, facial and limb edema, and external and internal abscesses in some experimentally infected cats. In addition, *T. evansi* causes leukopenia, which may result in immunosuppression and might decrease vaccine responses or exacerbate other conditions.

POST MORTEM LESIONS

The gross lesions tend to be nonspecific, and may include wasting or emaciation of the carcass, subcutaneous edema, signs of anemia, enlargement of the spleen, liver and lymph nodes, and petechiae on some internal organs. Muscle atrophy may be noted, particularly in the hindquarters. Icterus and nephritis may also be present. Fluid accumulation in other body cavities (e.g., ascites, hydrothorax) is sometimes seen. Cardiac lesions including hydropericardium, pericarditis and evidence of cardiomyopathy or myocarditis occur in some animals. The lungs may also be affected in some species; respiratory lesions (congestion, consolidation, edema, emphysema, hemorrhages and/or pneumonia) were reported in some *T. evansi*-infected cattle and water buffalo and some experimentally infected bandicoots, rats, mice and coatis.

In some horses with neurological signs, the cerebral hemispheres may be swollen and the gyri flattened. There may be severe edema and malacia, with the white matter becoming yellow, gelatinous and friable. Subpial hemorrhages may also be present.

DIAGNOSTIC TESTS

A presumptive diagnosis may be possible if organisms consistent with *T. evansi* are detected in the blood, lymph nodes, tissues (e.g., at necropsy) or edema fluid by direct examination, and other trypanosomes do not exist in the area. While *T. evansi* differs in morphology from some other trypanosomes, it cannot be distinguished from certain species such as *T. equiperdum*. In addition, atypical forms have been observed in some outbreaks (e.g., organisms that resembled *T. vivax* during the 2008 surra outbreak in Spain). Blood should be collected from live animals during a febrile period. The organism may be difficult to find, especially in mild or subclinical cases, and parasitemia is often intermittent in chronically infected animals. Repeated sampling may be necessary.

Microscopy specimens used to look for trypanosomes include wet blood films, used to detect the motile organisms, and thick or thin stained blood smears. Thick films have the advantage of being able to detect parasites in low numbers; however, the morphology of the parasite is difficult to determine. Detection can be improved with parasite concentration techniques including mini anion-exchange chromatography, hemolysis methods that use sodium dodecyl sulphate (SDS) to destroy the erythrocytes (i.e., wet blood film clarification or hemolysis centrifugation) hematocrit centrifugation (Woo method) or the dark-ground/phase-contrast buffy coat technique (Murray method). The latter two methods rely on the concentration of trypanosomes near the buffy coat after centrifugation.

Polymerase chain reaction (PCR) assays are used in some laboratories. They can identify the organism to the level of the subgenus *Trypanozoon*, but cannot distinguish it from *T. equiperdum*. Recombinant DNA probes may also be employed, but are not in routine use.

In some horses with neurological signs, immunohistochemical staining could detect parasites in the brain, even when they were not visible in hematoxylin and eosin stained sections. This technique has also been used to detect *T. evansi* in the brains of cattle, hog deer and buffalo. Other antigen detection tests have also been published; however, the most recent World Organization for Animal Health (OIE) Manual of Diagnostic Tests and Vaccines did not currently consider any method to be sufficiently developed for routine diagnosis using blood or serum.

Serological tests include ELISAs and card agglutination tests (CATT). The CATT detects IgM and is particularly useful early in the course of the disease. The trypanolysis test may be employed to confirm positive results, and immunofluorescent assays can be used with small numbers of samples. All serological tests have not been validated or standardized for each species, and cross-reactions can occur with other trypanosomes.

Some serological and molecular tests, including PCR, may not detect the type B *T. evansi* variants reported from parts of Africa. Assays that can recognize type B isolates and/or distinguish types A and B include mobile genetic element PCR (MGE-PCR) and loop-mediated isothermal amplification (LAMP).

Animal inoculation studies in rats or mice may be used, if necessary, to detect low levels of parasites, such as when importing an animal into a surra-free regions. They are not generally recommended unless the need is critical.

TREATMENT

Surra can be treated with antiparasitic (trypanocidal) drugs. The efficacy and toxicity of a particular drug may differ between species. Depending on the drug dose and other factors, treatment may be clinically curative without completely eliminating the parasite, and relapses are possible. Drug resistance also occurs. Cases with neurological signs are very difficult to treat, although some newer drugs may cross the blood-brain barrier to some extent.

Treatment may or may not be permitted in countries where *T. evansi* is not endemic.

CONTROL

Disease reporting

A quick response is vital for containing outbreaks in surra-free regions. Veterinarians who encounter or suspect a *T. evansi* infection should follow their national and/or local guidelines for disease reporting. In the U.S., state or federal veterinary authorities should be informed immediately.

Prevention

T. evansi is excluded from uninfected areas by quarantines and testing. This organism has often become endemic after its introduction into a new area, due to the large number of potential hosts and its ability to be transmitted mechanically by numerous biting insects. Nevertheless, eradication was successful in a few cases when the outbreak was recognized early. In some instances, such outbreaks were controlled by quarantines, movement controls and the slaughter of infected animals. In 2008, an outbreak among camels and equids on an isolated farm in Spain was eradicated by treating the infected camels, with isolation and monitoring in a closed stable for 6 years. Two equids were euthanized 4 months after treatment; however, treatment appeared to be effective in the camels. An outbreak in France in 2006 was also eradicated by isolating and treating camels but euthanizing seropositive sheep in the area.

In endemic areas, it is difficult to control the biting flies that transmit *T. evansi*; however, some animals may be protected with insecticides/repellents, traps, insect screens/netting in stables, and/or other controls. In one recent outbreak, most cases occurred among horses kept in open paddocks, while horses in nearby fly-proof stables were spared. Flies are most infective soon after feeding on an infected host (e.g., in the first half hour), and the highest probability of transmission is to nearby hosts. Because tabanids are persistent feeders and do not usually leave one animal to bite another more than 50 meters away, it is also considered advisable to separate highly susceptible animals, such as horses, from herds of cattle, water buffalo or other animals that may be subclinical hosts. In South America, animals should also be protected from vampire bats.

Antiparasitic drugs are used routinely to protect susceptible animals in some endemic regions. Carnivores and omnivores should not be allowed to eat the carcasses of infected animals. No vaccines are available.

MORBIDITY AND MORTALITY

The severity of the clinical signs can vary with the strain of *T. evansi* and with host factors including previous exposures, stress, concurrent infections and general health. Horses and camels are generally considered to be the most susceptible species, and often develop severe illness, with high case fatality rates, even in endemic regions. Donkeys and mules are reported to have less severe signs than horses. In camels, surra is most common soon after weaning, but can occur in all ages. Severe outbreaks are especially likely when *T. evansi* is introduced into disease–free areas or susceptible animals are moved into endemic regions. Morbidity rates of 50% or greater, with comparable mortality, can be seen in some herds. Chronically or subclinically infected animals may relapse with parasitemia under conditions of stress.

Infections are often milder in other species of mammals; nevertheless, severe cases and deaths have been documented in many species including water buffalo, cattle, other domesticated animals and captive wild animals. Why surra is much more likely to become clinical among cattle and water buffalo in Asia than Africa or Latin America is uncertain; however, mortality rates ranging from 10% to > 90% have sometimes been reported among bovids in Asia, especially where *T. evansi* was newly introduced. Among carnivores, clinical cases have been reported more often in dogs than cats, and can be severe. Some studies suggest that infections might be relatively common in this species. Approximately 2% of dogs tested by microscopic examination had trypanosomes in one endemic region in India, and 29% of dogs were seropositive in a survey in Brazil. Deaths are especially likely in untreated stray dogs, but can also occur despite treatment.

PUBLIC HEALTH

Humans possess innate resistance against many species of trypanosomes, including *T. evansi*, due to the trypanolytic activity of the serum protein apolipoprotein L-I. Nevertheless, there have been a small number of human infections with atypical trypanosomes, including a few infections caused by *T. evansi*. Whether illnesses caused by this organism are underestimated or occur very rarely and under unusual circumstances is currently unclear.

One *T. evansi* infection was reported in 1977, in a laboratory worker exposed to contaminated blood. The symptoms included insomnia, memory loss, tachycardia and an enlarged liver, spleen, and lymph nodes, and resolved after treatment with an antitrypanosomal drug. While the parasite was identified only by morphology (which is not definitive), the diagnosis appears likely in this case. A definitive diagnosis was established in two naturally-occurring cases. One occurred in 2005, in a 45-year-old Indian farmer who had a genetic defect in apolipoprotein L1. His symptoms included intermittent fever, chills, sweats and neurological signs. The diagnosis was established by PCR and antiparasitic treatment was successful. The other case occurred in Sri Lanka in 1999, in a patient who had a headache and intermittent fever. While this case was not published in the scientific literature, a recent review article reported that the identity of the parasite had been confirmed by PCR. Four additional suspected cases, diagnosed only by parasite morphology, were reported from India. They included one person who died 2 days after admission to a hospital. Another suspected case (2010) was a cattle farmer in Egypt who had recurrent episodes of fever. He was reported to have been hospitalized and "successfully treated."

In 2005, a study conducted in the village of the farmer with the apolipoprotein L1 defect did not detect trypanosomes in the blood of any other humans, although some people were seropositive. The serological test used has not been validated in humans. In a study from Egypt, published in 2013, there was no virological evidence of *T. evansi* infection in camel owners, using either PCR or microscopic examination of blood smears, although 10-46% of their camels had evidence of infection. A new organization, the Network on Atypical Human Infection by Animal Trypanosomes (NAHIAT) was established in 2011, and is coordinated by the Institute of Research for Development (IRD) and the Center for International Collaboration on Agricultural Research for Development (CIRAD). Its purpose is to coordinate information and research about various atypical trypanosomes, including *T. evansi,* in humans.

TICKS (EXOTIC SPECIES)

Amblyomma variegatum, Amblyomma hebraeum, Rhipicephalus microplus, Rhipicephalus annulatus, Rhipicephalus appendiculatus, Ixodes ricinus

IMPORTANCE

Tick bites can be irritating and/or painful. They also provide entry points for secondary bacterial invaders or screwworms. Heavy infestations can damage hides and may cause anemia, particularly when the animal is in poor condition. *Rhipicephalus appendiculatus*, the brown ear tick, damages the ears of cattle and other livestock, and some species of ticks cause tick paralysis. However, the most important risk with the introduction of exotic ticks is that they may carry the agents of exotic diseases. The greatest danger is when the tick acts as a biological vector, but pathogens carried mechanically can be introduced if they survive long enough.

Important tick species at risk for introduction into North America include *Amblyomma variegatum, Amblyomma hebraeum, Rhipicephalus microplus* (formerly *Boophilus microplus*)*, Rhipicephalus annulatus* (formerly *Boophilus annulatus*)*, Rhipicephalus appendiculatus* and *Ixodes ricinus.*

Disease risks

A. variegatum and *A. hebraeum* can transmit *Ehrlichia ruminantium* (formerly *Cowdria ruminantium*), the agent

of heartwater. These ticks can also carry *Rickettsia africae*, which causes African tick-bite fever, and other disease agents. *I. ricinus* transmits a number of pathogens including *Babesia divergens* (babesiosis), louping ill virus and tick-borne encephalitis virus, which are exotic to the Americas. *Rhipicephalus appendiculatus* can carry *Theileria parva*, the cause of East Coast fever, as well as Nairobi sheep disease virus and other disease agents.

R. microplus and *R. annulatus* are particularly important in transmitting babesiosis, which is caused by *Babesia bigemina* and *Babesia bovis,* and anaplasmosis, caused by *Anaplasma marginale*. Babesiosis or "cattle fever" was eradicated from the United States between 1906 and 1943, by eliminating these vectors. *R. annulatus* and *R. microplus* still exist in Mexico and further south, and a permanent quarantine zone is maintained along the U.S./Mexican border to prevent their reintroduction.

SPECIES AFFECTED AND LIFE CYCLE

Although ticks have host preferences, which may vary with the life stage, most species will feed on a wide variety of wild and domesticated animals, as well as humans.

Three-host ticks

Amblyomma variegatum, A. hebraeum, I. ricinus and *R. appendiculatus* are 3-host ticks. Three-host ticks can be found on the host while they feed, then they drop to the ground to develop to the next stage. Larvae, nymphs and adults all require a blood meal. Once the adult female has fed and mated, she deposits her eggs in the environment.

The life cycle for *Amblyomma variegatum, A. hebraeum* and *I. ricinus* usually takes more than a year, and up to a few years, to complete. Immature *Amblyomma* spp. and *I. ricinus* tend to be found on smaller mammals, birds and reptiles, while the adult stages usually feed on large mammals including both livestock and wildlife

R. appendiculatus can complete one to three life cycles in a year, depending on the environment. This tick mainly infests cattle, buffalo and large antelope, but it can occur on other species including sheep and goats. Immature ticks may also be seen on small antelope, carnivores, hares and other species. Adult *R. appendiculatus* prefer to feed in the ears, but some are found on the head. Immature stages feed in the ears, on the head, and on the legs. Large numbers of ticks may be found on an animal, and heavy infestations can damage the ears.

One-host ticks

Rhipicephalus microplus and *R. annulatus* are one-host ticks: all stages are spent on a single animal. The eggs hatch in the environment and the larvae crawl up plants to find a host. Newly attached larvae ("seed ticks") are usually found on the underside of the animal, particularly on the softer skin inside the thigh, flanks and forelegs. After feeding, the larvae molt twice, to become nymphs and then adults. Each developmental stage (larva, nymph and adult) feeds only once, but the feeding takes places over several days. Adult male ticks become sexually mature after feeding, and mate with feeding females. An adult female tick that has fed and mated detaches from the host and deposits a single batch of eggs in the environment. *R. microplus* and *R. annulatus* have a life cycle than can be completed in 3 to 4 weeks. This characteristic can result in a heavy tick burden on animals.

Cattle are the preferred hosts for *R. annulatus*. This tick is also found occasionally on other mammals, particularly large animals but also capybaras and other species. It rarely feeds on sheep and goats. *R. microplus* mainly infests cattle, deer and buffalo, but it can also be found on many other hosts including horses, donkeys, goats, sheep, pigs, dogs and wild animals.

GEOGRAPHIC DISTRIBUTION

A. variegatum, A. hebraeum, R. annulatus, R. microplus and *R. appendiculatus* are found in the tropics and subtropics. *Amblyomma variegatum, A. hebraeum* and *R. appendiculatus* are endemic in Africa. *A. variegatum* has also been found in southern Arabia, and in the Caribbean and on some other islands. An eradication program is in progress in the Caribbean. *R. annulatus* and *R. microplus* are more widely distributed. *R. annulatus* is endemic in parts of Africa and Asia, the southern regions of the former U.S.S.R., the Middle East, the Mediterranean, Mexico and parts of South and Central America. *R. microplus* occurs in large areas of Asia, as well as in Madagascar, Latin America including Mexico, the Caribbean, and parts of Africa and Australia. *R. annulatus* and *R. microplus* have been eradicated from the U.S., but they can be sometimes found in Texas or California, in a buffer quarantine zone along the Mexican border.

In contrast, *I. ricinus* is restricted to cool, relatively humid, shrubby or wooded areas. In addition to deciduous and mixed forests, this tick can be found in more open areas when the vegetation is dense and rainfall is abundant. It is endemic in most of Europe (with the exception of the Mediterranean region, which has a warm, dry climate). *I. ricinus* also occurs as far south as the Caspian Sea and northern Iran, as well as in northern Africa.

IDENTIFICATION

A. variegatum, A. hebraeum, R. microplus, R. annulatus, R. appendiculatus and *I. ricinus* are all members of the family Ixodidae (hard ticks). Hard ticks have a dorsal shield (scutum) and their mouthparts (capitulum) protrude forward when they are seen from above.

Amblyomma variegatum and *A. hebraeum* are large, ornate, variegated ticks with long, strong mouthparts. The bodies of female *A. variegatum* are brown, but the males are brightly ornamented with orange. When they are engorged, adult female *A. variegatum* are about the size of a nutmeg. *Rhipicephalus* spp. and *Ixodes* spp. have no ornamentation and

are less distinctive, but they may be identified at least to the genus level using tick keys.

Tick identification to the species level can be difficult, and ticks should be submitted to an expert for identification or confirmation. Ticks that are submitted in 70% ethanol can be examined morphologically, and if necessary, tested by PCR. Both male and female ticks, and ticks from different life stages, should be submitted if they can be found.

CONTROL

Disease reporting

Veterinarians who encounter or suspect the presence of an exotic tick should follow their national and/or local guidelines for disease reporting. In the U.S., state or federal authorities must be notified immediately.

Prevention

Measures used to exclude exotic ticks from a country include pre-export inspection and certification that the animals are free of ectoparasites, quarantines upon entry, and treatment with acaricides. Three-host ticks spend at least 90% of their life cycle in the environment rather than on the host animal, and can be very difficult to eradicate once they have become established. *R. microplus* and *R. annulatus*, which are one-host ticks, have been successfully eliminated from some countries. Eradication programs are based on animal identification and periodic acaricide treatment of livestock, as well as public education, surveillance, quarantines and movement restrictions.

In the U.S., *R. annulatus* and *R. microplus* incursions are controlled by USDA APHIS Fever Tick Eradication Program personnel, including mounted inspectors called "tick riders." Tick riders patrol the Rio Grande river, inspect ranches in the quarantine zone, and apprehend stray and smuggled livestock from Mexico. Before being moved from the quarantine zone, cattle and horses must be inspected and given a precautionary treatment with acaricides. Farms and ranches with infestations are placed under quarantine for 6 to 9 months, depending on the time of the year, and the animals are treated for ticks. The infested pasture must remain free of all livestock for 6 to 9 months or longer, to break the tick life cycle. Deer and exotic ungulates may maintain the ticks on vacated pastures; ivermectin-based feed and pesticide treatment protocols have been established to treat wild animals visiting the field.

In regions where *A. variegatum, A. hebraeum, R. microplus, R. annulatus, R. appendiculatus* or *I. ricinus* are already endemic, control methods include acaricide treatment, pasture rotation, environmental modification, and integrated biologic and chemical control strategies. Acaricides can eliminate the ticks from the animal, but they do not prevent reinfestation and must be repeated periodically. Ticks can become resistant to these chemicals. The use of resistant breeds is an important means of tick control in some countries. European (*Bos taurus*) breeds of cattle usually remain fairly susceptible to ixodid ticks, even after multiple exposures. However, some cattle such as zebu (*Bos indicus*) or zebu crosses can become resistant to *B. microplus* after exposure. Vaccines against *R. microplus* have recently been introduced.

PUBLIC HEALTH

Tick bites can be irritating or painful, and the wound may become infected. *Amblyomma* spp. cause particularly large wounds and are difficult to remove. Exotic ticks can transmit exotic diseases such as African tick bite fever and tick-borne encephalitis to humans.

VESICULAR STOMATITIS

Sore Mouth of Cattle and Horses, Indiana Fever

IMPORTANCE

Vesicular stomatitis is an important viral disease of livestock in the Americas. It can affect ruminants, horses and pigs, causing vesicles, erosions and ulcers on the mouth, feet and udder. Although deaths are rare, these lesions can result in pain, anorexia and secondary bacterial mastitis, and some animals may lose their hooves after developing laminitis. Vesicular stomatitis viruses are endemic from southern Mexico to northern South America, but regularly spread north and south from these regions, causing outbreaks and epidemics. While these viruses are no longer endemic in the U.S., they are introduced periodically into the southwestern states, and can sometimes spread farther north. These outbreaks end after freezing temperatures kill the insect vectors that transmit vesicular stomatitis; however, the introduced viruses may overwinter for a year or two, re-emerging in the spring. Vesicular stomatitis is clinically indistinguishable from several other vesicular diseases of livestock including foot-and-mouth disease (FMD). Prompt diagnosis is important not only for containing vesicular stomatitis outbreaks, which can restrict international trade, but also in preventing major livestock diseases such as FMD from spreading undetected. People who work with vesicular stomatitis viruses or come in close contact with infected animals sometimes become infected and develop an influenza-like illness.

ETIOLOGY

Vesicular stomatitis can be caused by four named viruses in the genus *Vesiculovirus* (family Rhabdoviridae): vesicular stomatitis New Jersey virus (VSV-NJ), vesicular stomatitis Indiana virus (VSV-IN), vesicular stomatitis Alagoas virus (VSV-AV) and Cocal virus. The viruses that cause vesicular stomatitis have been divided into two major serotypes, New

Jersey and Indiana. VSV-NJ belongs to the New Jersey serotype. The remaining three viruses are members of the Indiana serotype, which is currently subtyped serologically into 3 groups. VSV-IN belongs to the Indiana 1 subtype, Cocal virus to the Indiana 2 subtype, and VSV-AV to Indiana 3.

The genus *Vesiculovirus* also contains several related viral species, which, as of 2014, included Piry virus, Maraba virus, Isfahan virus and Chandipura virus. Chandipura virus has been associated with influenza-like illnesses and encephalitis in humans in India. This virus may also infect ruminants and pigs in the area, based on serological studies, although there is currently no evidence that it causes disease in these species. Isfahan virus may circulate between gerbils, sandflies and people in the Middle East, but it is not thought to infect domesticated animals. Piry and Maraba viruses were found in South America. Experimental infection with Piry virus caused vesicular lesions at the inoculation site in horses but not in any ruminant species. Maraba virus has only been isolated from insects. None of these viruses, including Chandipura virus, is currently considered to be an agent of the livestock disease vesicular stomatitis. However, they are thought to be pathogens or potential pathogens for people working in laboratories.

Additional vesiculoviruses have been reported in the literature, but have not yet been officially accepted as separate viral species.

SPECIES AFFECTED

Vesicular stomatitis mainly affects equids, cattle and swine. Sheep and goats can develop clinical signs, although this is uncommon, and South American camelids have also been affected. Antibodies to vesicular stomatitis viruses (VSV) have been found in many other species including deer, pronghorn (*Antilocapra americana*), bighorn sheep (*Ovis canadensis*), bats, raccoons (*Procyon lotor*), opossums (*Didelphis marsupialis*), anteaters (*Tamandua tetradactyla*), bobcats (*Lynx rufus*), bears, wild canids, dogs, non-human primates, rabbits, various rodents, fruit bats (*Artibeus* spp.), turkeys and ducks. Additional non-livestock species (e.g., guinea pigs, hamsters, mice, ferrets, opossums, chickens) have been infected experimentally.

Livestock are not thought to maintain vesicular stomatitis viruses long term, and their reservoir or amplifying hosts are unknown. Deer mice (*Peromyscus* sp.) can become viremic, and small rodents have been proposed as possible reservoir hosts; however, this remains speculative. Some authors have even suggested that vesicular stomatitis viruses might be plant viruses found in pastures, with animals at the end of an epidemiological chain.

Zoonotic potential

Humans can be infected with vesicular stomatitis viruses, and may become ill.

GEOGRAPHIC DISTRIBUTION

Vesicular stomatitis viruses are endemic in southern Mexico, Central America, and northern South America. VSV-NJ was also endemic on Ossabaw Island, Georgia in the U.S for decades; however, recent surveys could find no evidence for its presence. Reductions in the feral swine population on this island may have resulted in its eradication.

VSV-NJ and VSV-IN regularly cause outbreaks in areas of North and South America where they are not endemic. However, viruses are not maintained in these regions long term. VSV-AV and Cocal virus have been only been detected in limited areas of South America, to date.

Vesicular stomatitis is not thought to be endemic outside the Western Hemisphere, although other vesiculoviruses do circulate in the Eastern Hemisphere.

TRANSMISSION

The transmission of vesicular stomatitis is incompletely understood. The relative importance of the various transmission routes in each situation is also sometimes unclear.

Insect vectors are thought to introduce VSV into populations of domesticated animals. Sand flies (*Lutzomyia* sp.), blackflies (family Simuliidae) and *Culicoides* midges can act as biological vectors. Sand flies seem to be important vectors in endemic areas, but have a limited flight range and are not thought to spread these viruses long distances. Blackflies are believed to be particularly important vectors in parts of the western U.S. Where the virus originates, before entering livestock populations, is still uncertain. Once animals develop lesions, however, insects may become infected by feeding on viruses in these lesions or contaminated secretions. In addition, infected blackflies can transmit VSV to other blackflies feeding at the same time on a host, even if the host is not infected. Transovarial transmission has been demonstrated in sandflies and blackflies in the laboratory, and may be possible in *Culicoides*. It might contribute to virus overwintering in cold climates.

Vesicular stomatitis viruses have also been found in other insects including *Aedes* mosquitoes, Chloropidae (eye gnats), and flies in the genus *Musca* or family Anthomyiidae These insects may act as mechanical vectors. Migratory grasshoppers *(Melanoplus sanguinipes)* have been proposed to play a role in spreading VSV. In laboratory experiments, these grasshoppers could be infected from plants or other sources, and cattle that ate grasshoppers developed clinical signs. In the field, cattle may ingest large numbers of molting grasshoppers while grazing, as these insects are immobile during that stage.

Once it has been introduced into a herd, vesicular stomatitis can spread from animal to animal by direct contact. Broken skin or mucous membranes may facilitate entry of the virus. Infected animals shed VSV in vesicle material. Viruses from lesions in the mouth and on the muzzle can contaminate saliva, and to a lesser extent, nasal secretions. However, VSV has also been detected in the saliva of some experimentally infected horses that did not have oral lesions. Vesicular stomatitis viruses are not considered to be shed in feces, urine or milk, although they have been detected occasionally in the feces of symptomatic, experimentally infected swine. Livestock can be infected experimentally by aerosols in the laboratory, but this route did not result in skin lesions in most species. VSV does not appear to cross the placenta or cause fetal seroconversion.

Contaminated fomites such as food, water and milking machines are also thought to play a role in transmission. VSV in saliva was reported to survive for 3-4 days on milking pails, mangers and hay. Viruses dried onto glass, plastic or stainless steel in the laboratory lost a great deal of infectivity within the first 1-6 days at 22°C, although some infectious virus was still recovered after 2-8 days. However, survival in liquid medium that contained organic material (i.e., cell culture medium with 5% fetal bovine serum) was prolonged, especially at cold temperatures. These suspensions did not lose significant infectivity for at least 4 weeks at 4°C. Approximately 90% of infectious virus disappeared during the first 8 days in such suspensions incubated at 28°C, but some viable viruses were still present after 4 weeks. At 37°C, 90% of infectivity had been lost by 3 days, and no live viruses could be detected after 21 days. Only 10% of the viruses suspended in cell culture medium without serum were still viable by 4-12 days at 4°C.

People can be infected by contact with lesions or secretions from infected animals, particularly vesicular fluid and saliva, or when manipulating VSV in the laboratory. Aerosol transmission has been reported in laboratories, and some cases occurred after accidental inoculation (needlestick injuries). Some people are probably infected through insect bites, as antibodies to these viruses are common in endemic regions.

DISINFECTION

Vesicular stomatitis viruses are susceptible to numerous disinfectants including 1% sodium hypochlorite, 40-70% ethanol, 2-propanol, aldehydes (e.g., 0.5%-2% glutaraldehyde, formaldehyde), 1% cresylic acid, phenolic disinfectants and detergents. These viruses appear to be more susceptible to inactivation by acid (e.g., pH 2) than alkaline conditions. VSV are also susceptible to UV light including sunlight, or heat (e.g., 4 minutes at 55°C, or one minute at 60°C).

INFECTIONS IN ANIMALS

INCUBATION PERIOD

The incubation period is usually 3-7 days, but longer or shorter incubation periods have been reported. During one outbreak in California, the average incubation period was approximately 9 days. Lesions and/or fever developed in 1-3 days in some experimentally infected livestock.

CLINICAL SIGNS

Vesicular stomatitis is characterized by vesicles, papules, erosions and ulcers. These lesions occur mainly in and around the mouth, and on the feet, udder (especially the teats) and prepuce. The predominant sites affected may differ between outbreaks, and are probably influenced by the feeding preferences of the insect vectors. In the southwestern U.S., lesions are reported to be more common around the mouth than on the feet. Subclinical infections also seem to be common in livestock.

A transient fever can be seen early in clinical cases, but it may disappear by the time the animal is examined. Excessive salivation is often the first sign noticed. Closer examination may reveal blanched areas and the characteristic raised vesicles (blisters). Vesicles differ widely in size; while some are as small as a pea, others can cover the entire surface of the tongue. They quickly rupture to become erosions or ulcers, and vesicles may be absent by the time the animal is examined. The lips and tongue (especially the dorsal surface) are often affected in the mouth. However, lesions can also be present on the gums and palate. Ulcers and erosions in the mouth frequently coalesce to form large, denuded areas of mucosa with epithelial tags. Severe oral sloughing was unusually common in horses during one recent outbreak in the U.S. Lesions can also occur in other locations on the muzzle or snout, which may swell as a result of tissue damage. When foot lesions are present, they are usually located on the coronary band and/or the interdigital spaces of the hooves. Coronitis, with inflammation and edema extending up the lower leg, is the typical presentation. In pigs, lesions can sometimes appear first on the feet, although the mouth and snout are also affected frequently. In some horses, vesicles and erosions may go unnoticed and the disease may appear as crusting scabs that affect sites such as the muzzle, lips, ventral abdominal wall, prepuce and udder.

Vesicular stomatitis lesions are painful and can cause anorexia, refusal to drink and lameness. Some animals may develop a catarrhal nasal discharge, bleeding from ulcers, or a fetid mouth odor. Lesions on the coronary band may result in laminitis and even loss of the hoof (or claws in pigs). Teat lesions can lead to mastitis from secondary infections. Weight loss may be severe, and milk production can drop in dairy cows. Some infected cattle were reported to be normal but had a poor appetite. Unless secondary bacterial infections or other complications develop, animals usually recover within approximately 2-3 weeks. However, if recovering animals are transported, the stress may cause new lesions to develop.

There is limited information about other species; however, fever and oral lesions also occurred in experimentally infected pronghorn and deer. In one early study, experimental subcutaneous inoculation of VSV-NJ caused fatal illnesses with neurological signs in infant wild mice, hamsters, marmosets, anteaters and opossums. Vesicular lesions were not seen in these young animals. Adults remained asymptomatic when inoculated by the same protocol. In a recent study, opossums experimentally infected with VSV-NJ developed ulcers and erosions at the inoculation site on the tongue, and sometimes had petechiae, ecchymoses and ulcers on the cheeks. Opossums inoculated via snout lesions had inflammation of the nose and erosions on the nasal septum, with or without a serous nasal discharge. A litter of young, nursing opossums remained asymptomatic although their dam had lesions, and they may have been protected by maternal antibodies.

POST MORTEM LESIONS

Necropsy lesions resemble the lesions in live animals. Heart and rumen lesions, which may be seen in foot and mouth disease, do not occur in cases of vesicular stomatitis.

DIAGNOSTIC TESTS

Vesicular stomatitis viruses can be found in vesicle fluid, swabs of ruptured vesicles, the epithelium over unruptured vesicles, and epithelial flaps from freshly ruptured vesicles (e.g., epithelial tags from the mouth). Sedation is recommended before sample collection, as the lesions are very painful. If these samples are not available, esophageal/pharyngeal fluid can be collected with a probang cup from cattle, or throat swabs may be taken from pigs. VSV can be detected in oral and nasal secretions for up to 7 days after infection. Electron microscopy of tissue samples may be helpful in distinguishing VSV from some other viruses that cause vesicular lesions, such as foot and mouth disease virus or swine vesicular disease virus.

Many cell lines can be used to isolate VSV from clinical samples. Virus recovery is also possible in embryonated eggs, and animal inoculation (mice) was sometimes employed in the past. The identity of cultured virus can be confirmed with immunofluorescence, complement fixation or ELISAs to detect viral antigens, or with other tests such as reverse transcription polymerase chain reaction (RT-PCR) assays. Antigen capture (indirect sandwich) ELISAs are often used to identify the viral serotype. Some RT-PCR tests can also distinguish New Jersey and Indiana serotypes, and one group in Brazil reported using RT-PCR to confirm the identity of isolated VSV-AV and distinguish these viruses from Cocal virus.

VSV antigens can be detected in tissue samples or vesicle fluid with an antigen capture ELISA, complement fixation or virus neutralization. Descriptions of other antigen detection assays, including lateral flow devices, have been published. Some laboratories may use RT–PCR tests to detect viral nucleic acids directly in tissues. However, this does not seem to be common at present. Genetic identification is complicated by the variability in vesicular stomatitis viruses, including changes in epidemic viruses as they continue to circulate. Genetic assays may need to be standardized for each region where these viruses circulate. Some published multiplex RT-PCR assays can identify a wide range of vesicular stomatitis viruses, belonging to both serotypes, from North and Central America. Unexpected strains may, nevertheless, be missed.

Vesicular stomatitis can also be diagnosed by serology, using paired serum samples. A fourfold increase in titers is diagnostic. Animals usually develop serotype-specific antibodies to VSV 5-8 days after they are infected. ELISAs and virus neutralization (VN) are the preferred serological tests, according to the World Organization for Animal Health (OIE), but early antibodies can also be quantified by complement fixation. Complement fixation cannot detect antibodies for as long as ELISA or VN. Some ELISAs for VSV are quantitative (e.g., the liquid-phase blocking ELISA), but others only report the presence or absence of antibodies to this virus. Additional serological tests have been described and/ or used in the past, including agar gel immunodiffusion and counterimmunoelectrophoresis.

TREATMENT

Treatment is symptomatic. Cleansing the lesions with a mild antiseptic solution may aid healing and reduce secondary bacterial infections. Animals with mouth lesions should be provided with softened feed.

CONTROL

Disease reporting

Veterinarians who encounter or suspect that an animal is infected with a vesicular stomatitis virus should follow their national and/or local guidelines for disease reporting. In the U.S., state and federal veterinarians should be informed immediately of any suspected vesicular disease.

Prevention

Vesicular stomatitis can spread between animals by direct contact, as well as via insect-mediated transmission. During outbreaks, uninfected livestock should kept away from any animals that could be infected. Quarantines and animal movement restrictions can help reduce virus spread. There should be no movement of animals from a quarantined property for at least 21 days after all lesions are healed, unless the animals are going directly to slaughter. Isolating symptomatic animals may also be helpful within a herd. Horses appear to be most contagious for the first 6 days after infection. Good sanitation and disinfection can reduce the spread of the virus on fomites. Lower attack rates have been reported on dairies where feed and water troughs were cleaned regularly. Milking equipment should also be disinfected between uses, and cows with lesions should be milked last. The avoidance of hard or abrasive feeds may prevent oral abrasions that could facilitate infections.

Pastured livestock are more likely to become infected than animals with access to a shelter or barn. Stabling animals during outbreaks seems to decrease the risk of disease. During one outbreak in the U.S., animals were also more likely to develop vesicular stomatitis if there were sources of running water (e.g., streams, irrigation canals) within a quarter mile, probably because water sources encourage higher vector populations. If practical (and permitted), moving animals farther from such locations during outbreaks might reduce the risk of infection. Various insect control measures are also thought be helpful, though their efficacy is not absolute. Insecticide applications should include the inner surface of the pinna, where blackflies tend to feed.

Commercial vaccines are available in some endemic regions of Central and South America. Vaccines are not available in the U.S.

MORBIDITY AND MORTALITY

Outbreaks of vesicular stomatitis tend to occur each year in endemic areas. Both explosive epidemics and slowly spreading outbreaks with relatively few cases (an endemic pattern) can be seen in these regions. VSV-NJ is involved more often than VSV-IN, while VSV-AV is seen only in limited regions. Outbreaks caused by Cocal virus are reported to occur sporadically in Argentina and Southern Brazil. Vesicular stomatitis is seasonal. Although cases may occur throughout the year, they are particularly common at the end of the rainy season or early in the dry season.

Epidemics occur periodically outside endemic areas, spreading south in South America or north in North America. These outbreaks can sometimes involve hundreds or thousands of farms, as well as wildlife. Outbreaks in the U.S. tend to occur at approximately 5-10 year intervals. In the past, they were seen in the Southwest, the upper Mississippi, and the Rocky and Appalachian mountains; however, most recent epidemics have affected only the western states. These outbreaks appear to be caused by new introductions of viruses from endemic regions, often Mexico. They tend to begin in the spring or early summer in states bordering Mexico, then spread north, often along riverways and in valleys. Some epidemics may extend as far as Canada. The climatic and environmental factors affecting the extent of an outbreak are poorly understood, although transportation of animals has been shown to spread the virus in some cases. Epidemics usually end with the first frosts, but viruses sometimes overwinter outside endemic areas for up to 3 years, re-emerging in the spring. Until the early 1970s, VSV-NJ also affected animals in an endemic pattern in the Southeast; however, the remaining reservoirs of these viruses in wildlife or feral pigs seem to have disappeared.

The morbidity rate for vesicular stomatitis is highly variable, and ranges from 5% to more than 90%. Estimates of typical morbidity differ, and are likely to be affected by the animals' previous exposure to VSV and other factors. Some authors report that only 10-20% of the animals in a herd are usually symptomatic, with up to 100% seroconverting. In some nonendemic areas, however, morbidity rates may approach 40-60% in susceptible populations. Some outbreaks tend to affect cattle more often than horses, or vice versa. Most clinical cases occur in adults; young cattle and horses under a year of age are uncommonly affected. Deaths are very rare in cattle and horses, but higher mortality rates have been seen in some pigs infected with VSV-NJ. Cattle that develop mastitis or horses with laminitis may be culled due to these sequelae.

INFECTIONS IN HUMANS

INCUBATION PERIOD

Incubation periods of 1-6 days have been reported in the limited number of human cases described.

CLINICAL SIGNS

Some of the most thoroughly documented clinical cases are from a handful of published reports describing infections in laboratory workers. Symptomatic vesicular stomatitis has also been reported in people infected via the environment; however, laboratory confirmation in these reports is sometimes unavailable or inadequate.

In general, vesicular stomatitis is reported to be an acute illness that resembles influenza, with symptoms that may include fever, muscle aches, headache, malaise, enlarged lymph nodes and conjunctivitis. Some authors have suggested that conjunctivitis or cheilitis may be a common early sign. The fever is sometimes but not always biphasic. One person with a needlestick injury developed acute nausea, vomiting and diarrhea, in addition to nonspecific flu-like signs. The gastrointestinal signs resolved spontaneously within 24 hours. Some infected people also had vesicles in the mouth or on the lips or hands; in other cases, no vesicles were present. Most people are reported to recover without complications within 4-7 days. However, one case of severe encephalitis was attributed to VSV in a 3-year-old child in Panama.

Many or most infections with vesicular stomatitis viruses may be subclinical. Seroconversion without obvious signs of illness is reported to be common among laboratory workers, as well as in human populations in endemic regions.

DIAGNOSTIC TESTS

Most human cases have been diagnosed by serology, using tests such as serum neutralization and complement fixation. Virus isolation can be attempted from the blood, but viremia is very brief and this tends to be unsuccessful. If vesicles are present, attempts should be made to isolate the virus from vesicle fluid and epithelium.

TREATMENT

Treatment is supportive, as needed.

CONTROL

Protective clothing and gloves should be used when handling infected animals, and biological safety precautions should be taken in the laboratory.

MORBIDITY AND MORTALITY

Infections with VSV were seemingly common among laboratory workers and animal handlers before the advent of modern biological safety procedures and equipment. In one study, 54 of 74 laboratory workers or animal handlers had antibodies to these viruses. Some studies have reported that 48–100% of the population in Central America is seropositive, and one study detected antibodies in 25% of the people tested in southeastern Georgia, U.S. when outbreaks were common among livestock there in the 1950s. In contrast, a later study found that the infectivity of a VSV-NJ virus for veterinarians, laboratory workers and other risk groups was relatively low during the 1982-1983 epidemic in the U.S. Evidence of infection was only detected in 17 of 133 people exposed to the virus, and relatively close contact with sources of virus seemed to be necessary.

The percentage of human infections that become symptomatic is unknown. Although some sources suggest clinical cases are rare, others point out that human infections may be underreported as they can easily be misdiagnosed as influenza. In the study above, 31 of the 54 seropositive laboratory workers or animal handlers reported having had a mild, acute illness consistent with vesicular stomatitis. In most cases, clinical cases have had no serious consequences. Laboratory infections have resolved without complications, and no deaths have been reported. Nevertheless, there is one reported serious case, with encephalitis attributed to VSV in a young child.

WEST NILE VIRUS INFECTION

West Nile Fever, West Nile Neuroinvasive Disease, West Nile Disease, Near Eastern Equine Encephalitis, Lordige

IMPORTANCE

West Nile virus (WNV) is a mosquito-borne virus that circulates among birds, but can also affect other species, particularly humans and horses. Many WNV strains are thought to be maintained in Africa; however, migrating birds carry these viruses to other continents each year, and some strains have become established outside Africa. At one time, the distribution of WNV was limited to the Eastern Hemisphere, and it was infrequently associated with serious illness. Clinical cases usually occurred sporadically in humans and horses, or as relatively small epidemics in rural areas.

Most human infections were asymptomatic, and if symptoms occurred, they were typically mild and flu-like. Severe illnesses, characterized by neurological signs, seemed to be uncommon in most outbreaks. Birds appeared to be unaffected throughout the Eastern Hemisphere, possibly because they had become resistant to the virus through repeated exposure.

Since the 1990s, this picture has changed, and WNV has emerged as a significant human and veterinary pathogen in the Americas, Europe, the Middle East and other areas. Severe outbreaks, with an elevated case fatality rate, were initially reported in Algeria, Romania, Morocco, Tunisia, Italy, Russia and Israel between 1994 and 1999. While approximately 80% of the people infected with these strains were still asymptomatic, 20% had flu-like signs, and a small but significant percentage (< 1%) developed neurological disease. One of these virulent viruses entered the U.S. in 1999. Despite control efforts, it became established in much of North America, and spread to Central and South America and the Caribbean. Outbreaks were reported across North America in humans, horses and captive alligators; sporadic cases occurred in less susceptible mammals; and asymptomatic infections were recognized in a number of mammalian and several reptilian species. Although the introduction of an equine vaccine has helped control the disease in horses, there is currently no vaccine for humans, and recent experiences suggest that human outbreaks may continue to occur in North America at unpredictable intervals. Many North American species of birds were also affected, particularly when the virus first entered the continent. While some bird populations seem to have rebounded, the effect of WNV on threatened or endangered avian species continues to be a concern. California condors and greater sage grouse are among the species susceptible to this virus, and WNV introduction into Hawaii could have severe consequences for some native birds. Surprisingly, the effects of virus introduction seem to have been milder in South America, although the reason for this is still uncertain.

The epidemiology of WNV infections may also be changing in Eurasia. A number of outbreaks have been reported recently in Europe, Russia and parts of the Middle East. One virus affected significant numbers of wild and captive raptors in Hungary and Austria. This has led to a re-examination of the potential for West Nile viruses to cause illness or deaths in other European birds. Some viruses, which were not thought to persist from year to year in Europe, seem to have become endemic and are spreading.

ETIOLOGY

West Nile virus is an arbovirus in the *Flavivirus* genus of the family Flaviviridae. It belongs to the Japanese encephalitis virus complex or serogroup. The two most common genetic lineages of WNV are lineage 1, which contains 3 clades (1a, 1b and 1c), and lineage 2. Both lineages contain virulent

viruses, as well as strains that usually cause asymptomatic infections or mild disease. Many of the virulent viruses from recent outbreaks belonged to clade 1a, which is widespread. The strain that entered the United States in 1999, called NY99, appears to be related to a lineage 1a virus found in Israel from 1997 to 2000, and is among the most pathogenic strains. NY99 has continued to evolve in the Americas, where it has been replaced by its variants, especially WN02. Clade 1b consists of Kunjin viruses, a subtype of WNV found in Australia, and clade 1c consists of some West Nile viruses found in India.

Several additional WNV lineages also exist or have been proposed. Under some taxonomic schemes, it might be possible to classify this virus into as many as eight lineages by including Koutango virus, a related virus that circulates in Africa, and elevating clades 1b and 1c to lineages.

SPECIES AFFECTED

Birds

Wild birds are the main reservoir hosts for West Nile virus. Passeriformes (perching birds) are important in virus amplification. Some members of other orders including (but not limited to) Charadriiformes (shorebirds), Falconiformes (hawks, eagles, vultures and related species) and Strigiformes (owls) may also transmit the virus to mosquitoes.

Birds in the Western hemisphere

Overall, WNV-infections have been documented in more than 320 species of North American birds since 1999. Some species usually carry the virus asymptomatically, while others are more likely to become ill. Clinical cases have been reported in domesticated birds, wild birds, and captive wild species in zoos and collections.

Among domesticated birds, outbreaks have occurred in geese, and symptomatic infections have been reported in a number of psittacine species (although psittacine birds were relatively resistant to disease in one experimental study). Chickens and turkeys (order Galliformes) seroconvert but remain asymptomatic; however, outbreaks have occurred in farmed chukar partridges (*Alectoris chukar*) and Impeyan pheasants (*Lophophorus impeyanus*). Some wild gallinaceous birds have also been affected: greater sage grouse (*Centrocercus urophasianus)* are highly susceptible, and one case was reported in a wild turkey (*Meleagris gallopavo* ssp).

The effects of WNV on wild birds vary with the species. When this virus was first introduced to North America, corvids (e.g., crows, ravens, magpies and jays) were severely affected. Other affected wild birds have included American robins (*Turdus migratorius*), eastern bluebirds (*Sialia sialis*), chickadees (*Poecile* sp.), tufted titmice (*Baeolophus bicolor*), house finches (*Carpodacus mexicanus*), house sparrows (*Passer domesticus*), house wrens (*Troglodytes aedon*) and black-crowned night herons (*Nycticorax nycticorax*). Northern cardinals (*Cardinalis cardinalis*) also seem to be susceptible, although the population as a whole appears to be resilient and did not decline. High mortality rates have been reported in infected Falconiformes, and owls have also been killed. Emus, penguins, pigeons, flamingos, American white pelicans (*Pelecanus erythrorhyncos*) cormorants, gulls, sandhill cranes (*Grus canadensis*) and other species can also be affected. Although ducks are not thought to be highly susceptible, there have been reports of illness in several species, or their young.

Similarly to the pattern of disease in humans, birds in South and Central America, Mexico and the Caribbean seem to be less severely affected than birds in North America. However, this might vary with the viral strain and species of bird. One WNV isolate from Mexico was less virulent for crows, but not house sparrows, compared to a North American virus.

Birds in the Eastern Hemisphere

WNV outbreaks have been reported among domesticated geese in the Eastern Hemisphere, but generally there have been only sporadic reports of deaths in individual wild birds. It is uncertain whether this is related to the virulence of the viruses circulating in this region, host susceptibility, reduced transmission/amplification or lack of surveillance. One recently introduced lineage 2 virus in Central Europe has affected significant numbers of wild and captive raptors. Species known to be susceptible to this isolate include sparrow hawks (*Accipiter nisus*), goshawks (*Accipiter gentilis*) and gyrfalcons (*Falco rusticolus*). The same virus was isolated from a dead collared dove (*Streptopelia decaocto*) in Italy, during an outbreak of mortality in collared doves and other species including blackbirds. Lineage 1a or 2 viruses have also been found occasionally in other sick or dead birds including European robins (*Erithacus rubecula*), a raven (*Corvus corax*), common magpies (*Pica pica*), a Eurasian jay (*Garrulus glandarius*), house sparrows (*Passer domesticus*), a black redstart (*Phoenicurus ochruros*), a sedge warbler (*Acrocephalus schoenobaenus*) and a Savi's warbler (*Locustella luscinioides*).

European birds that became ill when infected experimentally with WNV outbreak strains from the Eastern Hemisphere included falcons that received European lineage 1 or lineage 2 viruses; red legged partridges (*Alectoris rufa*) infected with a European lineage 1 virus; house sparrows infected with European lineage 1 viruses; and wild carrion crows (*Corvus corone*) inoculated with lineage 1 isolates from Europe or Israel. Most European species have not yet been examined for susceptibility.

Mammals and marsupials

Among mammals, disease occurs mainly in equids (horses, donkeys and mules). Although serious illnesses in horses have mainly been attributed to lineage 1 viruses, lineage 2 isolates in Africa and Hungary also caused severe clinical signs or death.

A few clinical cases have been reported in other domesticated mammals including alpacas, sheep and

reindeer (*Rangifer tarandus*). Dogs and cats appear to be readily infected, but rarely become ill. Wild or captive wild species that have been affected include squirrels, harbor seals (*Phoca vitulina*), a killer whale (*Orcinus orca*), Indian rhinoceroses (*Rhinoceros unicornis*), wolf pups, a polar bear (*Ursus maritimus*), a Barbary macaque (*Macaca sylvanus*), mountain goats (*Oreamnos americanus*) and a white-tailed deer (*Odocoileus virginianus*). Experimental infections have been established in a variety of mammals: mice, hamsters, chipmunks, cats and rhesus monkeys developed mild to severe clinical signs, but rabbits, pigs, guinea pigs, dogs, raccoons and hedgehogs (*Erinaceus europaeus*) remained asymptomatic.

Antibodies to WNV have been found in many mammalian and some marsupial species including cattle, sheep, goats, pigs, camels, wild boar, deer, lemurs, bats, skunks, bears, coyotes, foxes, various big cats (e.g., tiger, lion, cougar), stone marten (*Martes foina*), a civet, raccoons (*Procyon lotor*), opossums, rabbits, non-human primates, killer whales, dolphins, seals, small rodents and insectivores. Due to the limitations of serological testing for WNV, some of these antibodies may represent infections with flaviviruses other than WNV.

Some species of mammals including squirrels (*Sciurus* sp.), eastern chipmunks (*Tamias striatus*) and eastern cottontail rabbits (*Sylvilagus floridanus*) may be capable of transmitting WNV to mosquitoes, although their importance as reservoir hosts is still uncertain. Individual animals of certain other species, such as raccoons (*Procyon lotor*), may develop moderate levels of viremia, even if the species overall is not considered to be of epidemiological significance in infecting mosquitoes.

Reptiles and amphibians

Among reptiles, clinical signs were mainly reported during outbreaks in alligators, although there is also a report of neurological signs associated with WNV infection in a crocodile monitor (*Varanus salvadori*) lizard. Some infections in garter snakes (*Thamnophis sirtalis*) experimentally inoculated with WNV were also fatal. Green iguanas (*Iguana iguana*) can be infected, and antibodies have been found in turtles, wild and farmed crocodiles, and alligators.

Amphibians including lake frogs (*Rana ridibunda*) and North American bullfrogs (*Rana catesbeiana*) can also be infected with WNV.

Some alligators (e.g., American alligators, *Alligator mississippiensis*) and frogs (e.g., *Rana ridibunda* in Russia) may develop viremia sufficient to infect mosquitoes. As with mammals, their importance as reservoir hosts is still uncertain.

Zoonotic potential

Humans usually acquire WNV in mosquito bites; however, some species of birds, mammals and reptiles can shed this virus in secretions and excretions. Tissues from infected animals, especially the brain, are also sources of exposure.

GEOGRAPHIC DISTRIBUTION

West Nile viruses have been found throughout much of the world including Africa, Europe, Asia, the Middle East, Australia, the Americas and the Caribbean. In some regions, the viruses do not seem to be endemic, but are re-introduced regularly by migratory wild birds. These viruses may either cause outbreaks, or circulate asymptomatically among birds during warm weather, and disappear with the onset of cold temperatures. Relatively little is known about the occurrence of WNV in Asia, where the presence of the closely-related Japanese encephalitis virus (JEV) complicates diagnosis. However, WNV is endemic in India, and it was recently reported from an outbreak in China that was originally thought to be caused by JEV.

Lineage 1 WNV

In the Eastern Hemisphere, lineage 1a viruses have been found in Africa, the Middle East, Europe and parts of Asia. Whether these viruses circulate in any avian populations in Europe, or are only introduced periodically by wild birds without overwintering, is still under investigation. Currently, it appears that many lineage 1 viruses do not overwinter, while others may persist from year to year in the Mediterranean region, but not in some other countries that have been examined (e.g., the U.K. and Germany). There is also evidence for the continuing endemic circulation of a lineage 1 virus in Romania between 1997 and 2009, after an epidemic in 1996. In the Western Hemisphere, lineage 1a viruses have been endemic in North America since 1999. Since spreading to South and Central America, they have been documented in several countries including Colombia, Argentina, Venezuela and Brazil. WNV has also spread to the Caribbean, but it is not yet present in Hawaii in 2013.

Lineage 1b (Kunjin virus) occurs in Australia, and lineage 1c viruses are found in India.

Lineage 2 WNV

Lineage 2 viruses have mainly been isolated south of the Sahara desert in Africa, where they co-circulate in some regions with lineage 1 viruses. They also occur in Madagascar. Virulent lineage 2 strains have been endemic in Central Europe (Hungary and Austria) since 2004, and seem to be spreading. Identical or closely related viruses were recently isolated from mosquitoes, a dead indigenous bird and two human patients in Italy, and from mosquitoes in Greece during a human WNV outbreak. Different lineage 2 viruses caused outbreaks in Russia in 2007, and viruses related to this strain were found in Romanian outbreaks in 2010. One genetic analysis suggested that the viruses originally identified in Hungary and Russia might have been introduced in 1999 and 2000, respectively.

TRANSMISSION

West Nile virus is primarily transmitted by mosquitoes. Members of the genus *Culex* are the main vectors worldwide, although other mosquito genera can also be infected. In North America alone, there is evidence of infection in more than 60 mosquito species. Transovarial transmission has been demonstrated in some species of mosquitoes, and is likely to important in overwintering. Dormant mosquitoes that survive the winter may also harbor WNV. Other arthropods might have minor roles in transmission. Infections have been documented in ticks in Asia, Europe and the Middle East, and soft (argasid) ticks have been shown to transmit WNV in the laboratory. Hippoboscid flies might be able to transmit this virus in North America, and infected lice (*Philopterus* spp.) have been collected from WNV-infected crows.

Birds are the primary vertebrate reservoir hosts for West Nile virus, but the level and duration of viremia varies with the species. In endemic regions, the virus is maintained in an enzootic cycle between culicine mosquitoes and birds. When environmental conditions favor high viral amplification, significant numbers of "bridge vector" mosquitoes (mosquitoes that feed on both birds and mammals) become infected in the late summer, and can transmit the virus to humans, horses and other incidental hosts. In some birds, viremia can persist for more than three months, possibly contributing to the overwintering of the virus. Whether birds harbor sufficient infectious virus to initiate a new cycle in mosquitoes, after the winter, is still under investigation. Migratory birds are thought to be important in introducing WNV into new areas, and can reintroduce viruses into some regions each year.

Some species of birds can shed WNV in oral and cloacal secretions, and may transmit the virus directly. Crows, jays, magpies, gulls, raptors and some other birds, including domesticated chickens and turkeys, are known to excrete WNV for varying periods of time, and evidence for horizontal transmission was reported during an outbreak in domesticated geese. However, not all birds that shed WNV seem to transmit the virus efficiently. Experimentally infected red-legged partridges (*Alectoris rufa*) excreted this virus in oral and cloacal secretions, but there was no evidence of transmission to birds in contact. WNV also occurs in the skin of geese and the blood-feather pulp of crows, possibly contributing to transmission by cannibalism and feather picking. Raptors and crows may become infected when they eat other animals, and insectivorous species might eat infected mosquitoes. WNV does not seem to persist very long in the environment: the infectivity of virus in avian feces decreases dramatically after 24 hours.

Mosquito bites are the usual source of WNV for mammals, reptiles and amphibians. Most animals, including horses, appear to be dead-end hosts that do not transmit WNV to mosquitoes, but a few species have higher levels of viremia, and might be able to act as amplifying or maintenance hosts. In some animals, there is also evidence for transmission by other routes. Carnivorous mammals and reptiles (e.g., cats and alligators) can be infected by eating contaminated tissues. WNV-contaminated horsemeat was implicated in one outbreak in alligators. Direct transmission during close contact has also been reported in alligators, possibly via fecal shedding of virus. Chipmunks, squirrels and raccoons can also shed WNV in feces, oral secretions and/or urine. WNV has been found in the urine of experimentally infected hamsters, and in very small amounts in the oral and/or cloacal fluids of experimentally infected North American bullfrogs (*Rana catesbeiana*) and green iguanas (*Iguana iguana*). Transplacental transmission was reported in experimentally infected sheep and mice, as well as in a horse that was fatally infected with a lineage 1 virus in Africa, and aborted in the final stage of the disease. The epidemiological significance (if any) of mammalian, reptilian and amphibian hosts in the maintenance or amplification of WNV remains to be established.

Humans are usually infected by mosquito bites, but a few cases have been linked to accidental inoculation through breaks in the skin. These cases frequently occurred in people who handled infected tissues (often brains) from various animals. One recent infection occurred in a person who had removed the brain of an infected horse, using only latex gloves for protection. Whether the gloves had an unnoticed small puncture, or there was another source of the virus, is uncertain. An outbreak among workers on a turkey farm may have resulted from fecal-oral transmission, exposure of broken skin or mucous membranes to virus, or exposure to aerosolized virus. Humans do not develop viremia sufficient to transmit WNV to mosquitoes, and do not appear to shed significant levels of infectious virus in secretions or excretions. While WNV RNA is often found in patients' urine, infectious virus was only isolated from one encephalitis patient who had a very high viral load, and other isolation attempts on urine have been unsuccessful. For this reason, a recent article concluded that human urine is probably not a risk for virus transmission. However, WNV can be transmitted between people in blood transfusions and organ transplants. Rare cases of transplacental transmission and probable transmission in breast milk have also been reported.

In mammals, WNV is usually cleared from the body during the illness. A few studies have suggested that this virus or its RNA might persist for up to several months, or perhaps even years, in some mammals including humans. The evidence is currently conflicting, and this issue has not yet been resolved.

DISINFECTION

West Nile virus can be destroyed by many disinfectants including sodium hypochlorite solutions (500-5000 ppm available chlorine), 2-3% hydrogen peroxide, 2% glutaraldehyde, 3-8% formaldehyde, ethanol, 1% iodine and phenol iodophors. It is also inactivated by UV light and gamma irradiation, as well as exposure to temperatures of 56-60°C (133-140 °F) for 30 minutes.

INFECTIONS IN ANIMALS

INCUBATION PERIOD

The incubation period in horses is 3 to 15 days. Infections in other mammals are uncommon, and the incubation period is unknown. Clinical cases are reported to occur in birds, on average, approximately 5 days after experimental inoculation.

CLINICAL SIGNS

Birds

Some species of birds carry WNV asymptomatically, while others develop clinical signs. Trauma (e.g., as a consequence of neurological signs) or concurrent bacterial, fungal or viral infections may also complicate the course of the disease.

On poultry or game bird farms, outbreaks have been reported in geese, chukar partridges and Impeyan pheasants. Only young geese were affected during outbreaks in North America and Israel; older birds did not become ill. The clinical signs in goslings included weight loss, decreased activity, depression, and neurological signs such as torticollis, opisthotonos and rhythmic side-to-side head movements. Myocarditis was seen in some birds at necropsy. Many infections were fatal. Illness has also been reported in chukar partridges and Impeyan pheasants. In one outbreak, hundreds of 6-8-week-old chukar partridges were either found dead without previous clinical signs, or displayed incoordination for less than a day before dying. Incoordination and diarrhea, followed by death, were reported in Impeyan pheasants. Naturally or experimentally infected chickens and turkeys are asymptomatic regardless of age.

A variety of clinical signs have been reported in zoo birds, pet psittacines and captive raptors. The predominant signs and course of the disease can vary with the species. Nonspecific signs such as anorexia, rapid weight loss, weakness, lethargy and ruffled feathers are common; some birds display only nonspecific signs before death. Neurological signs also occur in some birds; ataxia, incoordination, paresis or paralysis, disorientation, tremors, nystagmus, impaired vision or blindness, circling and seizures have been reported. Myocarditis is sometimes seen at necropsy. Sudden death also occurs. In contrast, one great horned owl had intermittent, mild clinical signs for more than five months, and a vulture with neurological signs exhibited progressive deterioration over the course of three weeks. In early reports, most clinically affected birds died or were euthanized due to their deteriorating condition. However, some birds, including those with neurological signs, can recover with supportive care. Full recovery can sometimes take longer than 6 months in raptors. Sequelae that have been reported in recovered birds of prey include relapses of neurological signs (e.g., ataxia), abnormal molting and persistently abnormal feathers.

Affected wild birds are usually found dead, and the clinical signs in many species have not been well described. Neurological signs have been reported in some moribund birds, and myocarditis, encephalitis or other lesions are sometimes found at necropsy. Experimentally infected sage grouse developed a profuse, clear, watery oral and nasal discharge. Affected birds ruffled their feathers, shivered, isolated themselves from the group, and showed signs of weakness or lethargy. These signs were followed by drooping wings, ataxia, copious oral and nasal secretions, and labored breathing. The grouse became moribund within hours.

Mammals

Most horses are infected asymptomatically with WNV. In clinical cases, the illness is characterized by anorexia, depression and neurological signs, which may include ataxia, weakness or paralysis of one or more limbs, teeth grinding, aimless wandering, convulsions and/or circling. Tremors of the face and neck muscles are very common. Some animals have cranial nerve deficits, particularly weakness or paralysis of the face and tongue, which may lead to difficulty in swallowing. Attitudinal changes including somnolence, apprehension, hyperesthesia or periods of hyperexcitability are also common. Some horses with severe depression and facial paralysis may hang their heads; this can result in severe facial edema. Coma, impaired vision and head pressing can be seen, but tend to be less common than in cases of encephalitis caused by alphaviruses. Colic and urinary dysfunction (from mild straining to stranguria) have also been reported. Fever is present in some but not all cases. Fatal hepatitis was seen in a donkey with neurological signs in France. Injuries, pulmonary infections acquired during prolonged recumbency, and other secondary effects can complicate the course of the disease in equids. Some animals die spontaneously, but many severely affected animals are euthanized for humane reasons. Horses that recover usually begin to show improvement within seven days of the onset of clinical signs. Most but not all horses return to full function; approximately 10-20% horses are estimated to have residual defects such as weakness in one or more limbs, decreased exercise tolerance, muscle atrophy or behavioral changes. Studies from outbreaks in Hungary suggest that the lineage 2 virus circulating in Central Europe causes similar clinical signs and mortality as lineage 1a strains in horses.

Clinical cases have also been reported in ruminants and cervids, although they seem to be uncommon. In many cases, only a single animal was affected on a farm. Occasionally, a few other animals became ill around the same time. Most affected sheep, alpacas, reindeer and white-tailed deer have had neurological signs, which were often the first signs observed in the animal. However, a prodromal syndrome of fever, anorexia and depression was reported in one alpaca; the fever disappeared by the time the neurological signs appeared. Sudden death without prior clinical signs was seen in a reindeer. Another reindeer had diarrhea for 1-2 weeks before the onset of neurological signs. Most affected animals have died, but one alpaca recovered from mild head tremors and ataxia. Death often occurs within 1-2 days, particularly in reindeer, but some animals were ill for several days to a week. Experimentally infected sheep did not develop systemic signs, but some pregnant ewes aborted, had stillborn lambs, or gave birth to lambs that died soon after birth.

Neurological signs, sometimes accompanied by other clinical signs, have been reported from rare clinical cases in dogs and wolf pups. In one dog, the first signs were episodes of uncontrolled rolling, which quickly progressed to generalized tremors, ataxia and intermittent fever. Other neurological signs reported in dogs were decreased conscious proprioception, a stiff gait, neck pain, paresis, depressed mentation, muscle atrophy and head tilt. Fever, inappetence, oculonasal discharge, conjunctivitis, excessive salivation, polydypsia, diarrhea, abdominal pain, myocarditis, dyspnea and polyarthritis have also been seen. Asymptomatic infections appear to be common, and only mild recurrent myopathy was reported in experimentally infected dogs. Oculonasal discharge, vomiting, anorexia, and lethargy, progressing to ataxia, were reported in a 4-month-old wolf cub. This animal died 24 hours after the onset of neurological signs. West Nile virus was also recovered from the brain of a cat with CNS signs. Experimentally infected cats were transiently lethargic and had fluctuating fevers, but neurological signs were not seen.

Cases in other animals have also been characterized mainly by neurological signs or sudden death, with systemic signs in some instances. Some infected squirrels circled, chewed at their feet, were lethargy or ataxic; other squirrels have been found dead. Incoordination, tremors and head tilt were reported in one of ten experimentally infected fox squirrels (*Sciurus niger*); the other nine squirrels remained asymptomatic. Acute paraparesis was the presentation in an aged polar bear at a zoo, while a fatal infection in a harbor seal was characterized by progressive neurological signs, inappetence and weakness, with intermitted diarrhea and vomiting, and labored breathing. Tremors and twitching were seen in another captive seal for four days, but this animal recovered. Sudden death occurred in a captive killer whale that had fulminant secondary bacteremia and septicemia, together with primary WNV encephalitis. West Nile virus was also suspected as the cause of depression, lethargy, partial anorexia and a drooping lip in two Indian rhinoceroses during a WNV outbreak at a zoo. Both animals recovered. Infections in some experimentally infected mice, hamsters and rhesus monkeys were characterized by fatal encephalitis. Experimentally infected pigs remained asymptomatic.

W

Reptiles

In alligators, the clinical signs included anorexia, lethargy, weakness and neurological signs including tremors, unresponsiveness, slow reflexes, head tilt, anisocoria and opisthotonos. Some alligators were unable to submerge and stranded in dry parts of the pen, dragged their hind feet, or swam on their sides or in circles. Animals usually died 24-48 hours after the onset of clinical signs. A strong association between WNV infection and lymphohistiocytic proliferative cutaneous lesions has also been reported in this species.

Neurological signs in one naturally infected crocodile monitor were also linked to WNV. Fatal illness was reported in experimentally infected garter snakes. Some snakes died suddenly, while others exhibited unusual aggression and immobility of the caudal part of the body, or weakness and cachexia, which may have been caused by inappetence.

POST MORTEM LESIONS

Birds

A wide variety of gross and microscopic lesions, which are often nonspecific, have been reported in birds. Some birds may be thin or emaciated, but others are in good body condition. The most common macroscopic lesions, in addition to emaciation and dehydration, are multiorgan hemorrhages, petechiae and congestion. Splenomegaly, hepatomegaly, myocardial pallor and pale mottling of the liver, spleen or kidney have also been observed in various species. Several reports described cerebral atrophy and malacia in raptors. Gross lesions seem to be minimal or absent in some infected birds, including some psittacines. No macroscopic lesions appear to be pathognomonic for WNV, and reported lesions are not necessarily consistent between species, even when the birds belong to the same family. The limited number of samples from some species may contribute to the seeming high variability in gross lesions.

Histopathologic lesions have been detected in most organs, but in most families of birds, lesions are usually concentrated in the CNS (e.g., encephalitis), heart, spleen, liver and kidney. Frequently reported findings include lymphoplasmacytic and histiocytic infiltrates, cellular degeneration and necrosis, and hemorrhages. The pattern and severity of microscopic lesions vary with the species of bird and the length of time it has been ill. In birds that die quickly, the lesions may be acute and have minimal inflammatory reactions. Birds that have been ill longer, such as raptors, can have chronic lesions, including lesions in the CNS. Severe CNS lesions are not always found in birds with neurological signs.

Mammals

Gross lesions are uncommon in horses. If they occur, they are usually limited to small multifocal areas of discoloration and hemorrhage in the spinal cord, brain stem and midbrain. The meninges may be congested in acute cases. Meningeal hemorrhages have also been described. Gross lesions in tissues other than the CNS are uncommon. The histopathologic lesions are characterized by lymphocytic or histiocytic poliomeningoencephalitis with perivascular cuffing of mononuclear cells, neuronal degeneration, neuronophagia and focal gliosis. These lesions are particularly apparent in the lower brain stem and spinal cord, and may also occur in the midbrain. They are less common in the cerebral and cerebellar cortices. Mild nonsuppurative myocarditis, scattered hemorrhages in the renal medulla, and lymphoid depletion of the spleen have been seen in some horses.

Few or no gross lesions have been reported in most other mammals including reindeer, squirrels, sheep and alpacas. In one sheep, multifocal hemorrhagic and malacic foci were found in the lumbar spinal cord. A wolf pup was emaciated, with mucoid nasal exudate, and unclotted blood was found in the small and large intestinal lumen. This animal also had vascular lesions in the kidneys, and to a lesser extent, in the cerebral cortex. The liver, which was mildly enlarged, was yellow and friable; hepatic lipidosis was partly attributed to anorexia. In a harbor seal, gross lesions included decreased blubber thickness and hyperemia of the brainstem and spinal cord blood vessels. In mammals, histological lesions in the CNS have generally resembled those seen in horses. Lymphocytic and necrotizing myocarditis, granulomatous inflammation of the kidneys, renal tubular epithelial cell necrosis, pancreatitis, synovitis (polyarthritis) and acute, diffuse, moderate hepatic necrosis were also reported in affected dogs. Mild to moderate lymphocytic myocarditis, myocardial necrosis and mild focal hepatic necrosis were seen in some squirrels.

Reptiles

During an outbreak in alligators, moderately sized fat bodies and approximately 3–5 ml of clear yellow fluid were found in the coelomic cavity. The liver was mottled red to yellow, and slightly enlarged with rounded edges. Tan to red mottling was also seen in the spleen and myocardium.

DIAGNOSTIC TESTS

WNV infections can be diagnosed by isolating the virus, detecting viral antigens or RNA, or using serological methods. The usefulness of the various techniques varies with the level of virus replication in the host. In horses, viremia is short-lived and low, and clinical cases are usually confirmed by serology, or by detecting WNV in the brain and spinal cord at necropsy. Both serology and tests to detect the virus are useful in live birds, with the caveat that the amount of virus can vary between avian species. There is limited information about other animals; however, virus replication seems to be widespread in affected alligators, while viremia appears to be low in ruminants.

Isolation of West Nile virus can be used for diagnosis, especially when disease is suspected in a species not previously known to be susceptible. WNV is often recovered in African green monkey kidney (Vero) cells or rabbit kidney (RK-13) cells. Mosquito cell lines and embryonating chicken eggs may also be used. The identity of the virus can be confirmed by tests such as immunofluorescence or RT-PCR. In birds, WNV is sometimes found in the blood, and it can often be isolated from the CNS and/or major organs (e.g., heart and liver) at necropsy. This virus was also recovered from plasma and several tissues in affected alligators. In one outbreak, viral titers were reported to be higher in the liver of alligators than the CNS. In horses, WNV is difficult to isolate from the blood, but it can sometimes be found in the brain and spinal cord at necropsy. Disadvantages to virus isolation are that it is time-consuming, requires level 3 biosafety (BL 3) containment, and is not widely available at diagnostic laboratories.

RT-PCR assays are valuable as both antemortem and postmortem tests in birds. In some live birds, this test may be able to detect West Nile virus RNA in oral and cloacal swabs and/or serum samples. Viral RNA was also found in plasma samples from sick alligators. In horses, RT-PCR is most useful with brain and spinal cord samples taken at necropsy. Although viral RNA can sometimes be found in the blood of subclinically infected horses, it has usually disappeared by the time the neurological signs appear. In addition, RT-PCR has been used to diagnose WNV infections in other animal species. Some commercial assays may not detect lineage 2 viruses.

Several tests can be used to detect WNV antigens. Immunohistochemistry is often used on tissue samples collected at necropsy. Equine CNS does not contain large quantities of virus, and immunohistochemistry can detect some, but not all, infected animals. In contrast, this test may detect antigens in multiple organs, as well as the CNS, in alligators and some species of birds. One study found that the spleen, liver, kidney and duodenum contained antigens in almost all crows infected in the wild. Antigen-capture ELISA tests can also be used to find antigens in avian tissues; however, they are not useful in horses, which have much lower levels of virus. An antigen capture dipstick assay is valuable for rapid testing of oral or cloacal swabs from live birds, and tissue homogenates from dead birds. The antigen-capture ELISA and the antigen-capture dipstick assay are also used for mosquito surveillance. Cross-reactions with closely related flaviviruses can occur in antigen tests.

Serological tests for WNV include various ELISAs, hemagglutination inhibition (HI), virus neutralization assays (the plaque reduction neutralization, or PRN assay) and other tests. Cross-reactive antibodies to closely related flaviviruses are also detected by the ELISAs, HI and some other tests, but can be distinguished with the PRN test. This test is also used to confirm positive or equivocal ELISAs in horses. A disadvantage to the PRN test is that it must be performed in a BL 3 laboratory, and it is not available at all diagnostic laboratories. Serological tests are particularly valuable in live horses, where they are often used to diagnose clinical cases. A four-fold or greater increase in WNV-specific antibodies in serum, the detection of specific IgM in CSF, or the detection of specific IgM in serum confirmed by specific IgG in the same or a later sample are diagnostic. If clinical signs have not been present long enough for IgG to develop, the presence of IgM alone in serum is suggestive. Serology is also valuable in birds, as well as some mammals other than horses; however, it should be noted that some ELISAs can only be used in the species for which they have been standardized. Vaccination history must be considered when interpreting serological tests in horses and in some birds (e.g., geese and California condors).

TREATMENT

No specific treatment is available, but animals may recover on their own if they are given supportive care. Supportive treatment has the goal of reducing inflammation in the CNS, preventing self-inflicted injuries and adverse effects from recumbency, and providing supportive nutrition and fluids. Therapy is empiric, and similar to the treatment of other causes of viral encephalomyelitis. Mild cases have sometimes recovered without treatment.

CONTROL

Disease reporting

Veterinarians who encounter or suspect a West Nile virus infection should follow their national and/or local guidelines for disease reporting.

Animal cases are a warning that humans may be at risk from mosquito-borne transmission. Although West Nile virus is endemic in the U.S., infections are reportable in many states. Some states require that all horses with signs of encephalomyelitis be reported.In some countries, authorities collect dead birds for West Nile virus surveillance. In the U.S., state and/or wildlife agencies should be contacted for information about the current programs.

Prevention

Commercial WNV vaccines are available for horses in the U.S. and other countries, and for geese in Israel. Vaccines are sometimes used "off label" to protect sensitive birds (e.g., endangered California condors) or other species.

Topical repellents can reduce the risk of WNV during the mosquito season. Repellents should be approved for the species; products that are safe in one species (including humans) can sometimes be toxic in others. Housing susceptible species indoors or in screened barns, cages or other screened areas can also decrease mosquito bites. Fans can be helpful in barns, as mosquitoes are not strong flyers. Insecticides or mosquito traps may also be used. Areas around barns, paddocks and pastures should be kept free of weeds, feces and other organic materials that could shelter

W

adult mosquitoes. Standing or stagnant water should be eliminated to prevent them from breeding. Water tanks and buckets should be cleaned at least weekly, and containers (e.g. flower pots and used tires) should be removed or emptied of water. In some areas, ponds may be stocked with mosquito fish (*Gambusia affinis*), which feed on mosquito larvae. The inconveniences from mosquito control measures such as indoor housing can be weighed against the risk of infection in each species. For example, some species of birds are highly susceptible to WNV, but cases in dogs, cats and sheep are rare. In some areas, agencies conduct mosquito abatement programs using larvicides, adulticides and other measures to reduce mosquito populations.

Other measures, such as quarantines of infected animals, may be helpful in species suspected or known to transmit the virus horizontally. Carnivores and omnivores should not be allowed to eat any meat that might be contaminated with WNV. One outbreak occurred in alligators that had been fed WNV-infected horsemeat. Tissues from some birds are also known to contain high levels of virus.

MORBIDITY AND MORTALITY

Clinical cases caused by WNV usually occur seasonally. Birds are mainly affected from summer to late fall, and cases in horses peak in late summer and fall. Occasional outbreaks may be seen when mosquitoes are absent, in species that can transmit the virus horizontally. In the U.S., one outbreak occurred among crows during the winter. WNV isolates differ in their virulence for birds, and only some viruses cause severe illness or death. Different patterns of disease have been reported among avian species in the Eastern and Western Hemispheres.

Birds in North America

With minor exceptions (e.g., some individual animals in zoos), birds in the Western Hemisphere were first exposed to WNV in 1999. Some North American populations of wild birds experienced high mortality rates. Corvids were severely affected. Overall, the number of crows in the U.S. fell by an estimated 30%, with much greater decreases in some localized areas. Declines were also measured in populations of blue jays (*Cyanocitta cristata*). Greater sage grouse are also highly susceptible to WNV, and some local populations of these birds were severely affected. Nearly all of the breeding birds died in some areas. In the Powder River basin of Montana and Wyoming, the minimum mortality rate from WNV-infection in sage grouse was 2-13% in 2003-2005, and the maximum possible mortality rate was 8-29%. In raptors, one study estimated the annual mortality rate from WNV infections to be 7-15%. Other affected populations included American robins, eastern bluebirds, chickadees, tufted titmice, house sparrows, house wrens, house finches and black-crowned night herons, with declines either after intense epidemics or over longer periods. In some cases, the number of birds fell across their entire range; in others, the decreases were regional. With time, some species (for example, crows, blue jays and house wrens) have apparently recovered or are recovering; other populations remained smaller than normal. In contrast, the abundance of some birds does not seem to have been affected by WNV. While some of these unaffected species may not be very susceptible to WNV, this is not necessarily true in all cases. For example, a wild population of northern cardinals was shown to be affected by the virus, although this population as a whole appeared to be resilient and did not decline. WNV may also affect some age groups more than others. It appears to cause significant mortality in American white pelican chicks in North America, although adults are not severely affected.

In zoos and rehabilitation centers, WNV has affected a wide variety of avian species. During one outbreak at a New York zoo, the overall morbidity rate among infected birds was estimated to be 14%; it was higher among species found in the Western Hemisphere (20%) than species indigenous to Eastern Hemisphere (5%). In this outbreak, the morbidity rate was high in corvids, owls and penguins, but only 9% of infected gallinaceous birds became ill. Most clinical cases ended in death; the case fatality rate was 69% overall, and in most orders, it reached 100%. A high case fatality rate was also reported during an outbreak at Kansas zoos: only one of 11 affected birds, a sandhill crane, survived. Among raptors, symptomatic infections have been documented in both falconiformes and owls. Widely varying mortality rates have been reported among owls at rehabilitation centers, with some species experiencing mortality rates of greater than 90%, while others suffered no deaths.

Among poultry, young geese seem to be particularly susceptible to WNV, and have been affected in both Western and Eastern Hemispheres. In Israel, disease was reported in 3-8-week-old goslings, with morbidity and mortality rates of approximately 40%. During an outbreak in Canada, the mortality rate was 25% in 6-week-old goslings, but 15-month-old and 5-year-old geese seroconverted with no clinical signs. In experimental infections, up to 50–75% of geese may die. Ducks are not thought to be highly susceptible to WNV; however, an outbreak among captive lesser scaup (*Aythya affinis*) ducklings resulted in 70% mortality. During other outbreaks, the morbidity and mortality rates were 100% in Impeyan pheasants, and the mortality rate was 25% in chukar partridges. Similarly to geese, young partridges and pheasants seem to be more susceptible to disease. In contrast, both young and old chickens and turkeys are infected asymptomatically.

A limited number of bird species have been experimentally infected with North American strains of WNV. These studies demonstrate that susceptibility varies greatly between avian species. Mortality rates as high as 100% have been reported in American crows (*Corvus brachyrhynchos*), black-billed magpies (*Pica hudsonia*), ring-billed gulls, house finches and greater sage grouse. Mortality was 75% in blue jays (*Cyanocitta cristata*), 53% in fish crows (*Corvus ossifragus*), 16% in house sparrows and 0% in cliff swallow nestlings. In addition to the species, factors that may affect the severity of disease include pre-existing immunity to WNV, co-existing conditions and general health, and possibly the route of exposure.

Birds in South and Central America

Few detailed studies have been conducted on WNV mortality among birds in South and Central America, Mexico and the Caribbean. Overall, these birds are thought to have been less severely affected than birds in North America.

Birds in the Eastern Hemisphere

In areas where WNV has been endemic for decades, the prevalence of infection in wild birds ranges from 10% to greater than 50%. While WNV outbreaks have been reported among domesticated geese in the Eastern Hemisphere, there have generally been only sporadic reports of deaths in wild birds, and no major mortality events have been reported. It is uncertain whether this is related to the virulence of the viruses circulating in this region, lower host susceptibility (including immunity from repeated exposure), reduced transmission/ amplification or lack of surveillance. However, one recently introduced lineage 2 virus in Central Europe has affected significant numbers of wild and captive raptors. Species known to be susceptible to this isolate include sparrow hawks (*Accipiter nisus*), goshawks (*Accipiter gentilis*) and gyrfalcons (*Falco rusticolus*). Dead songbirds of various species have also been diagnosed occasionally with WNV in this area. The same virus was isolated from a dead collared dove in Italy, during an outbreak of mortality in collared doves and other species including blackbirds. Other lineage 1a or 2 viruses have also been found occasionally in sick or dead birds. For example, lineage 1a viruses have killed raptors in Spain, and a lineage 1a virus was detected in a dead magpie and a moribund wild house sparrow with torticollis and tremors during a WNV outbreak in France. No unusual mortality was otherwise observed in birds during the latter outbreak, but systematic examinations of bird populations were not carried out.

A few European species have been shown to be susceptible to illness after experimental inoculation of WNV. Red-legged partridges infected with two European lineage 1 viruses had mortality rates of 30% or 70%. Both lineage 1 and lineage 2 European viruses caused illness and some deaths in experimentally infected falcons, with both viruses causing a similar clinical picture. In one study, the illness was fatal in a third of the falcons inoculated with an Austrian lineage 2 WNV strain. In other experiments using European birds, the mortality rates were 0-25% in house sparrows inoculated with WNV isolates from Italy or Spain, 33% in wild carrion crows inoculated with a lineage 1 equine isolate from France, and 100% in wild carrion crows inoculated with an avian (stork) lineage 1 isolate from Israel.

Equids

Among domesticated mammals, West Nile outbreaks occur mainly in equids. Many infections in horses are asymptomatic. While seroprevalence rates vary greatly between studies (and cross-reactivity with other flaviviruses can be a concern), up to 90% of horses are reported to be seropositive in some parts of Africa. During outbreaks, 10-43% of infected horses are estimated to develop neurological signs. The reported case fatality rate ranges from 23% to 57%. It is approximately 30-40% in the U.S., and was 30% during a lineage 2 outbreak in Hungary. Although some horses that recover have residual neurological defects, approximately 80-90% (60-100% in individual studies) are estimated to return to full function. As with other species, the impact of WNV on horses seems to have been greater in North America than in other parts of the Americas.

Ruminants and other livestock

Livestock are uncommonly affected by WNV, although seropositive animals are relatively common in some regions. A few clinical cases have been reported in sheep, alpacas and reindeer, but even in North America, clinical signs have been limited to one to a few animals in the herd. However, approximately 26% of camels, 20% of sheep, 18% of goats and 6% of cattle in Nigeria had antibodies to WNV in the HI test, while 29% of camels in Morocco were confirmed to be seropositive by virus neutralization (44% were seropositive by HI). In the Astrakhan region of Russia, antibodies were confirmed by virus neutralization in small numbers of cattle, sheep, pigs and camels; in all species, the seroprevalence rate was less than 6.5% by HI and less than 5% by virus neutralization. Similarly, less than 1% of cattle in Croatia, < 1% to 6% of cattle in Belarus, and 1% of sheep in eastern Slovakia were seropositive. One study reported that 4% of cattle and 1% of sheep in Turkey had WNV antibodies, while a report from northern Turkey found antibodies in 3% of goats, and no cattle, sheep or water buffalo. Symptomatic infections have not been reported in pigs, but approximately 3-10% of domesticated pigs in India, 3% of domesticated pigs in Nepal, 3% of pigs in Spain and 22% of feral pigs in Florida, Georgia, and Texas were seropositive.

Dogs and cats

Only rare clinical cases have been reported in dogs and cats, and they develop few or no clinical signs after experimental infection. However, asymptomatic infections may be common, as significant numbers of dogs and cats have antibodies to WNV. The seroprevalence among dogs was reported to be 8-37% in South Africa, 38% in Turkey, 5% in Shanghai, China and 2-56% in localized areas of the U.S. In two studies from the U.S. studies, the seroprevalence rates were 9-10% in cats, while another U.S. study detected no antibodies among 12 cats. In Shanghai, China, 15% of cats had antibodies to WNV.

Wild mammals

Antibodies have also been reported in many species of wild mammals, and infections may be common in the members of some species. In the U.S., up to 63% of striped skunks, up to 46% of raccoons and up to 49% of squirrels in some areas may have antibodies to WNV. In Spain, antibodies to WNV or closely related flaviviruses were detected by ELISA in 13% of wild boars and 20% of red foxes (*Vulpes vulpes*). Only a few of the approximately 650 samples could also be analyzed by virus neutralization, but 43% of 21 samples from wild boars and the one sample analyzed from a fox were found to contain antibodies to WNV. High seroprevalence rates were also reported in a recent study of wild lemurs in Madagascar. The susceptibility of most species to WNV is unknown, but occasional clinical cases have been reported in a wide variety of species in zoos. Squirrels may be especially susceptible. In some regions, sick and dead squirrels have been seen during periods of high WNV activity, and the morbidity rate in experimentally infected fox squirrels was 10%.

Case fatality rate in mammals other than horses

Once a mammal develops neurological signs, the case fatality rate seems to be high. Most clinically affected animals, which included sheep, alpacas, reindeer, dogs, cats, wolves, deer and a bear, have died, although one alpaca with relatively mild neurological signs recovered. Both rhinoceroses affected in a zoo and one of two seals also recovered.

Reptiles

Among reptiles, disease has been reported only in alligators, one lizard (a crocodile monitor) and experimentally infected garter snakes. At one U.S. alligator farm with more than 10,000 animals, 250 alligators died in an outbreak one year, and more than 1,000 died the following year. Young alligators were more severely affected than adults.

INFECTIONS IN HUMANS

INCUBATION PERIOD

The incubation period is approximately 2 to 14 days. It is reported to be longer in transplant patients than in people who are not immunocompromised.

CLINICAL SIGNS

Human illness has been classified into two forms: West Nile fever, which is a flu-like illness, and West Nile neuroinvasive disease, which encompasses all cases with neurological signs. Many WNV infections are asymptomatic.

West Nile fever is the most common form of the disease. This form resembles influenza, and is characterized by fever, malaise, weakness, headache and body aches. Anorexia, lymphadenopathy, nausea, diarrhea, vomiting, sore throat and conjunctivitis may be seen in some patients. An erythematous, nonpruritic macular, papular or morbilliform skin rash occasionally develops on the neck, trunk, arms or legs. Most uncomplicated infections resolve in 2 to 6 days, but in some severe cases, persistent fatigue can last for a month or more.

Although many cases of West Nile fever are mild, there have also been reports of severe illness, and death is possible, though rare. In the U.S., fatal West Nile fever has occurred mainly in elderly patients, who frequently had underlying health conditions. In most cases, the illness appears to have exacerbated or precipitated an underlying medical condition, resulting in death from acute myocardial infarction, cardiac arrhythmia, respiratory failure, stroke, cancer or other conditions. Death was often the result of cardiac or respiratory complications.

A few patients with West Nile fever develop West Nile neuroinvasive disease. This form can be severe, and in some cases, it is life-threatening. Three syndromes - encephalitis, meningitis, and acute flaccid paralysis – are seen. Symptoms of more than one syndrome often occur in the same patient. West Nile meningitis is characterized by fever, headache, a stiff neck and photophobia. Patients with West Nile encephalitis have changes in consciousness, disorientation and/or focal neurological signs, which may include ataxia, incoordination, tremors, involuntary movements, and signs that resemble Parkinson's disease (rigidity, postural instability and bradykinesia). Concurrent signs of meningitis are common, and seizures or coma may also occur. Some patients who recover have persistent neurological dysfunction.

Acute flaccid paralysis (sometimes called West Nile poliomyelitis) is seen in some patients. The paralysis, which resembles polio, appears suddenly and progresses rapidly, usually reaching a plateau within hours. It is typically asymmetrical and can affect one or more limbs, often the legs. The weakened limbs become darker than normal at the peak of the paralysis. This syndrome may be accompanied by muscle aches in the lower back and/or abnormalities in bladder and bowel function. Some patients develop respiratory distress, which may require mechanical ventilation. Sensory functions are usually normal or minimally affected. Some patients with flaccid paralysis have prodromal signs of West Nile fever, sometimes with signs of meningitis or encephalitis; however, many patients are asymptomatic before the onset of paralysis. Late in the illness, the muscles may become atrophied. Recovery is highly variable: some patients recover completely within weeks, while others remain paralyzed.

Cranial nerve abnormalities in patients with neuroinvasive disease may result in facial weakness, dizziness, vertigo or nystagmus. Rhabdomyelitis, myositis, polyradiculitis and other syndromes have also been seen. Many individuals complain of blurred or impaired vision and photophobia; ocular syndromes that have been reported include chorioretinitis, uveitis, vitritis and optic neuritis.

Other syndromes have occasionally been reported. Myocarditis, pancreatitis, orchitis and fulminant hepatitis are uncommon, but have been seen in some outbreaks. A life-threatening hemorrhagic syndrome occurred in a few West Nile cases in Africa, and was reported in a patient in the U.S. Acute kidney disease has been seen in some patients with WNV encephalitis. Possible associations between West Nile neurological disease and chronic kidney disease have also been suggested by some authors, but a causative role remains to be confirmed.

DIAGNOSTIC TESTS

In humans, West Nile virus infections are often diagnosed by serology. Serological tests used in humans include ELISAs, a rapid microsphere-based fluorescence immunoassay (MIA), the plaque reduction neutralization (PRN) test, indirect immunofluorescence (IFA) and hemagglutination inhibition. Diagnostic criteria include a rising titer or the presence of IgM in serum or cerebrospinal fluid (CSF). In the serum, anti-WNV IgM can occasionally persist for more than a year. Serum IgM is thus suggestive of recent infection, but not definitive. This is not a concern for IgM in CSF. As in animals, cross-reactions can occur with closely related flaviviruses (e.g., yellow fever, Japanese encephalitis, St. Louis encephalitis or dengue viruses) in some serological tests. Positive reactions in other serological tests may be confirmed with the PRN test, if available.

Infectious viruses, viral antigens or nucleic acids can sometimes be detected in human tissues, CSF, blood, urine and other body fluids. This virus can usually be found in the blood of patients with West Nile fever during the first few days after the onset of illness. However, viremia usually disappears before the onset of neurological signs in immunocompetent patients, and viral RNA is often absent from the serum of patients with neuroinvasive disease. In these patients, nucleic acids may be detected in the CSF, using RT-PCR tests, during the acute stage of CNS signs. Immunohistochemistry to detect viral antigens is mainly used postmortem in fatal cases. Virus isolation requires level 3 biosafety containment, and is rarely performed.

TREATMENT

There is no specific recommended treatment, other than supportive care, at present. Intensive care and mechanical ventilation may be required in some cases. Various therapies including interferon, antisense nucleotides and intravenous immunoglobulins (passive immunization) are being tested in clinical trials. While a few case reports suggest that some of these treatments may be promising, larger studies are still lacking. Some antiviral drugs were promising *in vitro*, but most have been ineffective when tested in animal models or given to humans with severe disease. Screening for new drugs that may inhibit WNV is underway.

CONTROL

In most cases, WNV infections can be prevented by preventing mosquito bites. Outdoor activities should be limited when mosquitoes are active, particularly during the peak biting times of dusk and dawn. Mosquito repellents should be used when avoidance is impractical. Long pants and long-sleeved shirts are helpful; specialized fine mesh clothing (e.g., mesh head coverings and jackets) is also available. Measures to reduce mosquito populations include rational application of adulticides and larvicides, as well as environmental modifications such as emptying containers that may hold standing water. Surveillance in sentinel birds, dead birds and mosquitoes can help predict human exposure. Dead or sick birds should be reported to health, agriculture or mosquito-control agencies. In some cases, only certain species or groups of birds, such as corvids, may be tested for WNV. Dead animals should never be handled without gloves and sanitary precautions, as feces and body fluids may be infectious in some species (and may also contain pathogens other than WNV).

Veterinarians, wildlife rehabilitators, wildlife biologists, laboratory workers and others should practice good biosecurity and hygiene when handling either tissues or birds, mammals, reptiles and amphibians that may shed WNV in feces, oral secretions or urine. Mucous membranes and skin should be protected from contact with infectious material, such as tissues or secretions and excretions. Under some conditions, respiratory protection might be needed. Protective clothing and gloves should be used when performing necropsies.

How soon a human vaccine might become available is uncertain, but some vaccines have entered or completed clinical trials. Blood products are screened for WNV in some countries, to prevent transfusion-associated cases.

MORBIDITY AND MORTALITY

West Nile infections usually occur in humans during warm weather, when mosquitoes are active. Outbreaks of West Nile disease appear to be sporadic, as well as geographically focal in their distribution, with shifts in their locations from year to year. Some of the factors that might affect the occurrence of outbreaks include weather patterns, the number and distribution of mosquitoes, and herd immunity in amplifying hosts; however, the interactions of these factors in producing outbreaks are likely to be complex, and outbreaks are difficult or impossible to predict.

The epidemiology of WNV infections appears to differ between geographic regions, although differences in surveillance and diagnostic testing may also play a part in this perception. In some parts of Africa, there seems to be relatively little mortality in people. Although severe disease can occur, it is thought that people tend to become infected as children, and are immune by the time they become more susceptible to neuroinvasive disease as adults. In many parts of Europe, the usual pattern of WNV epidemiology has been that of occasional, self-limited outbreaks affecting very few people. Larger and more severe outbreaks are also reported

W

occasionally. For example, nearly 200 cases of neuroinvasive disease were documented during an outbreak in Greece in 2010. This and other recent outbreaks, together with evidence that some viruses may have become endemic, has led to the suggestion that the epidemiology of WNV infections may be changing in Eurasia. In North America, large numbers of West Nile fever cases, and much fewer cases of neuroinvasive disease, have been seen: more than 13,000 cases of West Nile fever were reported to the CDC between 2002 and 2006. Based on the pattern of infections in North America so far, including a peak in the number of cases in 2002-2003, followed by declines, then another upsurge in 2012, periodic outbreaks and epidemics may be expected in the future. Surprisingly, far fewer clinical cases or deaths have been reported in Central and South America. The reason for this is not known; however, it might involve protective immunity to cross-reactive flaviviruses, the occurrence of WNV isolates with decreased virulence, decreased surveillance and diagnosis, or other causes. In areas where dengue is present, some West Nile infections could be misdiagnosed as this disease.

Most human infections with WNV are asymptomatic. Approximately 20% of those infected during recent outbreaks in the U.S., Europe and Israel developed West Nile fever, and less than 1% had West Nile neuroinvasive disease. Neuroinvasive disease is more likely to occur in people over 50 years of age and patients who are immunocompromised. In a study from North Dakota, the risk varied from 1 in 54, in people over the age of 65, to 1 in more than 1,200 in young, low risk individuals. A study from Ohio estimated approximately 1 case of neuroinvasive disease for every 4,000 infected children, 154 infected adults under the age of 65 years, or 38 infected adults who were more than 65. Recipients of organ transplants are estimated to have a 40% chance of developing neuroinvasive disease. Underlying diseases such as diabetes and autoimmune syndromes are also associated with more severe clinical signs.

Case fatality rates reported during outbreaks have ranged from 3% to 15%, but the case fatality rate varies with the form of the disease. West Nile fever is typically self-limited, and many cases are mild. However, more severe illnesses have also been reported, and deaths are possible, though uncommon. In a recent analysis of cases in the U.S., approximately 0.2% of West Nile fever cases reported to the CDC between 2002 and 2006 were fatal. (Milder cases are likely to be underdiagnosed, and are probably underrepresented in this database.) Of the fatal cases, 78% occurred in patients who were older than 70 years of age. Many affected patients had underlying health conditions, and most of these deaths appeared to result from the exacerbation or precipitation of these illnesses, similarly to the effects of influenza on the elderly. For West Nile neuroinvasive disease, the overall case fatality rate is approximately 10%. Death is more likely to occur in older patients; case fatality rates of 15-29% have been seen in people who are more than 70 years old. Some patients with neuroinvasive disease may suffer substantial long-term morbidity after recovery from the acute syndrome. Patients with encephalitis are more likely to have a poor prognosis and long term sequelae than those with meningitis alone.

SECTION
3

Transboundary and Emerging Diseases of Animals
IMAGES OF DISEASES

Authors:

Claire B. Andreasen, DVM, PhD, Diplomate ACVP

Steven D. Sorden, DVM, PhD, Diplomate ACVP

Department of Veterinary Pathology
College of Veterinary Medicine
Iowa State University
Ames, IA 50011

We are grateful to the many institutions and individuals that made this project possible by contributing images, technical assistance, editing, and feedback. Project directors include: Dr. Steve Sorden and Dr. Claire Andreasen, Department of Veterinary Pathology (VPTH), College of Veterinary Medicine (CVM), Iowa State University (ISU) who had responsibility for annotation and collection of images with assistance from Dr. Aaron Lehmkuhl, USDA-APHIS, Ames, IA; and Dr. James Roth, Director of the Center for Food Security and Public Health (CFSPH) CVM ISU. Additional collaborators (former location) include: Dr. Terrell Blanchard and Dr. Dale Dunn, Armed Forces Institute of Pathology (AFIP); Dr. Samia Metwally (USDA-APHIS), Dr. Thomas McKenna (formerly USDA-APHIS), and Dr. Beth Lautner (USDA-APHIS, Director, NVSL, IA.; and prior Director, Plum Island Animal Disease Center, N.Y.). For technical assistance: The staff of the CFSPH, Ms. Deb Hoyt, student assistants, and numerous faculty in VPTH. Image acquisition was funded by a USDA Cooperative State Research, Education, and Extension Service (CREES) Higher Education Challenge Grant "A Digital Image Database to Enhance Foreign Animal Disease Education" (grant # 2005-38411-15859).

We are grateful to the following institutions for contributing images. In the subsequent pages, each institution is acknowledged for image contribution (abbreviations listed below). Where appropriate, the individual who contributed the image also is acknowledged. Armed Forces Institute of Pathology (AFIP), Education Branch, Division of Research and Education, Department of Veterinary Pathology, Washington, D.C. California Animal Health and Food Safety Laboratory System (CAHFSLS), CA. Canadian Cooperative Wildlife Health Centre (CCWHC), University of Saskatchewan, Saskatoon, Saskatchewan, Canada. Central Livestock Hygiene Service Center, Saitama pref., Japan. Commonwealth Scientific and Industrial Research Organisation (CSIRO), Australia. Animal Health Laboratory, East Geelong, Victoria, Australia. Cornell University, CVM, Aquatic Animal Health Program, Ithaca, NY. Cornell University, CVM, Department of Clinical Sciences, Ithaca, NY. Elizabeth Macarthur Agricultural Institute (EMAI), NSW, Australia. Federal Research Institute for Animal Health, Riems, Germany. Kansas State University, Department of Diagnostic Medicine and Pathobiology, College of Veterinary Medicine (KSU CVM), Manhattan, KS. Kasetsart University, Department of Pathology, Faculty of Veterinary Medicine, Bangkok, Thailand. Institute of Animal Pathology, University of Bern, Switzerland. Iowa State University, College of Veterinary Medicine (ISU CVM), Ames, IA. Department of Veterinary Pathology (VPTH), ISU CVM, Ames, IA. Veterinary Diagnostic Laboratory (VDL), ISU CVM, Ames, IA. National Institute of Animal Health, Aomori, Japan. Noah's Arkive, University of Georgia, Athens, GA. USDA Plum Island Animal Disease Center (PIADC), Greenport, NY. USDA-ARS Southeast Poultry Research Laboratory, Athens, GA. University of Edinburgh, Scotland. University of Kentucky, Lexington, KY. University of Melbourne, Australia

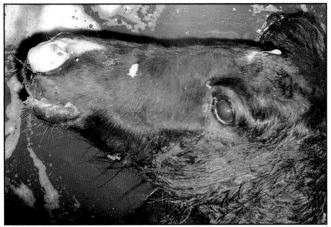

African Horse Sickness

Horse. Abundant froth draining from the nostrils reflects severe pulmonary edema.
Source: PIADC

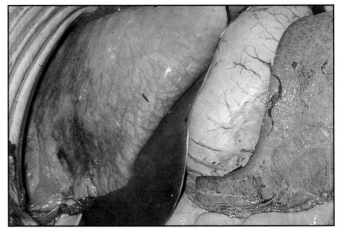

African Horse Sickness

Horse. The lung exhibits severe interlobular edema. There are petechiae on the pulmonary pleura and the splenic capsule.
Source: PIADC

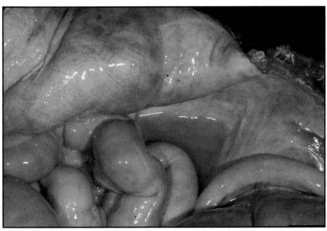

African Horse Sickness

Horse, peritoneal cavity. There is excessive straw-colored fluid (hydroperitoneum).
Source: PIADC

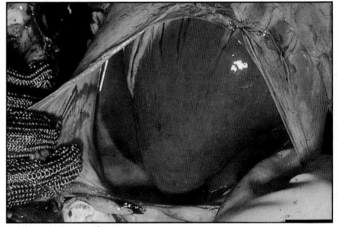

African Horse Sickness

Horse, heart. The pericardial sac contains excessive, slightly turbid straw-colored fluid (hydropericardium).
Source: PIADC

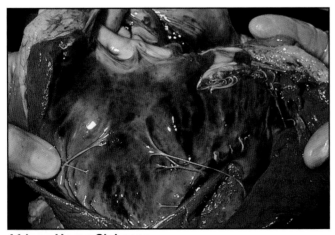

African Horse Sickness

Horse, heart. There are many subendocardial hemorrhages.
Source: PIADC

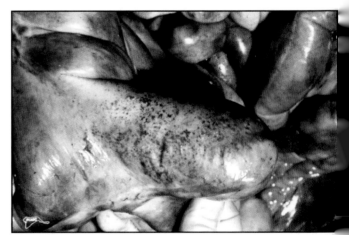

African Horse Sickness

Horse, cecum. There are serosal petechiae on the apex of the cecum.
Source: Noah's Arkive, PIADC

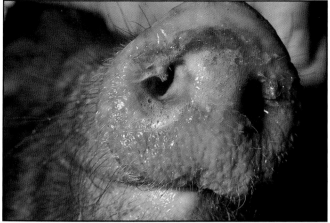

African Swine Fever

Pig. There is bloody, mucoid, foamy nasal discharge.
Source: PIADC

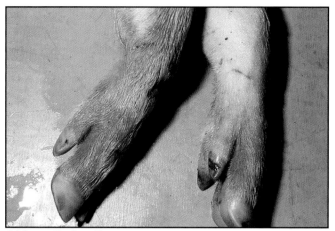

African Swine Fever

Pig, limbs. There is marked hyperemia of the distal limbs.
Source: PIADC

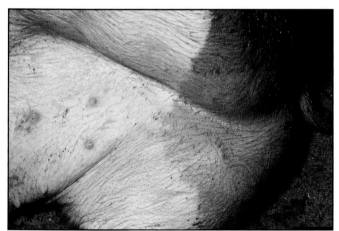

African Swine Fever

Pig, perineal skin. There is a large sharply demarcated zone of hyperemia.
Source: PIADC

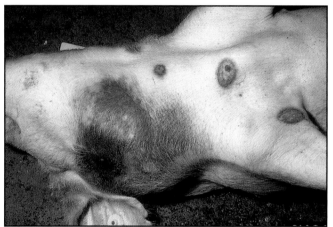

African Swine Fever

Pig. There are multiple sharply demarcated foci of cutaneous hemorrhage and/or necrosis; hemorrhagic lesions may contain dark red (necrotic) centers.
Source: PIADC

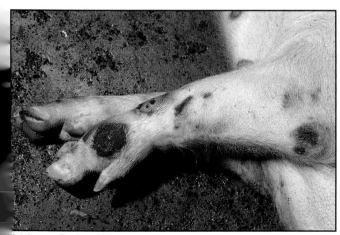

African Swine Fever

Pig. There are multiple sharply demarcated foci of cutaneous hemorrhage and/or necrosis; hemorrhagic lesions may contain dark red (necrotic) centers.
Source: PIADC

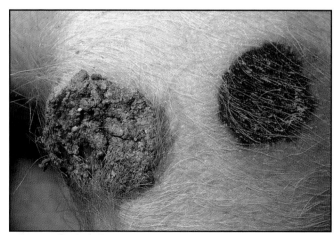

African Swine Fever

Pig, skin. Necrotic exudate is sloughing from the lesion on the left. There is a rim of hyperemia around the focus of hemorrhage and necrosis (infarct) on the right.
Source: PIADC

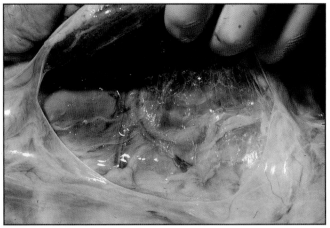

African Swine Fever

Pig, kidney. There is moderate perirenal (retroperitoneal) edema.
Source: PIADC

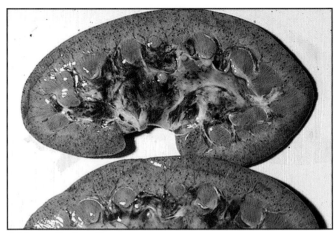

African Swine Fever

Pig, kidney. Petechiae are disseminated throughout the cortex, and there are larger coalescing pelvic hemorrhages.
Source: PIADC

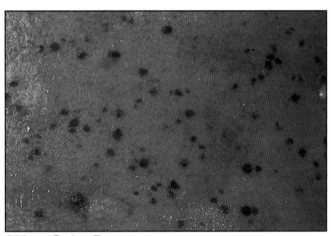

African Swine Fever

Pig, kidney. Close-up of cortical petechiae.
Source: PIADC

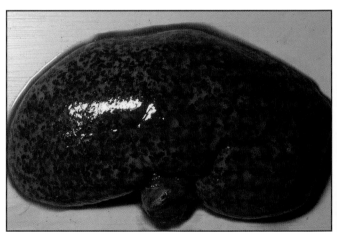

African Swine Fever

Pig, kidney. The cortex contains numerous coalescing petechiae and ecchymoses.
Source: PIADC

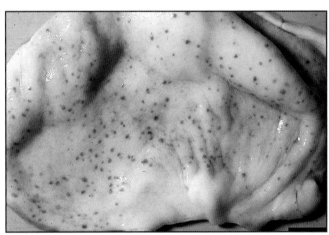

African Swine Fever

Pig, urinary bladder. There are disseminated mucosal petechiae.
Source: PIADC

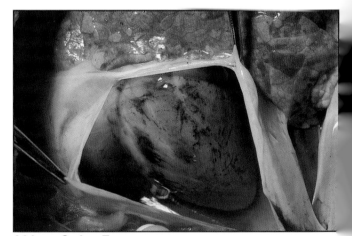

African Swine Fever

Pig, heart. There is abundant straw-colored pericardial fluid (hydropericardium), and multifocal epicardial hemorrhage.
Source: PIADC

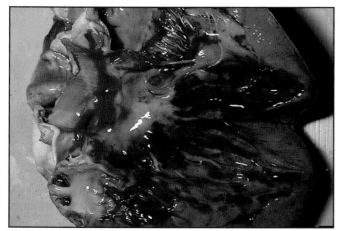

African Swine Fever

Pig, heart. Subendocardial hemorrhage.
Source: PIADC

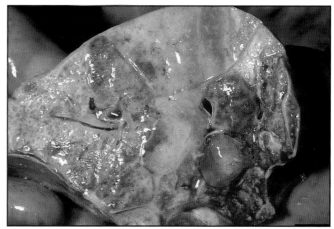

African Swine Fever

Pig, lung. The lung is noncollapsed and edematous; there is dorsal hemorrhage and ventral tan consolidation.
Source: PIADC

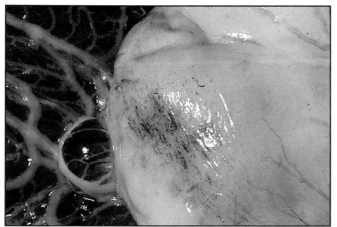

African Swine Fever

Pig, stomach. There is "paintbrush" hemorrhage on the serosa.
Source: PIADC

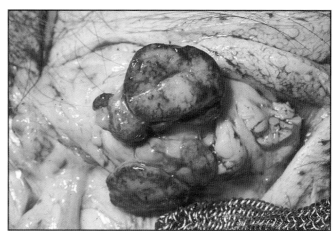

African Swine Fever

Pig, mandibular lymph node. There is moderate peripheral (medullary) hemorrhage.
Source: PIADC

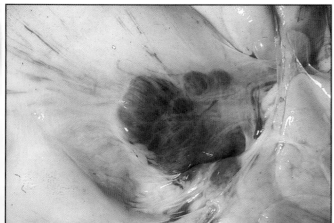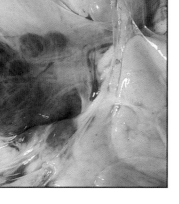

African Swine Fever

Pig, stomach. The hepatogastric lymph node is markedly enlarged and hemorrhagic, and the adjacent lesser omentum is edematous.
Source: PIADC

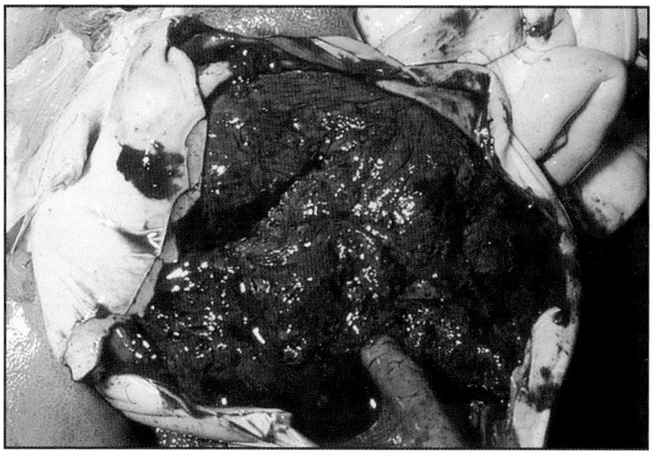

African Swine Fever

Pig, stomach. The stomach is filled with clotted blood, and the wall is markedly edematous.
Source: PIADC

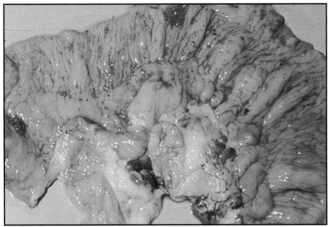

African Swine Fever

Pig, cecum. Mucosa is markedly edematous and hyperemic, and lymph nodes are hemorrhagic.
Source: PIADC

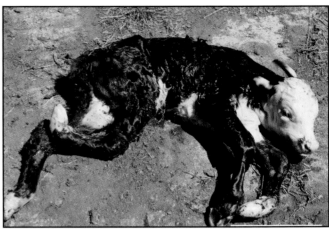

Akabane

Bovine neonate. This live calf cannot stand due to severe arthrogryposis, primarily affecting the hindlimbs.
Source: Dr. P. Mansell, University of Melbourne

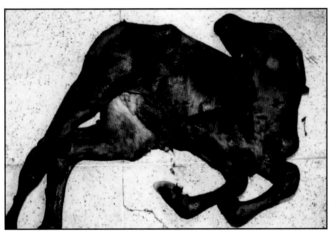

Akabane

Bovine neonate (Aino). This stillborn calf exhibits torticollis and arthrogryposis.
Source: Dr. K. Kawashima, National Institute of Animal Health, Japan

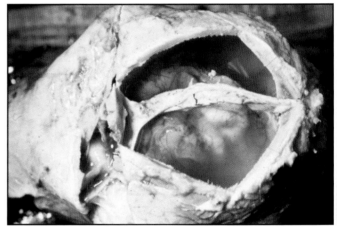

Akabane

Bovine neonate, brain. The entire brain is reduced in size (microencephaly), and surrounded by cerebrospinal fluid.
Source: Dr. K. Kawashima, National Institute for Animal Health, Japan

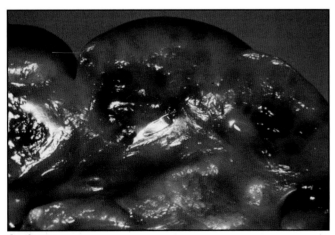

Anthrax

Bovine, lymph node. The node is hyperemic and contains multiple dark foci of hemorrhage.
Source: AFIP

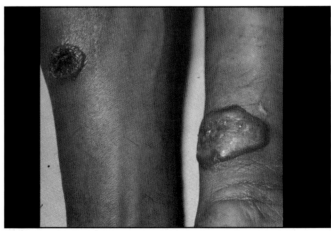

Anthrax

Human, skin. Lesions are raised and have necrotic centers.
Source: AFIP

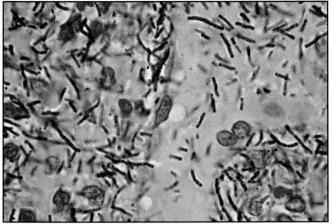

Anthrax

Bacillus anthracis is a large, blunt- to square-ended bacterial rod that forms short chains.
Source: ISU CVM

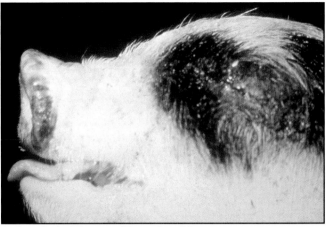

Aujeszky's Disease/Pseudorabies

Pig, head. The mucosal membranes around the eye and nares are crusted, and the eye has periorbital serous exudate.
Source: AFIP

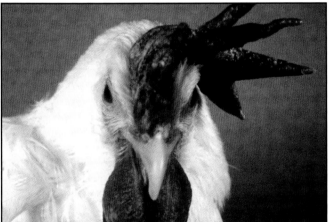

Avian Influenza

Chicken, head. The comb and wattles are congested and markedly edematous.
Source: Dr. D. Swayne, USDA

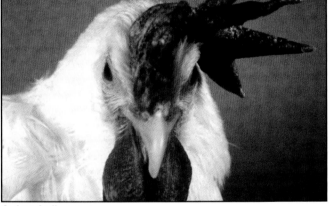

Avian Influenza

Chicken, shanks. The shanks are swollen (edema) and extensively reddened (hemorrhage).
Source: Dr. D. Swayne, USDA

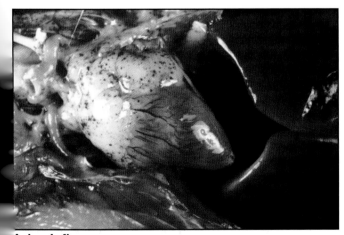

Avian Influenza

Chicken, heart. There are numerous epicardial petechiae.
Source: Dr. D. Swayne, USDA

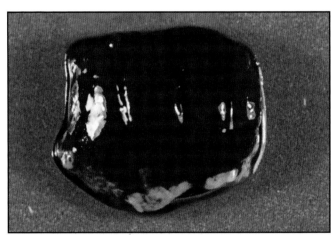

Avian Influenza

Chicken, lung. The lung is diffusely reddened, wet, and swollen (congestion and edema).
Source: Dr. D. Swayne, USDA

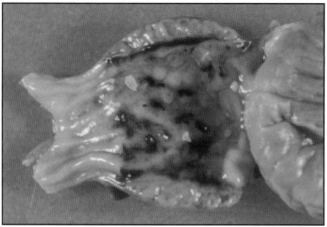

Avian Influenza

Chicken, proventriculus. There are multiple hemorrhages on the mucosal surface of the proventriculus.
Source: Dr. D. Swayne, USDA

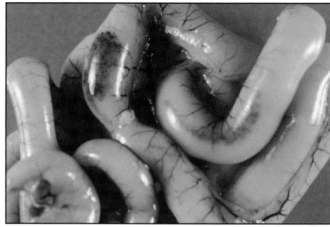

Avian Influenza

Chicken, intestine. There are serosal hemorrhages over the Peyer's patches.
Source: Dr. D. Swayne, USDA

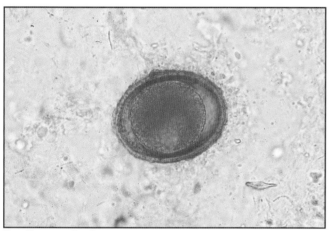

Baylisascariasis

Raccoon, feces. *Baylisascaris procyonis* eggs are typical ascarid eggs with thick, finely pitted shells; slightly smaller than *Toxocara canis* eggs.
Source: PIADC

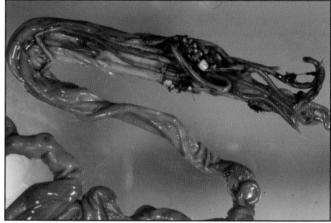

Baylisascariasis

Raccoon, intestine. A partially opened small intestine contains many adult *B. procyonis*.
Source: Dr. A. Hamir, ARS, USDA

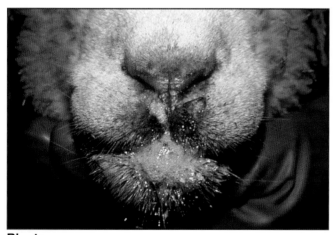

Bluetongue

Sheep. There is bilateral nasal exudate, erosion of the nasal planum, and excessive salivation.
Source: PIADC

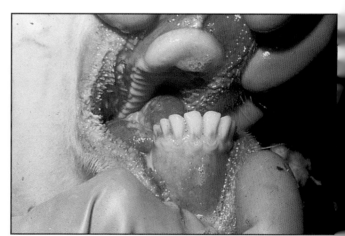

Bluetongue

Sheep, mouth. There is linear erosion and reddening of the right buccal mucosa.
Source: PIADC

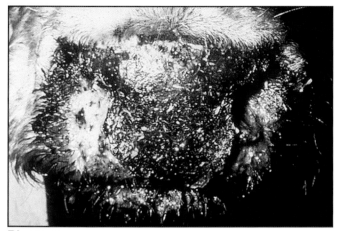

Bluetongue

Bovine. The muzzle is covered by an adherent crust, and the underlying (eroded) tissue is hyperemic.
Source: PIADC

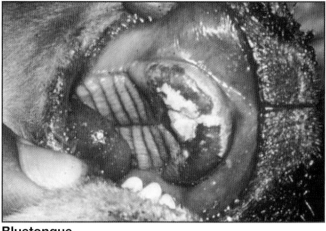

Bluetongue

Sheep, mouth. Most of the dental pad is eroded; the remaining pale mucosa is necrotic.
Source: AFIP

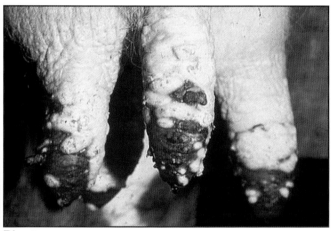

Bluetongue

Bovine, mammary gland. There is extensive coalescing ulceration of the teat skin.
Source: PIADC

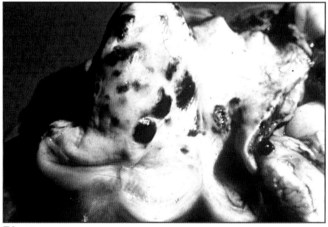

Bluetongue

Sheep, pulmonary artery. There are multiple ecchymoses on the intimal surface.
Source: AFIP

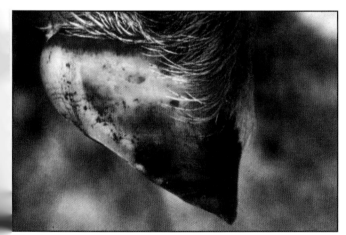

Bluetongue

Sheep, foot. There are multiple petechiae in the hoof wall, and there is marked hyperemia of the coronary band.
Source: AFIP

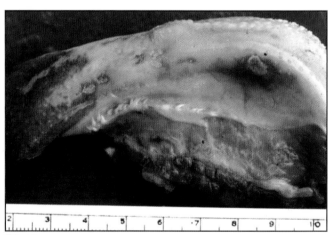

Bluetongue

Sheep, tongue. The lateral mucosa contains several ulcers that are covered by exudate and surrounded by zones of hyperemia.
Source: PIADC

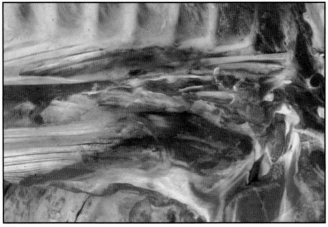

Bluetongue

Sheep, skeletal muscle. There is a focus of hemorrhage on the tendons. Pale areas are consistent with myodegeneration.
Source: AFIP

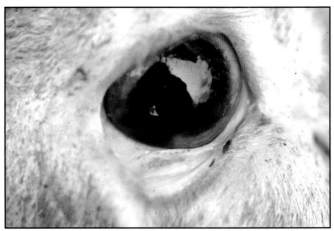

Bluetongue

Sheep, eye. There are foci of bulbar and palpebral conjunctival hemorrhage.
Source: AFIP

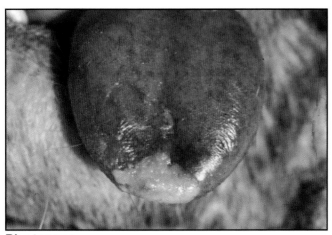

Bluetongue

Sheep, tongue. There are disseminated mucosal petechiae, and a single large vesicle on the tip.
Source: AFIP

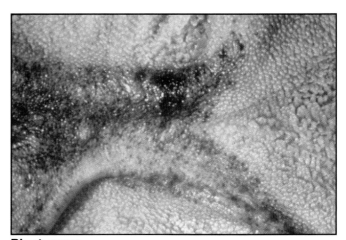

Bluetongue

Sheep, rumen. There are multiple mucosal hemorrhages centered on the pillars.
Source: AFIP

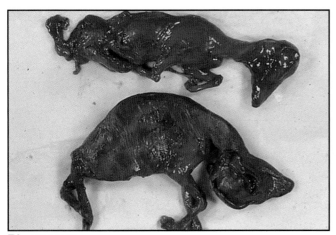

Bluetongue

Sheep, fetuses. The larger of these aborted macerated fetuses exhibits torticollis.
Source: PIADC

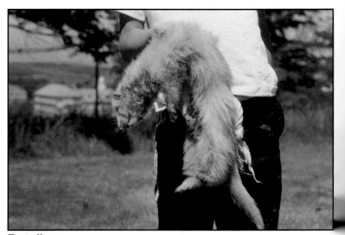

Botulism

Mink. Flaccid paralysis characteristic of botulism.
Source: AFIP

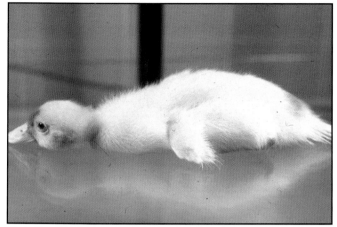

Botulism

Duck. Flaccid paralysis characteristic of botulism.
Source: AFIP

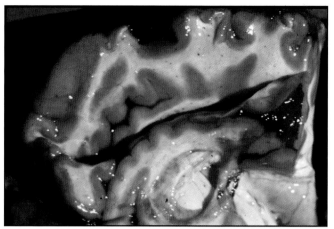

Bovine Babesiosis

Bovine, brain. The cerebral cortex is diffusely reddened
("cerebral flush").
Source: AFIP

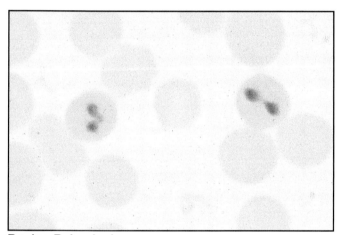

Bovine Babesiosis

Bovine, blood smear. Two erythrocytes contain pairs of ovoid
Babesia bovis.
Source: AFIP

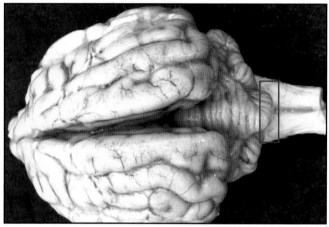

Bovine Spongiform Encephalopathy

Brain. The red box indicates the region of the obex, the portion
of the brainstem that is required for BSE diagnosis.
Source: Dr. S. Sorden, ISU CVM, VPTH

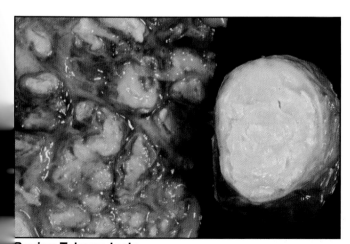

Bovine Tuberculosis

Elk, lung and lymph node. Lung contains multiple coalescing
foci of caseous necrosis surrounded by thin pale fibrous tissue
capsules (tubercles).
Source: Dr. G. Wobeser, CCWHC

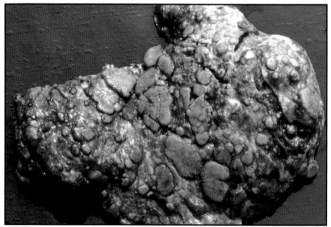

Bovine Tuberculosis

Bovine, lung. Lung parenchyma is almost entirely replaced by
variably-sized, coalescing, raised pale nodules.
Source: AFIP

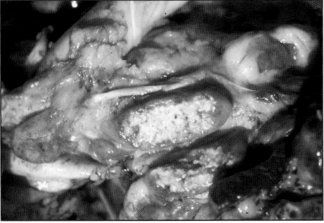

Bovine Tuberculosis

Pig, tracheobronchial lymph nodes. The center of the sectioned node is replaced by caseous, mineralized debris.
Source: AFIP

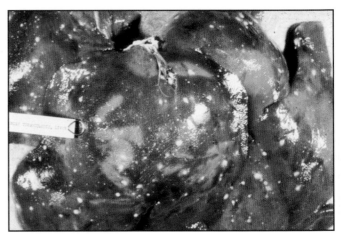

Bovine Tuberculosis

Pig, liver. Pale, slightly raised granulomas are disseminated throughout all liver lobes.
Source: AFIP

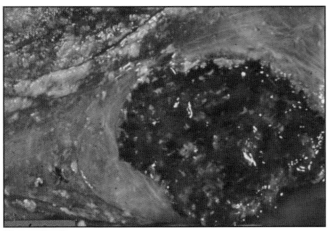

Brucellosis

Bovine, placenta. Numerous pale clumps of exudate are scattered over the cotyledon and adjacent chorion.
Source: AFIP

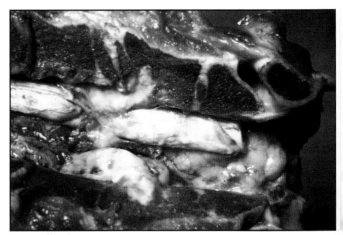

Brucellosis

Bovine, vertebrae. Purulent exudate within a vertebra extends into the adjacent spinal canal.
Source: AFIP

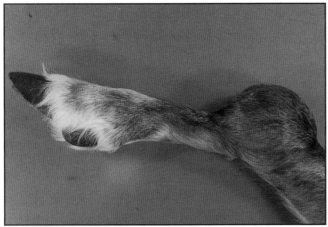

Brucellosis

Caribou, carpus, *B. suis* biovar 4. The carpal bursa is markedly swollen and fluctuant.
Source: Dr. G. Wobeser, CCWHC

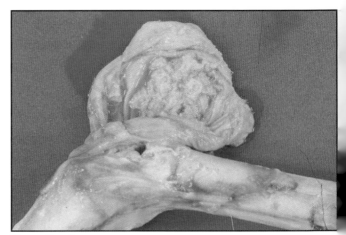

Brucellosis

Caribou, carpus, *B. suis* biovar 4. The carpal bursa contains purulent exudate.
Source: Dr. G. Wobeser, CCWHC

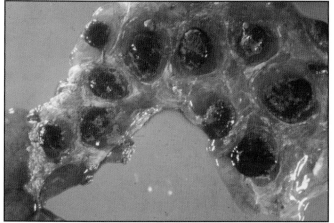

Brucellosis

Bovine, placenta. The placenta contains numerous hemorrhagic cotyledons.
Source: AFIP

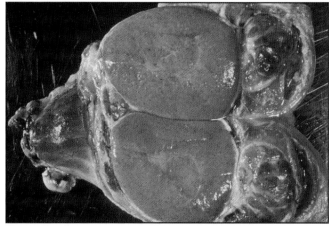

Brucellosis

Sheep, testis (bisected). The epididymis is markedly enlarged and contains bands of fibrous tissue (chronic epididymitis). In this case, the testis itself is relatively unaffected.
Source: AFIP

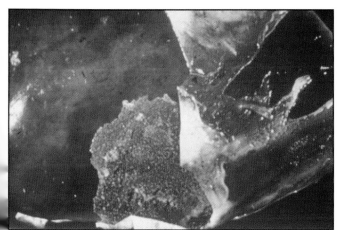

Chlamydiosis, avian

Avian, liver. Sheets of fibrinous exudate partially cover the capsular surface of the liver.
Source: AFIP

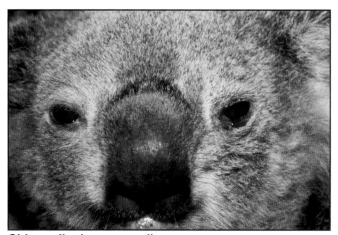

Chlamydiosis, mammalian

Koala, eye. Reddened conjunctiva with a focal erosion and serous exudate.
Source: AFIP

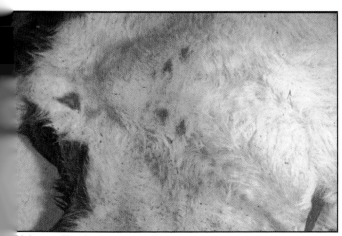

Chlamydiosis, mammalian

Bovine, skin, fetus. Ulcerated reddened foci on the skin of an aborted fetus due to *Chlamydia psittaci*.
Source: AFIP

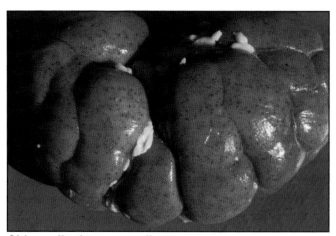

Chlamydiosis, mammalian

Bovine, kidney. Diffuse petechial hemorrhages are present in the kidney.
Source: AFIP

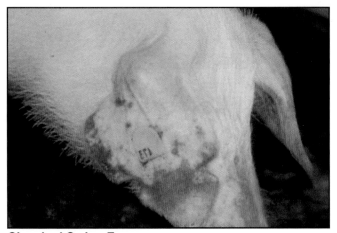

Classical Swine Fever

Pig. The distal pinnae contain coalescing dark red foci of hemorrhage and necrosis (infarction).
Source: USDA

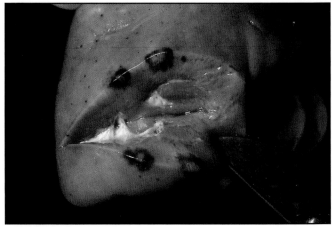

Classical Swine Fever

Pig, kidney. The cortex contains multiple petechiae and pale infarcts surrounded by hemorrhage.
Source: PIADC

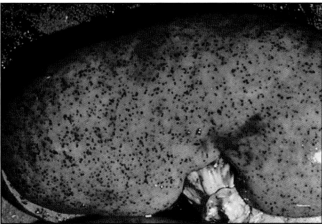

Classical Swine Fever

Pig, kidney. There are numerous disseminated cortical petechiae ("turkey egg kidney").
Source: PIADC

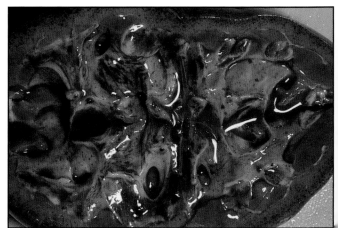

Classical Swine Fever

Pig, kidney. The cortex contains disseminated petechiae. Calyces are moderately dilated (hydronephrosis) andcontain hemorrhages.
Source: PIADC

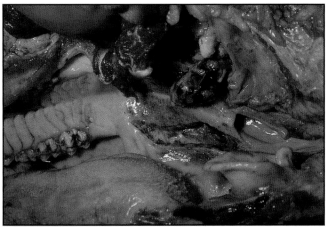

Classical Swine Fever

Pig, retropharyngeal lymph node. The lymph node is markedly enlarged and hemorrhagic; the tonsil contains multiple poorly demarcated hemorrhages.
Source: PIADC

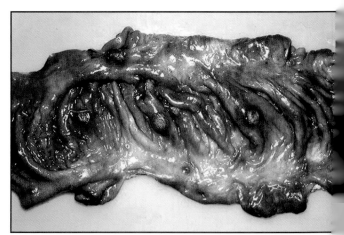

Classical Swine Fever

Pig, colon. The mucosa is reddened and contains multiple discrete ("button") ulcers surrounded by zones of hemorrhage
Source: Dr. R. Panciera, Noah's Arkive, Oklahoma State University

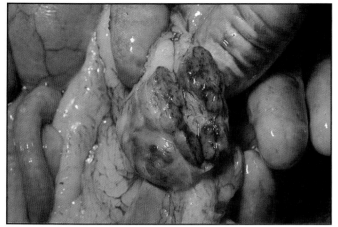

Classical Swine Fever

Pig, inguinal lymph node. There are petechial and peripheral (medullary sinus) hemorrhages.
Source: PIADC

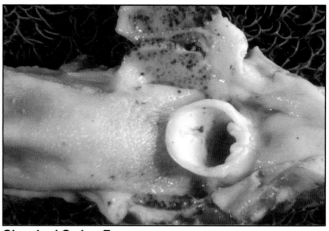

Classical Swine Fever

Pig, pharynx and larynx. There are coalescing foci of petechial hemorrhage (and necrosis) in the palatine tonsils and adjacent pharyngeal and laryngeal mucosa.
Source: Dr. W. Wajjwalku, Kasetsart University, Thailand

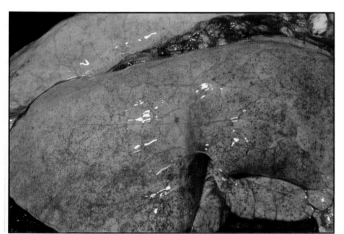

Classical Swine Fever

Pig, lungs. There are numerous disseminated pleural petechiae, and there is mild interlobular edema.
Source: PIADC

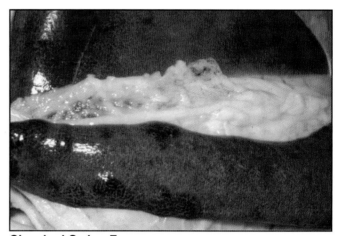

Classical Swine Fever

Pig, spleen. There are multiple coalescing, swollen dark red infarcts along the margins.
Source: Dr. D. Gregg, Noah's Arkive, PIADC

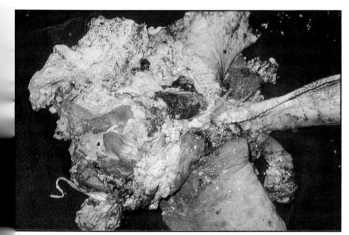

Contagious Bovine Pleuropneumonia

Bovine, lung. Most of the pleural surface is covered by abundant fibrin and fibrous tissue.
Source: PIADC

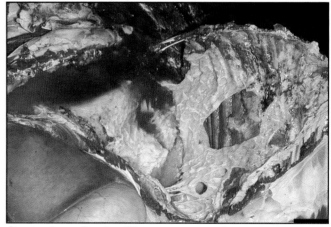

Contagious Bovine Pleuropneumonia

Bovine, pleural cavity. Large sheets of fibrin cover the costal and diaphragmatic pleura, and form pockets containing straw-colored fluid.
Source: PIADC

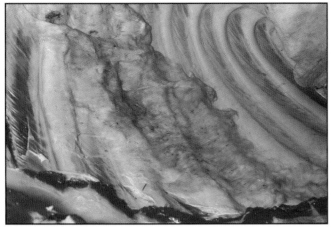

Contagious Bovine Pleuropneumonia

Bovine, pleural cavity. There is a thick plaque (adhesion) of fibrous tissue on the costal pleura.
Source: PIADC

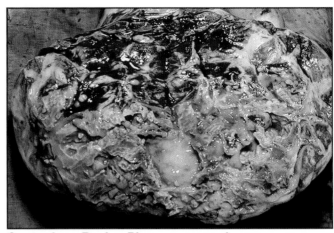

Contagious Bovine Pleuropneumonia

Bovine, lung. Most of the parenchyma is dull and tan (necrotic); partially surrounded by a fibrous capsule, this necrotic zone is termed a sequestrum.
Source: PIADC

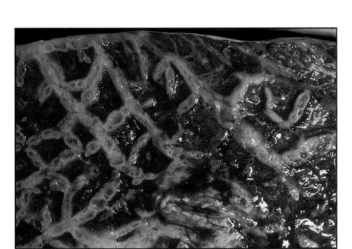

Contagious Bovine Pleuropneumonia

Bovine, lung. Interlobular septa are markedly thickened by fibrous tissue, and also contain small depressions (air pockets = emphysema).
Source: PIADC

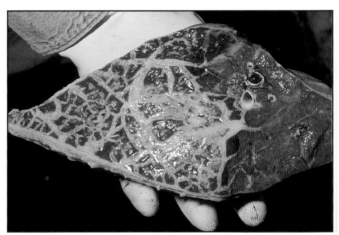

Contagious Bovine Pleuropneumonia

Bovine, lung. In the ventral portion of this lung (left side of the image), interlobular septa and the pleura are markedly thickened with fibrous tissue.
Source: PIADC

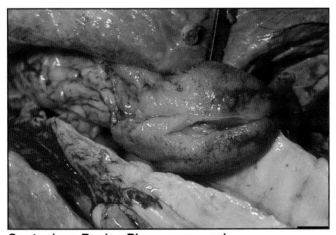

Contagious Bovine Pleuropneumonia

Bovine, tracheobronchial lymph node. This bisected node is enlarged (hyperplasia) and contains a focal area of hemorrhage.
Source: PIADC

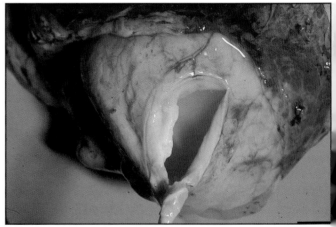

Contagious Bovine Pleuropneumonia

Bovine, heart. The pericardial wall is markedly thickened and the pericardial sac contains abundant pale tan, turbid fluid.
Source: PIADC

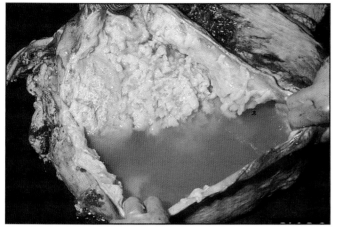

Contagious Bovine Pleuropneumonia

Bovine, heart. The pericardial sac is distended with abundant turbid, tan fluid, and abundant fibrin coats the pericardial surfaces.
Source: PIADC

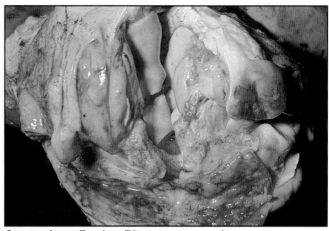

Contagious Bovine Pleuropneumonia

Bovine, carpus. The joint capsule and extensor tendon sheath are thickened and contain excessive fluid.
Source: PIADC

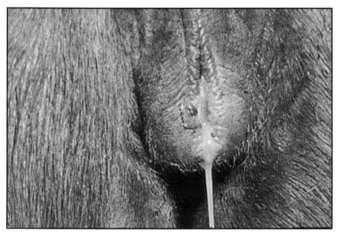

Contagious Equine Metritis

Horse, vulva. Mucopurulent exudate drains from the vulva.
Source: PIADC

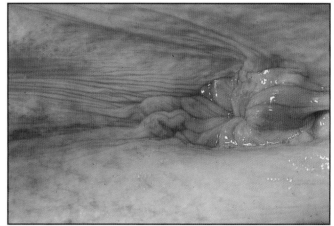

Contagious Equine Metritis

Horse, vagina. There is straw-colored fluid within the cranial vagina.
Source: PIADC

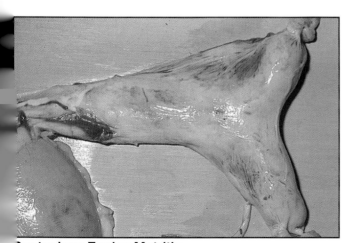

Contagious Equine Metritis

Horse, uterus. The uterine horns and body are mildly distended with mucopurulent exudate).
Source: PIADC

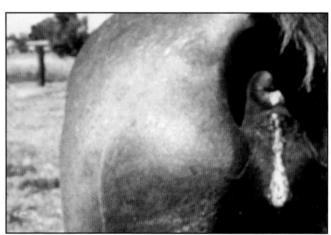

Dourine

Horse, rump. Vulvar thickening and edema, often gelatinous, due to *Trypanosoma equiperdum*.
Source: AFIP

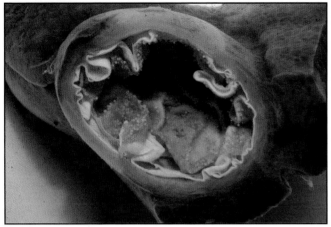

Echinococcosis

Liver. Cross-section of cyst due to echinococcosis.
Source: ISU CVM, VPTH

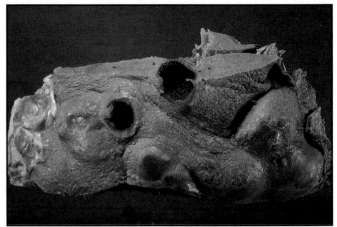

Echinococcosis

Skunk, liver. The inner surface of the cyst is lined by hydatid sand and surrounded by a thick capsule of fibrous connective tissue.
Source: ISU, CVM

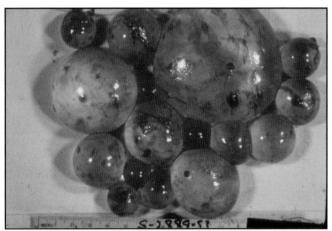

Echinococcosis

Human, liver. Multiple thin-walled hydatid cysts project from the capsular surface of the liver.
Source: AFIP

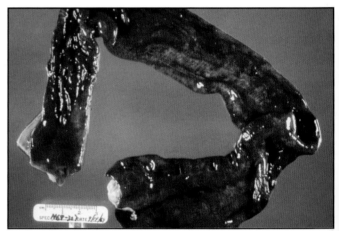

Enterohemorrhagic *Escherichia coli*

Canine, small intestine. hemorrhagic enteritis due to *E. coli 0157:H7*.
Source: AFIP

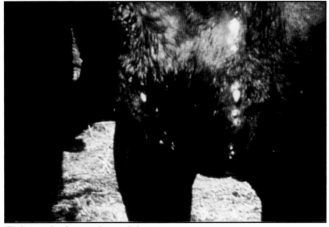

Epizootic Lymphangitis

Horse, skin. The thoracic (brisket area) skin and subcutaneous tissue are thickened with purulent foci (abscesses).
Source: AFIP

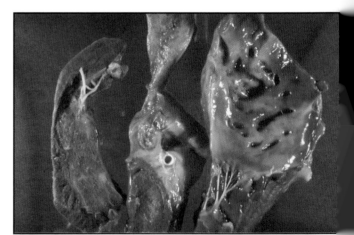

Equine Infectious Anemia

Horse, heart. Pale cardiac muscle, focal white areas of myocardial degeneration, and reddened hemorrhagic areas (possible hypoxia during death).
Source: ISU CVM

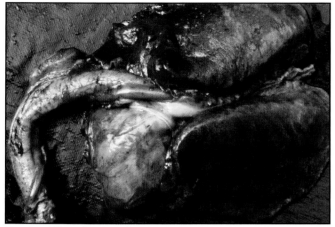

Equine Piroplasmosis

Horse, heart and lungs. The trachea and pericardial fat are icteric. Lungs are irregularly congested with consolidation of the right cranioventral lung.
Source: AFIP

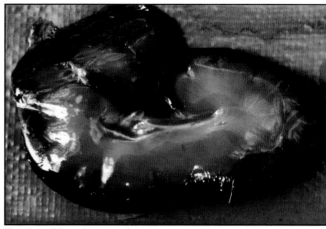

Equine Piroplasmosis

Horse, kidney. The cortex is dark red due to hemoglobinemia; medulla and pelvis are icteric.
Source: AFIP

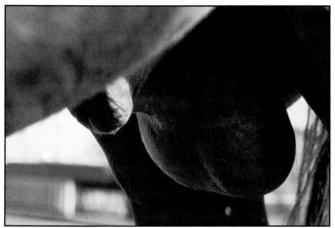

Equine Viral Arteritis

Horse scrotum. Scrotal edema occurring in equine viral arteritis.
Source: Dr. R.C. Giles, University of Kentucky, Noah's Arkive

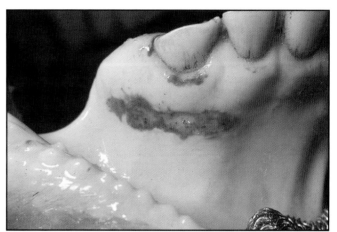

Foot and Mouth Disease

Bovine, gingiva. There is an elongate erosion (ruptured vesicle) ventral to the incisors.
Source: PIADC

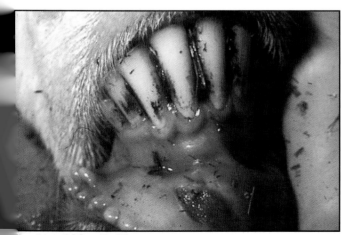

Foot and Mouth Disease

Goat, oral mucosa. There is a large erosion (ruptured vesicle) on the rostral mandibular buccal mucosa.
Source: PIADC

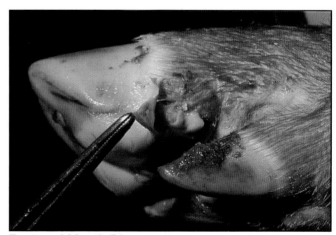

Foot and Mouth Disease

Pig, foot. There is a ruptured vesicle on the caudal-lateral coronary band, with undermining of the heel.
Source: PIADC

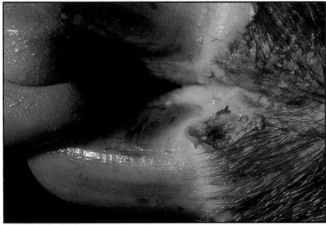

Foot and Mouth Disease

Pig, foot. A ruptured vesicle of the coronary band extends into the interdigital skin.
Source: PIADC

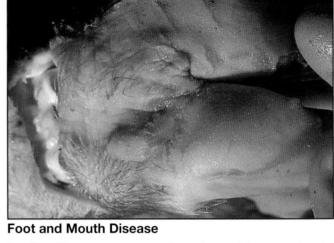

Foot and Mouth Disease

Pig, foot. There is an intact vesicle on the caudal coronary band of the left claw, and a cleft (ruptured vesicle) on the heel bulb of the right claw.
Source: PIADC

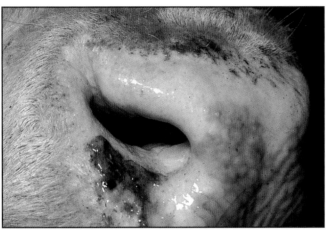

Foot and Mouth Disease

Bovine, muzzle. Within the naris, the ventromedial mucosa contains an intact vesicle.
Source: PIADC

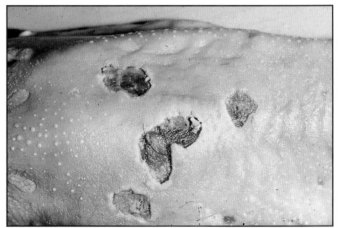

Foot and Mouth Disease

Bovine, tongue. There are multiple large mucosal erosions and ulcers.
Source: PIADC

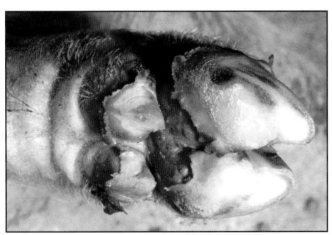

Foot and Mouth Disease

Pig, foot. Large clefts at the coronary bands precede sloughing of the claws.
Source: Dr. D. Gregg, Noah's Arkive, PIADC

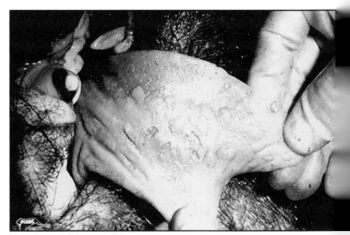

Foot and Mouth Disease

Pig, tongue. Many ("dry") vesicles are ruptured and lack fluid.
Source: Foreign Animal Diseases "The Grey Book" USAHA

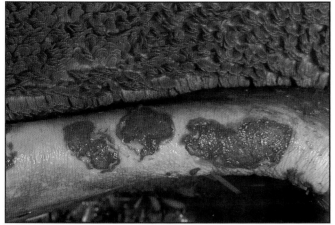

Foot and Mouth Disease

Rumen mucosa, higher magnification. There are several irregularly shaped erosions (ruptured vesicles) on the pillar.
Source: PIADC

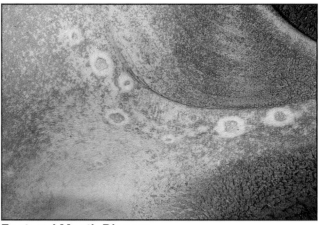

Foot and Mouth Disease

Rumen mucosa, dorsal sac, low magnification. There are several erosions (ruptured vesicles) on the pillars. The pale margins are undermined epithelium.
Source: PIADC

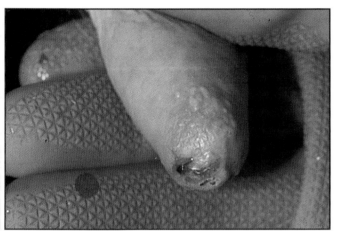

Foot and Mouth Disease

Bovine, teat. There is a ruptured vesicle on the end of the teat.
Source: PIADC

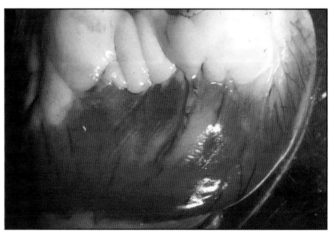

Foot and Mouth Disease

Sheep, heart. There is a pale area of myocardial necrosis visible from the epicardial surface.
Source: Dr. D. Gregg, Noah's Arkive, PIADC

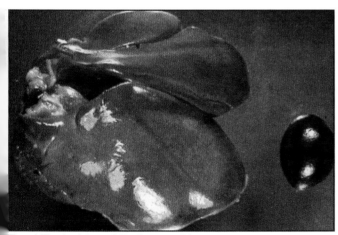

Fowl Typhoid and Pullorum Disease

Avian liver, spleen. Liver is pale with diffuse yellow-brown (bronze) discoloration; splenic congestion and enlargement.
Source: Dr. Andreasen, CVM

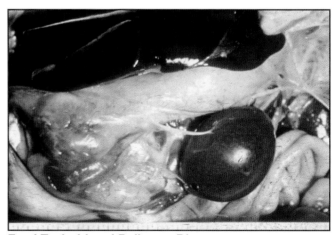

Fowl Typhoid and Pullorum Disease

Avian, abdominal cavity. Liver with focal pale edges (top of abdominal cavity) and enlarged, rounded spleen with white pinpoint multifocal lesions due to *Salmonella gallinarum*.
Source: AFIP

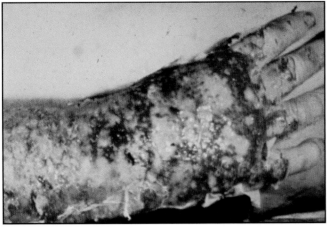

Glanders

Human, skin. There is extensive ulceration and sloughing of the skin of the forearm and hand. Ulcers may be connected by lymphatic vessels ("Farcy pipes") full of thick purulent exudate.
Source: AFIP

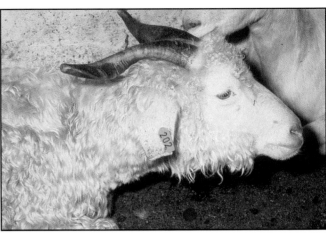

Heartwater

Goat. The neck is extended, consistent with dyspnea.
Source: PIADC

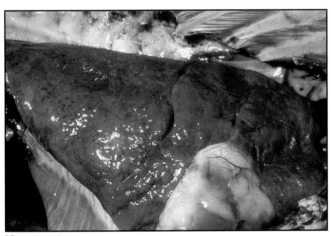

Heartwater

Goat, thoracic viscera. There are many pleural hemorrhages, and the lung is moderately noncollapsed (edema).
Source: PIADC

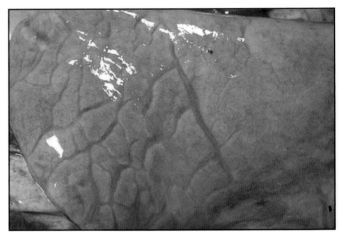

Heartwater

Sheep, lung. There is severe interlobular edema.
Source: PIADC

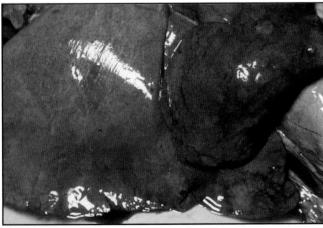

Heartwater

Sheep, lung. Interlobular septa are distended with edema fluid.
Source: PIADC

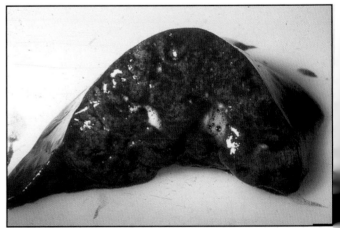

Heartwater

Sheep, lung. The lung is noncollapsed and hyperemic, and the bronchi contain frothy fluid (pulmonary edema).
Source: PIADC

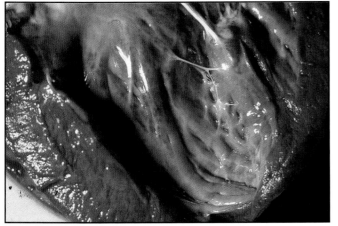

Heartwater

Goat, heart. There are many small hemorrhages on the endocardial surface.
Source: PIADC

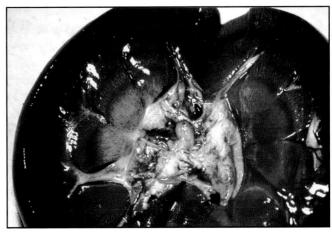

Heartwater

Sheep, kidney. Section reveals numerous fine linear radial hemorrhages; hemorrhages coalesce in the papillae.
Source: PIADC

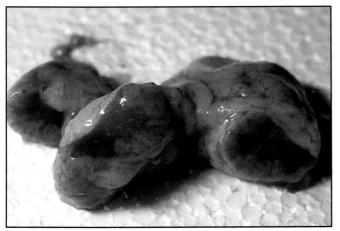

Heartwater

Goat, prescapular lymph node. There are multiple barely discernable petechiae in the cortex.
Source: PIADC

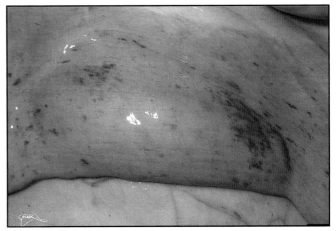

Heartwater

Goat, abomasum. There are multiple petechial and paintbrush serosal hemorrhages.
Source: PIADC

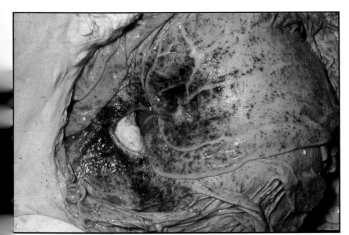

Heartwater

Small ruminant, abomasum. The mucosa contains disseminated petechial and coalescing ecchymotic hemorrhages.
Source: PIADC

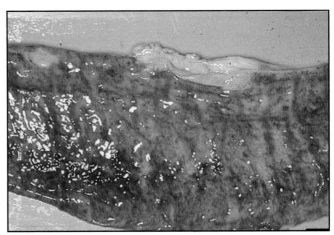

Heartwater

Small ruminant, small intestine. The mucosa contains numerous petechiae and ecchymoses.
Source: PIADC

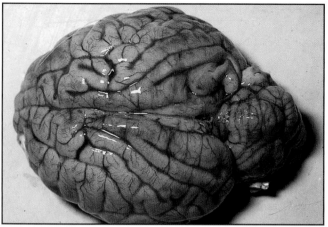

Heartwater

Sheep, brain. The leptomeninges are congested and contain many small hemorrhages. Gyri are flattened (cerebral edema).
Source: PIADC

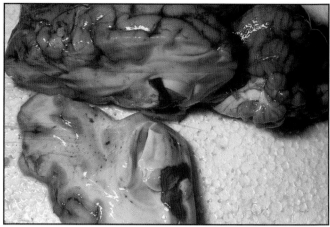

Heartwater

Goat, brain. The cerebrum contains multiple petechiae and a few ecchymoses. The swollen, hemorrhagic choroid plexus protrudes from the lateral ventricle.
Source: PIADC

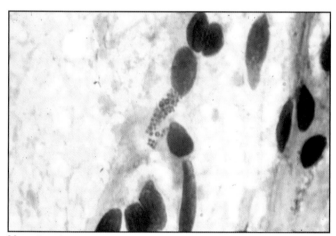

Heartwater

Goat, brain smear. An endothelial cell contains a morula (cluster) of *Ehrlichia ruminantium*.
Source: PIADC

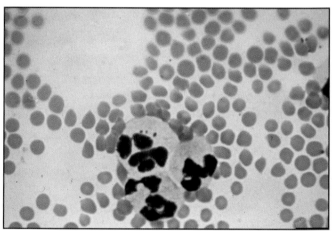

Heartwater

Goat, peripheral blood smear. A neutrophil contains a few *Ehrlichia ruminantium*.
Source: PIADC

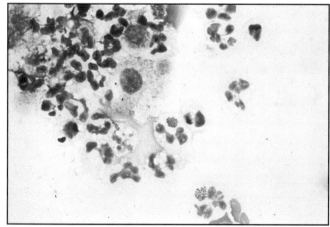

Heartwater

Goat, buffy coat smear. Several neutrophils contain *E. ruminantium* morulae.
Source: PIADC

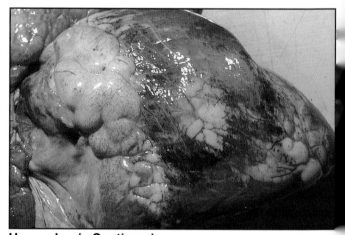

Hemorrhagic Septicemia

Bovine, heart. There are numerous often coalescing petechiae on the epicardium.
Source: PIADC

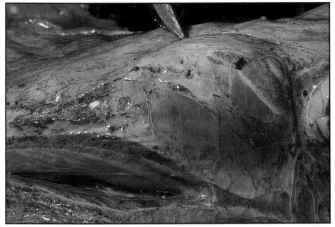

Hemorrhagic Septicemia

Bovine, submandibular region. There is severe subcutaneous/ fascial edema and multifocal hemorrhage. The parotid gland exhibits interlobular edema.
Source: PIADC

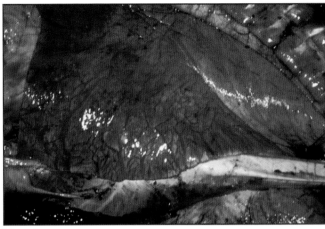

Hendra

Horse, lung. There is severe interlobular edema.
Source: Dr. M. Williamson, CSIRO, Australia

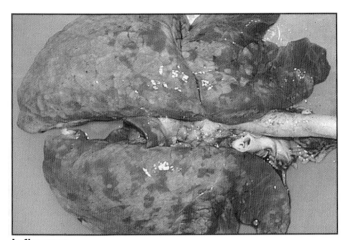

Influenza

Pig, lungs. There is diffuse tan consolidation of cranial lobes, and multifocal lobular consolidation of the caudal lobes.
Source: Dr. B. Janke, ISU CVM, VDL

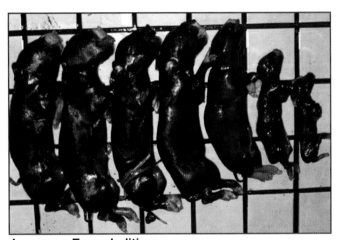

Japanese Encephalitis

Pig, fetuses. The litter consists of five large (full-term) stillborn fetuses and two small mummified fetuses.
Source: Dr. K. Kawashima, Central Livestock Hygiene Service Center Saitama pref., Japan

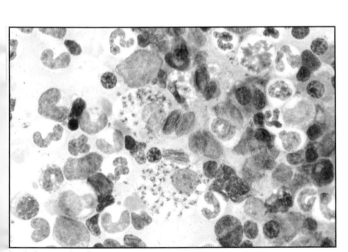

Leishmaniasis

Dog, bone marrow. The bone marrow contains hematopoietic precursors and macrophages with numerous intracytoplasmic *Leishmania sp.*
Source: Dr. C. Andreasen, ISU CVM, VPTH

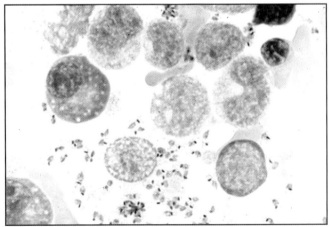

Leishmaniasis

Dog, bone marrow. Higher magnification of bone marrow demonstrating intracellular and extracellular *Leishmania sp.*
Source: Dr. C. Andreasen, ISU CVM, VPTH

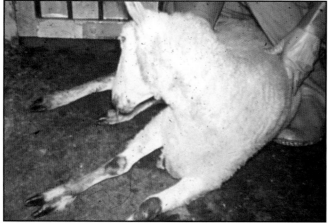

Louping III

Sheep. Sheep with neurologic deficits that is unable to stand.
Source: AFIP

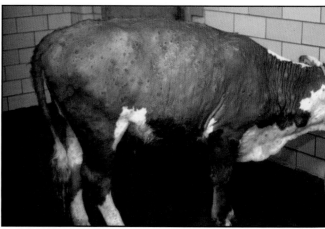

Lumpy Skin Disease

Bovine, skin. There are disseminated cutaneous papules with necrotic centers (sitfasts).
Source: Noah's Arkive, PIADC

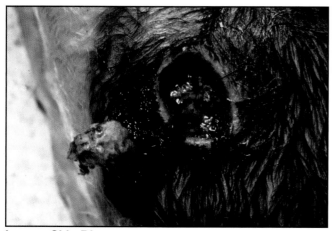

Lumpy Skin Disease

Bovine, skin. There is hemorrhagic exudate subjacent to the necrotic center (sitfast) of a papule.
Source: Noah's Arkive, PIADC

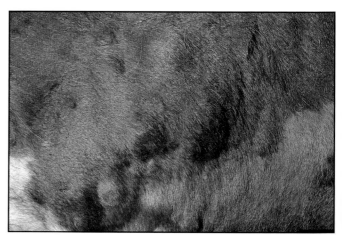

Lumpy Skin Disease

Bovine, skin. Multiple subcutaneous nodules elevate the skin.
Source: PIADC

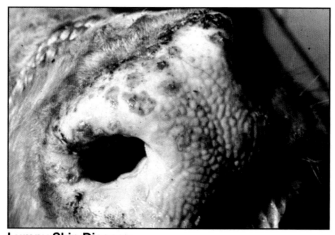

Lumpy Skin Disease

Bovine, muzzle. There are multiple sharply-demarcated slightly raised papules, often with eroded surfaces, that extend into the nares.
Source: Noah's Arkive, PIADC

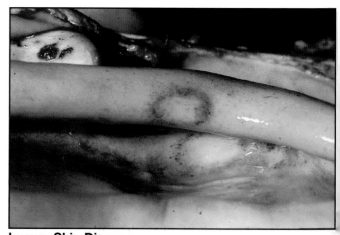

Lumpy Skin Disease

Bovine, nasal turbinate. Early pox lesions are slightly pale round foci rimmed by petechiae.
Source: PIADC

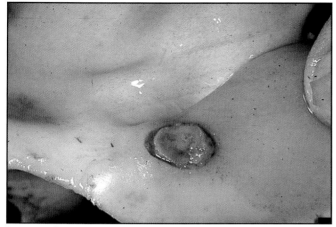

Lumpy Skin Disease

Bovine, nasal turbinate. The centers of well-developed pox are necrotic.
Source: PIADC

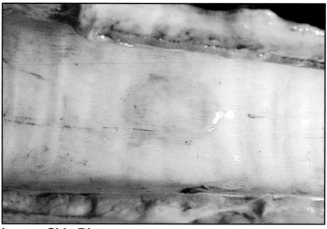

Lumpy Skin Disease

Bovine, trachea. The mucosa contains a poorly demarcated round focus rimmed by mild hemorrhage (early pox lesion).
Source: PIADC

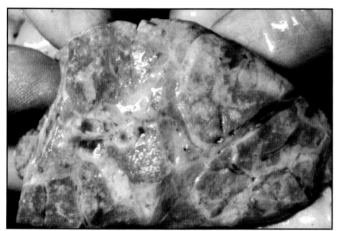

Lumpy Skin Disease

Bovine, lung. There is marked generalized interlobular edema, and there is a small cluster of red nodules on the left side of the specimen.
Source: Noah's Arkive, PIADC

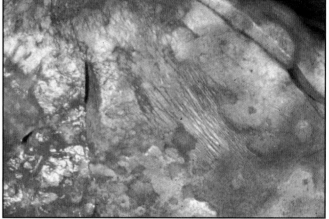

Maedi-Visna

Sheep, lung. Lung fails to deflate and contains coalescing multifocal gray-white nodules/plaques (proliferative lymphocytes and pneumocytes) with adjacent atelectatic depressed parenchyma (red-pink).
Source: AFIP

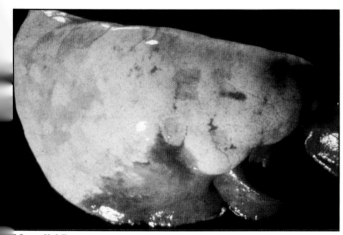

Maedi-Visna

Sheep, lung. Lung fails to deflate with pale gray coalescing proliferative areas and cranioventral atelectasis (reddish area).
Source: AFIP

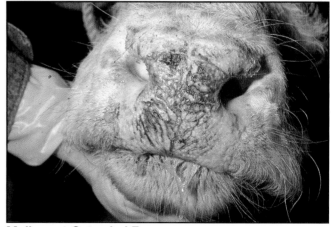

Malignant Catarrhal Fever

Bovine, muzzle. Multiple shallow erosions are filled with dried nasal exudate.
Source: PIADC

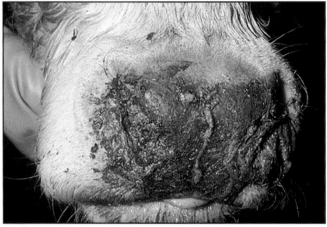

Malignant Catarrhal Fever

Bovine. There is diffuse superficial necrosis of the muzzle.
Source: PIADC

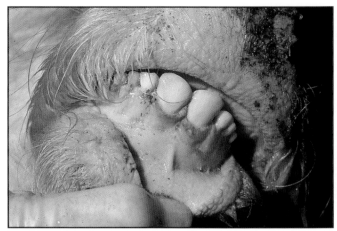

Malignant Catarrhal Fever

Bovine, oral mucosa. There is gingival hyperemia and focal erosion.
Source: PIADC

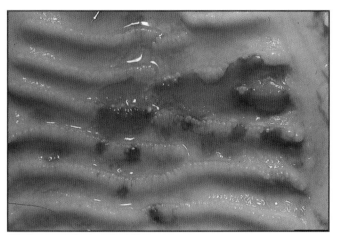

Malignant Catarrhal Fever

Bovine, hard palate. There are multiple coalescing mucosal erosions.
Source: PIADC

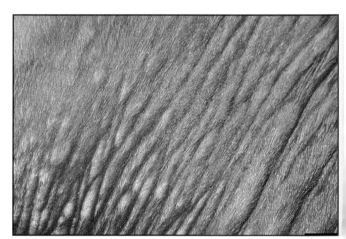

Malignant Catarrhal Fever

Bovine, skin. There are numerous raised plaques (multifocal dermatitis).
Source: PIADC

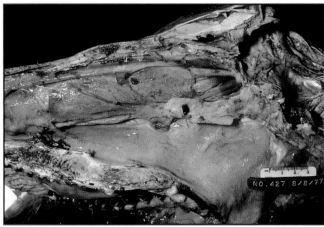

Malignant Catarrhal Fever

Bovine, head, sagittal section. Mucoid exudate multifocally covers the nasal and pharyngeal mucosa.
Source: PIADC

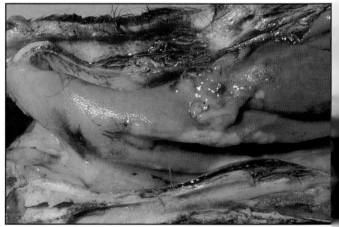

Malignant Catarrhal Fever

Bovine, nasal turbinate. There is a small amount of mucoid exudate.
Source: PIADC

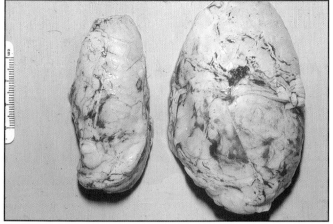

Malignant Catarrhal Fever

Bovine, prescapular lymph nodes: Moderately (left) to markedly enlarged (right) due to MCF.
Source: PIADC

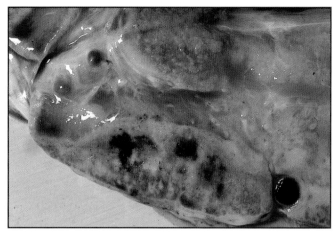

Malignant Catarrhal Fever

Bovine, prescapular lymph node. There are foci of hemorrhage (and necrosis) in the cortex, and the medulla is edematous.
Source: PIADC

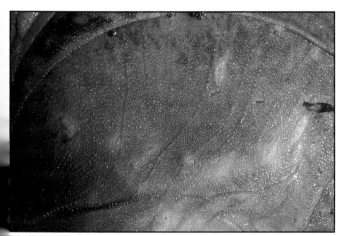

Malignant Catarrhal Fever

Bovine, omasum. Omasal leaves contain multiple pale foci of necrosis; on the right there are several ulcers.
Source: PIADC

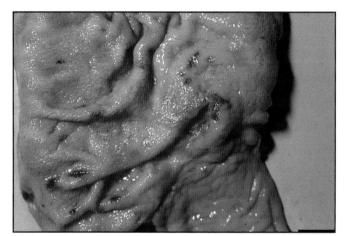

Malignant Catarrhal Fever

Bovine, cecum and ileum. There are scattered small foci of mucosal hemorrhage and erosion.
Source: PIADC

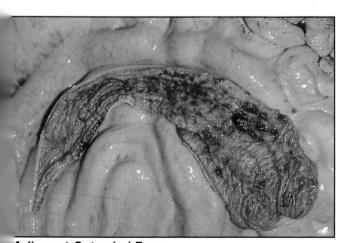

Malignant Catarrhal Fever

Bovine, spiral colon. There are multiple mucosal hemorrhages.
Source: PIADC

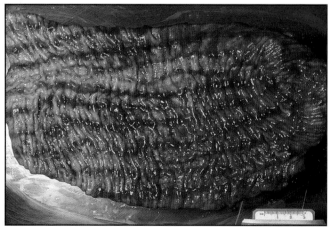

Malignant Catarrhal Fever

Bovine, colon. There is severe longitudinal linear congestion of the mucosa.
Source: PIADC

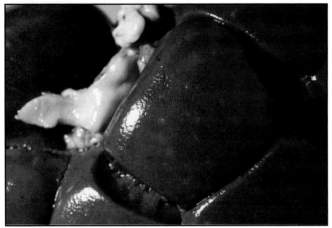

Malignant Catarrhal Fever

Bovine, kidney. Multiple pale foci in the cortex are foci of
interstitial nephritis.
Source: PIADC

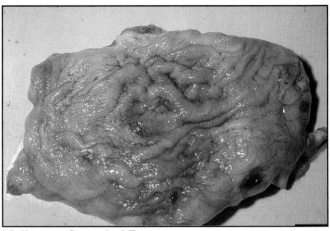

Malignant Catarrhal Fever

Bovine, urinary bladder. The mucosal surface contains several
small erosions and one large hemorrhagic ulcer.
Source: PIADC

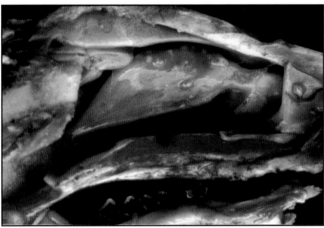

Melioidosis

Goat, nasal turbinates. There are multiple raised pale nodules
(abscesses) on the nasal mucosa.
Source: Dr. K. Kawashima, National Institute of Animal Health, Japan

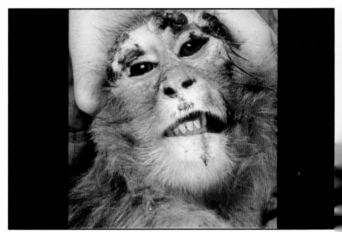

Monkeypox

Rhesus macaque, monkeypox. There are multiple hemorrhagic
papules on the forehead and eyelids.
Source: AFIP

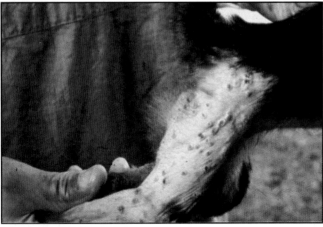

Monkeypox

Primate, hindlimb, monkeypox. There are numerous discrete
papules with red, depressed centers.
Source: AFIP

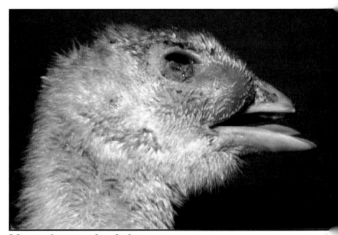

Mycoplasmosis, Avian

Turkey, head. Purulent sinusitis.
Source: Dr. N. Cheville, ISU CVM.

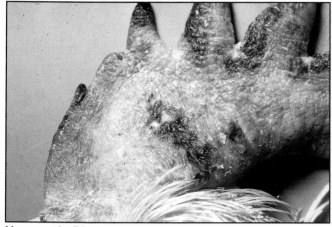

Newcastle Disease

Chicken, comb. The comb is markedly edematous and contains multiple foci of hemorrhage.
Source: PIADC

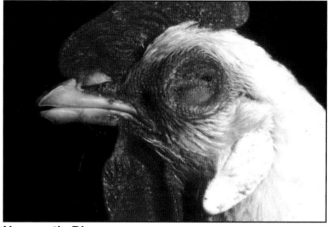

Newcastle Disease

Chicken. There is a marked hemorrhage of the comb, wattle, and adjacent skin.
Source: AFIP

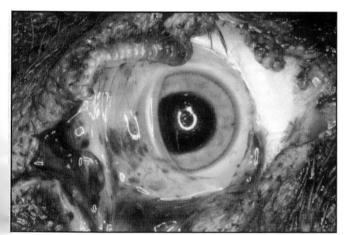

Newcastle Disease

Chicken, eye. Conjunctival hemorrhage is most severe in the nictitans.
Source: CAHFSLS

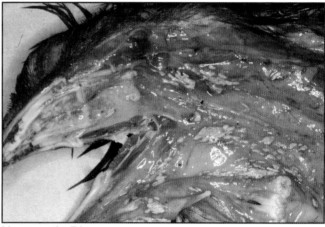

Newcastle Disease

Chicken, oral cavity. Numerous clumps of fibrinonecrotic exudate adhere to foci of necrosis in the oral, pharyngeal, and esophageal mucosa.
Source: CAHFSLS

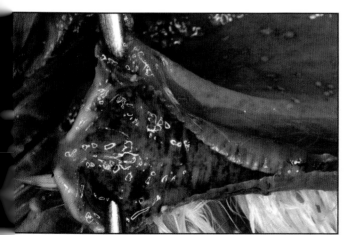

Newcastle Disease

Chicken, trachea. Tracheal and laryngeal mucosa contain many foci of hemorrhage and small clumps of fibrinonecrotic exudate.
Source: CAHFSLS

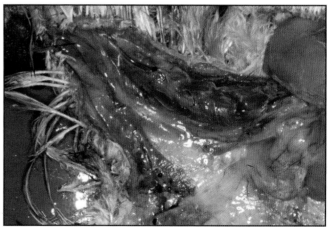

Newcastle Disease

Chicken, subcutis. There is marked subcutaneous edema in the neck, extending to the thoracic inlet.
Source: CAHFSLS

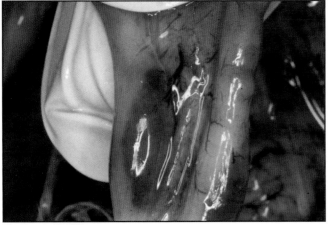

Newcastle Disease

Chicken, ceca. Hyperemic, necrotic cecal tonsils are visible from the serosal surface.
Source: CAHFSLS

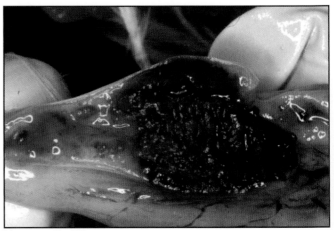

Newcastle Disease

Chicken, ceca. The cecal tonsil is red-brown, thickened, and friable (necrotic).
Source: CAHFSLS

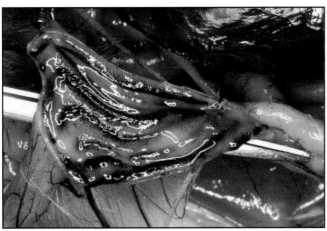

Newcastle Disease

Chicken, rectum. There are multiple linear mucosal hemorrhages.
Source: CAHFSLS

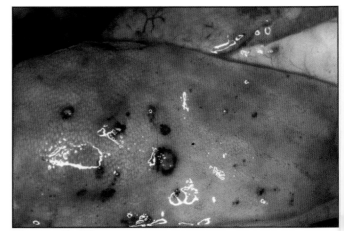

Newcastle Disease

Chicken, colon. The mucosa contains multiple sharply demarcated foci of hemorrhage and necrosis.
Source: CAHFSLS

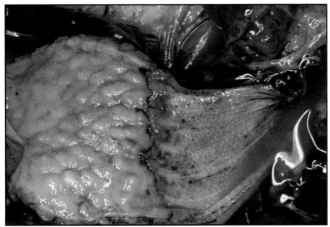

Newcastle Disease

Chicken, proventriculus. The proximal mucosa is eroded and covered by a fibrinonecrotic (diptheritic) membrane.
Source: CAHFSLS

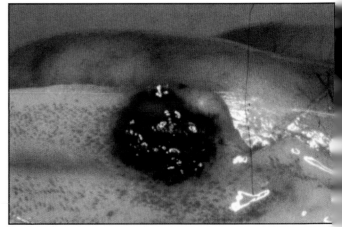

Newcastle Disease

Chicken, cecal tonsil necrosis.
Source: CAHFSLS

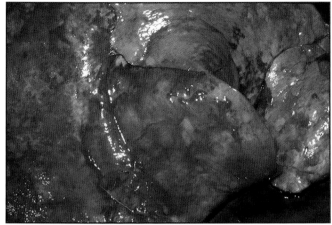

Ovine Pulmonary Adenocarcinoma (Adenomatosis)

Sheep, lung. The lungs fail to deflate and are mottled with coalescing to diffuse proliferative areas (pale pink) with red areas of atelectasis.
Source: Dr. C. Clarke, University of Edinburgh, Noah's Arkive.

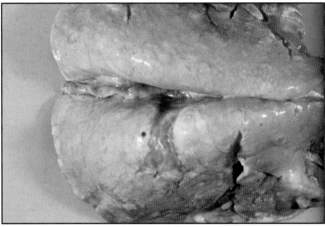

Ovine Pulmonary Adenocarcinoma (Adenomatosis)

Sheep, lung. The lungs fail to deflate and the ventral edges of the lungs contain multiple white proliferative and fibrotic coalescing nodules.
Source: Dr. C. von Tscharner, Institute of Animal Pathology, Vetsuisse Faculty, University of Bern, Switzerland, Noah's Arkive

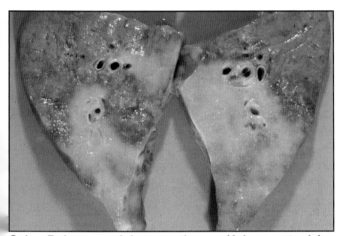

Ovine Pulmonary Adenocarcinoma (Adenomatosis)

Sheep, lung. The cut surface of the lung has large, firm, gray coalescing proliferative and fibrotic masses that are sharply demarcated.
Source: Dr. C. von Tscharner, Institute of Animal Pathology, Vetsuisse Faculty, University of Bern, Switzerland, Noah's Arkive

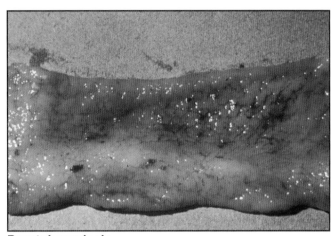

Paratuberculosis

Sheep, intestine. The mucosal surface of the intestine contains a roughened cobblestone appearance due to granulomatous infiltrates.
Source: AFIP

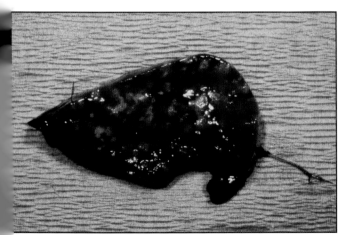

Plague

Primate, liver. The liver has multifocal to coalescing white lesions due to *Yersinia pestis*.
Source: AFIP

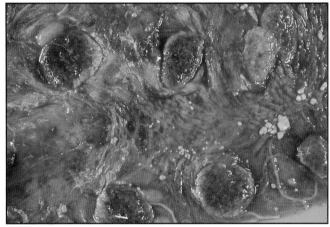

Q Fever

Goat, placenta. The intercotyledonary placenta is thickened, opaque, and multifocally covered by tan exudate. Margins of several cotyledons are tan (necrosis), and centers are mottled red-brown (congestion and exudation).
Source: Dr. J. Arzt, PIADC

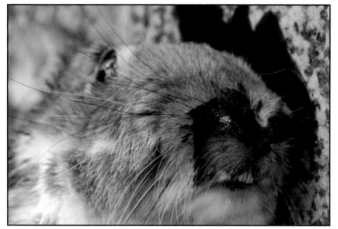

Rabbit Hemorrhagic Disease

Rabbit. Severe epistaxis.
Source: Dr. J.P. Teifke, Federal Research Institute for Animal Health Riems, Germany

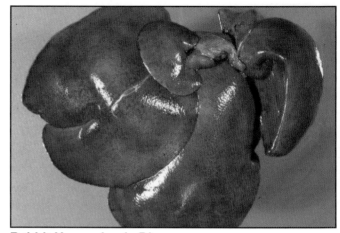

Rabbit Hemorrhagic Disease

Rabbit, liver. All liver lobes are swollen, pale and have a reticular pattern.
Source: Dr. J.P. Teifke, Federal Research Institute for Animal Health Riems, Germany

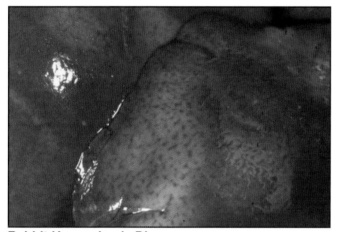

Rabbit Hemorrhagic Disease

Rabbit, liver. There is a large area of pallor (necrosis) with a prominent reticular pattern.
Source: Dr. J.P. Teifke, Federal Research Institute for Animal Health Riems, Germany

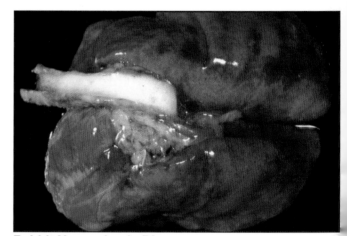

Rabbit Hemorrhagic Disease

Rabbit, lungs. The trachea is filled with foam, and the lungs are mottled and noncollapsed (severe pulmonary edema).
Source: Dr. J.P. Teifke, Federal Research Institute for Animal Health Riems, Germany

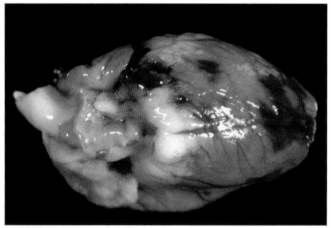

Rabbit Hemorrhagic Disease

Rabbit, heart. There are multiple epicardial hemorrhages.
Source: Dr. J.P. Teifke, Federal Research Institute for Animal Health Riems, Germany

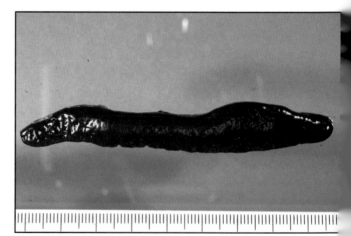

Rabbit Hemorrhagic Disease

Rabbit, spleen. The spleen is markedly enlarged and congested.
Source: Dr. J.P. Teifke, Federal Research Institute for Animal Health Riems, Germany

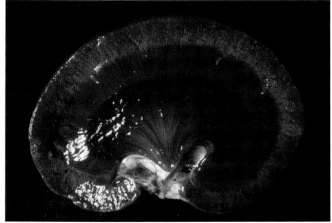

Rabbit Hemorrhagic Disease

Rabbit, kidney. There are petechiae throughout the cortex, and the medulla is severely congested.

Source: Dr. J.P. Teifke, Federal Research Institute for Animal Health Riems, Germany

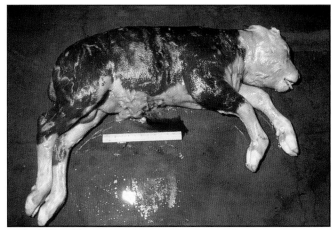

Rift Valley Fever

Bovine, fetus. The skin of this emphysematous fetus is stained with meconium.

Source: PIADC

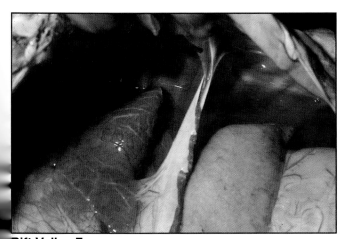

Rift Valley Fever

Sheep, fetus. Both the pleural and peritoneal cavities contain excessive clear, straw-colored fluid.

Source: PIADC

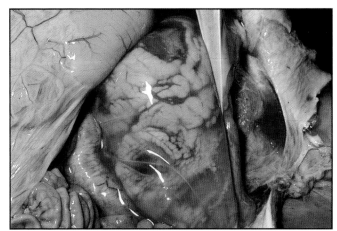

Rift Valley Fever

Sheep, fetus, kidney. There is severe perirenal edema.

Source: PIADC

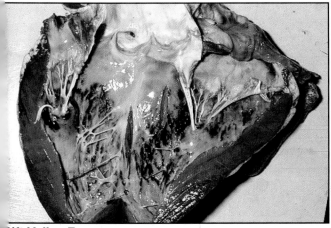

Rift Valley Fever

Sheep, heart. The ventricular endocardium contains many hemorrhages.

Source: PIADC

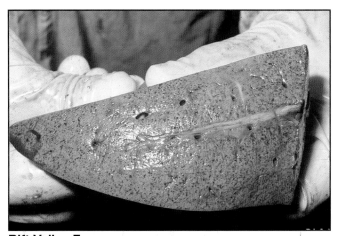

Rift Valley Fever

Sheep, liver. The cut surface of this swollen liver is pale and contains many petechiae.

Source: PIADC

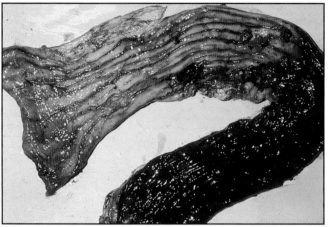

Rift Valley Fever

Sheep, colon. There is severe locally extensive mucosal hemorrhage.
Source: PIADC

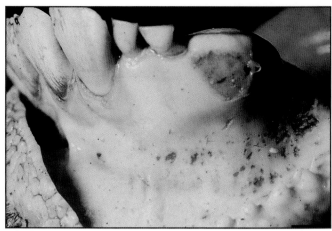

Rinderpest

Bovine, oral mucosa. There are numerous small gingival erosions.
Source: PIADC

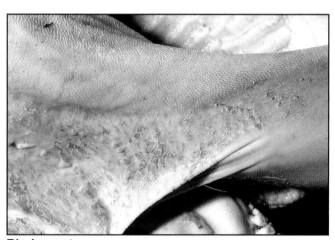

Rinderpest

Bovine, oral mucosa. There are numerous coalescing erosions on the ventrolateral lingual mucosa.
Source: PIADC

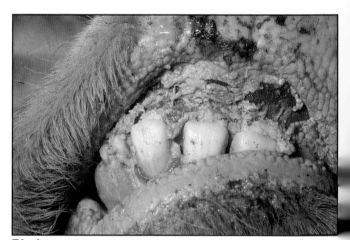

Rinderpest

Bovine, oral mucosa. There is severe diffuse necrosis/coalescing ulceration of the dental pad; mandibular mucosa contains smaller erosions.
Source: PIADC

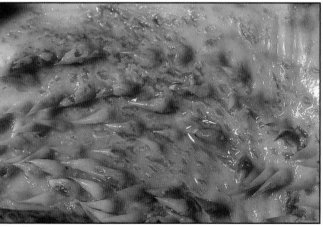

Rinderpest

Bovine, oral mucosa. There are numerous erosions on and between the buccal papillae.
Source: PIADC

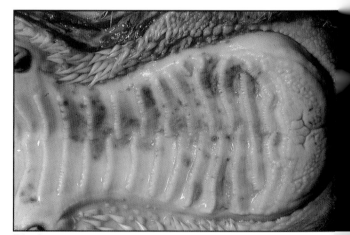

Rinderpest

Bovine, hard palate. The mucosa contains many small, coalescing, pale to dark red erosions or foci of necrosis.
Source: PIADC

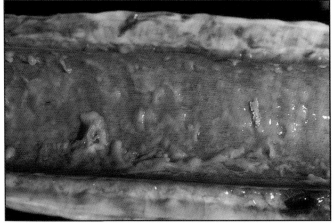

Rinderpest

Bovine, trachea. The mucosa is hyperemic and covered by abundant mucopurulent exudate.
Source: PIADC

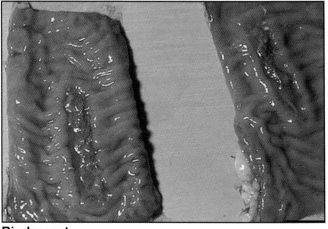

Rinderpest

Bovine, ileum. Peyer's patches are depressed and covered by fibronecrotic exudate.
Source: PIADC

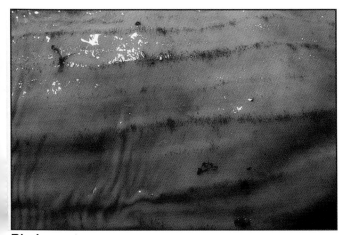

Rinderpest

Bovine, colon. There are many petechiae on the crests of the mucosal folds, and there are several small blood clots on the mucosal surface.
Source: PIADC

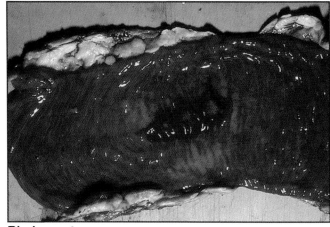

Rinderpest

Bovine, ileum. The mucosa is hemorrhagic and edematous, and the Peyer's patch is depressed (necrosis).
Source: PIADC

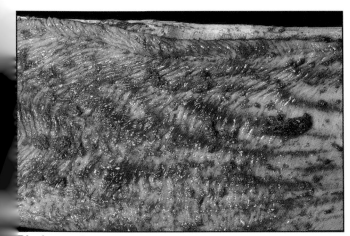

Rinderpest

Bovine, colon. The mucosa contains multiple longitudinal linear hemorrhages.
Source: PIADC

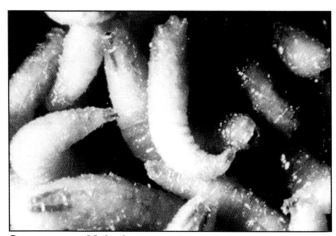

Screwworm Myiasis

Screwworm. Third instar screwworm larvae have dark tracheal tubes.
Source: Foreign Animal Diseases "The Grey Book" USAHA

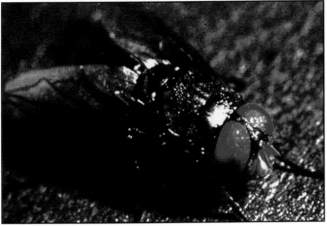

Screwworm Myiasis

Screwworm fly. The head of the adult fly is red-orange.
Source: Foreign Animal Diseases "The Grey Book" USAHA

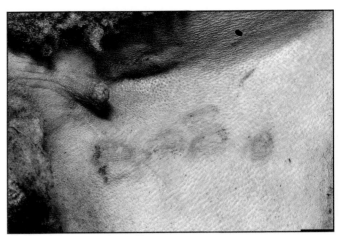

Sheep Pox and Goat Pox

Sheep, inguinal skin. Several coalescing macules contain petechiae.
Source: PIADC

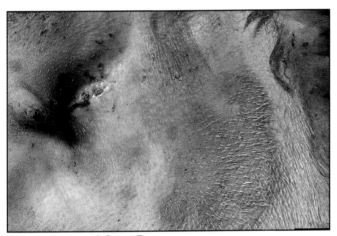

Sheep Pox and Goat Pox

Sheep, inguinal skin. There are several coalescing macules.
Source: PIADC

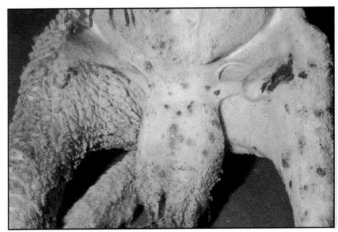

Sheep Pox and Goat Pox

Sheep, scrotum and inguinal skin. There are multiple red brown papules. There are two hemorrhagic ulcers on the medial aspect of the stifle.
Source: PIADC

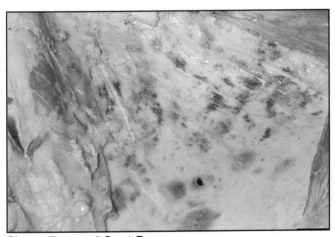

Sheep Pox and Goat Pox

Sheep, subcutis. There are numerous hemorrhages, and several dark red round foci of hemorrhage and necrosis (beneath cutaneous pox).
Source: PIADC

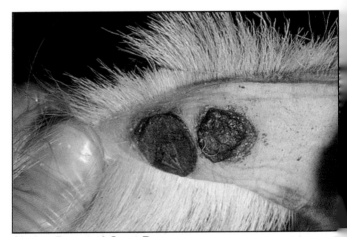

Sheep Pox and Goat Pox

Goat. Two pox on the ventral tail have dessicated, dark red, undermined (necrotic and sloughing) centers.
Source: PIADC

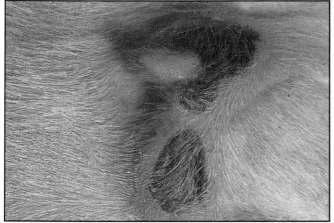

Sheep Pox and Goat Pox

Goat, udder. The skin contains two sharply demarcated necrotic foci (subacute pox).
Source: PIADC

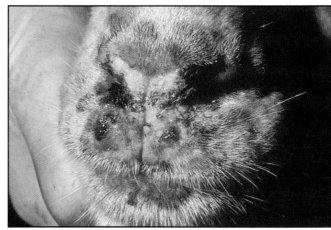

Sheep Pox and Goat Pox

Goat, muzzle. The muzzle contains several papules and is partially covered by hemorrhagic nasal exudate.
Source: PIADC

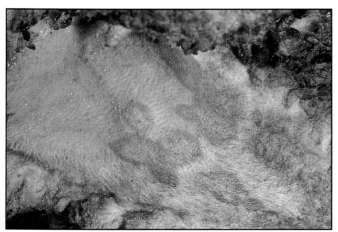

Sheep Pox and Goat Pox

Sheep, skin. Several coalescing pox have pale tan (necrotic) centers.
Source: PIADC

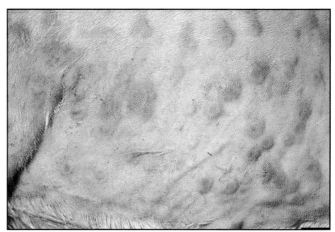

Sheep Pox and Goat Pox

Goat, skin. There are multiple coalescing papules (pox) that often have tan, dry (necrotic) centers.
Source: PIADC

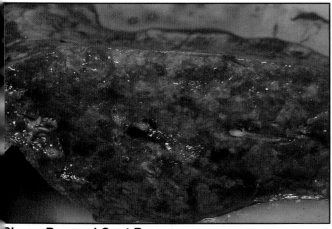

Sheep Pox and Goat Pox

Small ruminant, lung. There are numerous, small, coalescing, red-tan, consolidated foci (pneumonia).
Source: PIADC

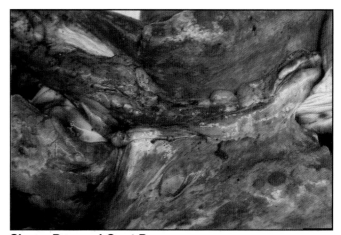

Sheep Pox and Goat Pox

Small ruminant, lungs. The lungs contain multiple discrete tan to red-brown nodules (multifocal interstitial pneumonia). Mediastinal lymph nodes are enlarged.
Source: PIADC

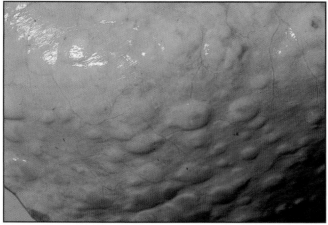

Sheep Pox and Goat Pox

Small ruminant, lung. There are numerous raised pale nodules (multifocal pneumonia).
Source: PIADC

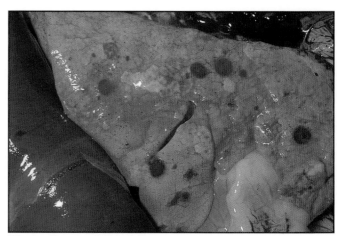

Sheep Pox and Goat Pox

Small ruminant, lung. There are multiple discrete, round, red-brown foci of consolidation (pneumonia).
Source: PIADC

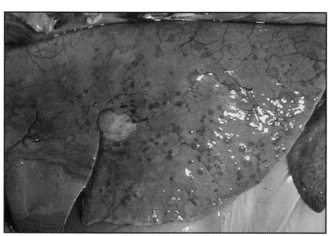

Sheep Pox and Goat Pox

Sheep, lung. The numerous widely disseminated discrete round tan foci are foci of pneumonia; a few have pale (necrotic) centers.
Source: PIADC

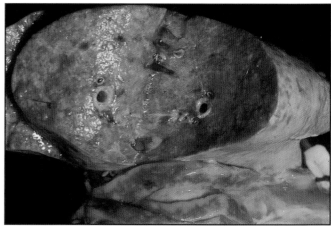

Sheep Pox and Goat Pox

Goat, lung. There are multiple coalescing tan foci of consolidation (pneumonia), and the adjacent lymph node is markedly enlarged.
Source: PIADC

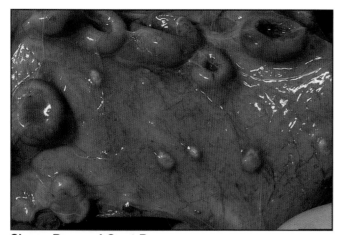

Sheep Pox and Goat Pox

Small ruminant, uterus. The endometrium contains several tan papules (pox) among the caruncles.
Source: PIADC

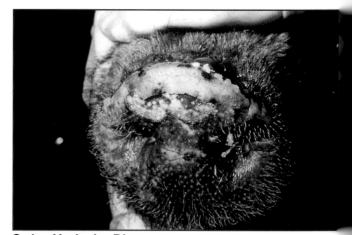

Swine Vesicular Disease

Pig, skin. There is a deep ulcer on the dorsum of the snout.
Source: ISU CVM

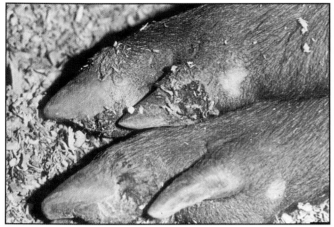

Swine Vesicular Disease

Pig, feet. There are multiple large erosions/ulcers of the coronary bands.
Source: PIADC

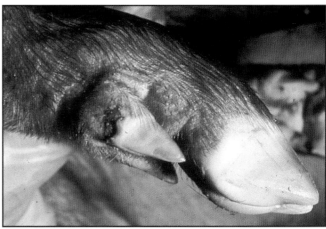

Swine Vesicular Disease

Pig, foot. The wall of the dewclaw is undermined adjacent to an ulcer at the coronary band.
Source: PIADC

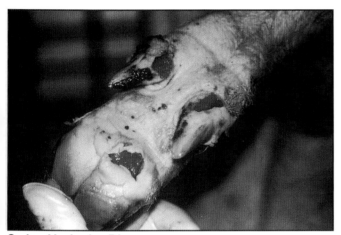

Swine Vesicular Disease

Pig, foot. A claw and both dewclaws have ulcers at the coronary bands.
Source: ISU CVM

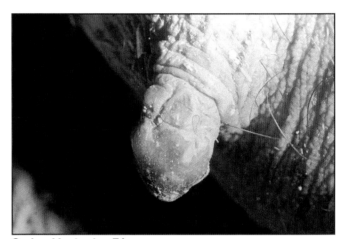

Swine Vesicular Disease

Pig, skin. There are coalescing erosions on the teat.
Source: ISU CVM

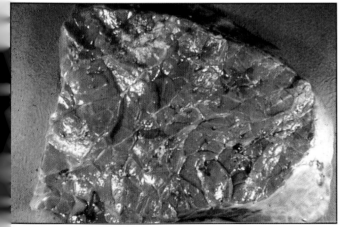

Theileriosis

Bovine, lung. The lung tissue is diffusely tan-brown, and lobules are noncollapsed and rubbery (interstitial pneumonia).
Source: PIADC

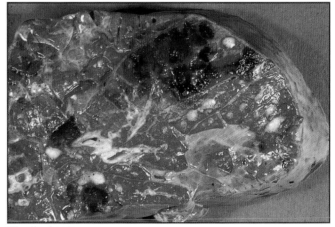

Theileriosis

Bovine, lung. Lung tissue is noncollapsed, contains multiple foci of hemorrhage, and there is fluid/foam within bronchi and interlobular septa.
Source: PIADC

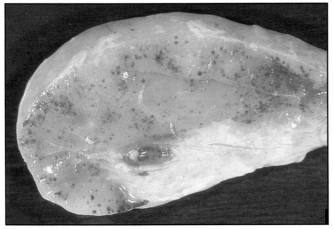

Theileriosis

Bovine, popliteal lymph node. The node is enlarged and diffusely pale, and contains numerous petechiae.
Source: PIADC

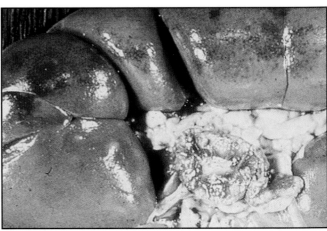

Theileriosis

Bovine, kidney. There are multiple petechiae on the surface of the cortex. The lymph node near the hilus is markedly enlarged.
Source: PIADC

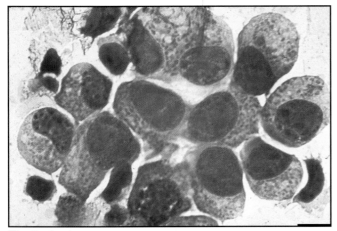

Theileriosis

Bovine lymphoblasts contain intracytoplasmic *Theileria parva*.
Source: PIADC

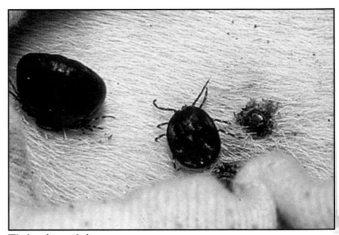

Ticks (exotic)

Amyblyomma variegatum - Ticks, skin. Ticks feeding on goat skin. Can transmit the agent of heartwater (*Ehrlichia ruminantium*).
Source: PIADC

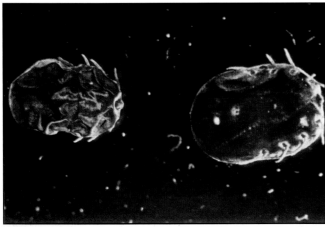

Ticks (exotic)

Rhipicephalus annulatus (Boophilus annulatus) - Cattle tick, arthropod. Known to transmit babesiosis and anaplasmosis.
Source: AFIP

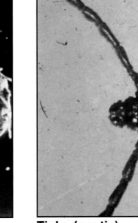

Ticks (exotic)

Rhipicephalus appendiculatus - Tick, arthropod. Brown ear tick and vector of theileriosis.
Source: PIADC

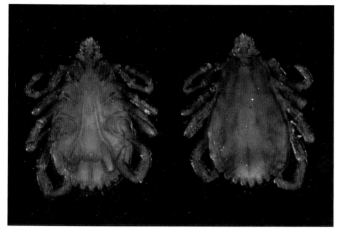

Ticks (exotic)

Rhipicephalus microplus - Tick, arthropod. Known to transmit babesiosis and anaplasmosis.
Source: Dr. J. Ostojic, ISU, CVM, VPTH

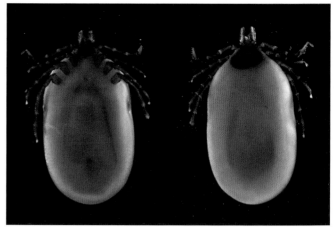

Ticks (exotic)

Ixodes ricinus - Tick, arthropod. Can transmit agents of babesiosis, louping ill, and other diseases.
Source: Dr. J. Ostojic, ISU, CVM, VPTH

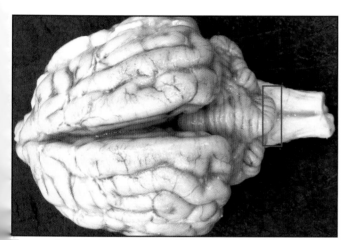

Transmissible Spongiform Encephalopathies

Brain. The red box indicates the region of the obex, the portion of the brainstem that is required for TSE diagnosis.
Source: Dr. S. Sorden, ISU CVM, VPTH

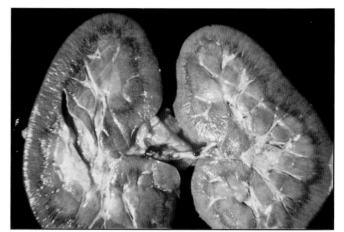

Trypanosomiasis, African

Horse, kidney. Cortex is pale and there are multiple petechial hemorrhages at the corticomedullary junction.
Source: AFIP

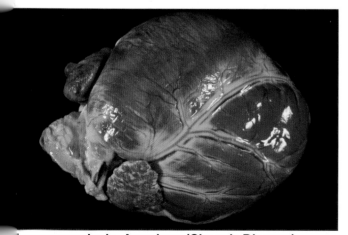

Trypanosomiasis, American (Chaga's Disease)

Dog, heart. There are multiple white linear streaks on the surface of the right and left ventricles corresponding to myocardial necrosis and myocarditis.
Source: Dr. S. Barr, Cornell University, CVM, Dept of Clinical Sciences

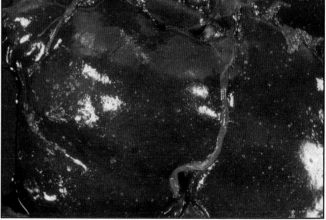

Tularemia

Beaver, liver. There are disseminated small pale foci of necrotizing hepatitis.
Source: Dr. G. Wobeser, CCWHC

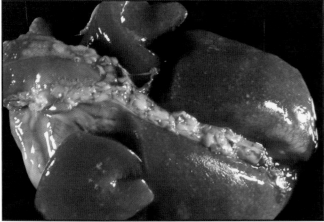

Tularemia

Cat, lung. Numerous <1 mm diameter pale foci are disseminated throughout all lung lobes.
Source: Dr. J. Nietfeld, KSU CVM

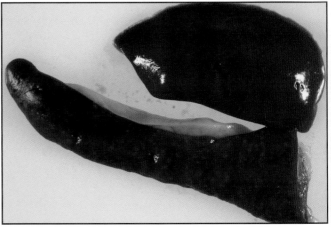

Tularemia

Cat, spleen and liver. Numerous ~1 mm diameter pale foci are disseminated throughout the spleen; fewer pale foci are discernible in the liver lobe.
Source: Dr. J. Nietfeld, KSU CVM

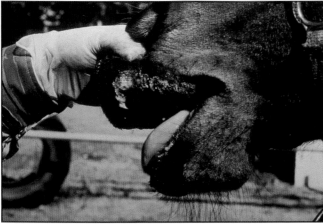

Vesicular Stomatitis

Horse, mouth. There is extensive erosion of the lips at the mucocutaneous junction.
Source: ISU CVM

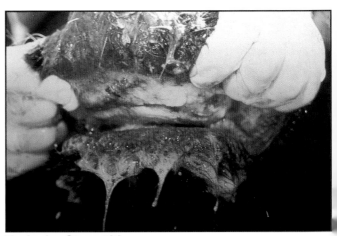

Vesicular Stomatitis

Bovine, mouth. There is extensive ulceration of the dental pad, and severe salivation.
Source: ISU CVM

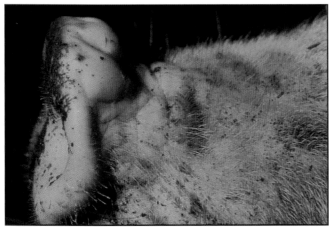

Vesicular Stomatitis

Pig, skin. There is a large vesicle (bulla) on the dorsal snout.
Source: ISU CVM

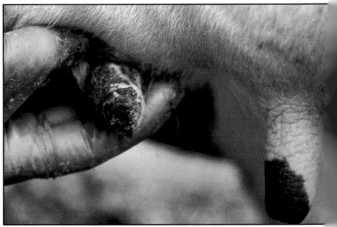

Vesicular Stomatitis

Bovine, mammary gland. The distal teat is severely eroded and hemorrhagic.
Source: ISU CVM

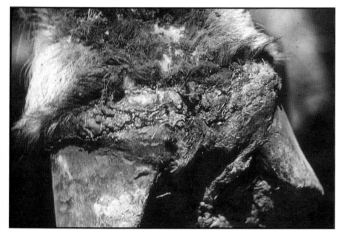

Vesicular Stomatitis

Bovine, foot. The coronary band at the heels is thickened, multifocally eroded, and covered by dried necrotic exudate.
Source: PIADC.

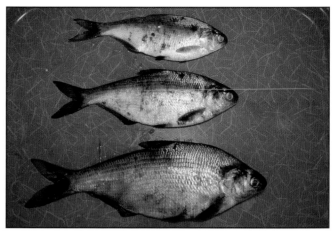

Viral Hemorrhagic Septicemia

Fish, whole body. The external surface of the fish (gizzard shad) contains numerous ecchymotic hemorrhages.
Credit: Dr. P. Bowser, Aquatic Animal Health Program, CVM, Cornell University

SECTION
4

Transboundary and Emerging Diseases of Animals
REFERENCE CHARTS

Disease From Potential
  Bioterrorist Agents — Animal

Disease From Potential
  Bioterrorist Agents — Human

Additional High Consequence
  Livestock Pathogens

Disease From Potential Bioterrorist Agents

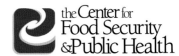

the Center for
Food Security
& Public Health

www.cfsph.iastate.edu • cfsph@iastate.edu • 515.294.7189

Severity of disease in potentially affected species
■ Mild ▲ Moderate ● Severe

CDC Category	Animal — Disease or Agent	Cattle	Sheep	Goats	Pigs	Horses	Dogs	Cats	Birds	Other	Incubation Period	Prominent Clinical Signs
A	**Anthrax** *Bacillus anthracis*	●	●	●	▲	●	▲	▲		wild herbivores and carnivores, guinea pigs	3-7 days	Sudden death from septicemia with lack of rigor mortis; blood fails to clot; excitement followed by depression or stupor; blood from mouth, nose, anus; edema, especially neck, throat and shoulders
A	**Botulism** *Clostridium botulinum toxin*	●	●	●	■	●	●	■	●	foxes, mink	24-72 hours	Muscle paralysis - progressive symmetrical to flaccid; disturbed vision; unable to swallow or chew; death from respiratory or cardiac paralysis
A	**Plague** *Yersinia pestis*						■	●		rodents, rock and ground squirrel, prairie dog	Variable; several days	High fever; extremely swollen lymph nodes—"buboes"; severe pneumonia; septicemia
A	**Tularemia** *Francisella tularensis*		●		■	▲	■	■		rabbits, rodents, aquatic animals	1-10 days	Sudden high fever with lethargy and anorexia; stiffness; reduced mobility; tachycardia; tachypnea; prostration and death; miliary white necrotic foci of liver, spleen or lymph node
A	**Viral Hemorrhagic Fevers** *Ebola, Marburg, Lassa, Machupo*									nonhuman primates, guinea pigs	2-16 days	Fever; petechiae; bleeding from orifices and internal organs; skin rash; splenomegaly
B	**Brucellosis** *Brucella melitensis*	■	●	●						wild ruminants	Variable	Abortions; stillborn or weak newborns; retained placentas; placentitis; orchitis; epididymitis; arthritis; lameness; Goats: may also have mastitis
B	**Brucellosis** *Brucella abortus, B. ovis, B. suis, B. canis*	●	●	●	●	■	▲			wild ruminants, buffalo, bison, elk	Variable	Abortions; stillborn or weak newborns; placentitis; orchitis; epididymitis; arthritis; lameness; Horses: suppurative bursitis ("fistulous withers")
B	**Glanders** *Burkholderia mallei*				■	●	■	▲		donkeys, mules, camels, guinea pigs, hamsters	2 weeks	Ulcerated nodules on skin, upper respiratory tract, lungs; septicemia; high fever; thick mucopurulent nasal discharge; respiratory signs
B	**Melioidosis** *Burkholderia pseudomallei*	■	●	●	●	▲	▲	■		rodents, rabbits, kangaroos, other zoo animals, fish	Variable; latency	Signs vary with site of lesion; suppurative or caseous lesions in lymph nodes, lungs, and viscera; pneumonia; possibly nasal discharge, arthritis or lameness; Horses: neurological; colic; Goats: mastitis
B	**Psittacosis** *Chlamydophila psittaci*								■	parakeets, parrots, love birds	3-10 days	Nasal and ocular discharges; conjunctivitis; yellow–green droppings; inactivity; ruffled feathers; inappetence; weight loss
B	**Q Fever** *Coxiella burnetii*	▲	▲	▲			■	■		rodents, rabbits	1-3 weeks	Typically asymptomatic. Sheep, Goats: abortion; anorexia; Cattle: infertility; sporadic abortion; Dog, Cat: subclinical; abortions
B	**Typhus Fever** *Rickettsia prowazekii*									flying squirrels	12 days	Asymptomatic

Disease From Potential Bioterrorist Agents

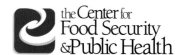

the **Center** for **Food Security** & **Public Health**

www.cfsph.iastate.edu • cfsph@iastate.edu • 515.294.7189

CDC Category	Disease or Agent	Severity of disease in potentially affected species ■ Mild ▲ Moderate ● Severe									Incubation Period	Prominent Clinical Signs
		Cattle	Sheep	Goats	Pigs	Horses	Dogs	Cats	Birds	Other		
B	**Viral Encephalitis** *VEE, EEE, WEE*					●		■		rodents	1-14 days	CNS dysfunction: altered behavior; impaired vision; wandering; head pressing; circling; unable to swallow; ataxia, paresis; paralysis; convulsions; death
B	**Toxins** *Clostridium perfringens, Ricinus communis, Staph. aureus*	●	●	●	●	●	●	●	●	nonhuman primates	12-72 hours	Ricin: violent vomiting; bloody diarrhea; salivation; trembling; incoordination; Clostridium: necrotic enteritis; bloody diarrhea; septicemia; acute death, esp. in young; Staph: diarrhea; vomiting; pulmonary edema
C	**Nipah** *Nipah virus*			▲	●	■	▲	▲			7-14 days	Severe respiratory distress; harsh "barking" cough; open mouth breathing; possibly neurological signs; head pressing
C	**Hantavirus** *Hantavirus*									rodents		Asymptomatic carriers
	West Nile Fever *West Nile virus*	■	■	■		●	■	■	●	many mammals and reptiles	3-14 days	Fever; encephalitis; altered behavior; impaired vision; circling; head pressing; ataxia; weakness of limbs; partial paralysis; death
	Hendra *Hendra virus*					●	■	▲		guinea pigs	6-18 days	Acute respiratory syndrome; nasal discharge; head pressing; ataxia
	Rift Valley Fever *Rift Valley fever virus*	●	●	●		▲	▲			camels, monkeys	12-36 hours in young	High mortality in newborn animals: fever, hemorrhagic diarrhea, abdominal pain, bloody nasal discharge; abortion storms in adults

Chart created by: Glenda Dvorak, DVM, MS, MPH, DACVPM

References available at www.cfsph.iastate.edu/WallChartReferences/
Technical factsheets for these diseases are available at www.cfsph.iastate.edu/Factsheets/

NOTE: Bioterrorism pathogens may have atypical routes of transmission and clinical manifestations. The information provided in this chart is intended to alert the public and medical professionals to the presence of possible bioterrorism agents. The information should not be used to rule out a diagnosis, and should not take the place of advice provided by your physician or veterinarian.

Disease From Potential Bioterrorist Agents

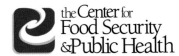

the Center for Food Security & Public Health

www.cfsph.iastate.edu • cfsph@iastate.edu • 515.294.7189

CDC Category	Human — Disease or Agent	Person-to-Person / Vector Transmitted / Zoonotic — Route of Transmission	Septicemia	Respiratory	Intestinal	Cutaneous	Ocular	Neurological	Incubation Period (days)	Prominent Clinical Signs
A	**Anthrax** *Bacillus anthracis*	Zoonotic — infected animal; inhalation; contaminated food	●	●	●	●			1-7	Flu–like signs; pustules; scabs; respiratory distress; wide mediastinum on x–ray; bloody vomit and diarrhea; abdominal distress; sepsis; shock; death
A	**Botulism** *Clostridium botulinum toxin*	Zoonotic — contaminated food; inhalation	●	●	●	●		●	1-5	Weakness; dizziness; dry mouth; nausea; vomiting; cranial nerve deficits; double vision; drooping eyes; slurred speech; symmetrical paralysis; respiratory paralysis; death
A	**Plague** *Yersinia pestis*	Person-to-Person / Vector / Zoonotic — fleas; infected animal; inhalation	●	●					1-6	Flu–like signs; enlarged tender lymph nodes "buboes"; rapid pneumonia; respiratory failure; toxemia; shock; death
A	**Smallpox** *Variola major*	Person-to-Person — direct contact with infected human; inhalation				●			7-17	Flu–like signs; vomiting; rash to pustules (skin, throat, mouth); death
A	**Tularemia** *Francisella tularensis*	Vector / Zoonotic — arthropods: tick, deer fly, mosquito; inhalation; infected animal tissue; contaminated food, water	●	●	●	●	●		1-14	Flu–like signs; exhaustion; ulcerative lesions; enlarged painful lymph nodes; painful purulent conjunctivitis; abdominal pain; diarrhea; vomiting; chest pain; respiratory distress; pneumonia; sepsis; death
A	**Viral Hemorrhagic Fevers** Ebola, Marburg, Lassa, Machupo	Person-to-Person / Zoonotic — varies with virus: direct contact with infected humans or animal reservoirs	●		●	●		●	2-21	Flu–like signs; fever; headache; vomiting; diarrhea; petechiae; maculopapular to hemorrhagic rash; hepatic damage; renal failure; seizures; shock; coma; death
B	**Brucellosis** *Brucella species*	Person-to-Person / Zoonotic — contact with infected animal tissue; inhalation; contaminated food	●					●	1-21	Flu–like signs; cyclic fever; arthritis; orchitis; epididymitis; hepatomegaly; Chronic: neurological; endocarditis
B	**Glanders** *Burkholderia mallei*	Person-to-Person / Zoonotic — infected animal; inhalation; wound contamination	●	●	●	●	●		1-14	Flu–like signs; diarrhea; chest pain; pulmonary signs; pustules; ulcerations; swollen lymph nodes; photophobia
B	**Melioidosis** *Burkholderia pseudomallei*	Person-to-Person / Zoonotic — inhalation; infected body fluids; wound contamination	●	●		●			2 days to years	Flu–like signs; pustules; chronic abcesses; chest pain; pneumonia; bronchitis; acute sepsis; death
B	**Psittacosis** *Chlamydophila psittaci*	Zoonotic — inhalation of dust from infected bird dander, droppings or secretions		●		●		●	7-28	Flu–like signs; rash; extensive pneumonia; endocarditis; myocarditis; encephalitis
B	**Q Fever** *Coxiella burnetii*	Vector / Zoonotic — tick; inhalation; infected animal body fluids (urine, milk, blood, birthing)		●			●	●	10-40	Flu–like signs; severe sweats; weakness; retrobulbar headache; pneumonitis but no cough or chest pain; granulomatous hepatitis; osteomyelitis; arteritis; endocarditis; neurologic signs; thrombocytopenia; in-utero death; placentitis
B	**Typhus Fever** *Rickettsia prowazekii*	Person-to-Person / Vector — human body louse; fleas from flying squirrels	●	●	●	●			7-14	Flu–like signs; macular eruptions on upper trunk then body, not face, palms or soles of feet; cough; chest pain; pneumonia; abdominal pain; toxemia

Disease From Potential Bioterrorist Agents

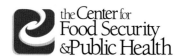

the Center for Food Security & Public Health

www.cfsph.iastate.edu • cfsph@iastate.edu • 515.294.7189

CDC Category	Human — Disease or Agent	Person-to-Person / Vector Transmitted / Zoonotic — Route of Transmission	Septicemia	Respiratory	Intestinal	Cutaneous	Ocular	Neurological	Incubation Period (days)	Prominent Clinical Signs
B	**Viral Encephalitis** *VEE, EEE, WEE* (Vector Transmitted; Zoonotic)	mosquito			●		●	●	2-6	Flu–like signs; nausea; vomiting; conjunctival congestion; encephalitis; disorientation; seizures; coma; death
B	**Toxins** *Clostridium perfringens, Ricinus communis, Staph. aureus*	contaminated food; inhalation	●	●	●	●	●		<1	Flu–like signs; vomiting; bloody diarrhea; abdominal cramps; kidney failure; shock; death
C	**Nipah** *Nipah virus* (Person-to-Person; Zoonotic)	direct contact with infected animal; ingestion; inhalation		●				●	3-18	Flu–like signs; drowsy; disoriented; neurological signs; seizures; respiratory distress; death
C	**Hantavirus** *Hantavirus* (Person-to-Person; Zoonotic)	inhalation of aerosolized rodent urine, feces or saliva	●	●	●	●	●		4-42	HPS: Flu–like signs; back pain; myalgia; cough; shortness of breath; dyspnea; tachypnea; tachycardia; death; HFRS: Febrile; hypotension; petechiae; conjunctival injection; oliguria followed by polyuria; shock; convalescence
	West Nile Fever *West Nile virus* (Person-to-Person; Vector Transmitted; Zoonotic)	mosquito			●		●	●	3-12	Flu–like signs; vomiting; lymphadenopathy; periocular pain; conjunctivitis; encephalitis; death
	Hendra *Hendra virus* (Zoonotic)	unknown; possible direct contact		●				●	3-14	Flu–like signs; severe acute respiratory signs; neurological signs; death
	Rift Valley Fever *Rift Valley fever virus* (Vector Transmitted; Zoonotic)	Mosquitoes; other insects, ticks ; direct contact with infected tissues or aerosol				●	●	●	3-12	Flu–like signs; petechiae; hemorrhagic fever; retinopathy; encephalitis; death

Legend: = Potential System Affected

Chart created by: Glenda Dvorak, DVM, MS, MPH, DACVPM

References available at www.cfsph.iastate.edu/WallChartReferences/
Technical factsheets for these diseases are available at www.cfsph.iastate.edu/Factsheets/

NOTE: Bioterrorism pathogens may have atypical routes of transmission and clinical manifestations. The information provided in this chart is intended to alert the public and medical professionals to the presence of possible bioterrorism agents. The information should not be used to rule out a diagnosis, and should not take the place of advice provided by your physician or veterinarian.

Additional High Consequence Livestock Pathogens

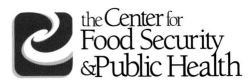

www.cfsph.iastate.edu • cfsph@iastate.edu • 515.294.7189

Disease or Agent	Humans Affected / Species Affected	Incubation Period	Mode of Transmission	Prominent Clinical Signs in Livestock
Tier 1: Diseases of national concern that pose the most significant threat (highest risk and consequence) to animal agriculture in the U.S.				
African swine fever virus	domestic and wild pigs	5-15 days	direct contact with body fluids (blood); contaminated objects; ticks	High fever; recumbency; skin reddening; cyanotic blotching on ear, tail or legs; enlarged friable spleen; hemorrhagic lymph nodes; swollen tonsils; petechiae; fibrinous pericarditis; death
Classical swine fever virus (hog cholera)	pigs	2-14 days	ingestion (uncooked meat); contaminated objects; aerosol; direct contact	Variable. Fever, dullness; ataxia; constipation followed by diarrhea; cyanosis of abdomen and ears; abortions, stillbirths, mummification, congenital malformations; death
Foot-and-mouth disease virus	Rare / cattle, sheep, goats, pigs	1-5 days	aerosol; direct contact; ingestion; contaminated objects	Fever, vesicles and erosions in mouth, nares, muzzle, and feet (coronary band, interdigital) or teats; depression, anorexia; salivation; nasal discharge; sloughing of hoof, abortion
Avian influenza virus (highly pathogenic)	👤 / chicken, turkey, pigs, waterfowl, cats, dogs	3-7 days	aerosol; direct contact with body fluids; ingestion; contaminated objects	Depression; respiratory signs (coughing, sneezing, nasal discharge); ataxia, green watery diarrhea, swollen, cyanotic combs and wattles; edema of eyes and neck, hemorrhage of legs, decreased egg production, death.
Newcastle disease virus (virulent)	👤 / poultry, other avian species	2-15 days	direct contact with feces and respiratory droplets; fomites,	Respiratory signs (coughing, gasping); neurological signs (muscle tremors, circling, paralysis), green watery diarrhea, decreased egg production
Tier 2: Diseases transmitted primarily by pests; disease spread depends largely on the presence of pests in the environment and ability to transmit disease between animals				
Heartwater *Ehrlichia (Cowdria) ruminantium*	cattle, sheep, goats, wild ruminants	7-16 days	*Amblyomma* ticks	Fever, respiratory distress, lacrimation, neurologic signs (tongue protrusion, circling, high stepping gait); convulsions, death. Post mortem lesions: hydropericardium, ascites, hydrothorax, petechiae
New World Screwworm *Cochliomyia hominivorax*	👤 / mammals, birds	5-7 days	eggs laid in wounds	Variable diameter openings containing migrating larvae; death can occur from toxicity or secondary infections
Rift Valley fever	👤 / cattle, sheep, goats, dogs, cats, camels	12-36 hours in young	mosquitoes; other insects, ticks ; in utero; direct contact with infected tissues or aerosol	High mortality in newborn animals: fever, hemorrhagic diarrhea, abdominal pain, bloody nasal discharge; abortion storms in adults
Venezuelan equine encephalitis	👤 / horses, wild rodents, wild birds	1-5 days	mosquitoes	Fever; tachycardia; neurological signs indicative of encephalitis (altered behavior, hypersensitivity, involuntary muscle movement, impaired vision, paresis, paralysis, convulsions); death; disease can be mild or asymptomatic

Additional High Consequence Livestock Pathogens

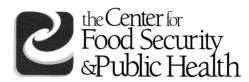

the Center for
Food Security
&Public Health

www.cfsph.iastate.edu • cfsph@iastate.edu • 515.294.7189

Disease or Agent	Humans Affected / Species Affected	Incubation Period	Mode of Transmission	Prominent Clinical Signs in Livestock
Tier 3: Diseases and pests that pose less risk and fewer consequences but still have potential negative impact on animal or human health				
African horse sickness virus	horses, zebras, donkeys, mules, camels	5-7 days	*Culicoides* midges, mechanically by other vectors	Variable forms; fever; severe dyspnea; spasmodic cough; serosanguinous nasal discharge; edema of supraorbital fossa, head, neck, and chest; profuse sweating; hydrothorax; hydropericardium
Contagious bovine pleuropneumonia *Mycoplasma mycoides mycoides*	cattle	20-123 days	close contact with respiratory droplets and other body fluids	Dyspnea, tachypnea, cough, fever; calves may have polyarthritis with or without pneumonia. Post mortem lesions: fibrinous, thickened, hyperemic "marbled" lung tissue; thickened interlobular septa
Contagious caprine pleuropneumonia *Mycoplasma capricolum/M. F38/M. mycoides capri*	goats	6-10 days	direct contact with respiratory droplets	Respiratory signs (coughing, labored respiration, frothy nasal discharge); fever; septicemia, lethargy; anorexia; death. Post mortem lesions: fibrinous pneumonia, no thickening of interlobular tissue
Glanders *Burkholderia mallei*	🖤 horses, dogs, goats, cats	14 days	direct contact, fomites, inhalation, ingestion, reproductive	Ulcerated nodules on skin, upper respiratory tract, lungs; septicemia; high fever; thick mucopurulent nasal discharge; respiratory signs
Hendra virus	🖤 horses, cats, dogs	6-18 days	ingestion, inhalation, close contact; fomites	Acute respiratory syndrome; nasal discharge; head pressing; ataxia
Melioidosis *Burkholderia pseudomallei*	🖤 sheep, goats, pigs, horses, dogs, cattle, cats	Variable latency	ingestion, inhalation, entry through wounds or abrasions	Signs vary with site of lesion; suppurative or caseous lesions in lymph nodes, lungs, and viscera; pneumonia; possibly nasal discharge, arthritis or lameness; Horses: neurological; colic; Goats: mastitis
Nipah virus	🖤 pigs, goats, dogs, cats, horses	7-14 days	aerosol, direct contact with respiratory secretions	Severe respiratory distress; harsh "barking" cough; open mouth breathing; possibly neurological signs; head pressing
Peste des petits ruminants virus	goats, sheep	3-10 days	close contact with body fluids; aerosol; contaminated objects	Sudden death; fever; restless; nasal discharge; respiratory distress; bronchopneumonia; necrotic stomatitis; diarrhea; death
Rinderpest virus	cattle, sheep, goats, pigs	3-15 days	direct or close contact with body fluids	High fever; tachypnea; tachycardia; oculonasal discharge; oral erosions and necrosis; watery to hemorrhagic diarrhea; abdominal pain; weakness; recumbency; sudden death
Tropical bont tick *Amblyomma variegatum*	🖤 cattle, sheep, goats, horses, dogs		direct contact (bite) of tick	Large wounds can damage skin and secondary infections; can transmit agents for heartwater and African tick-bite fever

Chart created by: Glenda Dvorak, DVM, MS, MPH, DACVPM

References available at www.cfsph.iastate.edu/WallChartReferences/
Technical factsheets for these diseases are available at www.cfsph.iastate.edu/Factsheets/

NOTE: This chart provides information on possible signs of foreign animal diseases. If you suspect a foreign animal disease, contact your state or federal veterinarian immediately. USDA High Consequence Foreign Animal Diseases and Pests list: https://www.aphis. usda.gov/publications/animal_health/2013/fs_hc_diseases.pdf

Transboundary and Emerging Diseases of Animals **335**

Index

Bold page numbers refer to disease fact sheets found in Section 2.

Bold/Italicized numbers refer to images in Section 3.